AF715261

Immunobiology of Dendritic Cells

Immunobiology of Dendritic Cells

Editor: Jeremy Collins

AMERICAN
MEDICAL PUBLISHERS
www.americanmedicalpublishers.com

AMERICAN
MEDICAL PUBLISHERS
www.americanmedicalpublishers.com

Cataloging-in-Publication Data

Immunobiology of dendritic cells / edited by Jeremy Collins.
p. cm.
Includes bibliographical references and index.
ISBN 979-8-88740-202-4
1. Dendritic cells. 2. Dendritic cells--Immunology. 3. Immunology. I. Collins, Jeremy.
QR185.8.D45 I46 2023
616.079--dc23

© American Medical Publishers, 2023

American Medical Publishers,
41 Flatbush Avenue,
1st Floor, New York,
NY 11217, USA

ISBN 979-8-88740-202-4 (Hardback)

This book contains information obtained from authentic and highly regarded sources. Copyright for all individual chapters remain with the respective authors as indicated. All chapters are published with permission under the Creative Commons Attribution License or equivalent. A wide variety of references are listed. Permission and sources are indicated; for detailed attributions, please refer to the permissions page and list of contributors. Reasonable efforts have been made to publish reliable data and information, but the authors, editors and publisher cannot assume any responsibility for the validity of all materials or the consequences of their use.

Trademark Notice: Registered trademark of products or corporate names are used only for explanation and identification without intent to infringe.

Contents

Preface

The purpose of the book is to provide a glimpse into the dynamics and to present opinions and studies of some of the scientists engaged in the development of new ideas in the field from very different standpoints. This book will prove useful to students and researchers owing to its high content quality.

Dendritic cells (DCs) refer to antigen-presenting cells of the mammalian immune system. The major job of the dendritic cells is to process antigen material and present it on the cell surface to the T cells of the immune system. They serve as messengers among the adaptive and innate immune systems. Dendritic cells are found in those tissues that come in contact with the external environment, such as the skin and the inner lining of the stomach, nose, intestines and lungs. They can also be detected in the blood in an immature form. Dendritic cells are obtained from hematopoietic bone marrow progenitor cells, which first develop into immature dendritic cells and communicate continuously with other cells in the body. The communication can occur in the form of direct cell–cell contact on the basis of interaction between cell-surface proteins. This book aims to understand the immunobiology of dendritic cells. The topics included herein are of utmost significance and bound to provide incredible insights to the readers. Researchers and students engaged in the study of dendritic cells will be assisted by this book.

At the end, I would like to appreciate all the efforts made by the authors in completing their chapters professionally. I express my deepest gratitude to all of them for contributing to this book by sharing their valuable works. A special thanks to my family and friends for their constant support in this journey.

Editor

1

Endocytic Recycling of MHC Class I Molecules in Non-Professional Antigen Presenting and Dendritic Cells

Sebastian Montealegre [1,2,3] and Peter M. van Endert [1,2,3]**

[1] *Institut National de la Santé et de la Recherche Médicale, Unité 1151, Paris, France,* [2] *Université Paris Descartes, Faculté de Médecine, Paris, France,* [3] *Centre National de la Recherche Scientifique, UMR8253, Paris, France*

***Correspondence:**
Sebastian Montealegre
sebastian.montealegre@inserm.fr
Peter M. van Endert
peter.van-endert@inserm.fr

Major histocompatibility complex class I (MHC I) molecules are glycoproteins that display peptide epitopes at the cell surface of nucleated cells for recognition by $CD8^+$ T cells. Like other cell surface receptors, MHC class I molecules are continuously removed from the surface followed by intracellular degradation or recycling to the cell surface, in a process likely involving active quality control the mechanism of which remains unknown. The molecular players and pathways involved in internalization and recycling have previously been studied in model cell lines such as HeLa. However, dendritic cells (DCs), which rely on a specialized endocytic machinery that confers them the unique ability to "cross"-present antigens acquired by internalization, may use distinct MHC I recycling pathways and quality control mechanisms. By providing MHC I molecules cross-presenting antigens, these pathways may play an important role in one of the key functions of DCs, priming of T cell responses against pathogens and tumors. In this review, we will focus on endocytic recycling of MHC I molecules in various experimental conditions and cell types. We discuss the organization of the recycling pathway in model cell lines compared to DCs, highlighting the differences in the recycling rates and pathways of MHC I molecules between various cell types, and their putative functional consequences. Reviewing the literature, we find that conclusive evidence for significant recycling of MHC I molecules in primary DCs has yet to be demonstrated. We conclude that endocytic trafficking of MHC class I in DCs remains poorly understood and should be further studied because of its likely role in antigen cross-presentation.

Keywords: major histocompatibility, endosome, dendritic cell, recycling, antigen presentation, cross-presentation, Arf6, Rab11

INTRODUCTION

MHC I molecules present pathogen, tumor and self-antigens to CD8+ T cells through the endogenous or direct and the exogenous or cross-presentation (1, 2) pathways. The spatio-temporal separation of these pathways (3) implies that intracellular transport of MHC-I molecules must be regulated, and that MHC I trafficking may vary according to cell type and particularly to the presence or absence of cross-presentation capacity. Mechanisms regulating trafficking likely are intertwined with mechanisms of quality control and act at various places in the cell: the endoplasmic reticulum (ER), the Golgi apparatus, the cell surface, and the endosomal system. A vast amount of information is available about the quality control steps selecting properly folded class I molecules in the secretory pathway (4–7). In contrast, the endocytic transport of class I molecules and the mechanisms of quality control in it are much less understood.

Analysis of endocytic trafficking is complicated by the fact that MHC I molecules exist in various forms presumably sensed by mechanisms of quality control, and that may follow distinct intracellular trafficking pathways: trimers made of a heavy chain, beta-2 microglobulin (β_2m), and high affinity peptides; trimers made of heavy chain, β_2m, and low affinity peptides; dimers without any bound peptides; and free heavy chains (FHC). For simplicity, we will refer to the trimers with high-affinity peptide as "fully conformed," and the other forms as "sub-optimally loaded," unless otherwise specified. Distinguishing complexes with high and low affinity peptides is important, since the affinity of the peptide-MHC interaction is the first determinant of the lifetime of class I molecules at the cell surface (8–10). It also determines the dissociation of β_2m, the binding of which acts as signal preventing degradation of class I complexes (9). The picture becomes even more complex considering that different class I allotypes have different half-lives at the cell surface (11). Thus, putative quality control mechanisms should sense correctly structural variants for more than 5,500 class I allotypes (12) to discriminate between degradation and recycling.

As we will describe in detail, a large amount of information about the recycling pathways followed by class I molecules has been obtained in HeLa cells and H-2L^d-expressing L cell fibroblasts. Available data suggest quantitative and mechanistic differences relative to the speed and efficacy of class I recycling between model cell lines. In contrast, very limited information is available on MHC I trafficking in professional antigen presenting cells (pAPCs). It is ironic that recycling has mainly been studied in cell lines unable to cross-present, given that the likely biological role of recycling concerns cross-presentation in DCs priming T cell responses to tumors and pathogens.

While some discrepancies between published studies may be derived from methodological approaches, many will be due to variation between cell types studied. In this review we will not only emphasize differences between model cell lines and pAPCs, but also examine the methods that have been used to obtain quantitative data on recycling efficacy and kinetics. Moreover, we will highlight knowledge on trafficking of fully conformed and sub-optimally loaded class I molecules obtained studying non-immune, non-phagocytic cell lines. Finally, we will relate these observations to existing and lacking knowledge on MHC I trafficking in pAPCs and its role in antigen cross-presentation. As we discuss key data on endocytic trafficking and evidence for differential sorting of distinct MHC I conformers, it needs to be kept in mind that the molecular players and chaperones mediating quality control in this context remain unknown. We anticipate that identification of such players will be required to fully understand endocytic trafficking and recycling of class I molecules, and conclusively answer the questions discussed below.

ENDOCYTOSIS IN A NUTSHELL

Proteins that are destined to be recycled to the cell surface need, by definition, first to be internalized from the cell surface. Internalization of cell surface components is a constitutive event in all cell types and important in nutrient uptake, signal transduction, cell adhesion, and in renewal and recycling of plasma membrane components, among others (2, 13). Internalization of membrane proteins requires the formation of endocytic vesicles delivering cargo to the cell. The formation of such vesicles can be mediated by clathrin, a protein forming a lattice around the newly generated vesicle in the form of triskelions (14), or can be clathrin-independent. Clathrin-mediated endocytosis (CME) and clathrin-independent endocytosis (CIE) are commonly distinguished as the two main routes of endocytosis (15, 16). Proteins that are internalized via CME typically harbor the motif Y-X-X-Φ at their cytosolic tail, where Φ is any bulky hydrophobic amino acid and X is any amino acid. MHC I molecules do not possess such a motif, although a sequence in the cytoplasmic tail of HLA-A and B molecules has been postulated to represent a non-canonical motif for CME endocytosis (17). CIE pathways are named according to the morphology of the vesicle coat or cargo (e.g., caveolae, or lipid raft endocytosis), or to key intracellular proteins regulating trafficking (18). One of the latter CIE pathways is named for the small GTPase Arf6 and has been widely described as the mechanism of endocytosis of MHC I molecules in model cell lines. In this pathway, hydrolysis of Arf6-GTP is required twice, first after internalization of cargo (19) to change the phosphoinositide composition of the early endosomes and allow fusion with EEA-1 vesicles (13, 19), and a second time to promote recycling from tubular recycling endosomes (described below) (19, 20). Regardless of the mode of internalization, after 5 to 10 min, internalized proteins arrive to a shared station, the early sorting endosomes (21, 22). Typical markers of the sorting endosomes, with a luminal pH in the range of 6.3 to 6.8, are the GTPase Rab5 and its effector EEA-1 (23). From these vesicles, internalized cargo can be sorted to late endosomes and lysosomes for degradation or be re-directed to the cell surface using various routes of recycling. At least three recycling pathways have been described for model cell surface receptors and in model cell lines: direct recycling from the sorting endosomes to the cell surface ("fast recycling"), the route followed by the transferrin receptor; transport from sorting endosomes to the Trans Golgi Network (TGN) and then to the cell surface ("retrograde transport") (24); and transport from the sorting endosomes to the endocytic recycling compartment (ERC) and then to the cell surface ("slow recycling"). Fast recycling is in the order of 5–10 min (25), whereas slow recycling is in the order of 30–60 min (2). For an extensive review of the mechanistic regulation of each pathway we refer the reader to two excellent recent reviews (22, 26). For MHC I molecules, a fourth pathway from late endosomes to the surface (discussed below) has also been suggested. We will focus mainly on the pathway involving the ERC, the main route taken by recycling MHC I molecules in non-professional APCs according to literature data.

Recycling endosomes are dynamic, tubulo-vesicular structures of nearly neutral pH in charge of sorting and re-exporting internalized membrane material (2, 26). The most widely used though by no means exclusive marker of recycling endosomes is the small GTPase Rab11. Rab11 localizes mostly to a perinuclear region that defines the ERC. Rab11 also localizes to the TGN (27) and to vesicular structures. Rab22 is another small GTPase involved in endosomal membrane trafficking (28) found both in the ERC and in tubular recycling endosomes (TRE) (29). Activation of Rab22 is required for the formation of TREs from the ERC, and inactivation is required for the final fusion of the tubules with the surface (29). Apart from Rab22, the biogenesis and maintenance of the TRE is in part regulated by the actin regulatory redox enzyme MICAL-L1(30), the family of Eps15 homology domain-containing 1-4 proteins (EHD-1 to 4) (31), and the small GTPases Arf6 (see above), Rab35, and Rab8a (32, 33). MICAL-L1 is a central protein required for the *de novo* generation of TREs (32) since it can bind directly phospholipids, and can form tubules *in vitro* and *in vivo* (34). MICAL-L1 serves as a hub for multiple proteins to regulate the formation of the TREs: it binds to EHD-1 via Rab8, as well as to Arf6 or Rab35 (33). Arf6 positively regulates recycling by aiding to localize Rab8 to the forming TREs, as well as by activating phospholipase D and PIP5 kinase, thereby providing the necessary lipids for the generation of recycling vesicles (35). Rab35, on the other hand, works as a negative regulator of TRE formation, by binding to MICAL-L1 and promoting GTP hydrolysis of Arf6 by the GTPase activating protein (GAP) ACAP2 (35, 36).

RECYCLING OF FULLY CONFORMED MHC CLASS I MOLECULES: METHODS AND EVIDENCE

Fully conformed and sub-optimally loaded MHC I molecules can be distinguished by monoclonal antibodies. We will first discuss work performed using antibodies recognizing the former category of class I molecules, which represents the vast majority of published studies (**Figure 1**). Early work from the groups of Watts and Jondal showed that upon internalization, class I molecules recycle to the cell surface (37, 38). Making use of a surface iodination assay in B lymphoblastoid cells, Reid and Watts were able to show that after accumulation of peptide-bound class I molecules in intracellular compartments by incubation with the inhibitor primaquine for 30 min, removal of primaquine resulted in recycling of nearly all the internalized class I to the cell surface within 16 min. Using the TAP-deficient thymoma cell line RMA-S, Abdel-Mottal et al. loaded class I molecules with glycopeptides and antibodies against the glycopeptide, then allowed for internalization, removed the remaining cell-surface complexes by a protease, and finally found that, depending on the peptide sequence, 36 to 63% of the class I molecules bound to the glycopeptides recycled to the surface. The re-appearance of the class I molecules was sensitive to chloroquine and leupeptin, indicating trafficking of the complexes via endosomal compartments. Although these experiments were performed using the thymoma line RMA-S, the findings of Abdel-Mottal et al. were a first indication that internalized peptides, and by extrapolation possibly antigens, might be loaded on recycling MHC I molecules in a "vacuolar" pathway.

Other work corroborated the conclusions of these early studies that class I molecules can recycle to the cell surface in model cell lines. The seminal work by Radakhrishna and Donaldson (20) showed for the first time the involvement of the small GTPase Arf6 in the recycling of MHC I molecules. As in most of the pertinent literature, the experimental system was HeLa cells, and the antibody used to detect class I was W6/32, which detects HLA heavy chains bound to β_2m. In this system, class I localized to tubulo-vesicular structures decorated with Arf6. Moreover, in HeLa and Jurkat cells where the constitutively active mutant Arf6 Q67L was overexpressed, internalized class I molecules accumulated in PIP_2 rich endosomes, thereby preventing their further degradation or recycling (13, 39, 40). Furthermore, overexpression of an effector domain mutant of Arf6 (N48I) in HeLa cells decreased recycling of class I molecules by 60% relative to control cells (35).

Subsequent studies of class I recycling in HeLa cells showed that 10–15 min after internalization, class I molecules reached tubular structures, presumably the TRE, the formation of which required EHD-1 among other players (see above) (29, 41). The quantitative assay to examine the role of EHD-1 in the recycling of class I was a "CELISA": the authors seeded HeLa cells onto ELISA plates, incubated them with biotinylated MHC I antibodies at 37°C for 5 min, washed out free antibodies, and incubated the cells at 37°C for various time points. When EHD-1 was overexpressed, the number of cell surface class I molecules bound by biotinylated antibodies increased by 50% relative to the cell surface population present at the end of internalization (41).

The description of the role of Rab22 in endocytic recycling introduced the most widely used recycling assay so far (29). In a seminal study, HeLa cells were pulsed with mAb W6/32, allowed to internalize for 30 min at 37°C, acid-stripped to remove remaining cell surface complexes, and then chased at 37°C for various lengths of time. Quantification was based on the re-appearance of class I at the cell surface in unpermeabilized cells, as detected with a secondary antibody, compared to the internal class I signal, which was detected by removing the recycled class I with a second acid treatment, permeabilization of the cells, and detection with a secondary antibody. The read-out used microscopy or flow cytometry. In untransfected cells, 30% of the internalized class I population recycled to the surface by 30 min (29). Overexpression of wt Rab22 reduced recycling by 50%, an inhibitory effect that became even more pronounced upon overexpression of the dominant negative Rab22 S19N and the constitutively active Rab22 Q64L mutants. Using the same experimental system, the authors found that overexpression of the dominant negative mutant Rab11 S25N reduced class I recycling by nearly 80% relative to control cells, confirming a role for Rab11 in class I recycling in HeLa cells.

More recently, using the same recycling assay and HeLa cells, it was shown that the enzyme diacylglycerol kinase alpha (DGKα) was required for formation of tubular recycling endosomes by interacting with MICAL-L1 and generating phosphatidic acid

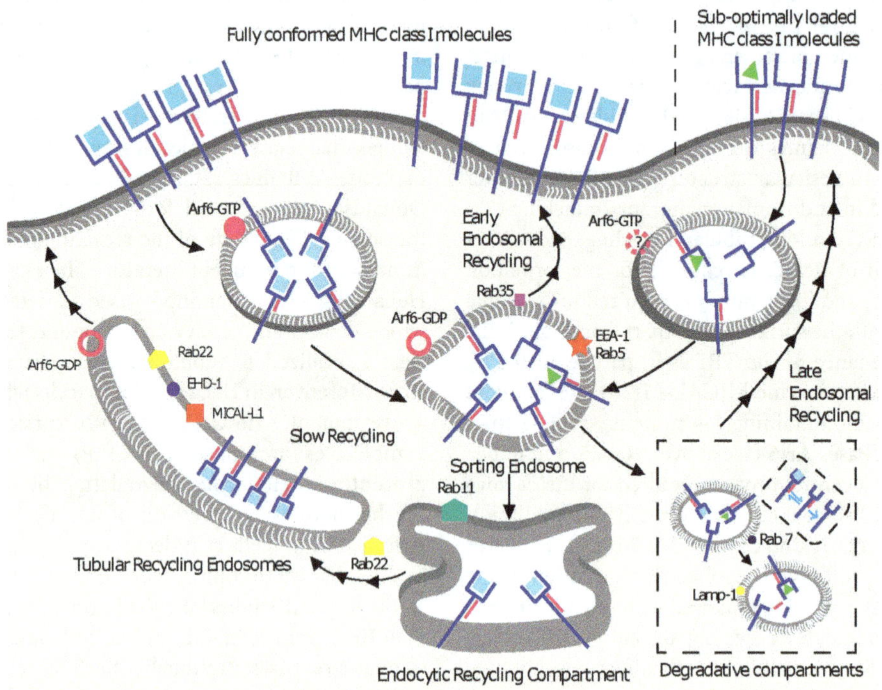

FIGURE 1 | MHC I recycling pathways in non-professional APCs. Fully conformed and sub-optimally loaded class I molecules partition in different domains at the cell surface. Fully conformed class I molecules are internalized by CIE in vesicles decorated by Arf6-GTP and reach EEA1$^+$/Rab5$^+$ sorting endosomes. From here, they can follow an early endosomal recycling route regulated by Rab35 or enter into the slow recycling pathway. Upon arrival to the ERC, fully conformed molecules are incorporated into tubular recycling endosomes, which are formed by the proteins MICAL-L1, EHD-1, Rab8, Rab22, and Arf6. Vesicles derived from the tubular recycling endosomes finally fuse with the plasma membrane with the help of Arf6, delivering fully conformed class I molecules to the cell surface. Upon internalization, sub-optimally loaded class I molecules reach sorting EEA-1$^+$/Rab5$^+$ endosomes; the role of Arf6 in this is not known. From there, sub-optimally loaded class I molecules travel to degradative compartments, in which peptides and β_2m will dissociate from the heavy chain, promoting the degradation of most molecules. However, a fraction may be able to recycle to the cell surface using a late endosomal recycling pathway independent of Rab11. Lines with single arrowheads represent internalization steps, whereas lines with multiple arrowheads represent recycling steps. Note that the ER is not represented.

(42). In turn, knockdown of DGKα delayed recycling of class I. Remarkably, after 30 min of internalization and 3 h of chase (recycling), the authors detected up to 40% recycled class I in wt Hela cells.

A putative alternative class I recycling pathway is mediated by Rab35, experimentally demonstrated in Cos-7 cells. Knockdown of Rab35 resulted in formation of enlarged EHD-1 negative endosomes (43). The authors proposed that Rab35 mediates "fast" direct recycling of class I from early endosomes to the cell surface, in a pathway distinct from the Rab22-Rab11 recycling axis. However, this conclusion was based on an assay that does not provide unequivocal evidence for recycling. The assay consisted in two 20-min incubations each followed by acid stripping to remove cell surface class I molecules. The first stripping removed MHC I not internalized after the initial 20-min pulse with an anti-MHC I antibody, and the second molecules "recycled" to surface after the second 20-min period. An increase in the number of labeled MHC-I molecules, detected by staining of permeabilized cells with a secondary antibody, was then interpreted as intracellular retention and lack of recycling. However, a role of Rab35 in degradation of internalized MHC-I molecules would equally well explain the increase by 60% of "retained" class I observed upon Rab35 knockdown.

Reviewing the different assays, some discrepancies are apparent, which may be biological or methodological. While the role of the different endocytic regulators is undisputed in the cell lines evaluated, the reported recycling kinetics of fully conformed class I molecules vary significantly from assay to assay and from cell line to cell line. The biochemical surface labeling assay (37) led to the conclusion that almost all fully conformed class I molecules that are internalized recycle very efficiently and fast. In contrast, the microscopy and FACS-based assays suggest that recycling of fully conformed class I recycling is slow and inefficient (**Table 1**). Perhaps the simplest explanation is that fully conformed class I can recycle via two different pathways, a fast one and a slow one. However, among the published pathways reviewed here, the "fastest" recycling pathway described implicates Rab35. In this pathway, recycling was detected after 20 min, which is already in the range of the slower recycling pathway dependent on the Arf6-Rab22-Rab11-MICAL-L1 axis. Thus, there is presently no conclusive evidence for class I recycling through a truly fast pathway returning for example the transferrin receptor to the surface. Variations between cell lines may also play a role. For example, in CHO cells, the Arf6 pathway plays a role in the recycling of the transferrin receptor, which is normally endocytosed via clathrin-mediated

TABLE 1 | Published data on MHC-I recycling.

Allele	Cell type/line	Assay	Percent recycled of internalized pool	Time of maximal recycling	References	Observations
HLA-A/B/C	EBV A46 B lymphoblastoid	Surface biotinylation	100	16 min	(37)	First demonstration that MHC I proteins to recycle upon internalization.
H-2D^b	HeLa cells	CELISA	50	15 min	(41)	Recycling observed upon overexpression of EHD-1.
HLA-A/B/C	HeLa cells	mAb uptake-Microscopy	30	60 min	(29)	Rab22 overexpression decreases recycling to 50% relative to untransfected cells. Rab22 mutant overexpression reduces recycling to 15-25% relative to untransfected cells.
H-2L^d, folded	L-L^d cells	mAb uptake-FACS	30	20 min	(44)	Recycling of unfolded H-2L^d was not detected with this assay. However, the authors could detect it in Mahmutefendić et al. (46) with a modification of the assay.
H-2L^d, folded	L-L^d cells	mAb uptake-FACS	25–30	20 min	(45)	Recycling of several folded MHC I molecules was evaluated. The authors did not observe recycling of unfolded molecules.
H-2L^d, folded	HeLa-L^d	mAb uptake-FACS				
HLA-CW6	J26Cw6	mAb uptake-FACS				
HLA-B7	J26B7	mAb uptake-FACS				
HLA-A/B/C	HeLa cells	mAb uptake-microscopy	40	3 h	(42)	The absence of the enzyme diacylglycerol kinase alpha inhibits recycling of folded human class I molecules.
H-2L^d, unfolded	L-L^d cells	mAb uptake-FACS	15–20	30 min	(46)	To observe recycling of unfolded H-L^d from late endosomes, the authors accumulated antibody-antigen complexes for 3h in late endosomal compartments, and then proceeded to evaluate recycling.
H-2K^b, folded	JAWS DCs	mAb uptake-FACS	40	10 min	(47)	First quantitative demonstration of MHC I recycling in a DC-like cell line. Knocking down Rab22 reduces recycling efficiency to 10% of the internalized pool.

The superscript letter indicates the allele of the gene indicated by the capital letter preceding it - no explanation required for any immunologist.

endocytosis (15), indicating that different recycling pathways might operate in different cells. Also, Rab22 is necessary for internalization of class I in Jurkat but not in HeLa cells (29, 40). As mentioned above, published data show remarkable variation with respect to the kinetics of class I recycling. Thus, in HeLa cells, the model system most frequently, recycling of W6/32 positive molecules ranges from 30 min to 3 h. At the same time, the authors of various publications agree on an estimated rate of 30–40% recycling class I molecules using the microscopy-based assay. How can the same rate of recycling be obtained in such divergent time spans? One possible explanation would be a mechanism of quality control that keeps the number of recycling class I molecules on the cell surface at any time below a certain threshold. For example, fully conformed class I molecules reaching the cell surface using the Arf6-Rab22-Rab11-MICAL-L1 axis within 30 min could rapidly be internalized again. It is unknown how many rounds of recycling a single class I molecule can undergo. It is also unclear whether and to what extent a peptide exchange occurs during class I recycling in non-professional APCs.

Differences between class I allotypes might also lead to diversion into a different recycling pathway. In the secretory pathway, where the molecular players mediating quality control such as tapasin and calreticulin are well characterized, class I polymorphism is well known to affect quality control. For example, class I allotypes differing by a single amino acid, such as HLA-B*44:02 and B*44:05 or HLA-B*27:05 and B*27:09, differ greatly with respect to dependence on tapasin in order to acquire high affinity peptide ligands and leave the ER (48, 49). Similar differences might be revealed in endocytic quality control once the relevant chaperones will be identified. One candidate for such a role is the tapasin homolog TAPBPR, which can operate in a pH range of 6.0–7.2 and may therefore be able to mediate peptide exchange in endosomes. Interestingly, very recent data suggest that TAPBPR also acts in an MHC I allele-specific manner (50). In conclusion, the recycling pathways of fully conformed class I molecules in non-professional APCs still require clarification and additional investigation.

RECYCLING OF SUB-OPTIMALLY LOADED MHC CLASS I MOLECULES

Heavy chain-β_2m empty dimers and FHC constitute a minor population out of the total pool of class I molecules present at the cell surface and can be identified by a number of monoclonal antibodies. The precise relative proportion of FHC and empty dimers among surface class I molecules are not known but likely vary according to the cell type and state as well as to the class I allotype considered. For example, among the two murine allotypes studied most frequently, H-2K^b and H-2L^d, cell surface L^d is known to comprise a larger proportion of FHC due to its lower stability relative to K^b. FHC have been found at the cell surface of T and B lymphocytes under inflammatory conditions (51, 52) and in β_2m deficient cells at resting conditions (53). While the function of the FHC is starting to be elucidated and may reside mainly in their binding to particular KIR receptors on NK cells (54–58), there is limited mechanistic evidence about their endosomal regulation and recycling.

Recent results provide initial insight into how sub-optimally loaded dimers are internalized, recycled, and degraded. The best evidence comes from the work of Lucin and co-workers, who have systematically evaluated the constitutive internalization of the murine class I allotype H-2L^d in their fully conformed and sub-optimally loaded forms (44, 59), as well as the early and late endosomal recycling of H-2L^d molecules (45, 46). This allotype is particularly suited for studying the different class I conformers because of the availability of the monoclonal antibodies 30.5.7 and 64.3.7, originally produced by Hansen et al. with a well-studied and exquisite specificity for the two conformers (60–62). As mentioned above, H-2L^d is less stable than other allotypes, resulting in a higher proportion of sub-optimally loaded or empty molecules, adding another argument in support of studying trafficking of different class I conformers using L^d as a model. The experimental system established by this group consists mainly, but not only, in L cell fibroblasts expressing L^d, which constitutively express high levels of sub-optimally loaded dimers; monoclonal antibodies 30.5.7 and 64.3.7 distinguishing fully conformed class I trimers and β_2m-bound heavy chains devoid of peptides, respectively; and a quantitative flow cytometry recycling assay based on the principle of the assay by Weigert et al. (29). Using these tools, they found that fully conformed internalized H-2L^d molecules that had accumulated during 1 h in a Rab11$^+$compartment, presumably the ERC (45, 46), recycled with an efficiency of 20–30 %, reaching a plateau at 30 min. In contrast, sub-optimally loaded H-2L^d molecules were not detected in the Rab11$^+$ ERC and could not recycle (44). They extended these results to other class I allotypes, such as HLA-Cw6 and HLA-B7, and cell lines, obtaining similar recycling rates (45). Whether recycling of fully conformed H-2L^d molecules was Arf6 dependent or not was not investigated. However, considering the recycling rates matching those observed in some of the HeLa-W6/32 recycling assays, and the involvement of the Rab11$^+$ ERC, it is likely that they followed the Arf6 pathway. Since recycling of sub-optimally loaded class I molecules was not detected using the conventional methods, they modified the assay by internalizing sub-optimally loaded molecules bound to 64.3.7 for 3 h instead of 1 h, and comparing the signal for internalized vs. total labeled class I by flow cytometry (46). Surprisingly, they were able to detect recycling sub-optimally loaded molecules that had passed through Rab7$^+$ late endosomes, with an efficiency of 15–20% after 30 min of chase.

So far, this is the sole quantitative evidence for recycling of sub-optimally loaded class I molecules, which may implicate a special pathway originating from late endosomes. In TAP-deficient fibroblasts pre-incubated at 26°C bearing relatively large numbers of sub-optimally loaded class I molecules at the cell surface (63, 64), FHCs, but not dimers, are rapidly removed from the cell surface (9). It is conceivable that a late endosomal pathway provides recycling dimers at low temperature, which at physiological temperature are degraded upon dissociation of β_2m (9). Importantly, the cellular compartment where class I molecules are sorted for a round of recycling using the ERC-dependent recycling pathway or the late endosomal recycling pathway is not known. Whether these processes depend on Arf6, or whether they can be extrapolated to other cell lines or cell types, are other open questions.

MHC CLASS I RECYCLING AND ANTIGEN PRESENTATION

While MHC I recycling has been subjected to some cell-biological scrutiny, there is surprisingly little published evidence on its role in antigen presentation. Given that the endocytic pathway plays a mandatory role in cross-presentation of internalized antigens, it may not surprise that the available literature concerns exclusively this pathway. Indeed, a role of recycling class I molecules in peptide loading of class I molecules in the ER appears little likely. However, class I molecules can also be loaded with endogenous peptides in post-ER compartments potentially accessible for recycling class I molecules. For example, Hsc70-coupled endogenous antigens can be processed through chaperone mediated autophagy (65), and HSV-1 antigens through a non-canonical pathway of macro-autophagy (66), both presumably implicating antigen degradation in endolysosomal compartments. Moreover, peptide fragments of endogenous transmembrane proteins can be produced and loaded in the same type of compartment (67). However, whether recycling MHC I molecules were responsible for presentation in these studies is not known.

As discussed above, there appears to exist significant variation regarding the pathways and type of class I molecules able to recycle in non-immune cells. The scenario in pAPCs, e.g., cells derived through differentiation from monocytes or from bone marrow precursors *in vitro*, or primary DCs obtained from mice or humans is even less understood. In DCs but probably also some macrophage types capable of cross-presentation, class I molecules need to have access to peptides from internalized antigens. This can occur in the perinuclear ER through a cytosolic pathway of cross-presentation, or in non-ER compartments, following either the ER-phagosome pathway or vacuolar pathways (2). In the two latter scenarios, cross-presenting pAPCs may require an alternative source of class I molecules independent of the secretory pathway. It is in this context that recycling class I molecules emerge as a candidate source of MHC I molecules provided to the ER-phagosome and the vacuolar pathway of cross-presentation (**Figure 2**).

One of the first indications of potential pathways operating in professional antigen presenting cells [for the subtypes of DCs, the reader is referred to other reviews (68, 69)], was curiously obtained in a melanoma cell line. Grommé et al. fractionated MelJuSo melanoma cells and identified HLA class I molecules in a fraction also containing acidic HLA class II loading compartments. A significant proportion of HLA class I-peptide complexes remained stable and could be immunoprecipitated at pH=5 using W6/32. This implied the existence of a compartment

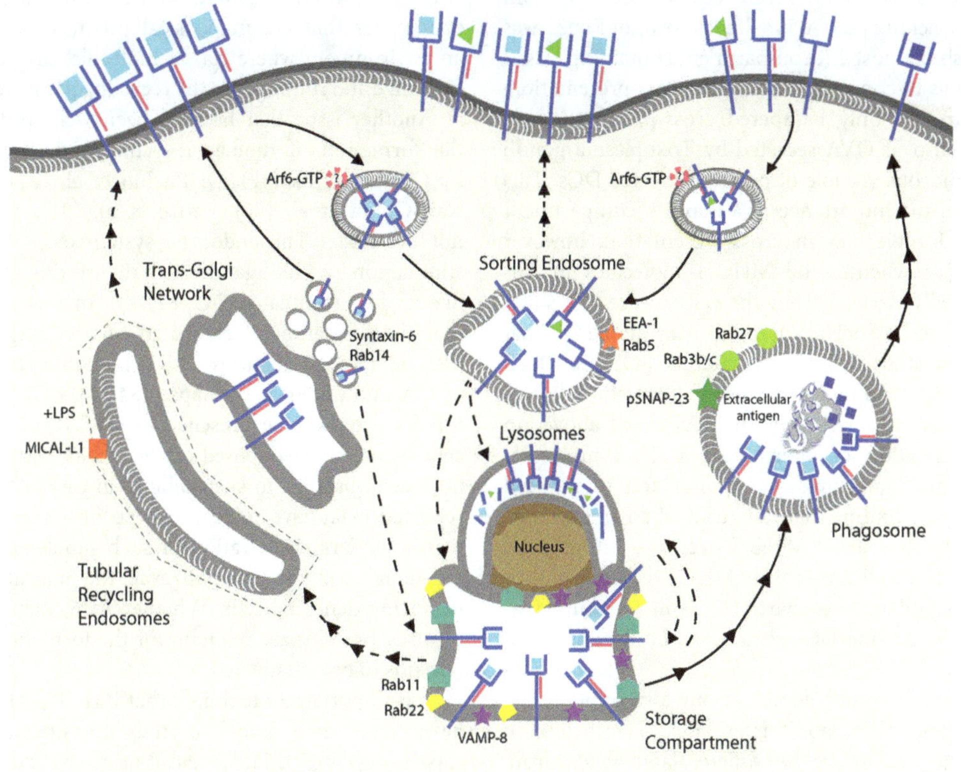

FIGURE 2 | MHC I recycling in pAPCs. Fully conformed and sub-optimally loaded class I molecules are internalized and reach sorting endosomes presumably by CIE. It is not known whether Arf6 is involved for internalization of one or both conformers. Under resting conditions, fully conformed class I molecules reside in a post-ER compartment positive for Rab11/Rab22/VAMP8. Class I molecules might be provided to this compartment from the sorting endosomes, from the secretory pathway using TGN derived vesicles positive for Syntaxin 6/Rab14, or from lysosomes. Given that the origin of the MHC I molecules in this compartment remains to be clarified, we prefer the term "storage compartment" to "ERC." Upon stimulation by TLR ligands, fully conformed class I molecules are recruited from the storage compartment to phagosomes positive for Rab3b/c, Rab27, and pSNAP23, and then travel to the cell surface via an uncharacterized mechanism. Peptide exchange may occur in the phagosome although formal proof is lacking. Tubular recycling endosomes bearing MICAL-L1 have been observed upon stimulation with LPS, but class I molecules have not been detected so far within the tubules. Lines with single arrowheads represent internalization and lines with multiple arrowheads recycling steps. Dashed lines represent hypothetical transport steps. Note that the ER is not represented.

potentially acidic enough to promote peptide exchange, but not enough to degrade class I molecules (70). More direct evidence for peptide exchange in presumably recycling MHC I molecules was provided by studies on TAP-deficient macrophages. Pre-incubation with peptide ligands stabilized a pool of class I molecules on these cells which then allowed for cross-presentation of a bacterial antigen through a vacuolar pathway, most likely involving peptide exchange in an acidic compartment (71). Coming back to a more physiologic setting, various groups have reported the existence of a post-ER compartment containing presumably fully conformed class I molecules in different types of (TAP-sufficient) DCs (72–74). A common characteristic of the latter studies is that upon incubation with primaquine, cross-presentation of soluble antigens is blocked (3, 75, 76). A possible interpretation is that class I molecules are located in a mildly acid endosomal compartment from which they are unable to recycle upon inhibition of acidification by primaquine.

Do class I molecules recycle in pAPCs? And if so, do they use the pathways described in non-immune cell lines? The recent studies from Nair-Gupta et al. and Cebrian et al. built on the knowledge gained from the studies of non-immune cell lines to identify players in the cross-presentation pathways. The former study characterized a post-ER Rab11^{+}/VAMP8^{+} compartment containing MHC I molecules in bone marrow-derived DCs (BM-DCs) and suggested that this compartment constituted an important source of cross-presenting MHC I molecules. Upon stimulation by TLR-2/4 ligands, class I molecules derived from the Rab11 compartment were recruited to phagosomes. Knockdown of Rab11 in BM-DCs had a profound detrimental effect on antigen cross-presentation. Remarkably, the authors showed that primary type 1 conventional DCs (cDC1), but not cDC2 harbor the class I/Rab11^{+} compartment, suggesting that cDC2s may have a different source of class I molecules for cross-presentation (77). It is puzzling that pDCs, which also have the post-ER compartment (73) have shown to be less efficient than their cDC1 and cDC2 counterparts in antigen cross-presentation.

Consistent with observations made in HeLa cells, the study by Cebrian et al. (47) showed that Rab22 partially co-localizes with Rab11 and with fully conformed class I molecules in BM-DCs and in JAWS-II cells, an immortalized cell line derived from C57BL/6 BM-DCs lacking p53. A 50% knockdown of Rab22 was sufficient to abolish the post-ER compartment containing class I molecules, as well as to compromise antigen cross-presentation. Rab22 knockdown not only hampered cross-presentation of soluble OVA but also of OVA secreted by Toxoplasma gondii into the parasitophorous vacuole of parasite-infected DCs. This result corroborated the importance of a Rab11+ compartment containing MHC I molecules in cross-presentation, however it remained unclear whether the MHC I molecules in this compartment actually derived from the cell surface. To study recycling, Cebrian and associates used an assay similar to that used by Allaire to study the role of Rab35 (43), in which an increase in MHC I molecules "retained" intracellularly was interpreted as evidence of lack recycling. As noted above, an intracellular accumulation of internalized MHC I molecules can be due both to compromised recycling and to reduced degradation. Thus, the finding that Rab22 knockdown inhibited "disappearance" of internalized MHC I over a 40-min period almost completely may indicate a role in MHC I recycling and/or in routing to a degradative compartment. Thus, in our view, MHC I recycling in murine DCs remains to be demonstrated conclusively.

Our review of the literature, as well as our own unpublished observations, suggests that monitoring MHC I recycling in primary DC-like populations, be they differentiated *in vitro* from bone marrow or monocytes, or isolated as primary *in vivo* DC populations, remains challenging. Considering the specialization but also plasticity of DCs, as well as the variation already existing between non-immune cell lines, it would not be surprising to find distinct recycling rates and pathways in primary DC populations. The role of recycling MHC I molecules might also be limited to specific antigen types. As an example, in a study including an assay directly measuring internalized MHC I molecules re-appearing at the cell surface, van den Eynde et al. recently showed that cross-presentation by human monocyte-derived DCs (mo-DCs) of a synthetic long peptide (an antigen type of interest for tumor vaccination) involved peptide exchange on MHC I molecules, however these molecules were nascent rather than recycling (78).

OUTLOOK

Although the cited papers provide solid evidence for an important role of Rab11 and Rab22 in cross-presentation, important mechanistic issues remain unresolved. Identification of the Rab11/Rab22/VAMP8 compartment containing fully conformed class I molecules may suggest that the class I molecules detected originate from the cell surface, where they return to through recycling. However, as discussed above, there is no formal proof that this is the case. Several alternative scenarios could be considered. The TGN might feed this compartment with fully conformed class I molecules arriving through the secretory pathway, using, for example, Syntaxin 6^{+} and $Rab14^{+}$ TGN-derived vesicles (79, 80). Another hypothesis is the adaptation of the late endosomal recycling pathway described by Lucin and coworkers, where lysosomes would communicate with recycling endosomes that are in physical proximity, thereby providing an environment where class I molecules are sorted for peptide exchange and routing into the recycling pathway, or degradation.

Another issue that has not been well studied in pAPCs is the formation of tubular recycling endosomes. In the work by Cebrian et al. (47), Di Puchio et al. (73), Zou et al. (74), Nair-Gupta et al. (77), Croce et al. (81), such tubules were not described. The endocytic system of DCs remodels upon stimulation by TLR ligands, such that resting DCs do not behave like an LPS stimulated DC (82, 83). In this context, it appears that the formation of elongated tubules originating from the ERC in moDCs requires TLR stimulation and the formation of the immunological synapse (84, 85). The formation of the tubules requires the presence of MICAL-L1 (86), as in HeLa cells. However, as opposed to HeLa cells, class I molecules have not been observed in such tubules in pAPCs. The observations reported so far have made use of specimens treated with fixation, which renders visualization of such tubules difficult (26). Live cell-imaging methods might reveal the presence of such tubules in resting dendritic cells. Whether Arf6, Rab8, Rab35, ACAP1, or other proteins are required for the formation of such tubules remains to be investigated.

It is important to highlight that BM-DCs and moDCs, which have served as a model to study cross-presentation (but not class I recycling so far) *in vitro*, might not reflect the pathways of class I recycling and cross-presentation operating *in vivo* (87, 88). Unfortunately, the typical cell biological and cross-presentation assays require a substantial number of cells that can be difficult to obtain for primary pAPC subsets. Since BM-DCs and moDCs reflect most closely the properties of inflammatory dendritic cells and macrophages found *in vivo* (89), and the latter ones use in some cases a purely vacuolar cross-presentation pathway (90), it is important to study recycling of class I molecules in primary cells. We anticipate that there will be significant variation and plasticity in the recycling pathways and rates of class I molecules in primary pAPC populations. Identifying the molecular machinery in charge of endocytic quality control will be essential in order to fully decipher MHC I endocytic trafficking, recycling and cross-presentation. Finally, the functional impact of MHC I recycling is almost entirely unexplored. Previous studies have been limited to examining presentation of the model antigen OVA to a CD8+ T cell line. The ultimate challenge for the field will be explore the impact of MHC I recycling in T cell responses to pathogens and tumors.

AUTHOR CONTRIBUTIONS

All authors listed have made a substantial, direct and intellectual contribution to the work, and approved it for publication.

ACKNOWLEDGMENTS

Work in the authors' laboratory was supported by grant 14-CE11-0014 from the *Agence Nationale de Recherche*. We are grateful to Maria Camila Montealegre for assistance with graphic design.

REFERENCES

1. Adiko AC, Babdor J, Gutiérrez-Martínez E, Guermonprez P, Saveanu L. Intracellular transport routes for MHC I and their relevance for antigen cross-presentation. *Front Immunol.* (2015) 6:335. doi: 10.3389/fimmu.2015.00335
2. van Endert P. Intracellular recycling and cross-presentation by MHC class I molecules. *Immunol Rev.* (2016) 272:80–96. doi: 10.1111/imr.12424
3. Burgdorf S, Schölz C, Kautz A, Tampé R, Kurts C. Spatial and mechanistic separation of cross-presentation and endogenous antigen presentation. *Nat Immunol.* (2008) 9:558–66. doi: 10.1038/ni.1601
4. Springer S. Transport and quality control of MHC class I molecules in the early secretory pathway. *Curr Opin Immunol.* (2015) 34:83–90. doi: 10.1016/j.coi.2015.02.009
5. Neerincx A, Boyle LH. Properties of the tapasin homologue TAPBPR. *Curr Opin Immunol.* (2017) 46:97–102. doi: 10.1016/j.coi.2017.04.008
6. Blees A, Januliene D, Hofmann T, Koller N, Schmidt C, Trowitzsch S, et al. Structure of the human MHC-I peptide-loading complex. *Nature* (2017) 551:525–8. doi: 10.1038/nature24627
7. Thomas C, Tampé R. Structure of the TAPBPR-MHC I complex defines the mechanism of peptide loading and editing. *Science* (2017) 358:1060–4. doi: 10.1126/science.aao6001
8. Howarth M, Williams A, Tolstrup AB, Elliott T. Tapasin enhances MHC class I peptide presentation according to peptide half-life. *Proc Natl Acad Sci USA* (2004) 101:11737–42. doi: 10.1073/pnas.0306294101
9. Montealegre S, Venugopalan V, Fritzsche S, Kulicke C, Hein Z, Springer S. Dissociation of β2-microglobulin determines the surface quality control of major histocompatibility complex class I molecules. *FASEB J.* (2015) 29:2780–8. doi: 10.1096/fj.14-268094
10. Arshad N, Cresswell P. Tumor-associated calreticulin variants functionally compromise the peptide loading complex and impair its recruitment of MHC-I. *J Biol Chem.* (2018) 293:9555–69. doi: 10.1074/jbc.RA118.002836
11. Su RC, Miller RG. Stability of surface $H\text{-}2K^b$, $H\text{-}2D^b$, and peptide-receptive $H\text{-}2K^b$ on splenocytes. *J Immunol.* (2001) 167:4869–77. doi: 10.4049/jimmunol.167.9.4869
12. Robinson J, Halliwell JA, Hayhurst JD, Flicek P, Parham P, Marsh SGE. The IPD and IMGT/HLA database: allele variant databases. *Nucleic Acids Res.* (2015) 43:D423–31. doi: 10.1093/nar/gku1161
13. Grant BD, Donaldson JG. Pathways and mechanisms of endocytic recycling. *Nat Rev Mol Cell Biol.* (2009) 10:597–608. doi: 10.1038/nrm2755
14. Kaksonen M, Roux A. Mechanisms of clathrin-mediated endocytosis. *Nat Rev Mol Cell Biol.* (2018) 19:313–26. doi: 10.1038/nrm.2017.132
15. Sandvig K, Pust S, Skotland T, van Deurs B. Clathrin-independent endocytosis: mechanisms and function. *Curr Opin Cell Biol.* (2011) 23:413–20. doi: 10.1016/j.ceb.2011.03.007
16. Sandvig K, Kavaliauskiene S, Skotland T. Clathrin-independent endocytosis: an increasing degree of complexity. *Histochem Cell Biol.* (2018) 150:107–18. doi: 10.1007/s00418-018-1678-5
17. Lizée G, Basha G, Tiong J, Julien J-P, Tian M, Biron KE, et al. Control of dendritic cell cross-presentation by the major histocompatibility complex class I cytoplasmic domain. *Nat Immunol.* (2003) 4:1065–73. doi: 10.1038/ni989
18. Watanabe S, Boucrot E. Fast and ultrafast endocytosis. *Curr Opin Cell Biol.* (2017) 47:64–71. doi: 10.1016/j.ceb.2017.02.013
19. Eyster CA, Higginson JD, Huebner R, Porat-Shliom N, Weigert R, Wu WW, et al. Discovery of new cargo proteins that enter cells through clathrin-independent endocytosis. *Traffic* (2009) 10:590–9. doi: 10.1111/j.1600-0854.2009.00894.x
20. Radhakrishna H, Donaldson JG. ADP-ribosylation factor 6 regulates a novel plasma membrane recycling pathway. *J Cell Biol.* (1997) 139:49–61.
21. Maxfield FR, McGraw TE. Endocytic recycling. *Nat Rev Mol Cell Biol.* (2004) 5:121–32. doi: 10.1038/nrm1315
22. Naslavsky N, Caplan S. The enigmatic endosome - sorting the ins and outs of endocytic trafficking. *J Cell Sci.* (2018) 131:jcs216499. doi: 10.1242/jcs.216499
23. Jovic M, Sharma M, Rahajeng J, Caplan S. The early endosome: a busy sorting station for proteins at the crossroads. *Histol Histopathol.* (2010) 25:99–112. doi: 10.14670/HH-25.99
24. Johannes L, Popoff V. Tracing the retrograde route in protein trafficking. *Cell* (2008) 135:1175–87. doi: 10.1016/j.cell.2008.12.009
25. Mellman I. Endocytosis and molecular sorting. *Annu Rev Cell Dev Biol.* (1996) 12:575–625. doi: 10.1146/annurev.cellbio.12.1.575
26. Goldenring JR. Recycling endosomes. *Curr Opin Cell Biol.* (2015) 35:117–22. doi: 10.1016/j.ceb.2015.04.018
27. Welz T, Wellbourne-Wood J, Kerkhoff E. Orchestration of cell surface proteins by Rab11. *Trends Cell Biol.* (2014) 24:407–15. doi: 10.1016/j.tcb.2014.02.004
28. Kauppi M, Simonsen A, Bremnes B, Vieira A, Callaghan J, Stenmark H, et al. The small GTPase Rab22 interacts with EEA1 and controls endosomal membrane trafficking. *J Cell Sci.* (2002) 115:899–911.
29. Weigert R, Yeung AC, Li J, Donaldson JG. Rab22a regulates the recycling of membrane proteins internalized independently of clathrin. *Mol Biol Cell.* (2004) 15:3758–70. doi: 10.1091/mbc.E04-04-0342
30. Frémont S, Romet-Lemonne G, Houdusse A, Echard A. Emerging roles of MICAL family proteins - from actin oxidation to membrane trafficking during cytokinesis. *J Cell Sci.* (2017) 130:1509–17. doi: 10.1242/jcs.202028
31. Naslavsky N, Caplan S. EHD proteins: key conductors of endocytic transport. *Trends Cell Biol.* (2011) 21:122–31. doi: 10.1016/j.tcb.2010.10.003
32. Sharma M, Giridharan SSP, Rahajeng J, Naslavsky N, Caplan S. MICAL-L1 links EHD1 to tubular recycling endosomes and regulates receptor recycling. *Mol Biol Cell* (2009) 20:5181–94. doi: 10.1091/mbc.E09-06-0535
33. Rahajeng J, Giridharan SSP, Cai B, Naslavsky N, Caplan S. MICAL-L1 is a tubular endosomal membrane hub that connects Rab35 and Arf6 with Rab8a. *Traffic* (2012) 13:82–93. doi: 10.1111/j.1600-0854.2011.01294.x
34. Rahajeng J, Giridharan SSP, Cai B, Naslavsky N, Caplan S. Important relationships between Rab and MICAL proteins in endocytic trafficking. *World J Biol Chem* (2010) 1:254–64. doi: 10.4331/wjbc.v1.i8.254
35. Jovanovic OA, Brown FD, Donaldson JG. An effector domain mutant of Arf6 implicates phospholipase D in endosomal membrane recycling. *Mol Biol Cell* (2006) 17:327–35. doi: 10.1091/mbc.E05-06-0523
36. Dutta D, Donaldson JG. Sorting of clathrin-independent cargo proteins depends on Rab35 delivered by clathrin-mediated endocytosis. *Traffic* (2015) 16:994–1009. doi: 10.1111/tra.12302
37. Reid PA, Watts C. Cycling of cell-surface MHC glycoproteins through primaquine-sensitive intracellular compartments. *Nature* (1990) 346:655–7. doi: 10.1038/346655a0
38. Abdel Motal UM, Zhou X, Joki A, Siddiqi AR, Srinivasa BR, Stenvall K, et al. Major histocompatibility complex class I-binding peptides are recycled to the cell surface after internalization. *Eur J Immunol.* (1993) 23:3224–9. doi: 10.1002/eji.1830231227
39. Naslavsky N, Weigert R, Donaldson JG. Convergence of non-clathrin- and clathrin-derived endosomes involves Arf6 inactivation and changes in phosphoinositides. *Mol Biol Cell* (2003) 14:417–31. doi: 10.1091/mbc.02-04-0053
40. Johnson DL, Wayt J, Wilson JM, Donaldson JG. Arf6 and Rab22 mediate T cell conjugate formation by regulating clathrin-independent endosomal membrane trafficking. *J Cell Sci.* (2017) 130:2405–15. doi: 10.1242/jcs.200477
41. Caplan S, Naslavsky N, Hartnell LM, Lodge R, Polishchuk RS, Donaldson JG, et al. A tubular EHD1-containing compartment involved in the recycling of major histocompatibility complex class I molecules to the plasma membrane. *EMBO J.* (2002) 21:2557–67. doi: 10.1093/emboj/21.11.2557
42. Xie S, Naslavsky N, Caplan S. Diacylglycerol kinase α regulates tubular recycling endosome biogenesis and major histocompatibility complex class I recycling. *J Biol Chem.* (2014) 289:31914–26. doi: 10.1074/jbc.M114.594291
43. Allaire PD, Marat AL, Dall'Armi C, Di Paolo G, McPherson PS, Ritter B. The Connecdenn DENN domain: a GEF for Rab35 mediating cargo-specific exit from early endosomes. *Mol Cell* (2010) 37:370–82. doi: 10.1016/j.molcel.2009.12.037
44. Mahmutefendić H, Blagojević G, Tomaš MI, Kučić N, Lučin P. Segregation of open Major Histocompatibility Class I conformers at the plasma membrane and during endosomal trafficking reveals conformation-based sorting in the endosomal system. *Int J Biochem Cell Biol.* (2011) 43:504–15. doi: 10.1016/j.biocel.2010.12.002
45. Zagorac GB, Mahmutefendić H, Tomaš MI, Kučić N, Le Bouteiller P, Lučin P. Early endosomal rerouting of major histocompatibility class I conformers. *J Cell Physiol.* (2012) 227:2953–64. doi: 10.1002/jcp.23042

46. Mahmutefendić H, Blagojević Zagorac G, Grabušić K, Karleuša L, Maćešić S, et al. Late endosomal recycling of open MHC-I conformers. *J Cell Physiol.* (2017) 232:872–87. doi: 10.1002/jcp.25495
47. Cebrian I, Croce C, Guerrero NA, Blanchard N, Mayorga LS. Rab22a controls MHC-I intracellular trafficking and antigen cross-presentation by dendritic cells. *EMBO Rep.* (2016) 17:1753–65. doi: 10.15252/embr.201642358
48. Garstka MA, Fritzsche S, Lenart I, Hein Z, Jankevicius G, Boyle LH, et al. Tapasin dependence of major histocompatibility complex class I molecules correlates with their conformational flexibility. *FASEB J.* (2011) 25:3989–98. doi: 10.1096/fj.11-190249
49. Abualrous ET, Fritzsche S, Hein Z, Al-Balushi MS, Reinink P, Boyle LH, et al. F pocket flexibility influences the tapasin dependence of two differentially disease-associated MHC Class I proteins. *Eur J Immunol.* (2015) 45:1248–57. doi: 10.1002/eji.201445307
50. Ilca FT, Neerincx A, Hermann C, Marcu A, Stefvanovic S, Deane JE, et al. TAPBPR mediates peptide dissociation from MHC class I using a leucine lever. *Elife* (2018) 7:40126. doi: 10.7554/eLife.40126
51. Grassi F, Meneveri R, Gullberg M, Lopalco L, Rossi GB, Lanza P, et al. Human immunodeficiency virus type 1 gp120 mimics a hidden monomorphic epitope borne by class I major histocompatibility complex heavy chains. *J Exp Med.* (1991) 174:53–62.
52. Schnabl E, Stockinger H, Majdic O, Gaugitsch H, Lindley IJ, Maurer D, et al. Activated human T lymphocytes express MHC class I heavy chains not associated with beta 2-microglobulin. *J Exp Med.* (1990) 171:1431–42.
53. Martayan A, Sibilio L, Tremante E, Lo Monaco E, Mulder A, Fruci D, et al. Class I HLA folding and antigen presentation in beta 2-microglobulin-defective Daudi cells. *J Immunol.* (2009) 182:3609–17. doi: 10.4049/jimmunol.0802316
54. Goodridge JP, Lee N, Burian A, Pyo C-W, Tykodi SS, Warren EH, et al. HLA-F and MHC-I open conformers cooperate in a MHC-I antigen cross-presentation pathway. *J Immunol.* (2013) 191:1567–77. doi: 10.4049/jimmunol.1300080
55. Goodridge JP, Burian A, Lee N, Geraghty DE. HLA-F and MHC class I open conformers are ligands for NK cell Ig-like receptors. *J Immunol.* (2013) 191:3553–62. doi: 10.4049/jimmunol.1300081
56. Burian A, Wang KL, Finton KAK, Lee N, Ishitani A, Strong RK, et al. HLA-F and MHC-I open conformers bind natural killer cell Ig-Like receptor KIR3DS1. *PLoS ONE* (2016) 11:e0163297. doi: 10.1371/journal.pone.0163297
57. Arosa FA, Esgalhado AJ, Padrão CA, Cardoso EM. Divide, conquer, and sense: CD8(+)CD28(-) T cells in perspective. *Front Immunol.* (2016) 7:665. doi: 10.3389/fimmu.2016.00665
58. Dulberger CL, McMurtrey CP, Hölzemer A, Neu KE, Liu V, Steinbach AM, et al. Human leukocyte antigen f presents peptides and regulates immunity through interactions with NK Cell Receptors. *Immunity* (2017) 46:1018–29.e7. doi: 10.1016/j.immuni.2017.06.002
59. Mahmutefendić H, Blagojević G, Kucić N, Lucin P. Constitutive internalization of murine MHC class I molecules. *J Cell Physiol.* (2007) 210:445–55. doi: 10.1002/jcp.20877
60. Yu YY, Myers NB, Hilbert CM, Harris MR, Balendiran GK, Hansen TH. Definition and transfer of a serological epitope specific for peptide-empty forms of MHC class I. *Int Immunol.* (1999) 11:1897–906.
61. Hansen TH, Lybarger L, Yu L, Mitaksov V, Fremont DH. Recognition of open conformers of classical MHC by chaperones and monoclonal antibodies. *Immunol Rev.* (2005) 207:100–11. doi: 10.1111/j.0105-2896.2005.00315.x
62. Mage MG, Dolan MA, Wang R, Boyd LF, Revilleza MJ, Robinson H, et al. The peptide-receptive transition state of MHC class I molecules: insight from structure and molecular dynamics. *J Immunol.* (2012) 189:1391–9. doi: 10.4049/jimmunol.1200831
63. Ljunggren HG, Stam NJ, Ohlén C, Neefjes JJ, Höglund P, Heemels MT, et al. Empty MHC class I molecules come out in the cold. *Nature* (1990) 346:476–80. doi: 10.1038/346476a0
64. Day PM, Esquivel F, Lukszo J, Bennink JR, Yewdell JW. Effect of TAP on the generation and intracellular trafficking of peptide-receptive major histocompatibility complex class I molecules. *Immunity* (1995) 2:137–47. doi: 10.1016/S1074-7613(95)80014-X
65. Reimann J, Schirmbeck R. Alternative pathways for processing exogenous and endogenous antigens that can generate peptides for MHC class I-restricted presentation. *Immunol Rev.* (1999) 172:131–52. doi: 10.1111/j.1600-065X.1999.tb01362.x
66. English L, Chemali M, Duron J, Rondeau C, Laplante A, Gingras D, et al. Autophagy enhances the presentation of endogenous viral antigens on MHC class I molecules during HSV-1 infection. *Nat Immunol.* (2009) 10:480–7. doi: 10.1038/ni.1720
67. Tiwari N, Garbi N, Reinheckel T, Moldenhauer G, Hämmerling GJ, Momburg F. A transporter associated with antigen-processing independent vacuolar pathway for the MHC class I-mediated presentation of endogenous transmembrane proteins. *J Immunol.* (2007) 178:7932–42. doi: 10.4049/jimmunol.178.12.7932
68. Segura E, Amigorena S. Cross-presentation in mouse and human dendritic cells. *Adv Immunol.* (2015) 127:1–31. doi: 10.1016/bs.ai.2015.03.002
69. Vendelova E, Ashour D, Blank P, Erhard F, Saliba A-E, Kalinke U, et al. Tolerogenic transcriptional signatures of steady-state and pathogen-induced dendritic cells. *Front Immunol.* (2018) 9:333. doi: 10.3389/fimmu.2018.00333
70. Grommé M, Uytdehaag FG, Janssen H, Calafat J, van Binnendijk RS, Kenter MJ, et al. Recycling MHC class I molecules and endosomal peptide loading. *Proc Natl Acad Sci USA.* (1999) 96:10326–31.
71. Chefalo PJ, Harding CV. Processing of exogenous antigens for presentation by class I MHC molecules involves post-Golgi peptide exchange influenced by peptide-MHC complex stability and acidic pH. *J Immunol.* (2001) 167:1274–82. doi: 10.4049/jimmunol.170.1.643
72. MacAry PA, Lindsay M, Scott MA, Craig JI, Luzio JP, Lehner PJ. Mobilization of MHC class I molecules from late endosomes to the cell surface following activation of CD34-derived human Langerhans cells. *Proc Natl Acad Sci USA.* (2001) 98:3982–7. doi: 10.1073/pnas.071477498
73. Di Pucchio T, Chatterjee B, Smed-Sörensen A, Clayton S, Palazzo A, Montes M, et al. Direct proteasome-independent cross-presentation of viral antigen by plasmacytoid dendritic cells on major histocompatibility complex class I. *Nat Immunol.* (2008) 9:551–7. doi: 10.1038/ni.1602
74. Zou L, Zhou J, Zhang J, Li J, Liu N, Chai L, et al. The GTPase Rab3b/3c-positive recycling vesicles are involved in cross-presentation in dendritic cells. *Proc Natl Acad Sci USA.* (2009) 106:15801–6. doi: 10.1073/pnas.0905684106
75. Spadaro F, Lapenta C, Donati S, Abalsamo L, Barnaba V, Belardelli F, et al. IFN-α enhances cross-presentation in human dendritic cells by modulating antigen survival, endocytic routing, and processing. *Blood* (2012) 119:1407–17. doi: 10.1182/blood-2011-06-363564
76. Fiegl D, Kägebein D, Liebler-Tenorio EM, Weisser T, Sens M, Gutjahr M, et al. Amphisomal route of MHC class I cross-presentation in bacteria-infected dendritic cells. *J Immunol.* (2013) 190:2791–806. doi: 10.4049/jimmunol.1202741
77. Nair-Gupta P, Baccarini A, Tung N, Seyffer F, Florey O, Huang Y, et al. TLR signals induce phagosomal MHC-I delivery from the endosomal recycling compartment to allow cross-presentation. *Cell* (2014) 158:506–21. doi: 10.1016/j.cell.2014.04.054
78. Ma W, Zhang Y, Vigneron N, Stroobant V, Thielemans K, van der Bruggen P, et al. Long-peptide cross-presentation by human dendritic cells occurs in vacuoles by peptide exchange on nascent MHC class I molecules. *J Immunol.* (2016) 196:1711–20. doi: 10.4049/jimmunol.1501574
79. Saveanu L, Carroll O, Weimershaus M, Guermonprez P, Firat E, Lindo V, et al. IRAP identifies an endosomal compartment required for MHC class I cross-presentation. *Science* (2009) 325:213–7. doi: 10.1126/science.1172845
80. De Angelis Rigotti F, De Gassart A, Pforr C, Cano F, N'Guessan P, Combes A, et al. MARCH9-mediated ubiquitination regulates MHC I export from the TGN. *Immunol Cell Biol.* (2017) 95:753–64. doi: 10.1038/icb.2017.44
81. Croce C, Mayorga LS, Cebrian I. Differential requirement of Rab22a for the recruitment of ER-derived proteins to phagosomes and endosomes in dendritic cells. *Small GTPases* (2017) 1–9. doi: 10.1080/21541248.2017.1384088
82. Alloatti A, Kotsias F, Pauwels A-M, Carpier J-M, Jouve M, Timmerman E, et al. Toll-like Receptor 4 engagement on dendritic cells restrains phago-lysosome fusion and promotes cross-presentation of antigens. *Immunity* (2015) 43:1087–100. doi: 10.1016/j.immuni.2015.11.006
83. Babdor J, Descamps D, Adiko AC, Tohmé M, Maschalidi S, Evnouchidou I, et al. IRAP+ endosomes restrict TLR9 activation and signaling. *Nat Immunol.* (2017) 18:509–18. doi: 10.1038/ni.3711

84. Boes M, Cerny J, Massol R, Op den Brouw M, Kirchhausen T, Chen J, et al. T-cell engagement of dendritic cells rapidly rearranges MHC class II transport. *Nature* (2002) 418:983–8. doi: 10.1038/nature01004
85. Compeer EB, Flinsenberg TWH, Boon L, Hoekstra ME, Boes M. Tubulation of endosomal structures in human dendritic cells by Toll-like receptor ligation and lymphocyte contact accompanies antigen cross-presentation. *J Biol Chem.* (2014) 289:520–8. doi: 10.1074/jbc.M113.511147
86. Compeer EB, Boes M. MICAL-L1-related and unrelated mechanisms underlying elongated tubular endosomal network (ETEN) in human dendritic cells. *Commun Integr Biol.* (2014) 7:e994969. doi: 10.4161/19420889.2014.994969
87. Helft J, Böttcher J, Chakravarty P, Zelenay S, Huotari J, Schraml BU, et al. GM-CSF mouse bone marrow cultures comprise a heterogeneous population of $CD11c^{+}MHCII^{+}$ macrophages and dendritic cells. *Immunity* (2015) 42:1197–211. doi: 10.1016/j.immuni.2015.05.018
88. Kretzer NM, Theisen DJ, Tussiwand R, Briseño CG, Grajales-Reyes GE, Wu X, et al. RAB43 facilitates cross-presentation of cell-associated antigens by CD8α+ dendritic cells. *J Exp Med.* (2016) 213:2871–83. doi: 10.1084/jem.20160597
89. Lutz MB, Inaba K, Schuler G, Romani N. Still alive and kicking: *in-vitro*-generated GM-CSF dendritic cells! *Immunity* (2016) 44:1–2. doi: 10.1016/j.immuni.2015.12.013
90. Tang-Huau T-L, Gueguen P, Goudot C, Durand M, Bohec M, Baulande S, et al. Human *in vivo*-generated monocyte-derived dendritic cells and macrophages cross-present antigens through a vacuolar pathway. *Nat Commun.* (2018) 9:2570. doi: 10.1038/s41467-018-04985-0

2

Neoadjuvant Radiochemotherapy Significantly Alters the Phenotype of Plasmacytoid Dendritic Cells and 6-Sulfo LacNAc^{+} Monocytes in Rectal Cancer

Felix Wagner[1†], *Ulrike Hölig*[1†], *Friederike Wilczkowski*[1†], *Ioana Plesca*[1,2], *Ulrich Sommer*[3], *Rebekka Wehner*[1,4,5], *Maximilian Kießler*[1], *Armin Jarosch*[3], *Katharina Flecke*[1,6], *Maia Arsova*[1,6], *Antje Tunger*[1,4], *Andreas Bogner*[7], *Christoph Reißfelder*[8], *Jürgen Weitz*[4,5,7], *Knut Schäkel*[9], *Esther G. C. Troost*[2,4,5,10,11], *Mechthild Krause*[2,4,5,10,11], *Gunnar Folprecht*[4,5,6], *Martin Bornhäuser*[4,5,6], *Michael P. Bachmann*[4,5,12], *Daniela Aust*[3,4,5], *Gustavo Baretton*[3,4,5] and *Marc Schmitz*[1,4,5*]

Institute of Immunology, Faculty of Medicine Carl Gustav Carus, Technische Universität Dresden, Dresden, Germany, Department of Radiotherapy and Radiation Oncology, University Hospital Carl Gustav Carus, Technische Universität Dresden, Dresden, Germany, [3] Institute of Pathology, University Hospital of Dresden, Dresden, Germany, [4] Partner Site Dresden, National Center for Tumor Diseases (NCT), Dresden, Germany, [5] Partner Site Dresden, German Cancer Consortium (DKTK), and German Cancer Research Center (DKFZ), Heidelberg, Germany, [6] Department of Medicine I, University Hospital Carl Gustav Carus, Technische Universität Dresden, Dresden, Germany, [7] Department of Gastrointestinal, Thoracic, and Vascular Surgery, University Hospital Carl Gustav Carus, Technische Universität Dresden, Dresden, Germany, [8] Department of Surgery, Mannheim University Medical Centre, University of Heidelberg, Mannheim, Germany, [9] Department of Dermatology, University Hospital of Heidelberg, Heidelberg, Germany, [10] OncoRay – National Center for Radiation Research in Oncology, Dresden, Germany, [11] Institute of Radiooncology – OncoRay, Helmholtz-Zentrum Dresden-Rossendorf, Dresden, Germany, [12] Department of Radioimmunology, Institute of Radiopharmaceutical Cancer Research, Helmholtz Center Dresden-Rossendorf, Dresden, Germany

***Correspondence:**
Marc Schmitz
marc.schmitz@tu-dresden.de

[†]These authors have contributed equally to this work

Neoadjuvant radiochemotherapy (nRCT) can significantly influence the tumor immune architecture that plays a pivotal role in regulating tumor growth. Whereas, various studies have investigated the effect of nRCT on tumor-infiltrating T cells, little is known about its impact on the frequency and activation status of human dendritic cells (DCs). Plasmacytoid DCs (pDCs) essentially contribute to the regulation of innate and adaptive immunity and may profoundly influence tumor progression. Recent studies have revealed that higher pDC numbers are associated with poor prognosis in cancer patients. 6-sulfo LacNAc-expressing monocytes (slanMo) represent a particular proinflammatory subset of human non-classical blood monocytes that can differentiate into DCs. Recently, we have reported that activated slanMo produce various proinflammatory cytokines and efficiently stimulate natural killer cells and T lymphocytes. slanMo were also shown to accumulate in clear cell renal cell carcinoma (ccRCC) and in metastatic lymph nodes from cancer patients. Here, we investigated the influence of nRCT on the frequency of rectal cancer-infiltrating pDCs and slanMo. When evaluating rectal cancer tissues obtained from patients after nRCT, a significantly higher density of pDCs in comparison to pre-nRCT tissue samples was found. In contrast, the density of slanMo was not significantly altered by nRCT. Further studies revealed that nRCT significantly enhances the proportion of rectal cancer-infiltrating CD8+ T cells expressing the cytotoxic effector molecule granzyme B. When exploring the impact of nRCT on the phenotype of rectal cancer-infiltrating pDCs and slanMo, we observed that nRCT markedly enhances the percentage of inducible nitric oxide synthase (iNOS)- or tumor necrosis factor (TNF) alpha-producing slanMo. Furthermore, nRCT significantly increased the percentage of mature CD83+ pDCs in rectal cancer tissues. Moreover, the proportion of pDCs locally expressing interferon-alpha, which plays a major role in antitumor immunity, was significantly higher in post-nRCT tissues compared to pre-nRCT tumor specimens. These novel findings indicate that nRCT significantly influences the frequency and/or phenotype of pDCs, slanMo, and CD8+ T cells, which may influence the clinical response of rectal cancer patients to nRCT.

Keywords: plasmacytoid dendritic cells, 6-sulfo LacNAc+ monocytes, CD8+ T cells, tumor immune architecture, radiochemotherapy, rectal cancer

INTRODUCTION

Colorectal cancer is one of the most common malignancies in the United States with an estimated incidence of 140,250 cases and an estimated number of 50,630 deaths in 2018 (1). Previous reports have provided evidence that the immune contexture plays a major role for the clinical outcome of colorectal cancer patients (2). Thus, it has been shown that high densities of CD45RO+ T helper (Th) 1 cells and CD8+ T cells are associated with improved survival of colorectal cancer patients (3, 4). However, patients with high expression of Th17 genes had a poor prognosis. These results led to the development of a so-called "immunoscore" for an optimized tumor classification (5).

Neoadjuvant radiochemotherapy (nRCT) followed by total mesorectal excision constitutes the current standard of care for locally advanced rectal cancers (6, 7). nRCT can efficiently reduce tumor size, resulting in a higher rate of sphincter-preserving surgical interventions, and an increased rate of R0-resections. In addition, this treatment modality decreases the local recurrence rate. Recent findings have revealed that nRCT can significantly influence the tumor immune contexture, affecting the tumor responsiveness to this treatment modality (2, 8–11). Thus, it has been reported that several chemotherapeutic agents as well as radiotherapy can efficiently stimulate antitumor immune responses by triggering immunogenic cell death in tumor cells (12, 13). This process is characterized by the translocation of intracellular calreticulin to the surface of tumor cells and the release of high-mobility-group box 1. Surface-exposed calreticulin markedly enhances the phagocytosis of tumor cells by dendritic cells (DCs) that play a crucial role in the induction and regulation of antitumor immunity (14). Released high-mobility-group box 1 from chemo- or radiotherapy-treated tumor cells promote the maturation and activation of DCs, resulting in an efficient processing and presentation of tumor-associated antigens and the stimulation of potent tumor-directed T-cell responses. In addition to immunogenic cell death induction, radiotherapy has been shown to reduce the surface expression of CD47, which acts as an antiphagocytosis signal to promote immune evasion (15). Inhibition of CD47 function significantly augments the engulfment of tumor cells by DCs, resulting in effective antitumor responses (16). In contrast to these immunostimulatory effects, radiotherapy, and chemotherapeutic agents can also induce immunosuppressive effects. They include the increase of tumor-infiltrating regulatory T cells and myeloid-derived suppressor cells, which produce immunosuppressive molecules (8, 9, 17). These immune cell subsets can profoundly impair the functional properties of effector T cells and can promote tumor growth and resistance.

Plasmacytoid DCs (pDCs) represent an important subset of human blood DCs that are capable of producing large amounts of interferon (IFN)-α upon stimulation (18, 19). In addition, pDCs can efficiently enhance the antitumoral capabilities of natural killer (NK) cells and T lymphocytes (20, 21). Based on these functional properties, stimulated pDCs can promote antitumor responses *in vivo*. Thus, the intratumoral administration of activated pDCs led to tumor regression in a B16 melanoma mouse model (22). Furthermore, it has been demonstrated in an orthotopic murine mammary tumor model that the intratumoral application of a toll-like receptor 7 ligand results in the activation of tumor-associated pDCs and tumor regression (23). In a clinical trial, intranodal injections of activated pDCs loaded with tumor-associated antigen-derived peptides in patients with metastatic melanoma induced specific CD8+ and CD4+ T cell responses (24). However, pDCs can also act as tolerogenic cells by suppressing T cell responses (19, 25). Previous studies have shown that pDCs infiltrate a variety of human cancers including head and neck, breast and ovarian cancer, and that a higher density is associated with poor clinical outcome (26–28). In addition, it has been demonstrated that tumor-infiltrating pDCs produce reduced amounts of IFN-α upon activation and can efficiently promote the expansion of regulatory T cells (29). 6-sulfo LacNAc (slan) monocytes (slanMo, formerly termed

M-DC8$^+$ DCs or slanDCs) are a subset of human non-classical blood monocytes, which can differentiate into DCs (30–40). Previously, we have reported that slanMo produce high levels of various proinflammatory cytokines and display a marked capability to handle IgG-complexed antigens (31, 32, 37). We have also demonstrated that slanMo mediate direct cytotoxicity against tumor cells (38, 39). Further studies have revealed that they efficiently induce neoantigen-specific CD4$^+$ T cells, activate tumor-reactive CD8$^+$ T cells, and promote the polarization of naïve CD4$^+$ T lymphocytes into Th1 or Th17/Th1 cells (30–32, 36). Moreover, slanMo have been shown to stimulate IFN-γ production and cytotoxic activity of NK cells (39, 40).

In the present study, we determined the impact of nRCT on the frequency of rectal cancer-infiltrating pDCs, slanMo, CD3$^+$ T cells, total CD8$^+$ T lymphocytes, and GrzB-expressing CD8$^+$ T cells. Furthermore, we analyzed the impact of nRCT on the percentage of rectal cancer-associated slanMo locally producing inducible nitric oxide synthase (iNOS) or tumor necrosis factor (TNF)-α, which play an important role in regulating tumor growth. Following recent findings, indicating that IFN-α essentially contributes to the antitumor effects mediated by RCT, the influence of nRCT on the proportion of rectal cancer-infiltrating pDCs locally expressing this cytokine was evaluated.

MATERIALS AND METHODS

Patients and Study Design

This is a retrospective study including 60 rectal cancer patients treated with nRCT followed by surgery at the University Hospital Carl Gustav Carus of Dresden between 2001 and 2013. From 20 of these patients, tumor biopsies prior to nRCT were available. Additionally, a cohort of 28 primarily resected rectal cancer patients without nRCT was matched according to gender, age, and TNM-stage. **Table 1** summarizes the clinicopathological characteristics of the study population.

Immunohistochemistry

Formalin-fixed and paraffin-embedded tissue sections were cut into 3–5 μm sections. Subsequently, these sections were deparaffinized in xylene (2 $\times$ 15 min, VWR International, Fontenay-sous-Bois, France) and hydrated by washes of graded ethanol (Berkel AHK, Ludwigshafen, Germany) to water (B. Braun, Melsungen, Germany). Tissue sections were boiled in citrate buffer (Zytomed Systems GmbH, Berlin, Germany) at pH 6.0 for 20 min for antigen retrieval. Subsequently, tissues were stained overnight at 4°C with either the polyclonal goat anti-BDCA-2 antibody (1:200, R&D Systems, Minneapolis, MN, USA) to evaluate pDCs (41) or the monoclonal mouse anti-slan antibody DD2 (1:10, Institute of Immunology, Faculty of Medicine Carl Gustav Carus, Technische Universität Dresden, Dresden, Germany) to analyze slanMo (32, 34–36). Then, tissues used for pDC staining were incubated with a mouse anti-goat antibody solution (Thermo Fisher Scientific, Rockford, IL, USA) for 60 min. Afterwards, all tissues were incubated with dextran-labeled antibodies against mouse immunoglobulins (Dako, Glostrup, Denmark) for 30 min. pDCs and slanMo were visualized by the alkaline phosphatase-based EnVision^{TM} detection system according to the manufacturer's instructions (Dako). All tissue sections were counterstained with Mayer's hematoxylin (Merck, Darmstadt, Germany). For pDC quantification, positively stained cells were counted in three different high power fields (HPF) of a section by using AxioVision 4.8.1.0 (Zeiss, Jena, Germany) and the mean value was determined. The mean number of pDCs per HPF (area: 0.237 mm^2) was converted to square millimeter. For slanMo, slides were digitized by an iScan Coreo slide scanner (Ventana Medical Systems, Oro Valley, AZ, USA) and evaluated using the same HPF method.

To determine the frequency of rectal cancer-infiltrating CD3$^+$ T cells, CD8$^+$ T cells, and granzyme B (GrzB)-expressing CD8$^+$ T cells, formalin-fixed, and paraffin-embedded tissue sections were deparaffinized in xylene BenchMark XT (Ventana Medical Systems) and then exposed to the Cell Conditioning 1 solution for antigen retrieval (Ventana Medical Systems). Two double immunohistochemical stainings were performed: CD3 / Ki67 and CD8 / GrzB. For the first double reaction, the monoclonal mouse anti-CD3 antibody (clone 2GV6, ready-to-use, Ventana Medical Systems) and the monoclonal mouse anti-Ki67 antibody (clone Mib-1, 1:50, Dako) were used. For the second double staining, the monoclonal mouse anti-CD8 antibody (clone C8/144B, 1:10, Dako) and the monoclonal mouse anti-GrzB antibody (clone GrzB-7, 1:10, Dako) were applied. All tissue sections were counterstained with Mayer's hematoxylin. Subsequently, the tissue sections were digitized by an iScan Coreo slide scanner, followed by T-cell quantification by using the Image viewer v. 3.1 (Ventana Medical Systems). Positively stained T lymphocytes were counted in three different HPF of a section and the mean value was determined. The mean number of T cells per HPF (area: 0.237 mm^2) was converted to square millimeter. To determine the percentage of GrzB-expressing CD8$^+$ T lymphocytes, between 65 and 576 CD8$^+$ T cells per tissue section were evaluated dependent on their frequency in the three HPF.

Immunofluorescence Staining

Tissues were deparaffinized, hydrated, and heat-treated as described above. After antigen retrieval, tissue sections were incubated overnight with primary antibody solutions containing goat anti-human BDCA-2 (1:50, R&D Systems) and either mouse anti-human CD83 (clone 1H4b, 1:100, Abcam, Cambridge, UK) or mouse anti-human IFN-α (clone F-7, 1:500, Santa Cruz Biotechnology, Heidelberg, Germany). Subsequently, tissue sections were incubated with a rabbit anti-goat antibody solution (1:100, Abcam) for 10 min. Afterwards, secondary antibody solution containing donkey anti-rabbit AF488 (1:100, Abcam) and donkey anti-mouse AF546 (1:100, Thermo Fisher Scientific) was applied for 30 min.

For staining of slanMo, tissue sections were incubated overnight with primary antibody solutions containing rabbit anti-human TNF-α (1:100, Abcam) and mouse anti-human DD2 (1:20), followed by 30 min of incubation with the secondary antibodies goat anti-mouse IgM biotin (1:100, SouthernBiotech, Birmingham, AL, USA) and fluorescence-labeled goat anti-rabbit IgG AF488 (1:100, Thermo Fisher Scientific). Finally,

TABLE 1 | Clinicopathological characteristics of the rectal cancer patients.

	nRCTx (*n* = 40)		Therapy-naïve (*n* = 28)		Matched group (*n* = 20)	
	Patients (*n*)	**%**	**Patients (*n*)**	**%**	**Patients (*n*)**	**%**
AGE						
Median (range)	61.1 years (44.1–78.2)		64.5 years (22.1–76.5)		59.5 years (40.7–72.6)	
GENDER						
Male	31	77.5	19	67.9	13	65.0
Female	9	22.5	9	32.1	7	35.0
pT						
1	2	5.0	3	10.7	0	0.0
2	9	22.5	9	32.1	6	30.0
3a	14	35.0	10	35.7	9	45.0
3b	12	30.0	6	21.4	4	20.0
4	3	7.5	0	0.0	1	5.0
pN						
0	25	62.5	20	71.4	17	85.0
1	9	22.5	8	28.6	1	5.0
2	6	15.0	0	0.0	2	10.0
nCT						
5-FU	30	75.0			14	70.0
5-FU + Oxaliplatin	6	15.0			2	10.0
Others	4	10.0			4	20.0
nRCT						
55.8 Gy	1	2.5			2	10.0
50.4 Gy	39	97.5			18	90.0

Streptavidin AF546 (1:500, Thermo Fisher Scientific) was applied for 15 min. To determine iNOS expression in rectal cancer-infiltrating slanMo, tissue sections were incubated with a mouse anti-human iNOS antibody (1:50, BD Biosciences, San Jose, CA, USA) for 60 min, followed by the application of a goat anti-mouse IgG (1:400, Abcam) and fluorescence-labeled donkey anti-goat AF488 antibody (1:100, Thermo Fisher Scientific), each for 20 min. Mouse serum (1:100, Dako) was applied for 10 min to prevent unspecific binding of the following antibody. For the detection of slanMo, mouse anti-human DD2 antibody (1:2) was applied for 60 min. Afterwards the tissues were incubated with a secondary antibody solution containing goat anti-mouse IgM Biotin (1:100, SouthernBiotech), followed by the application of fluorophore AF546 labeled Streptavidin (1:500, Thermo Fisher Scientific), each for 20 min. Then, tissues were mounted with 4,6 diamidino-2-phenylindole-containing AKLIDES® ANA plus medium (Medipan, Dahlewitz/Berlin, Germany), coverslipped, and analyzed with a Keyence fluorescence microscope BZ-9000 (Keyence, Osaka, Japan). To determine the percentage of CD83$^+$ and IFN-α^+ pDCs or iNOS$^+$ and TNF-α^+ slanMo, between 20 and 50 cells per tissue section were evaluated dependent on their frequency.

For additional experiments, immunofluorescence multiplex staining was accomplished by using the Opal kit and the Vectra imaging platform (Perkin Elmer, Hopkinton, MA, USA). Tissues were deparaffinized and hydrated as described above. Antigen retrieval was performed in AR6 or AR9 buffer (both from PerkinElmer) using microwave treatment. Afterwards, the Opal kit was used according to the manufacturer's instructions (PerkinElmer). Therefore, tissue sections were blocked for 10 min with the Antibody Dilutent/Block (PerkinElmer), then incubated with the primary antibody for one hour, followed by 10 min incubation with a horseradish peroxidase-conjugated secondary antibody (PerkinElmer). In case of goat anti-human primary antibodies, another 10 min incubation with a bridge mouse anti-goat antibody (1:100, Thermo Fisher Scientific) was required prior to the application of the secondary antibody. Finally, a TSA fluorophore was added to the tissue sections for 10 minutes. Subsequent stripping of the primary together with secondary antibodies was performed by microwave treatment. In between all the steps mentioned above, except prior to the primary antibody application, tissue sections were washed for 2 x 3 min in TBST buffer. Every incubation step took place in a humidified chamber on a rocking platform at room temperature. Blocking, incubation with primary and secondary antibody, visualization by a TSA fluorophore and microwave treatment were repeated for each primary antibody. Finally, all tissue slides were counterstained with spectral DAPI (PerkinElmer) for 5 min, washed with TBST buffer and with autoclaved water for 2 min, and then coverslipped with fluoromount medium (SouthernBiotech).

For the four-color Opal multiplex staining, primary antibodies directed against CD8 (clone C8/144B, 1:100, Dako, high pH retrieval), BDCA-2 (goat polyclonal, 1:100, R&D Systems, low pH retrieval), and panCK (clone AE1/AE3, 1:100, Thermo Fisher Scientific, low pH retrieval) were used and visualized by the TSA fluorophores 570 (1:100), 650 (1:100), and 690 (1:100, all from PerkinElmer), respectively. For the two-color Opal staining, the BDCA-2 primary antibody was used together with the polyclonal goat anti-human CXCL10, CCL4, or CCL5 primary antibody (1:100, all from R&D Systems, low pH retrieval) and combined with the TSA fluorophores 650 (1:100) and 570 (1:100), respectively. Acquisition of the multispectral images was performed with the Vectra 3.5 Automated Imaging System (Perkin Elmer). Spectral unmixing was done in inForm® using a library built from single stained tissue slides for each primary antibody-TSA fluorophore combination. ImageJ software was then used for final image processing.

Statistical Analysis

Statistical analysis was performed using unpaired student's t-test for the evaluation of pDCs and slanMo in non-matched tissues of untreated and nRCT-treated rectal cancer patients. Paired student's t-test was used for the analysis of pDCs, slanMo, and T cells in matched pre-nRCT and post-nRCT tumor tissues. Values of $^{*}p \leq 0.05$; $^{**}p \leq 0.01$; $^{***}\ p \leq 0.001$ were considered as significant.

RESULTS

nRCT Significantly Increases the Frequency of pDCs in Rectal Cancer

pDCs essentially contribute to the regulation of innate and adaptive immunity and may play an important role in the immune defense against tumors. Recently, it has been demonstrated that pDCs are present in a variety of primary

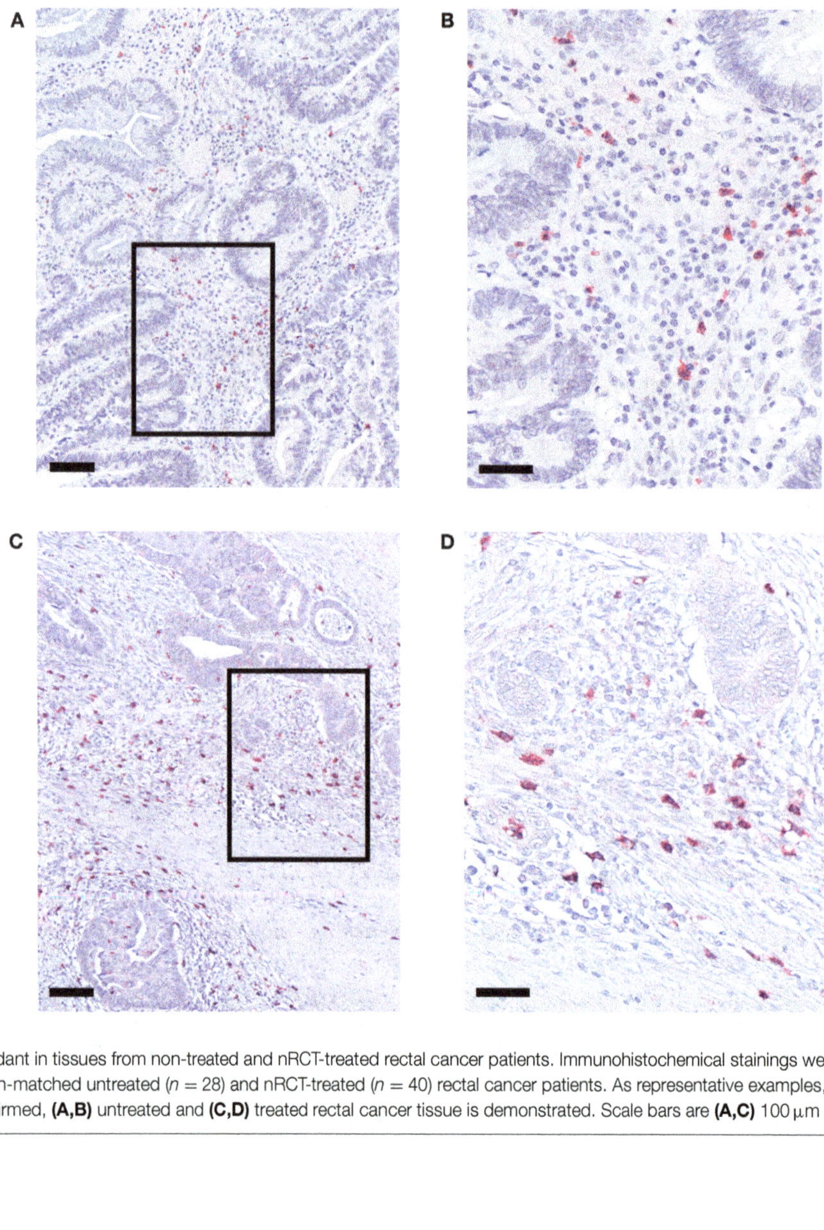

FIGURE 1 | pDCs are abundant in tissues from non-treated and nRCT-treated rectal cancer patients. Immunohistochemical stainings were performed to detect pDCs in tissue specimens from non-matched untreated ($n = 28$) and nRCT-treated ($n = 40$) rectal cancer patients. As representative examples, the presence of infiltrating pDCs in a histologically confirmed, **(A,B)** untreated and **(C,D)** treated rectal cancer tissue is demonstrated. Scale bars are **(A,C)** 100 μm or **(B,D)** 50 μm, respectively.

human tumor entities (26–28). However, little is known about the impact of nRCT on the density of tumor-infiltrating pDCs. Here, we address this issue by analyzing the frequency of pDCs in paraffin-embedded tissue specimens from non-treated ($n = 28$) and nRCT-treated ($n = 40$) rectal cancer patients (non-matched) with different clinicopathological characteristics (**Table 1**). BDCA-2^+ pDCs were present in all non-treated and nRCT-treated rectal cancer tissue specimens (**Figures 1A–D** and data not shown) at varying frequencies. pDCs were preferentially located in the tumor stroma, where they were not equally distributed. Whereas some regions are characterized by an accumulation of pDCs (**Figures 1A–D**), other regions contained only low pDC numbers. Interestingly, the number of pDCs was significantly higher in the nRCT-treated cohort (219.3 ± 106.6 pDCs/mm^2) than in the untreated cohort (160.3 ± 48.7 pDCs/mm^2) as depicted in **Figure 2A**. In further experiments, matched pre-nRCT and post-nRCT tumor specimens from 18 rectal cancer patients were analyzed. pDC infiltration increased >10% after nRCT in 15 out of 18 patients (**Figure 2B**). As shown in **Figure 2C**, the frequency of pDCs was significantly higher in the nRCT-treated cohort (172.0 ± 89.6 pDCs/mm^2) in comparison to the untreated cohort (99.2 ± 44.1 pDCs/mm^2), confirming the results obtained with the non-matched cohorts.

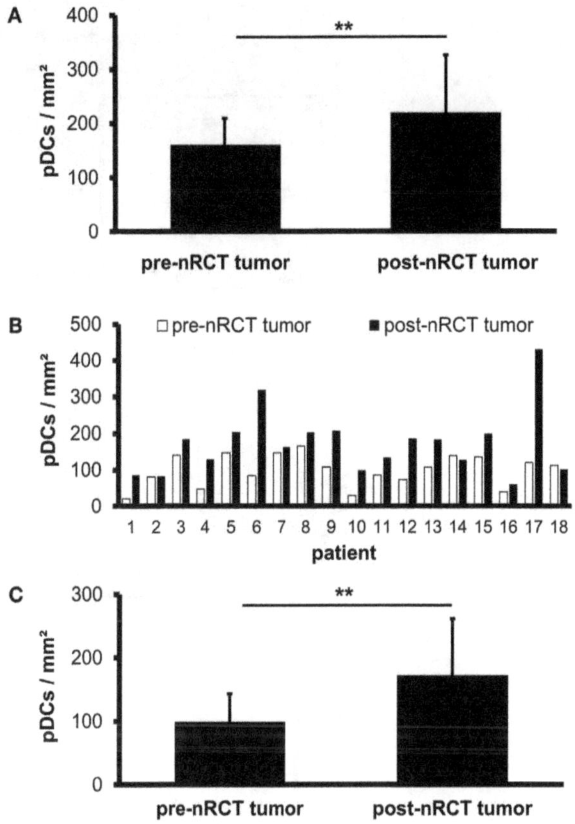

FIGURE 2 | pDC infiltration is significantly higher in nRCT-treated rectal cancer tissues. **(A)** Immunohistochemical stainings were performed to evaluate the frequency of infiltrating pDCs in tissue specimens from non-matched, untreated and nRCT-treated rectal cancer patients. **(B,C)** In addition, pDC density in matched pre-nRCT or post-nRCT tumor specimens from 18 rectal cancer patients was analyzed. **(A)** The number of pDCs in non-matched untreated ($n = 28$) compared to nRCT-treated ($n = 40$) rectal cancer tissues is depicted. The results are presented as mean value ± SD of rectal cancer-infiltrating pDCs. Asterisks indicate a statistically significant difference ($^{**}p < 0.01$). **(B)** pDC number in 18 matched pre-nRCT or post-nRCT tumor specimens is depicted for each patient. **(C)** pDC frequency in 18 matched pre-nRCT or post-nRCT tumor specimens is presented as mean value ± SD. Asterisks indicate a statistically significant difference ($^{**}p < 0.01$).

nRCT Does Not Significantly Modulate the Frequency of Rectal Cancer-Infiltrating slanMo

Previous studies have demonstrated that slanMo accumulate in primary tumor tissues of clear cell renal cell carcinoma (ccRCC) patients and in metastatic lymph nodes from cancer patients (42, 43). In the present study, we investigated whether infiltrating slanMo are detectable in rectal cancer tissues and whether nRCT can modulate their frequency. When analyzing the tissue specimens from non-treated and nRCT-treated rectal cancer patients (non-matched), we found that slanMo are present in 27 out of 28 non-treated and in all 40 nRCT-treated tissues (**Figures 3A–D** and data not shown) at varying frequencies. slanMo were preferentially located in the tumor stroma. In contrast to pDCs, nRCT only slightly increased the density of slanMo in the treated cohort (18 ± 13.8 slanMo/mm^2) compared to the untreated (13.4 ± 7.8 slanMo/mm^2) cohort (**Figure 3E**). These findings were confirmed when evaluating matched pre-nRCT and post-nRCT tumor specimens from 20 rectal cancer patients. Again, nRCT did not significantly modulate the frequency of rectal cancer-infiltrating slanMo (pre-nRCT: 12.4 ± 7.4 slanMo/mm^2, post-nRCT: 14.6 ± 6.6 slanMo/mm^2) as depicted in **Figure 3F**.

nRCT Significantly Enhances the Proportion of GrzB-Expressing CD8$^+$ T Cells in Rectal Cancer

Recent studies have demonstrated that tumor-infiltrating T cells play an important role for the clinical outcome of colorectal cancer patients (2–5). Based on these findings, we explored the impact of nRCT on the frequency of rectal cancer-infiltrating CD3$^+$ T lymphocytes, total CD8$^+$ T lymphocytes, and GrzB-expressing CD8$^+$ T cells in matched pre-nRCT and post-nRCT tumor samples of 18 patients. As demonstrated in **Figure 4A**, the number of rectal cancer-infiltrating CD3$^+$ T cells was not significantly altered by nRCT (pre-nRCT: 1598.1 ± 842.4 CD3$^+$ T cells/mm^2, post-nRCT: 1228.8 ± 671.6 CD3$^+$ T cells/mm^2). In contrast, nRCT significantly increased the frequency of total CD8$^+$ T cells in the nRCT-treated cohort (429.9 ± 284.2 CD8$^+$ T cells/mm^2) compared to the untreated cohort (286.8 ± 162.6 CD8$^+$ T cells/mm^2) as depicted in **Figure 4B**. The number of the CD8$^+$ T cells was increased in 14 out of 18 post-nRCT tumor samples (data not shown). In 12 out of these 14 tissues, a simultaneous accumulation of CD8$^+$ T cells and pDCs was detected. Within the total rectal cancer-infiltrating CD8$^+$ T cell compartment, CD8$^+$ T lymphocytes expressing the cytotoxic

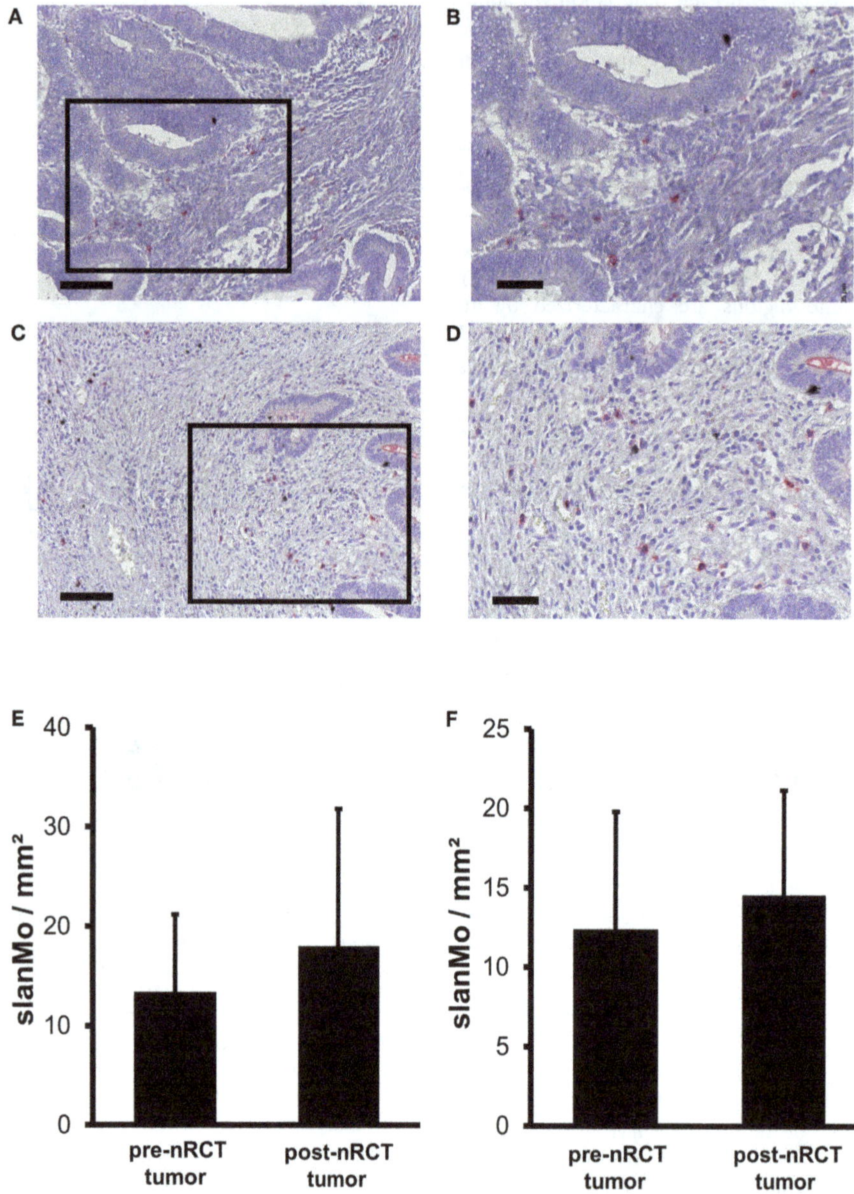

FIGURE 3 | nRCT does not significantly alter slanMo frequency in rectal cancer tissues. **(A–F)** Immunohistochemical stainings were conducted to determine the density of infiltrating slanMo in tissue specimens from non-matched and matched untreated and nRCT-treated rectal cancer patients. **(A–D)** As representative examples, the presence of infiltrating slanMo in an **(A,B)** untreated and **(C,D)** treated rectal cancer tissue is shown. Scale bars are **(A,C)** 100 μm or **(B,D)** 50 μm, respectively. **(E)** The number of slanMo in non-matched untreated ($n = 28$) compared to nRCT-treated ($n = 40$) rectal cancer tissues is depicted. The results are presented as mean value ± SD of rectal cancer-infiltrating slanMo. **(F)** The frequency of slanMo in 20 matched pre-nRCT or post-nRCT tumor specimens is demonstrated. The results are presented as mean value ± SD of rectal cancer-infiltrating slanMo.

effector molecule GrzB were also detectable (**Figures 4C–F**). Notably, the percentage of GrzB$^+$ CD8$^+$ T cells was significantly higher in the nRCT-treated cohort (57.5 ± 14.4% GrzB$^+$ CD8$^+$ T cells) in comparison to the untreated cohort (44.2 ± 9.4% GrzB$^+$ CD8$^+$ T cells) as shown in **Figure 4G**. Following these findings, we explored whether CD8$^+$ T cells co-localize with pDCs in four nRCT-treated rectal cancer tissues. As demonstrated in **Figure 5**, regions containing a high density of pDC and CD8$^+$ T cells were detectable in all analyzed rectal cancer tissues.

nRCT Increases the Proportion of iNOS- or TNF-α-Expressing slanMo in Rectal Cancer

iNOS and TNF-α were shown to mediate either tumor-promoting or antitumor effects and may therefore influence the efficacy of nRCT in cancer patients (44, 45). Following our previous findings that iNOS- and/or TNF-α-expressing slanMo are detectable in tissue specimens of patients with various inflammatory disorders (35, 36, 46), we investigated whether nRCT modulates the percentage of iNOS- or TNF-α-producing

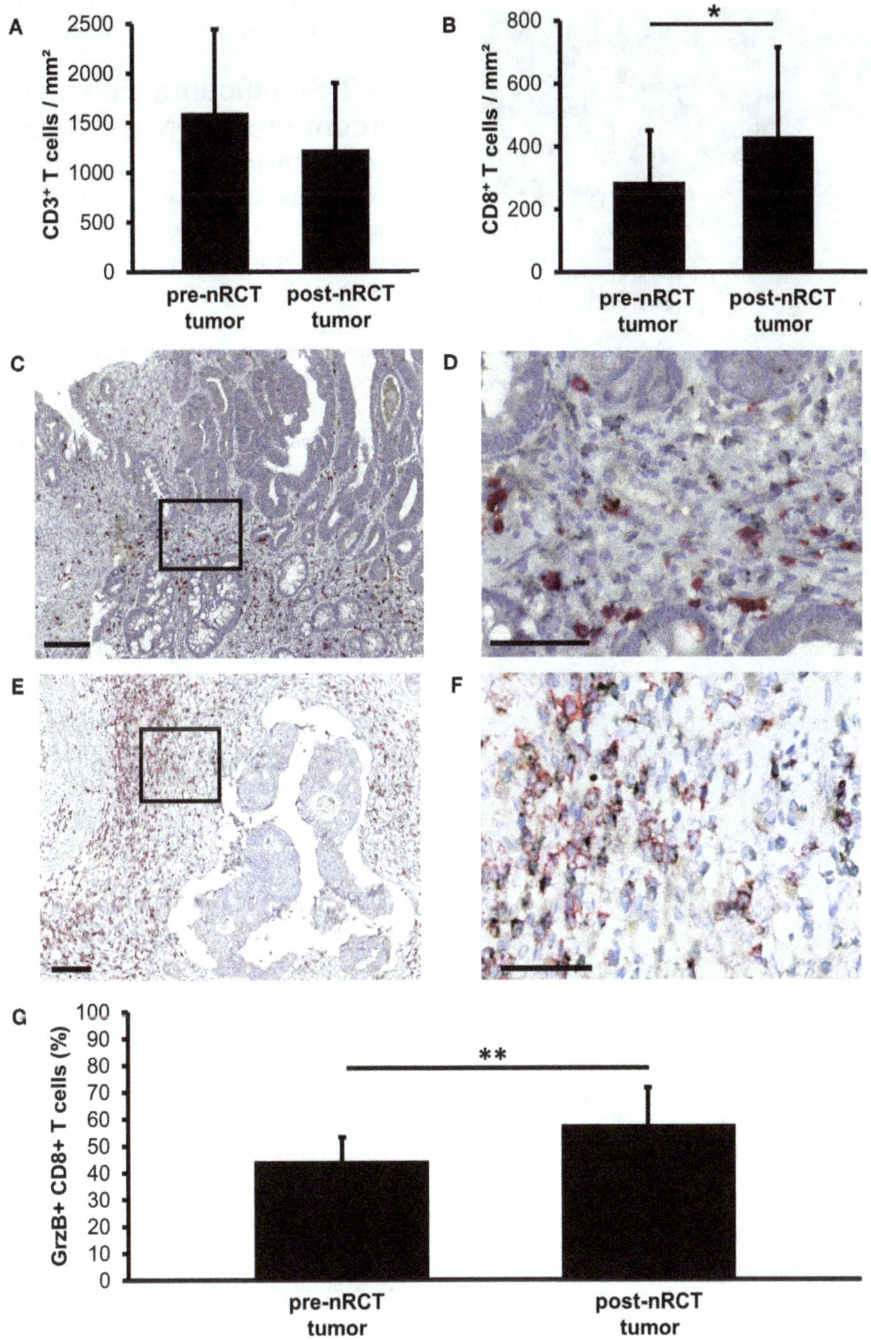

FIGURE 4 | nRCT significantly increases the proportion of rectal cancer-infiltrating GrzB$^+$ CD8$^+$ T cells. **(A–G)** Immunohistochemical stainings were performed to explore the frequency of rectal cancer-infiltrating CD3$^+$ T lymphocytes, total CD8$^+$ T lymphocytes, and GrzB$^+$ CD8$^+$ T cells in matched pre-nRCT and post-nRCT tumor samples. The frequency of **(A)** CD3$^+$ cells and **(B)** CD8$^+$ T cells in 18 matched pre-nRCT or post-nRCT tumor specimens is presented as mean value ± SD. Asterisks indicate a statistically significant difference (*$p < 0.05$). **(C–F)** As representative examples, the presence of infiltrating GrzB$^+$ CD8$^+$ T cells in an **(C,D)** untreated and **(E,F)** nRCT-treated rectal cancer tissue is demonstrated. Scale bars are **(C,E)** 100 μm or **(D,F)** 50 μm, respectively. **(G)** The percentage of GrzB-expressing CD8$^+$ T cells in 18 matched pre-nRCT or post-nRCT tumor specimens is presented as mean value ± SD. Asterisks indicate a statistically significant difference (**$p < 0.01$).

slanMo in matched pre-nRCT and post-nRCT tumor specimens of 10 patients. While iNOS$^+$ slanMo were present in 9 out of 10 post-nRCT rectal cancer tissues, TNF-α$^+$ slanMo were detectable in 7 out of 10 tumor tissues obtained after treatment at varying percentages (**Figures 6A–D**). In contrast, iNOS$^+$ slanMo were only found in 2 out of 10 pre-nRCT rectal cancer tissues, while

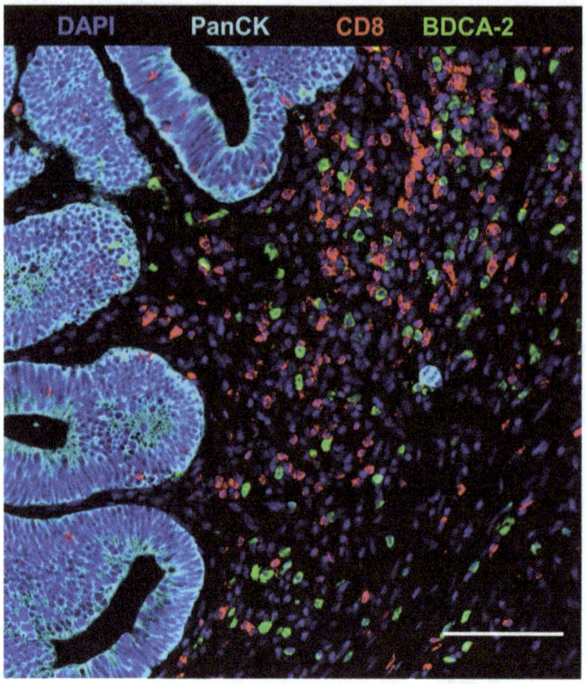

FIGURE 5 | Co-localization of pDC and CD8$^+$ T cells in nRCT-treated rectal cancer tissues. Immunofluorescence multiplex staining was performed to detect a co-localization of pDC and CD8$^+$ T cells in four post-nRCT tumor samples. As a representative example, an image of a tissue region containing high numbers of rectal cancer-infiltrating pDC and CD8$^+$ T cells is shown. Scale bar is 100 μm.

TNF-α$^+$ slanMo were absent in these tissues (**Figures 6C,D**). As depicted in **Figure 6E**, the proportion of iNOS$^+$ slanMo was significantly higher in post-nRCT tumor tissues (26 ± 24% iNOS$^+$ slanMo) compared to pre-nRCT tumor specimen (1 ± 2% iNOS$^+$ slanMo). In addition, nRCT significantly increased the percentage of slanMo locally expressing TNF-α in rectal cancer tissues (**Figure 6F**).

nRCT Significantly Increases the Proportion of CD83$^+$ pDCs in Rectal Cancer

To investigate whether nRCT influences the maturation status of rectal cancer-infiltrating pDCs, we analyzed the proportion of pDCs expressing the maturation marker CD83 in matched pre-nRCT and post-nRCT tumor samples of 18 patients. CD83$^+$ pDCs were detectable in all post-nRCT rectal cancer tissues, but only in 11 out of 18 tumor tissues before nRCT at varying percentages (**Figures 7A,B**). In 13 post-nRCT rectal cancer tissues, ≥30% of pDCs expressing CD83 were present, providing evidence that these tissues can contain a marked proportion of mature pDCs (**Figure 7B**). As shown in **Figure 7C**, the percentage of CD83$^+$ pDCs was significantly higher in post-nRCT tumor tissues (36.7 ± 18.9% CD83$^+$ pDCs) in comparison to pre-nRCT tumor specimens (3.2 ± 4.2% CD83$^+$ pDCs), indicating that nRCT can profoundly enhance the proportion of mature pDCs in rectal cancer tissues.

nRCT Significantly Enhances the Percentage of IFN-α-Expressing pDCs in Rectal Cancer

Activated pDCs are major producers of IFN-α, which may essentially contribute to the antitumor effects mediated by radio- and chemotherapy (18, 19). Following these findings, we determined the impact of nRCT on the proportion of IFN-α-expressing pDCs in matched pre-nRCT and post-nRCT tumor samples of 18 patients. Whereas, IFN-α$^+$ pDCs were only present in 11 out of 18 pre-nRCT rectal cancer tissues, infiltrating pDCs locally expressing IFN-α were found in all post-nRCT tumor samples at varying percentages (**Figures 8A,B**). In 16 post-nRCT rectal cancer tissues, ≥30% of IFN-α$^+$ pDCs were detectable (**Figure 8B**). The percentage of IFN-α$^+$ pDCs was significantly higher in post-nRCT tumor tissues (52.0 ± 20.5% IFN-α$^+$ pDCs) compared to pre-nRCT tumor specimen (5.5 ± 8.1% IFN-α$^+$ pDCs) as depicted in **Figure 8C**. These results provide evidence that nRCT can profoundly increase the proportion of pDCs locally expressing IFN-α in rectal cancer tissues.

Rectal Cancer-Infiltrating pDCs Express the Chemokines CXCL10 and CCL4

Recently, it has been shown that pDCs are able to produce various chemokines such as CCL4, CCL5, and CXCL10 (19, 47) that can promote the migration of T cells to tumor sites. Following these observations, we investigated the presence of pDCs expressing these chemokines in 9 pre-nRCT and 18 post-nRCT tumor specimens of the matched cohort. Whereas, CXCL10- or CCL4-expressing pDCs were not found in pre-nRCT tumor samples, CXCL10$^+$ pDCs were detectable in 14 out of 18 and CCL4$^+$ pDCs in 12 out of 18 post-nRCT tumor samples (**Figures 9A,B**). CCL5-expressing pDCs were not present in these tumor tissues (data not shown). These results imply that pDCs can contribute to the secretion of important chemokines for T-cell migration to rectal cancer tissues after nRCT.

DISCUSSION

Recent studies have revealed that DCs, as key regulators of innate and adaptive immunity, are a component of the immune architecture in colorectal cancer and may influence the clinical outcome of patients. When exploring the presence of human DCs in colorectal cancer, it has been reported that S-100$^+$ DCs are detectable in almost all colorectal specimens and are mainly located in the tumor stroma (48–50). Increasing numbers of S-100$^+$ DCs infiltrating tumor epithelium correlated with higher numbers of intraepithelial CD4$^+$ and CD8$^+$ T cells (49). Whereas, several studies provided evidence that a higher density of S-100$^+$ DCs was associated with improved survival of patients (48, 51–53), other studies did not find a statistically significant correlation between S-100$^+$ DC infiltration and a favorable clinical outcome (49, 50). In addition, it has been shown that DCs expressing the maturation marker CD83 are present in

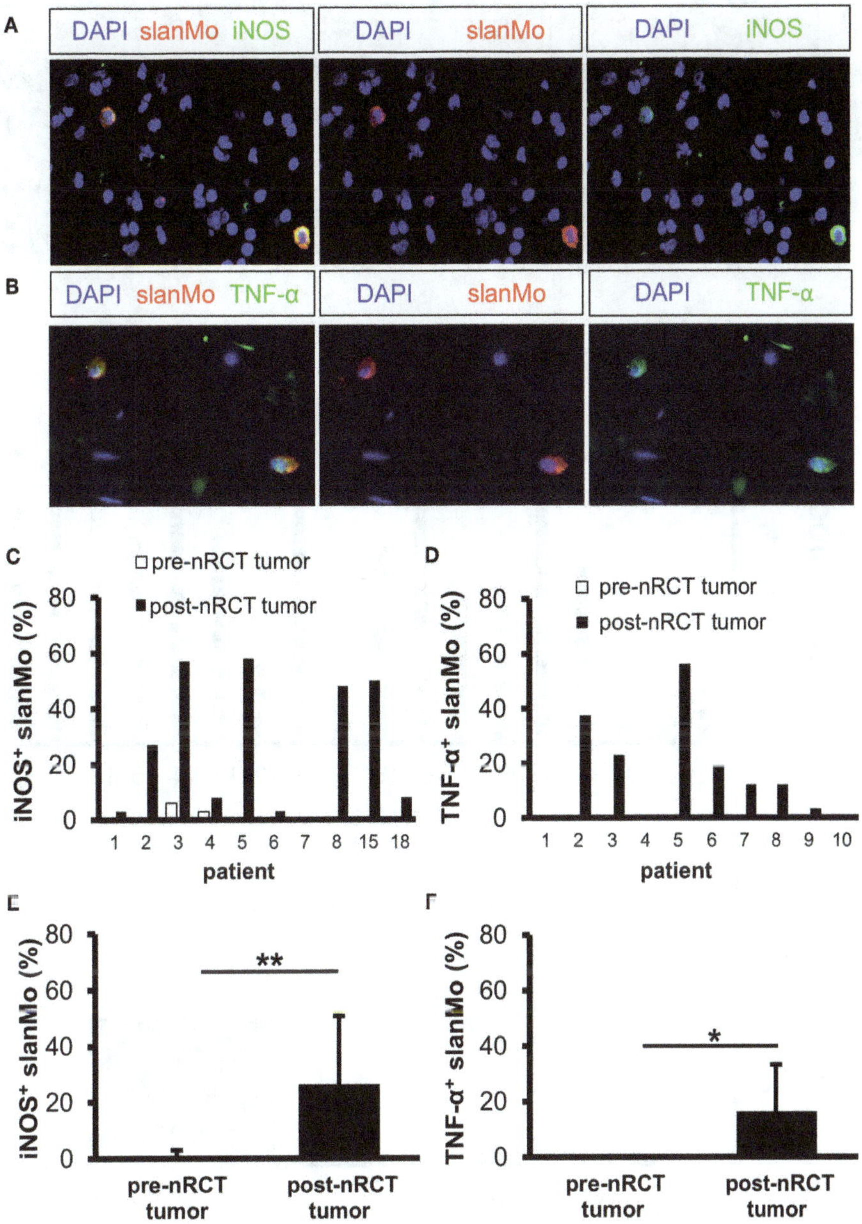

FIGURE 6 | nRCT significantly increases the proportion of iNOS- and TNF-α-producing slanMo in rectal cancer tissues. **(A–F)** Immunofluorescence stainings were performed to evaluate the presence and percentage of iNOS- and TNF-α-expressing slanMo in matched pre-nRCT or post-nRCT tumor specimens from 10 rectal cancer patients. **(A,B)** As representative examples, images of **(A)** single iNOS or slan and **(B)** single TNF-α or slan stainings as well as merged images are depicted. Original magnification was x400. **(C,D)** Percentage of **(C)** iNOS- and **(D)** TNF-α-expressing slanMo in matched pre-nRCT or post-nRCT tumor specimens is shown for each patient. The results are presented as mean value ± SD of the proportion of **(E)** iNOS- or **(F)** TNF-α-expressing slanMo in matched pre-nRCT or post-nRCT tumor specimens. Asterisks indicate a statistically significant difference (*$p < 0.05$, **$p < 0.01$).

colorectal cancer (53–55). These DCs were found predominantly in the invasive margin, often in clusters with lymphocytes (55). Gulubova et al. demonstrated that patients with locally advanced tumors had significantly lower infiltration of CD83+ DCs in tumor stroma and in the invasive margin (53). Whereas all these findings are based on the detection of general marker molecules for DCs, studies investigating the presence of distinct human DC subsets in colon cancer tissues are rather limited. When exploring the density and distribution of pDCs in rectal cancer, we found that pDCs are present in all non-treated rectal cancer specimens at varying frequencies and are preferentially located in the tumor stroma. These results further substantiate recent studies, indicating that pDCs are detectable in colorectal cancer (51, 56). Previously, we and others have determined the presence of slanMo in primary tumor samples and derived metastases. Vermi et al. have found an accumulation of slanMo in metastatic lymph

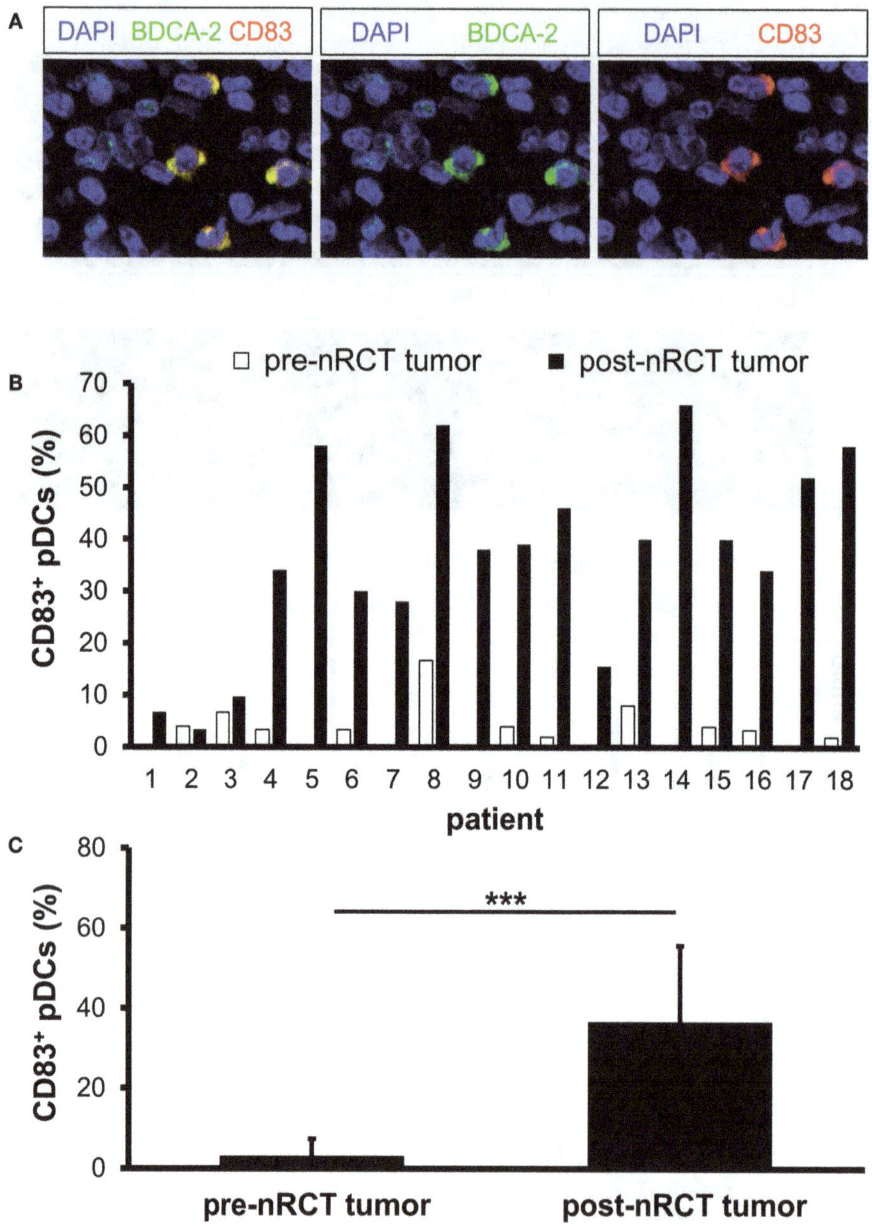

FIGURE 7 | nRCT increases the proportion of mature pDCs in rectal cancer tissues. **(A–C)** Immunofluorescence stainings were conducted to analyze the presence and percentage of CD83-expressing pDCs in matched pre-nRCT or post-nRCT tumor specimens from 18 rectal cancer patients. **(A)** As representative example, images of single CD83 or BDCA-2 stainings as well as merged images are depicted. Original magnification was x400. **(B)** Percentage of CD83-expressing pDCs in matched pre-nRCT or post-nRCT tumor specimens is depicted for each patient. **(C)** The results are presented as mean value ± SD of the percentage of CD83$^+$ pDCs in matched pre-nRCT or post-nRCT tumor specimens. Asterisks indicate a statistically significant difference (***$p < 0.001$).

nodes from cancer patients (42). In addition, we have detected slanMo in the majority of primary tumor specimens, metastatic lymph nodes, and distant metastases from ccRCC patients (43). Further findings have revealed that ccRCC-infiltrating slanDCs display a tolerogenic phenotype and that higher slanDC numbers are associated with a reduced survival of ccRCC patients (43). More recently, it has been shown that slanMo are also present in bone marrow specimens of multiple myeloma patients and in various types of non-Hodgkin lymphomas (57, 58). In the present study, we observed that slanMo are detectable in almost all non-treated rectal cancer specimens at varying frequencies and are preferentially located in the tumor stroma. The slanMo frequency is markedly lower in comparison to rectal cancer-infiltrating pDCs, but higher compared to RCC-infiltrating slanMo (43). So far, only little is known about the impact of nRCT on the frequency of tumor-infiltrating DCs. When exploring

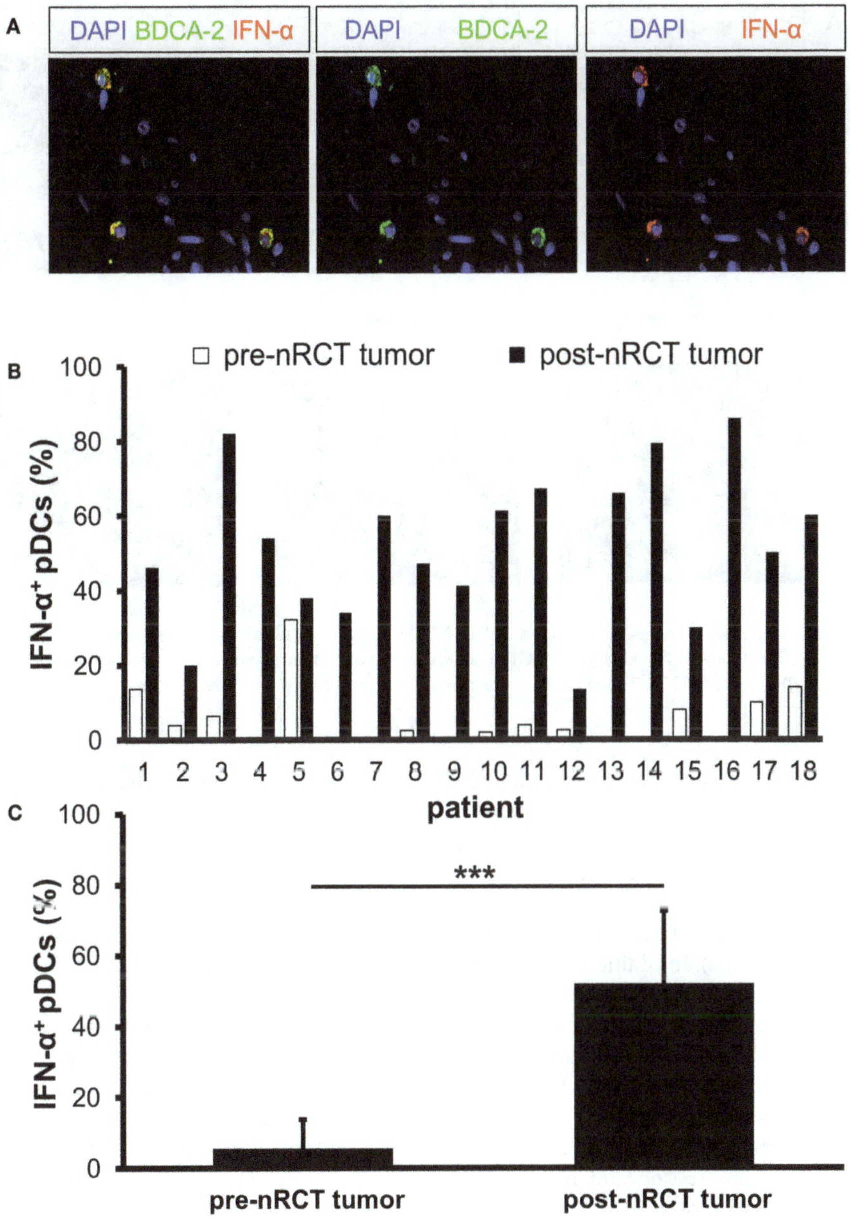

FIGURE 8 | nRCT significantly enhances the percentage of IFN-α-expressing pDCs in rectal cancer tissues. **(A–C)** Immunofluorescence stainings were performed to determine the presence and percentage of IFN-α-expressing pDCs in matched pre-nRCT or post-nRCT tumor specimens from 18 rectal cancer patients. **(A)** As representative example, images of single IFN-α or BDCA-2 stainings as well as merged images are shown. Original magnification was x400. **(B)** Percentage of IFN-α-expressing pDCs in matched pre-nRCT or post-nRCT tumor specimens is depicted for each patient. **(C)** The results are presented as mean value ± SD of the proportion of IFN-α^+ pDCs in matched pre-nRCT or post-nRCT tumor specimens. Asterisks indicate a statistically significant difference (***$p < 0.001$).

the influence of nRCT on the number of infiltrating pDCs and slanMo in rectal cancer, we found a significantly higher number of pDCs in nRCT-treated tissue specimens, whereas the frequency of slanMo remained stable after nRCT.

CD4$^+$ and CD8$^+$ T lymphocytes are important effector cells of adaptive antitumor immunity. CD8$^+$ effector T cells efficiently recognize and destroy tumor cells. CD4$^+$ effector T cells enhance the ability of DCs to induce CD8$^+$ T cell responses. They also provide help for the maintenance and expansion of CD8$^+$ T cells and can eliminate tumor cells directly. In addition, CD4$^+$ T cells are able to promote the differentiation of B cells into antibody-producing plasma cells. Based on these properties, tumor-infiltrating effector T cells efficiently influence tumor growth and play an essential role for the clinical outcome of colorectal cancer patients (2–5). Here, we explored the impact of nRCT on the frequency of rectal cancer-infiltrating T lymphocytes in matched pre-nRCT and post-nRCT tumor samples. We found that nRCT significantly increases the number of total CD8$^+$ T

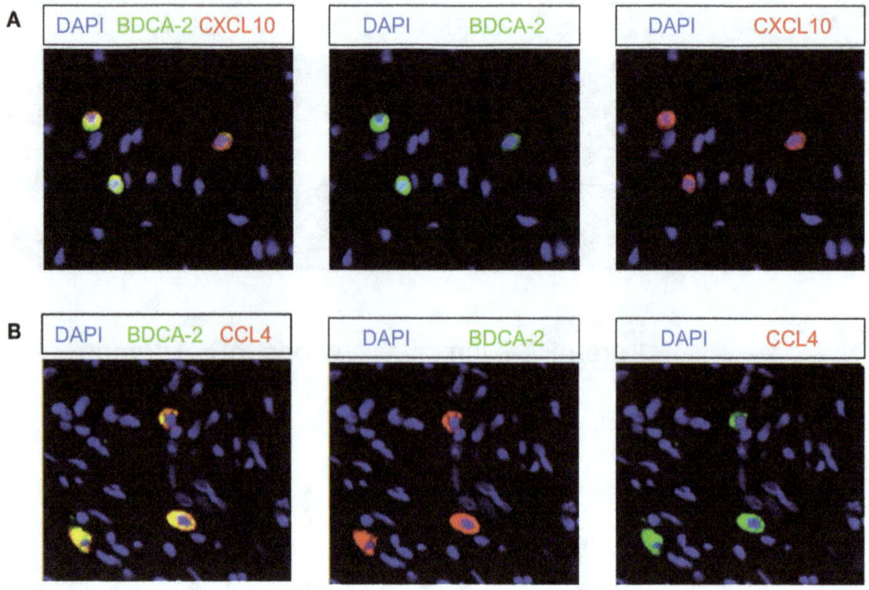

FIGURE 9 | Rectal cancer-infiltrating pDCs can express CXCL10 and CCL4. **(A,B)** Immunofluorescence stainings were conducted to analyze the presence of CXCL10- or CCL4-expressing pDCs in 9 pre-nRCT and 18 post-nRCT tumor specimens of the matched cohort. As representative examples, images of single **(A)** CXCL10 and BDCA-2 or single **(B)** CCL4 and BDCA-2 stainings as well as merged images are shown. Original magnification was x200.

cells as well as the percentage of $CD8^+$ T cells expressing GrzB in the nRCT-treated cohort. These results are in agreement with previous studies, indicating that nRCT can significantly enhance the density of infiltrating $CD8^+$ T cells in rectal cancer. Thus, it has been reported that the frequency of rectal cancer-infiltrating $CD8^+$ T cells and the proportion of $GrzB^+$ $CD8^+$ T cells is markedly increased by nRCT (59–62). In addition, a high density of $CD8^+$ T cells prior to treatment was associated with a good response to nRCT and was linked to a better clinical outcome (59–61). However, McCoy et al. did not observe an association between the frequency of rectal-cancer infiltrating $CD8^+$ T cells prior to treatment and response to nRCT (63).

iNOS and TNF-α are important molecules that have an impact on carcinogenesis and cancer progression and may influence the clinical response of patients to various treatment modalities. Both molecules play a dual role in cancer by mediating tumor-promoting or antitumor effects (44, 45). Thus, iNOS and TNF-α were shown to promote tumor proliferation, angiogenesis, invasiveness, and metastasis. Further studies have revealed that these molecules can also efficiently impair tumor growth by various mechanisms such as the inhibition of proliferation, the induction of apoptosis, and the recruitment of tumor-reactive T cells (44, 45). Previously, we have identified slanMo as inflammatory, iNOS- and/or TNF-α-expressing cells in tissues specimens of patients with psoriasis, lupus erythematosus, or graft-vs.-host disease (35, 36, 46). Here, we determined the impact of nRCT on the percentage of iNOS- or TNF-α-expressing slanMo in matched pre-nRCT and post-nRCT rectal cancer specimens. $iNOS^+$ or TNF-α^+ slanMo were rare or absent in pre-nRCT tissues. However, nRCT significantly augmented the proportion of infiltrating slanMo locally expressing iNOS- or TNF-α in rectal cancer. The nRCT-mediated increase of iNOS-producing slanMo is in line with a recent study, demonstrating that low dose irradiation induces iNOS expression in melanoma-infiltrating mouse macrophages, resulting in an enhanced recruitment of T cells (64). In addition, Klug et al. observed that low dose irradiation leads to an accumulation of $iNOS^+$ macrophages and intraepithelial T cells in tissue specimens of pancreatic cancer patients (64).

Type I IFN play a key role in antitumor immunity (65). They promote the maturation and antigen-presenting capacity of DCs as well as their migration to lymph nodes. Furthermore, type I IFN stimulate the release of proinflammatory cytokines by macrophages and improve the tumor-directed cytotoxic activity mediated by $CD8^+$ T cells and NK cells. Accumulating evidence indicates that type I IFN can essentially contribute to the beneficial effects mediated by chemotherapy and radiotherapy (9, 66). Thus, it has been demonstrated that the efficacy of anthracycline-based chemotherapy against established tumor in mice is critically dependent on type I IFN (66). Furthermore, it has been reported that radiotherapy increases the intratumoral type I IFN expression in mice (67). Type I IFN were shown to enhance the cross-priming and T-cell stimulatory capacity of tumor-infiltrating DCs leading to tumor regression (67). pDCs are major producers of type I IFN following stimulation with toll-like receptor 7 and 9 agonists (18, 19). However, recent studies have revealed that tumor-infiltrating pDCs are defective at producing type I IFN in response to toll-like receptor agonists (26, 28, 29). When analyzing matched pre-nRCT and post-nRCT rectal cancer specimens, we found that only a small proportion of IFN-α-expressing pDCs is detectable prior nRCT. Notably, nRCT profoundly increased the proportion of pDCs locally expressing IFN-α. Together with our finding that nRCT also enhances the percentage of $CD83^+$ pDCs, these results reveal that nRCT promotes the maturation and IFN-α production of rectal cancer-infiltrating pDCs.

pDCs are capable of producing various chemokines such as CCL4, CCL5, and CXCL10, which attract T cells to sites of infection and inflammation (19, 47). In addition, it has been reported that these chemokines play an essential role for the trafficking of T cells to tumor tissues. Thus, it has been shown that the expression of CCL4, CCL5, and CXCL10 in melanoma metastases is associated with the recruitment of $CD8^+$ T cells (68). Moreover, a recent study has revealed that CCL5 and CXCL10 expressed by colorectal cancer tissues promote the migration of $GrzB^+$ $CD8^+$ T cells (69). When investigating the expression of these chemokines by rectal cancer-infiltrating pDCs, we observed that CCL4- or CXCL10-expressing pDCs are present in the majority of post-nRCT tumor specimens, whereas they are absent in pre-nRCT tissue samples. These findings indicate that nRCT can induce CXCL10 and CCL4 expression in rectal cancer-infiltrating pDCs. In addition, they imply that pDCs can contribute to the production of important chemokines for T-cell migration to rectal cancer tissues after nRCT.

Taken together, we found that nRCT significantly increases the percentage of rectal cancer-infiltrating slanMo locally expressing iNOS and TNF-α, which can either mediate tumor-promoting or antitumor effects and may affect the efficacy of nRCT in rectal cancer patients. Moreover, we demonstrated for the first time that nRCT results in an accumulation of pDCs as well as an increased proportion of CD83- and IFN-α-expressing pDCs in rectal cancer. In addition, the density of infiltrating $GrzB^+$ $CD8^+$ T cells was significantly enhanced by nRCT. These findings indicate that nRCT can harness antitumor responses by converting immature, non-activated pDCs into mature, inflammatory cells and by increasing the frequency of $CD8^+$ T cells expressing the cytotoxic effector molecule GrzB. Activated pDCs and $GrzB^+$ $CD8^+$ T cells may contribute to the beneficial effect of nRCT in rectal cancer patients.

AUTHOR CONTRIBUTIONS

FeW, UH, FrW, and IP performed experiments, analyzed data, and wrote the manuscript. RW, MaK, KF, and MA performed experiments and analyzed data. US, AJ, and AT analyzed data and wrote the manuscript. AB, CR, JW, KS, ET, MeK, GF, MB, MPB, DA, and GB analyzed data and revised the article. MS designed research, interpreted the data, and wrote the manuscript.

ACKNOWLEDGMENTS

We thank Bärbel Löbel for excellent technical assistance.

REFERENCES

1. Siegel RL, Miller KD, Jemal A. Cancer statistics, 2018. *CA Cancer J Clin.* (2018) 68:7–30. doi: 10.3322/caac.21442
2. Fridman WH, Zitvogel L, Sautès-Fridman C, Kroemer G. The immune contexture in cancer prognosis and treatment. *Nat Rev Clin Oncol.* (2017) 14:717–34. doi: 10.1038/nrclinonc.2017.101
3. Galon J, Costes A, Sanchez-Cabo F, Kirilovsky A, Mlecnik B, Lagorce-Pagès C, et al. Type, density, and location of immune cells within human colorectal tumors predict clinical outcome. *Science.* (2006) 313:1960–4. doi: 10.1126/science.1129139
4. Pagès F, Kirilovsky A, Mlecnik B, Asslaber M, Tosolini M, Bindea G, et al. *In situ* cytotoxic and memory T cells predict outcome in patients with early-stage colorectal cancer. *J Clin Oncol.* (2009) 27:5944–51. doi: 10.1200/JCO.2008.19.6147
5. Pagès F, Mlecnik B, Marliot F, Bindea G, Ou FS, Bifulco C, et al. International validation of the consensus immunoscore for the classification of colon cancer: a prognostic and accuracy study. *Lancet.* (2018) 391:2128–39. doi: 10.1016/S0140-6736(18)30789-X
6. Kalyan A, Rozelle S, Benson A. Neoadjuvant treatment of rectal cancer: where are we now? *Gastroenterol Rep.* (2016) 4:206–9. doi: 10.1093/gastro/gow017
7. Li Y, Wang J, Ma X, Tan L, Yan Y, Xue C, et al. A review of neoadjuvant chemoradiotherapy for locally advanced rectal cancer. *Int J Biol Sci.* (2016) 12:1022–31. doi: 10.7150/ijbs.15438
8. Barker HE, Paget JT, Khan AA, Harrington KJ. The tumour microenvironment after radiotherapy: mechanisms of resistance and recurrence. *Nat Rev Cancer.* (2015) 15:409–25. doi: 10.1038/nrc3958
9. Weichselbaum RR, Liang H, Deng L, Fu YX. Radiotherapy and immunotherapy: a beneficial liaison? *Nat Rev Clin Oncol.* (2017) 14:365–79. doi: 10.1038/nrclinonc.2016.211
10. Derer A, Frey B, Fietkau R, Gaipl US. Immune-modulating properties of ionizing radiation: rationale for the treatment of cancer by combination radiotherapy and immune checkpoint inhibitors. *Cancer Immunol Immunother.* (2016) 65:779–86. doi: 10.1007/s00262-015-1771-8
11. Galluzzi L, Buqué A, Kepp O, Zitvogel L, Kroemer G. Immunological effects of conventional chemotherapy and targeted anticancer agents. *Cancer Cell.* (2015) 28:690–714. doi: 10.1016/j.ccell.2015.10.012
12. Obeid M, Tesniere A, Ghiringhelli F, Fimia GM, Apetoh L, Perfettini JL, et al. Calreticulin exposure dictates the immunogenicity of cancer cell death. *Nat Med.* (2007) 13:54–61. doi: 10.1038/nm1523
13. Apetoh L, Ghiringhelli F, Tesniere A, Obeid M, Ortiz C, Criollo A, et al. Toll-like receptor 4-dependent contribution of the immune system to anticancer chemotherapy and radiotherapy. *Nat Med.* (2007) 13:1050–9. doi: 10.1038/nm1622
14. Steinman RM, Banchereau J. Taking dendritic cells into medicine. *Nature.* (2007) 449:419–26. doi: 10.1038/nature06175
15. Vermeer DW, Spanos WC, Vermeer PD, Bruns AM, Lee KM, Lee JH. Radiation-induced loss of cell surface CD47 enhances immune-mediated clearance of human papillomavirus-positive cancer. *Int J Cancer.* (2013) 133:120–9. doi: 10.1002/ijc.28015
16. Liu X, Pu Y, Cron K, Deng L, Kline J, Frazier WA, et al. CD47 blockade triggers T cell-mediated destruction of immunogenic tumors. *Nat Med.* (2015) 21:1209–15. doi: 10.1038/nm.3931
17. Kanterman J, Sade-Feldman M, Biton M, Ish-Shalom E, Lasry A, Goldshtein A, et al. Adverse immunoregulatory effects of 5FU and CPT11 chemotherapy on myeloid-derived suppressor cells and colorectal cancer outcomes. *Cancer Res.* (2014) 74:6022–35. doi: 10.1158/0008-5472.CAN-14-0657
18. Gilliet M, Cao W, Liu YJ. Plasmacytoid dendritic cells: sensing nucleic acids in viral infection and autoimmune diseases. *Nat Rev Immunol.* (2008) 8:594–606. doi: 10.1038/nri2358
19. Swiecki M, Colonna M. The multifaceted biology of plasmacytoid dendritic cells. *Nat Rev Immunol.* (2015) 15:471–85. doi: 10.1038/nri3865
20. Salio M, Cella M, Vermi W, Facchetti F, Palmowski MJ, Smith CL, et al. Plasmacytoid dendritic cells prime IFN-gamma-secreting melanoma-specific

CD8 lymphocytes and are found in primary melanoma lesions. *Eur J Immunol.* (2003) 33:1052–62. doi: 10.1002/eji.200323676
21. Hanabuchi S, Watanabe N, Wang YH, Wang YH, Ito T, Shaw J, et al. Human plasmacytoid predendritic cells activate NK cells through glucocorticoid-induced tumor necrosis factor receptor-ligand (GITRL). *Blood.* (2006) 107:3617–23. doi: 10.1182/blood-2005-08-3419
22. Liu C, Lou Y, Lizée G, Qin H, Liu S, Rabinovich B, et al. Plasmacytoid dendritic cells induce NK cell-dependent, tumor antigen-specific T cell cross-priming and tumor regression in mice. *J Clin Invest.* (2008) 118:1165–75. doi: 10.1172/JCI33583
23. Le Mercier I, Poujol D, Sanlaville A, Sisirak V, Gobert M, Durand I, et al. Tumor promotion by intratumoral plasmacytoid dendritic cells is reversed by TLR7 ligand treatment. *Cancer Res.* (2013) 73:4629–40. doi: 10.1158/0008-5472.CAN-12-3058
24. Tel J, Aarntzen EH, Baba T, Schreibelt G, Schulte BM, Benitez-Ribas D, et al. Natural human plasmacytoid dendritic cells induce antigen-specific T-cell responses in melanoma patients. *Cancer Res.* (2013) 73:1063–75. doi: 10.1158/0008-5472.CAN-12-2583
25. Sharma MD, Baban B, Chandler P, Hou DY, Singh N, Yagita H, et al. Plasmacytoid dendritic cells from mouse tumor-draining lymph nodes directly activate mature Tregs via indoleamine 2, 3-dioxygenase. *J Clin Invest.* (2007) 117:2570–82. doi: 10.1172/JCI31911
26. Hartmann E, Wollenberg B, Rothenfusser S, Wagner M, Wellisch D, Mack B, et al. Identification and functional analysis of tumor-infiltrating plasmacytoid dendritic cells in head and neck cancer. *Cancer Res.* (2003) 63:6478–87.
27. Treilleux I, Blay J-Y, Bendriss-Vermare N, Ray-Coquard I, Bachelot T, Guastalla J-P, et al. Dendritic cell infiltration and prognosis of early stage breast cancer. *Clin Cancer Res.* (2004) 10:7466–474. doi: 10.1158/1078-0432.CCR-04-0684
28. Labidi-Galy SI, Sisirak V, Meeus P, Gobert M, Treilleux I, Bajard A, et al. Quantitative and functional alterations of plasmacytoid dendritic cells contribute to immune tolerance in ovarian cancer. *Cancer Res.* (2011) 71:5423–34. doi: 10.1158/0008-5472.CAN-11-0367
29. Sisirak V, Faget J, Gobert M, Goutagny N, Vey N, Treilleux I, et al. Impaired IFN-α production by plasmacytoid dendritic cells favors regulatory T-cell expansion that may contribute to breast cancer progression. *Cancer Res.* (2012) 72:5188–97. doi: 10.1158/0008-5472.CAN-11-3468
30. Schäkel K, Mayer E, Federle C, Schmitz M, Riethmüller G, Rieber EP. A novel dendritic cell population in human blood: one-step immunomagnetic isolation by a specific mAb (M-DC8) and *in vitro* priming of cytotoxic T lymphocytes. *Eur J Immunol.* (1998) 28:4084–4093. doi: 10.1002/(SICI)1521-4141(199812)28:12<4084::AID-IMMU4084>3.0.CO;2-4
31. Schäkel K, Kannagi R, Kniep B, Goto Y, Mitsuoka C, Zwirner J, et al. 6-Sulfo LacNAc, a novel carbohydrate modification of PSGL-1, defines an inflammatory type of human dendritic cells. *Immunity.* (2002) 17:289–301. doi: 10.1016/S1074-7613(02)00393-X
32. Schäkel K, von Kietzell M, Hänsel A, Ebling A, Schulze L, Haase M, et al. Human 6-sulfo LacNAc-expressing dendritic cells are principal producers of early interleukin-12 and are controlled by erythrocytes. *Immunity.* (2006) 24:767–77. doi: 10.1016/j.immuni.2006.03.020
33. Van Leeuwen-Kerkhoff N, Lundberg K, Westers TM, Kordasti S, Bontkes HJ, de Gruijl TD, et al. Transcriptional profiling reveals functional dichotomy between human slan^{+} non-classical monocytes and myeloid dendritic cells. *J Leukoc Biol.* (2017) 102:1055–68. doi: 10.1189/jlb.3MA0117-037R
34. Baran W, Oehrl S, Ahmad F, Döbel T, Alt C, Buske-Kirschbaum A, et al. Phenotype, function and mobilization of 6-sulfo LacNAc-expressing monocytes in atopic dermatitis. *Front Immunol.* (2018) 9:1352. doi: 10.3389/fimmu.2018.01352
35. Olaru F, Döbel T, Lonsdorf AS, Oehrl S, Maaş M, Enk AH, et al. Intracapillary immune complexes recruit and activate slan-expressing CD16+ monocytes in human lupus nephritis. *JCI Insight.* (2018) 3:96492. doi: 10.1172/jci.insight.96492
36. Hänsel A, Günther C, Ingwersen J, Starke J, Schmitz M, Bachmann M, et al. Human slan (6-sulfo LacNAc) dendritic cells are inflammatory dermal dendritic cells in psoriasis and drive strong Th17/Th1 T-cell responses. *J Allergy Clin Immunol.* (2011) 127:787–94. doi: 10.1016/j.jaci.2010.12.009
37. Döbel T, Kunze A, Babatz J, Tränkner K, Ludwig A, Schmitz M, et al. FcγRIII (CD16) equips immature 6-sulfo LacNAc-expressing dendritic cells (slanDCs) with a unique capacity to handle IgG-complexed antigens. *Blood.* (2013) 121:3609–18. doi: 10.1182/blood-2012-08-447045
38. Schmitz M, Zhao S, Schäkel K, Bornhäuser M, Ockert D, Rieber EP. Native human blood dendritic cells as potent effectors in antibody-dependent cellular cytotoxicity. *Blood.* (2002) 100:1502–4.
39. Schmitz M, Zhao S, Deuse Y, Schäkel K, Wehner R, Wöhner H, et al. Tumoricidal potential of native blood dendritic cells: direct tumor cell killing and activation of NK cell-mediated cytotoxicity. *J Immunol.* (2005) 174:4127–34. doi: 10.4049/jimmunol.174.7.4127
40. Wehner R, Löbel B, Bornhäuser M, Schäkel K, Cartellieri M, Bachmann M, et al. Reciprocal activating interaction between 6-sulfo LacNAc(+) dendritic cells and NK cells. *Int J Cancer.* (2009) 124:358–66. doi: 10.1002/ijc.23962
41. Dzionek A, Sohma Y, Nagafune J, Cella M, Colonna M, Facchetti F, et al. BDCA-2, a novel plasmacytoid dendritic cell-specific type II C-type lectin, mediates antigen capture and is a potent inhibitor of interferon alpha/beta induction. *J Exp Med.* (2001) 194:1823–34. doi: 10.1084/jem.194.12.1823
42. Vermi W, Micheletti A, Lonardi S, Costantini C, Calzetti F, Nascimbeni R, et al. slanDCs selectively accumulate in carcinoma-draining lymph nodes and marginate metastatic cells. *Nat Commun.* (2014) 5:3029. doi: 10.1038/ncomms4029
43. Toma M, Wehner R, Kloß A, Hübner L, Fodelianaki G, Erdmann K, et al. Accumulation of tolerogenic human 6-sulfo LacNAc dendritic cells in renal cell carcinoma is associated with poor prognosis. *Oncoimmunology.* (2015) 4:e1008342. doi: 10.1080/2162402X.2015.1008342
44. Burke AJ, Sullivan FJ, Giles FJ, Glynn SA. The yin and yang of nitric oxide in cancer progression. *Carcinogenesis.* (2013) 34:503–12. doi: 10.1093/carcin/bgt034
45. Waters JP, Pober JS, Bradley JR. Tumor necrosis factor and cancer. *J Pathol.* (2013) 230:241–8. doi: 10.1002/path.4188
46. Sommer U, Larsson B, Tuve S, Wehner R, Zimmermann N, Kramer M, et al. Proinflammatory human 6-sulfo LacNAc-positive dendritic cells accumulate in intestinal acute graft-versus-host disease. *Haematologica.* (2014) 99:e86–89. doi: 10.3324/haematol.2013.101071
47. Sozzani S, Vermi W, Del Prete A, Facchetti F. Trafficking properties of plasmacytoid dendritic cells in health and disease. *Trends Immunol.* (2010) 31:270–7. doi: 10.1016/j.it.2010.05.004
48. Ambe K, Mori M, Enjoji M. S-100 protein-positive dendritic cells in colorectal adenocarcinomas. Distribution and relation to the clinical prognosis. *Cancer.* (1989) 63:496–503. doi: 10.1002/1097-0142(19890201)63:3<496::AID-CNCR2820630318>3.0.CO;2-K
49. Dadabayev AR, Sandel MH, Menon AG, Morreau H, Melief CJM, Offringa R, et al. Dendritic cells in colorectal cancer correlate with other tumor-infiltrating immune cells. *Cancer Immunol Immunother.* (2004) 53:978–86. doi: 10.1007/s00262-004-0548-2
50. Sandel MH, Dadabayev AR, Menon AG, Morreau H, Melief CJ, Offringa R, et al. Prognostic value of tumor-infiltrating dendritic cells in colorectal cancer: role of maturation status and intratumoral localization. *Clin Cancer Res.* (2005) 11:2576–82. doi: 10.1158/1078-0432.CCR-04-1448
51. Nagorsen D, Voigt S, Berg E, Stein H, Thiel E, Loddenkemper C. Tumor-infiltrating macrophages and dendritic cells in human colorectal cancer: relation to local regulatory T cells, systemic T-cell response against tumor-associated antigens and survival. *J Transl Med.* (2007) 5:62. doi: 10.1186/1479-5876-5-62
52. Nakayama Y, Inoue Y, Minagawa N, Katsuki T, Nagashima N, Onitsuka K, et al. Relationships between S-100 protein-positive cells and clinicopathological factors in patients with colorectal cancer. *Anticancer Res.* (2003) 23:4423–26.
53. Gulubova MV, Ananiev JR, Vlaykova TI, Yovchev Y, Tsoneva V, Manolova IM. Role of dendritic cells in progression and clinical outcome of colon cancer. *Int J Colorectal Dis.* (2012) 27:159–69. doi: 10.1007/s00384-011-1334-1
54. Schwaab T, Weiss JE, Schned AR, Barth RJ Jr. Dendritic cell infiltration in colon cancer. *J Immunother.* (1991) 24:130–7. doi: 10.1097/00002371-200103000-00007

55. Suzuki A, Masuda A, Nagata H, Kameoka S, Kikawada Y, Yamakawa M, et al. Mature dendritic cells make clusters with T cells in the invasive margin of colorectal carcinoma. *J Pathol.* (2002) 196:37–43. doi: 10.1002/path.1018
56. Gai XD, Song Y, Li C, Lei YM, Yang B. Potential role of plasmacytoid dendritic cells for FOXP3+ regulatory T cell development in human colorectal cancer and tumor draining lymph node. *Pathol Res Pract.* (2013) 209:774–8. doi: 10.1016/j.prp.2013.08.011
57. Lamarthée B, de Vassoigne F, Malard F, Stocker N, Boussen I, Médiavilla C, et al. Quantitative and functional alterations of 6-sulfo LacNac dendritic cells in multiple myeloma. *Oncoimmunology.* (2018) 7:e1444411. doi: 10.1080/2162402X.2018.1444411
58. Vermi W, Micheletti A, Finotti G, Tecchio C, Calzetti F, Costa S, et al. slan+ monocytes and macrophages mediate CD20-dependent B-cell lymphoma elimination via ADCC and ADCP. *Cancer Res.* (2018) 78:3544–59. doi: 10.1158/0008-5472.CAN-17-2344
59. Shinto E, Hase K, Hashiguchi Y, Sekizawa A, Ueno H, Shikina A, et al. CD8+ and FOXP3+ tumor-infiltrating T cells before and after chemoradiotherapy for rectal cancer. *Ann Surg Oncol.* (2014) 21(Suppl 3):S414–21. doi: 10.1245/s10434-014-3584-y
60. Teng F, Mu D, Meng X, Kong L, Zhu H, Liu S, et al. Tumor infiltrating lymphocytes (TILs) before and after neoadjuvant chemoradiotherapy and its clinical utility for rectal cancer. *Am J Cancer Res.* (2015) 5:2064–74.
61. Teng F, Meng X, Kong L, Mu D, Zhu H, Liu S, et al. Tumor-infiltrating lymphocytes, forkhead box P3, programmed death ligand-1, and cytotoxic T lymphocyte-associated antigen-4 expressions before and after neoadjuvant chemoradiation in rectal cancer. *Transl Res.* (2015) 166:721–32.e1. doi: 10.1016/j.trsl.2015.06.019
62. Jarosch A, Sommer U, Bogner A, Reißfelder C, Weitz J, Krause M, et al. Neoadjuvant radiochemotherapy decreases the total amount of tumor infiltrating lymphocytes, but increases the number of CD8+/Granzyme B+ (GrzB) cytotoxic T-cells in rectal cancer. *Oncoimmunology.* (2017) 7:e1393133. doi: 10.1080/2162402X.2017.1393133
63. McCoy MJ, Hemmings C, Anyaegbu CC, Austin SJ, Lee-Pullen TF, Miller TJ, et al. Tumour-infiltrating regulatory T cell density before neoadjuvant chemoradiotherapy for rectal cancer does not predict treatment response. *Oncotarget.* (2017) 8:19803–13. doi: 10.18632/oncotarget.15048
64. Klug F, Prakash H, Huber PE, Seibel T, Bender N, Halama N, et al. Low dose irradiation programs macrophage differentiation to an iNOS^{+}/M1 phenotype that orchestrates effective T cell immunotherapy. *Cancer Cell.* (2013) 24:589–602. doi: 10.1016/j.ccr.2013.09.014
65. Zitvogel L, Galluzzi L, Kepp O, Smyth MJ, Kroemer G. Type I interferons in anticancer immunity. *Nat Rev Immunol.* (2015) 15:405–14. doi: 10.1038/nri3845
66. Sistigu A, Yamazaki T, Vacchelli E, Chaba K, Enot DP, Adam J, et al. Cancer cell-autonomous contribution of type I interferon signaling to the efficacy of chemotherapy. *Nat Med.* (2014) 20:1301–9. doi: 10.1038/nm.3708
67. Burnette BC, Liang H, Lee Y, Chlewicki L, Khodarev NN, Weichselbaum RR, et al. The efficacy of radiotherapy relies upon induction of type I interferon-dependent innate and adaptive immunity. *Cancer Res.* (2011) 71:2488–96. doi: 10.1158/0008-5472.CAN-10-2820
68. Harlin H, Meng Y, Peterson AC, Zha Y, Tretiakova M, Slingluff C, et al. Chemokine expression in melanoma metastases associated with CD8+ T-cell recruitment. *Cancer Res.* (2009) 69:3077–85. doi: 10.1158/0008-5472.CAN-08-2281
69. Zumwalt TJ, Arnold M, Goel A, Boland CR. Active secretion of CXCL10 and CCL5 from colorectal cancer microenvironments associates with GranzymeB+ CD8+ T-cell infiltration. *Oncotarget.* (2015) 6:2981–91. doi: 10.18632/oncotarget.3205

3

Dendritic Cell Subsets and Effector Function in Idiopathic and Connective Tissue Disease-Associated Pulmonary Arterial Hypertension

*Denise van Uden, Karin Boomars and Mirjam Kool**

Department of Pulmonary Medicine, Erasmus MC, Rotterdam, Netherlands

***Correspondence:**
Mirjam Kool
m.kool@erasmusmc.nl

Pulmonary arterial hypertension (PAH) is a cardiopulmonary disease characterized by an incurable condition of the pulmonary vasculature, leading to increased pulmonary vascular resistance, elevated pulmonary arterial pressure resulting in progressive right ventricular failure and ultimately death. PAH has different underlying causes. In approximately 30–40% of the patients no underlying risk factor or cause can be found, so-called idiopathic PAH (IPAH). Patients with an autoimmune connective tissue disease (CTD) can develop PAH [CTD-associated PAH (CTD-PAH)], suggesting a prominent role of immune cell activation in PAH pathophysiology. This is further supported by the presence of tertiary lymphoid organs (TLOs) near pulmonary blood vessels in IPAH and CTD-PAH. TLOs consist of myeloid cells, like monocytes and dendritic cells (DCs), T-cells, and B-cells. Next to their T-cell activating function, DCs are crucial for the preservation of TLOs. Multiple DC subsets can be found in steady state, such as conventional DCs (cDCs), including type 1 cDCs (cDC1s), and type 2 cDCs (cDC2s), AXL$^+$Siglec6$^+$ DCs (AS-DCs), and plasmacytoid DCs (pDCs). Under inflammatory conditions monocytes can differentiate into monocyte-derived-DCs (mo-DCs). DC subset distribution and activation status play an important role in the pathobiology of autoimmune diseases and most likely in the development of IPAH and CTD-PAH. DCs can contribute to pathology by activating T-cells (production of pro-inflammatory cytokines) and B-cells (pathogenic antibody secretion). In this review we therefore describe the latest knowledge about DC subset distribution, activation status, and effector functions, and polymorphisms involved in DC function in IPAH and CTD-PAH to gain a better understanding of PAH pathology.

Keywords: dendritic cell, dendritic cell subsets, pulmonary arterial hypertension, idiopathic pulmonary arterial hypertension, autoimmune disease, dendritic cell effector function, connective tissue disease

INTRODUCTION PULMONARY ARTERIAL HYPERTENSION

Pulmonary arterial hypertension (PAH) is characterized by a mean pulmonary arterial pressure (PAP) of $\geq$25 mmHg at rest and a mean capillary wedge pressure of $\leq$15 mmHg (1). The high PAP causes hypertrophy of the right ventricle (RV) leading eventually to RV dilatation, heart failure, and ultimately death. Particularly small pulmonary arteries (PAs) and arterioles are affected. They show a thickened vascular wall and formation of plexiform lesions due to endothelial dysfunction and proliferation of all three cell layers, the endothelium, smooth muscle cells (SMC), and the adventitia (2).

PAH patients can be subdivided into groups based on associated conditions and risk factors. However, in a substantial proportion of PAH patients no cause or associated condition can be identified: idiopathic PAH (IPAH). In another subgroup of patients, PAH is associated with autoimmune diseases (AD) such as connective tissue disease (CTD). CTD includes systemic sclerosis (SSc), systemic lupus erythematosus (SLE), rheumatoid arthritis (RA), and mixed connective tissue disease (MCTD). SSc is the most common AD associated with PAH, followed by SLE (3–6). PAH patients have a low 1-year survival rate: only 82% of SSc-PAH patients and 93% of IPAH patients are still alive after 1 year (6).

ROLE FOR IMMUNE ACTIVATION IN THE DEVELOPMENT OF PAH

The presence of PAH in a proportion of autoimmune patients suggests that activated immune cells (or their mediators) directly provoke pulmonary vascular remodeling. Local immune activation is also observed as tertiary lymphoid organs (TLOs or ectopic lymphoid structures) are present in the lungs of IPAH and CTD-associated PAH (CTD-PAH) patients (7, 8). TLOs are organized structures similar to lymph nodes (LNs), including distinct T-cell areas containing dendritic cells (DCs), organized B-cell follicles with germinal centers (GCs), high endothelial venules (HEV), and lymphatics. TLOs most likely develop due to long-lasting local immune activation and are considered a hallmark of chronic disease (9). In lungs of IPAH patients, TLOs are found in the vicinity of PAs, suggesting that they promote vascular remodeling (7). Not surprisingly, as TLOs are characteristic for ongoing/chronic immune activation, they are often found in target organs of several ADs. For instance, in SLE patients TLOs are present in the kidneys, and in SSc-PAH patients TLOs have even been found in the lungs (8, 10, 11). Even though the SSc-PAH patient group used in this study is small, it is conceivable that TLOs are present in the lungs of various CTD-PAH patients. In addition, it is very likely that immune activation in PAH patients will also occur in draining LNs.

During chronic antigenic stimulation, the lymphotoxin (LT)$\alpha1\beta2$-LTβ receptor axes is crucial for development of TLOs (12), whereby lymphoid tissue inducer (LTi) cells interact with lymphoid tissue organizer (LTo) cells. Repeated DC injection in the lungs of mice, mimicking chronic activation, provokes TLO development (13). Activated DCs can produce chemokines which attract T-cells and B-cells (e.g., CCL19/21 and CXCL13, respectively), as well as T- and B-cell survival factors (e.g., interleukin (IL)-15 and BAFF/IL-6, respectively) (13–17). They furthermore secrete cytokines creating a pro-inflammatory milieu and promote innate and adaptive responses. This milieu can also induce post-translational modifications of proteins, altering self-antigens into new antigens which could provoke autoimmune responses as seen in SLE (18). Within TLOs and LNs, tissue-migrated DCs present antigens to naïve T-cells, inducing their activation and differentiation. The main T helper (Th)-cell subsets are Th1, Th2, Th17, follicular Th-cells (Tfh), and regulatory T-cells (Tregs). Within the GC reaction in TLOs and LNs, Tfh-cells provide help to B-cells by producing cytokines that induce class switching, survival, proliferation, and antibody production.

The role of DC subsets and their effector function in pathogenesis of IPAH, AD, and CTD-PAH will be discussed in this review and is shown in **Table 1**.

DENDRITIC CELLS IN IPAH, CTD-PAH, AND AD

DCs are equipped with pathogen recognition receptors (PRRs) like toll-like receptors (TLR) to sense their surroundings. Antigen recognition leads to DC activation and migration toward LNs. Activated DCs upregulate co-stimulatory molecules like CD86, produce pro-inflammatory cytokines, and present antigen to T-cells using major histocompatibility complex class-II (MHC-II). In TLOs, DCs are mature, indicated by high CD86 expression and IL-12 production (37). The maintenance of TLOs in two lung infection models, has been shown to be dependent on DCs as they disintegrate when DCs are ablated (13, 38). Furthermore, impaired DC migration due to defects in the CCR7-signaling, has been shown to lead to the formation of bronchus-associated lymphoid tissue (39).

Under steady state conditions, several DC subsets with unique functions can be identified (40, 41). Conventional DCs (cDCs), identified by CD11c, and HLA-DR expression in humans, are a major DC subset and can be divided in two subtypes, type 1 cDCs (cDC1s) and type 2 cDCs (cDC2s). cDC1s express IRF8 and CD141 and excel in cross presentation (42). IRF4 and CD1c classify cDC2s, which are potent inducers of Th-cell responses. Plasmacytoid DCs (pDCs) produce interferons (IFN) and do not express CD11c, but express HLA-DR and CD123. Recently, within this HLA-DR$^+$CD123$^+$ population potent Th-cell inducers have been found, which

Abbreviations: PAH, Pulmonary arterial hypertension; PAP, pulmonary arterial pressure; RV, right ventricle; PAs, pulmonary arteries; SMC, smooth muscle cell; IPAH, idiopathic PAH; CTD, connective tissue diseases; CTD-PAH, CTD-associated PAH; AD, autoimmune disease; SSc, systemic sclerosis; SLE, systemic lupus erythematosus; RA, rheumatoid arthritis; MCTD, mixed connective tissue disease; SSc-PAH, Systemic sclerosis-PAH; TLOs, tertiary lymphoid organs, LNs, lymph nodes; DCs, dendritic cells; GCs, germinal centers; HEV, high endothelial venules; PH, pulmonary hypertensions; LT, lymphotoxin; LTi, lymphoid tissue inducers; LTo, lymphoid tissue organizer; Th, T helper; IL, interleukin; Tfh, follicular Th-cells; Tregs, regulatory T-cells; PRRs, pathogen recognition receptors; TLR, toll-like receptor; MHC-II, major histocompatibility complex class II; cDCs, conventional DCs; cDC1s, type 1 cDCs; cDC2s, type 2 cDCs; pDCs, Plasmacytoid DCs; IFN, interferons; AS-DCs, AXL$^+$Siglec6$^+$ DCs; mo-DCs, monocyte-derived dendritic cells; BM, bone marrow; IGS, interferon gene signature; PBMCs, peripheral blood mononuclear cells; LPS, lipopolysaccharide; ECs, endothelial cells; IPF, idiopathic pulmonary fibrosis; SSc-PF, pulmonary fibrosis associated SSc; NF-kB, nuclear factor-kappa B.

TABLE 1 | Involvement of DCs and monocytes in IPAH, AD, and CTD-PAH.

	Disease	Major finding	Tissue	References
cDC	IPAH SLE	cDCs are decreased in proportion and number	Blood	(19–23)
	SSc	cDC2s produce more IL-6, IL-10 and TNFα after TLR2 and TLR4 stimulation	Blood	(24, 25)
	SSc-PAH	• A *TLR2* polymorphism in AD patients is associated with PAH development • cDCs carrying this *TLR2* polymorphism produce more cytokines (e.g., IL-6)	Blood	(26)
	IPAH	cDCs numbers are increased	Lung	(27)
	IPAH AD[a]	cDCs are present in TLOs in target organs	Lung, Thyroid tissue	(7, 28)
pDC	IPAH	The number of pDCs is unaltered	Blood	(27)
	SLE SSc	pDCs are decreased in proportion and number	Blood	(22, 23, 29)
	SSc	pDCs predominantly secrete CXCL4	Blood, Skin	(30)
	IPAH	• pDC numbers are increased • pDCs are located around pulmonary vessels	Lung	(27)
	SLE SSc	pDCs are increased in diseased tissue	Skin	(29, 31)
Monocytes and mo-DCs	IPAH	hyporesponsive monocytes to TLR4 stimulation	Blood	(32)
	SSc-PAH	Monocytes show an activated profile (mRNA expression)	Blood	(33)
	SSc SSc-PAH	The number of non-classical monocytes is increased	Blood	(34)
	SSc	CXCL10, CXCL8, and CCL4-producing non-classical monocyte subset is increased	Blood	(24)
	IPAH	Monocytes have either a similar or decreased activation status, depending on the study	Blood	(19, 35)
	IPAH	*In vitro* generated mo-DCs have either an increased or decreased Th-cell stimulatory capability, depending on the study	Blood	(19, 35)
	SSc	mo-DCs carrying the *TLR2* polymorphism produce more cytokines (e.g., IL-6)	Blood	(26)
	IPAH	CD14+ cells are increased around pulmonary arteries	Lung	(36)

[a]*Graves disease and Hashimoto's thyroiditis, cDC, conventional dendritic cell; pDC, plasmacytoid dendritic cell; mo-DC, monocyte-derived-dendritic-cell; PAH, pulmonary arterial hypertension; IPAH, idiopathic pulmonary arterial hypertension; AD, autoimmune disease; CTD-PAH, connective tissue disease-associated PAH; SLE, systemic lupus erythematosus; SSc, systemic sclerosis; TLO, tertiary lymphoid organ; PAs, pulmonary arteries; TLR, toll-like receptor.*

additionally express AXL and Siglec6 ($AXL^+Siglec6^+$ (AS)-DCs) (43, 44). Under inflammatory conditions monocytes can differentiate into DCs, giving rise to monocyte-derived-DCs (mo-DCs).

Conventional Dendritic Cells

In IPAH patients, the proportion of circulating cDCs is decreased compared to controls (19). Numbers of circulating cDCs are also altered in several ADs associated with PAH. Both cDC1s and cDC2s are decreased in proportion and number in SLE patients compared to HCs, especially in patients with active disease (20–23). The decrease in circulating cDCs in PAH could indicate an increased cDC migration toward lung TLOs (**Figure 1**). In support of this idea, DCs can be found in lung TLOs of IPAH patients and cDC numbers were increased in total lung cell suspensions of these patients (7, 27). In IPAH TLOs, DCs are found inside T-cell zones, suggesting that they promote T-cell activation. In patients with ADs, cDCs in TLOs show increased expression of costimulatory molecules and a cDC2 phenotype, since they express CD1c and CD11c (28). Alternatively, the reduction in circulating cDCs might also be caused by alterations in cDC viability or DC progenitors resulting in a decreased output of cDCs from the bone marrow.

In addition to DC or DC precursors entering the affected tissue from the blood circulation, DCs may accumulate in tissue and contribute to TLO formation as they fail to go to LNs (39). Upon activation, DCs upregulate CCR7. The CCR7 allows the DC to respond to CCL19 and CCL21 expressed by the lymphatic endothelial cells and to enter the lymphatic vessels to migrate to the draining LN. Both CCL19 and CCL21 are expressed by lymphatic vessels in IPAH patients, which could facilitate DC attraction (7). Strikingly, CCR7-deficient mice develop lung TLOs and signs of PH, perhaps due to DC retention in the lungs (39, 45). DCs, amongst other cells, can produce CCL20 and CXCL13, which attract T-cells, B-cells, and immature DCs. CCL20 and CXCL13 mRNA expression are increased in IPAH lungs compared to controls (7), contributing to TLO formation. However, the cell responsible for this increased expression in IPAH is yet unknown.

Research into cDC subset activation is still limited in PAH and ADs. In SSc patients, circulating cDC2s produce more IL-6, IL-10, and TNF-α after TLR2 and TLR4 stimulation (24, 25). These

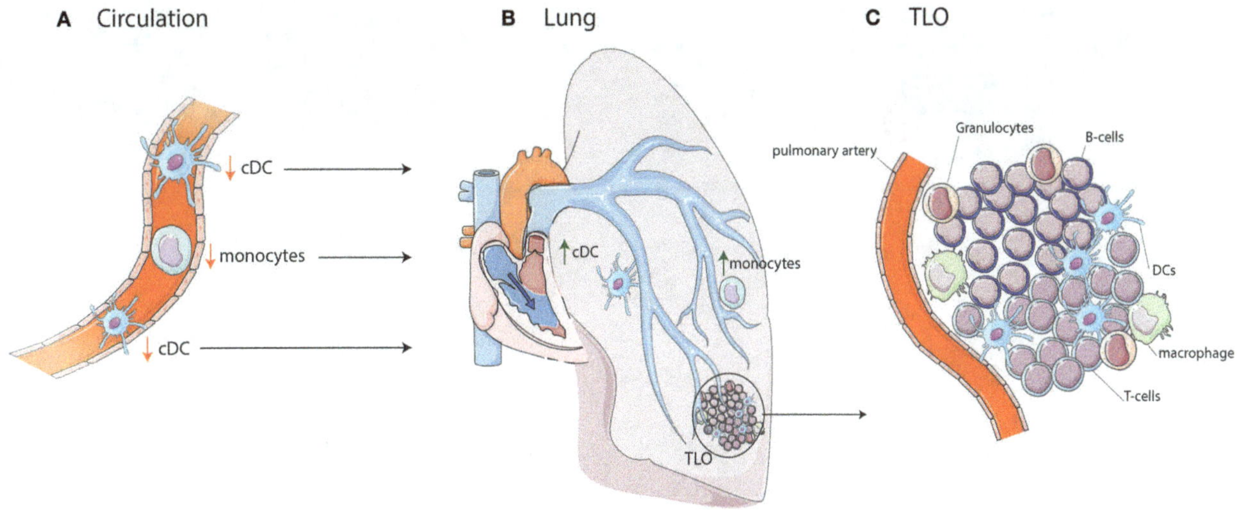

FIGURE 1 | cDC and monocyte migration toward lung TLOs. **(A)** cDCs and monocytes are decreased in circulation of IPAH patients due to migration to the lungs in which cDCs and monocytes are increased. **(B)** In the lung they can add to the development of TLOs surrounding PAs. **(C)** TLOs consist, besides DCs, of different immune cells such as T-cells, B-cells, macrophages, and granulocytes.

cytokines appear to play a central role in the immunopathology of PAH, as IL-6 and IL-10 are increased in the serum of IPAH patients and correlate with mortality (46). Especially IL-6 appears to be a crucial cytokine in PAH pathobiology, as mice overexpressing IL-6 develop signs of PH, while IL-6-deficient mice do not develop PH after hypoxia (47, 48). At this time, a phase II trial using Tocilizumab, an IL-6 receptor antagonist, is conducted in PAH patients (49).

In conclusion, in both IPAH and ADs circulating cDC proportions are decreased possibly due to migration to target organs, where they can both initiate adaptive immune responses and maintain TLOs (**Figure 2B**). Currently, only little is known about cDC subset distribution and function in IPAH, CTD-PAH, and ADs.

Plasmacytoid Dendritic Cells

Plasmacytoid DCs are predominantly found in lymphoid tissues and blood in steady state conditions. During inflammation, pDCs home toward peripheral tissues, produce type I IFNs, and promote activation of immune cells. In IPAH lungs pDC numbers are enhanced and pDCs are specifically located around the pulmonary vessels, while circulating pDC numbers are unaltered (27). In contrast, in SLE and SSc patients, circulating pDC number and frequency are decreased compared to controls, which could be due to emigration into diseased tissues (22, 23, 29, 31). Indeed, pDCs are present in diseased organs of SSc patients (29). Several ADs are associated with the interferon gene signature (IGS), to which different cells contribute. pDCs are major contributors to the IGS through their production of type I IFNs. One of the most strongly upregulated genes in pDCs within the IGS is CXCL10 (50). Augmented serum CXCL10 levels are associated with PAH in SSc patients (51). Likewise, in IPAH patients, serum CXCL10 is elevated and even associated with poor RV function (52), suggesting the possibility of a prominent role for pDCs in disease immunopathology. Next to IFNs, pDCs are also large producers of CXCL4 in SSc (30). CXCL4 can induce an influx of CD45^{+} cells in target tissues, perhaps leading to tissue remodeling and disease progression.

The associations of pDC with CTD-PAH and the increase in pDCs in lungs of IPAH patients suggest that type-I IFN and chemokine secretion by pDCs not only play an important role in several ADs, but also in CTD-PAH and IPAH pathology (**Figure 2A**).

Monocytes and Monocyte-Derived DCs

Monocytes are precursors of mo-DCs that arise under inflammatory conditions (40). Monocytes are heterogeneous and can be divided into 3 subsets based on CD14 and CD16 expression (53, 54). Classical monocytes, also called inflammatory monocytes, express CD14 and can infiltrate tissues, produce pro-inflammatory cytokines, and differentiate into inflammatory macrophages. Classical monocytes express several PRRs and are superior in phagocytosis. Monocytes expressing both CD14 and CD16 are termed intermediate monocytes, can also produce pro-inflammatory cytokines (55) and are unique in their ability to produce reactive oxygen species. Their gene expression signature indicates their ability to present antigens and induce T-cell activation (56). Intermediate monocytes specifically promote pro-inflammatory Th17-cell responses, which also contribute to PAH development, as discussed below (55). Finally, non-classical monocytes, expressing CD16, are known to survey the endothelium for danger signals (54). They differentiate into tissue-resident macrophages in steady state or into anti-inflammatory macrophages during inflammation, to repair damaged tissues.

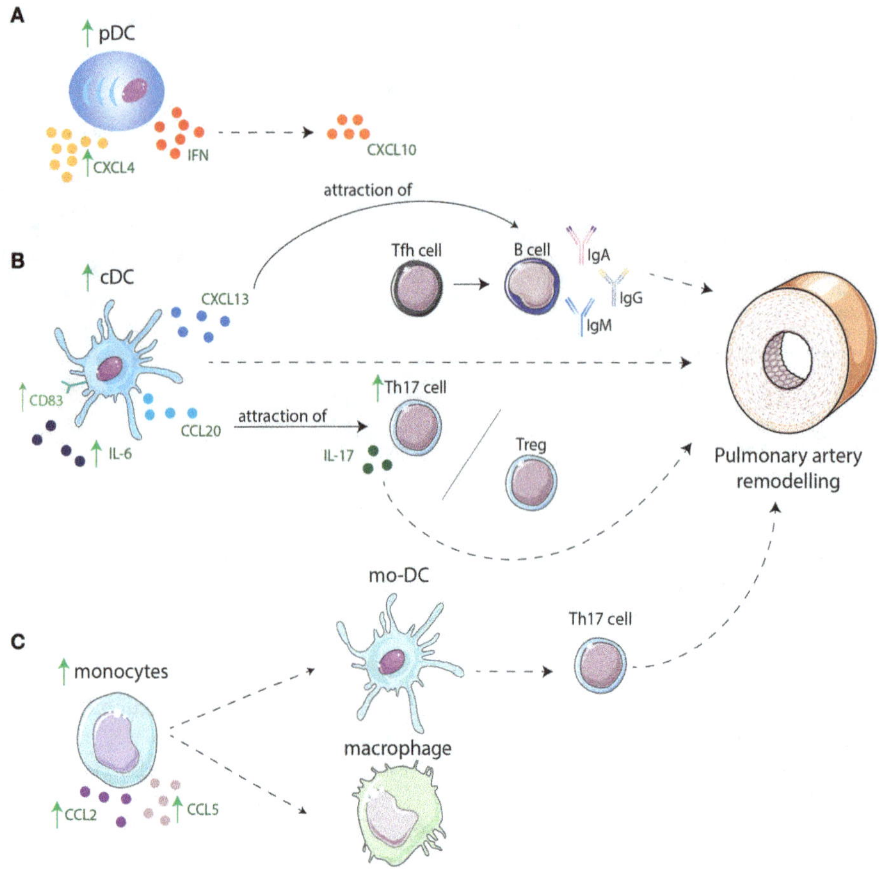

FIGURE 2 | Involvement of DCs and monocyte in lungs of IPAH and CTD-PAH patients. **(A)** pDCs are increased in lungs and might play a role in IPAH and CTD-PAH pathology by producing higher levels of CXCL4 and CXCL10 that is induced by IFNs. **(B)** cDC display higher levels of CD83 and have an enhanced cytokine production e.g., IL-6. cDCs are increased in lungs of PAH patients and can directly lead to PA remodeling or indirectly by production of CXCL13 and CCL20. CXCL13 leads to migration of B-cells toward the lungs, B-cells will produce pathogenic antibodies after interaction with Tfh cells, leading to remodeling of PAs. CCL20 attracts T-cells such as Tregs and Th17 cells leading to an increase in Th17 cells in the lung resulting in a Th17/Treg disbalance and by IL-17 production contributes to PA remodeling. **(C)** Monocytes are increased in the lung and produce CCL2 and CCL5 which might lead to attraction of other monocytes. Monocytes might differentiate in macrophages or mo-DCs. Mo-DCs induce Th17 cells adding to PA remodeling.

The number of non-classical monocytes is increased in SSc associated with PAH development, whereas there is no difference in the number of classical monocytes (34). The number of CTD-PAH patients in this study was very small, so this should be confirmed in a larger cohort. Increased numbers of $CD14^{+}$ cells, including classical/intermediate monocytes and macrophages, are observed around PAs of IPAH patients (36). Monocytes might be attracted to the PAs through their expression of CCR2 and CCR5 and an increased expression of their ligands CCL2 and CCL5 in lungs and serum of IPAH patients (57, 58). In SSc and CTD-PAH enhanced CCL2 is also observed in either skin or serum (59–61).

Strikingly, circulating monocytes of IPAH patients are hyporesponsive, as demonstrated by decreased cytokine production upon TLR4 stimulation (32). The local and/or systemic pro-inflammatory milieu in IPAH patients could provoke a feedback mechanism, resulting in hyporesponsive monocytes. However, the underlying mechanism is still unknown and further research is needed. In contrast to IPAH monocytes, monocytes from SSc-PAH patients are activated, as shown by their mRNA expression profile. This profile is even discriminative between SSc-PAH and SSc patients (33). Non-classical monocytes, expressing CXCL10, CXCL8, and CCL4 are involved in SSc pathology, and are found in increased numbers in SSc patients compared to controls (24).

Mo-DCs for *in vitro* assays, used to model and monitor human DC function, are commonly generated from monocytes. Contradictory results have been found using this model in IPAH. Decreased activation of monocytes together with lower T-cell stimulation (19), as well as a similar activation status with an increased Th-cell stimulatory capability have been observed (35). These opposite findings might be caused by the type of stimulation used to mature mo-DCs and different mo-DC:T-cell ratios in the T-cell stimulation assays.

Taken together, increased pulmonary expression of chemokines may attract monocytes to lungs of IPAH and CTD-PAH patients, where they become activated and alter their gene expression due to the pro-inflammatory environment. These altered monocytes may give rise to mo-DCs, which arise at places of inflammation and can induce T-cell activation (**Figure 2C**).

EFFECTOR FUNCTION OF DCS IN IPAH, CTD-PAH AND ADS

T-Cell Responses

DCs excel at antigen presentation to T-cells and together with their costimulatory molecule expression and cytokine production, they are pivotal for the succeeding T-cell response. Specifically, Th17-cells are implicated in the pathogenesis of many ADs and are observed inside mature TLOs of IPAH patients (7). Th17 differentiation from naïve Th-cells occurs in the presence of IL-1β, IL-6, and TGFβ (62), cytokines produced by activated DCs. Both IL-1β and IL-6 are elevated in serum of IPAH patients (46). Th17-cells are the main source of IL-17, IL-21, and IL-22. IL-21$^+$ cells are present in remodeled PAs of IPAH patients (63). In addition, IL-17 may affect structural remodeling observed in PAH, as IL-17 enhances fibroblast proliferation and collagen production *in vitro* (64). In SSc, IL-17 induces adhesion molecule expression and IL-1/chemokine production on endothelial cells (ECs) (65–67). Additionally, in IPAH PBMCs the IL-17 gene is hypo-methylated, indicating increased IL-17 transcription and supporting a possible role for Th17-cells in the pathology of IPAH (35). Indeed, IL-17 gene expression is enhanced in lungs of both IPAH and SSc-PAH compared to idiopathic pulmonary fibrosis (IPF) and pulmonary fibrosis associated SSc (SSc-PF) (68), this IL-17 may be expressed by cells in TLOs as well as in tissues outside of TLOs.

Furthermore, IL-23, also produced by DCs, stabilizes the phenotype of Th17-cells, but also promotes their pro-inflammatory potential (62). Th17-cells are also highly plastic cells and under the influence of IL-23 start co-expressing cytokines from the Th1-cell lineage. This leads to possibly pathogenic IFNγ-producing Th17-cells, also called Th17.1-cells. Enhanced expression of the IL-23 receptor on Th17(.1)-cells might contribute to their pro-inflammatory pathogenic phenotype (62, 69, 70). IL-23 is increased in exhale breath condensate of SSc patients, so perhaps Th17 plasticity plays a role in SSc pathology (71). Furthermore, IFNγ, IL-12, and TNFα can induce plasticity toward Th17.1-cells (62). Both serum IL-12 and TNFα are enhanced in IPAH patients and mRNA transcripts of these cytokines were increased in lungs rats in a PH model (46, 72). IL-17/IFNγ-double producing Th-cells are observed within the arteries of atherosclerosis patients, where they provoke pro-inflammatory cytokine production (e.g., IL-6, CXCL10) by vascular SMCs (73). This feedback loop could also exist within PAH, since IL-6 is highly produced by pulmonary ECs of IPAH patients. In addition, IL-6 promotes SMC proliferation in a hypoxia-induced PH model (74, 75). Blocking of IL-6 signaling improved PH physiology in a hypoxia-induced PH mouse model and prevented accumulation of Th17-cells (63). IL-6 also converts Th17-cells into IL-17+ Tregs, which are less suppressive than conventional Tregs (76). In SSc, IL-17+ Tregs are observed in the circulation and possibly also in the skin, indicated by IL-17 and FoxP3 positivity (64, 65, 77). The balance between pro-inflammatory Th17-cells and anti-inflammatory Tregs is crucial to control autoimmune features. IL-6 is a key cytokine in Th17/Treg balance, since TGF-β alone polarizes naïve Th-cells to Tregs, while TGF-β together with IL-6 induces Th17-cells (78). Active TGF-β signaling is very prominent in PAH and can be produced by different cells, like monocytes and DCs (79). However, whether DC-derived IL-6 plays a prominent role is unknown yet, as many cells can produce IL-6. In favor of a disturbed balance are the decreased number of Tregs observed in SLE, which correlates with disease severity (66). In CTD-PAH patients Th17-cells and Th17-related cytokines are elevated compared to AD patients without PAH (80). The disturbed Th17/Treg ratio even appears to correlate with PAH severity in APAH patients (80). This demonstrates that Th17-cells and Tregs are implicated not only in ADs but also in PAH (80).

Therefore, Th17 plasticity and Th17/Treg balance may contribute to ADs and PAH, potentially in part by modulating vascular remodeling.

Humoral Immune Response

Apart from their interaction with Th17-cells, DCs can induce (immature) Tfh-cells, which develop under the influence of IL-21, IL-6, IL-12, and IL-27 (78). In mature TLOs containing GCs, Tfh-cells interact with B-cells, leading to either antibody-producing plasma cells or memory B-cells. There is clear evidence for B-cell dysregulation in IPAH and CTD-PAH (81, 82). In IPAH patients circulating B-cells have an increased expression of genes involved in inflammatory mechanisms, host defense, and endothelial dysfunction, suggesting increased activation of B-cells (82). Also numbers of circulating plasmablasts are elevated in IPAH patients (83). Anomalies in B-cell homeostasis were also observed in SSc-PAH patients, with increased circulating IgD+ B-cell proportions (81). Tfh-cell numbers crucially control the development of auto-reactive B-cells, since an increase in Tfh-cell number can lead to increased autoantibody production (84, 85). In several ADs, Tfh-cells are increased in blood and target organs (86–89). Serum IgG, IgM, and IgA antibodies are elevated in IPAH patients, and EC-specific IgA promotes cytokine production and upregulation of adhesion molecules (83, 90–92). IgG and IgM antibodies directed against EC-surface antigens are also found in ADs and CTD-PAH, being most prevalent in SSc-PAH patients, followed by IPAH patients and SSc patients without PAH (92). IgG antibodies in SSc and SLE were directed against microvascular ECs antigens, while IgG in SSc, IPAH, and CTD-PAH recognized microvascular dermal and lung EC antigens, and vascular SMCs (90, 91, 93–95). Auto-reactive IgG provoked EC dysfunction, induced pro-inflammatory signals, and increased adhesiveness of T-cells to ECs, which also modulated migration and proliferation of SMC. These autoantibodies from SSc or CTD-PAH patients can directly cause signs of PH when injected into healthy mice (96). It is unknown where the autoantibodies found in IPAH and CTD-PAH patients are produced. TLO might be a likely location since Tfh-cells and B-cells, and perhaps antigens, are present in these TLOs. However, these autoantibodies can also be produced in the draining LNs.

In brief, pathogenic autoantibodies in CTD-PAH and IPAH might be produced by dysregulated B-cells that interact with Tfh-cells in TLOs. These autoantibodies recognize protein epitopes expressed by ECs, leading to endothelial dysfunction and vascular remodeling. So far, the role of Tfh-cells in IPAH is unknown and further research is needed.

GENETICS

Increased activation of the immune system in PAH is also supported by different polymorphisms observed in genome wide association studies. A polymorphism in *TLR2* of SSc patients is associated with PAH development (26). Functional analysis of mo-DCs and cDCs carrying the *TLR2* polymorphism showed enhanced cytokine production, including IL-6, compared to control DCs. As discussed above, IL-6 plays a prominent role in PAH pathology. Strikingly, a decreased IL-6 serum level was observed in healthy individuals and patients with a single nucleotide polymorphism in the promotor region of the *IL-6* gene, *IL-6-572C/G*, which correlated with decreased risk to develop IPAH (97). SNPs might not only be useful to determine disease susceptibility but also to determine disease onset or activity, as is seen for a specific SNP in *TGFB* gene in heritable PAH patients carrying a BMPR2 mutation (98). Another genetic association found in both PAH and SSc involving immune activation is a SNP in the *TNFAIP3* gene (99). *TNFAIP3* encodes for the ubiquitinating enzyme A20, which is crucial for down-regulation of the nuclear factor-kappa B (NF-κB) signaling pathway and thereby cell activation (100). Macrophages, pulmonary arterial ECs, and pulmonary arterial SMCs in end-stage IPAH patients showed an increased expression in NF-κB (101), suggesting an important role for the NF-κB pathway in IPAH.

This demonstrates that several SNPs and genes that are involved in DC function are present in PAH patients.

FUTURE DIRECTIONS

In conclusion, different DC subsets are involved not only in the pathobiology of ADs but appear to play a role in the pathobiology of IPAH and CTD-PAH as well. However, the exact role of these DCs in PAH development has not been fully elucidated. The increasing knowledge on DC biology obtained by advanced immunological techniques has led to a more unified method to identify DC subsets and the discovery of new DC subsets. Determining the role of all currently known DC populations, including AS-DCs, as well as their specific functions may help to unravel the pathobiology of PAH. This might lead to new opportunities for therapies targeting specific DC subsets, their activation, and/or their effector function.

AUTHOR CONTRIBUTIONS

DvU and MK wrote the manuscript. KB contributed to the review of the manuscript. All authors approved the manuscript for publication.

ACKNOWLEDGMENTS

We would like to thank O.B.J. Corneth for critically reading the manuscript.

REFERENCES

1. Galiè N, Humbert M, Vachiery JL, Gibbs S, Lang I, Torbicki A, et al. 2015 ESC/ERS Guidelines for the diagnosis and treatment of pulmonary hypertension: the joint task force for the diagnosis and treatment of pulmonary hypertension of the European Society of Cardiology (ESC) and the European Respiratory Society (ERS): endorsed by: Association for European Paediatric and Congenital Cardiology (AEPC), International Society for Heart and Lung Transplantation (ISHLT). *Eur Heart J.* (2016) 37:67–119. doi: 10.1093/eurheartj/ehv317
2. Humbert M, Montani D, Perros F, Dorfmüller P, Adnot S, Eddahibi S. Endothelial cell dysfunction and cross talk between endothelium and smooth muscle cells in pulmonary arterial hypertension. *Vascul Pharmacol.* (2008) 49:113–8. doi: 10.1016/j.vph.2008.06.003
3. McGoon MD, Miller DP. REVEAL: a contemporary US pulmonary arterial hypertension registry. *Eur Respir Rev.* (2012) 21:8–18. doi: 10.1183/09059180.00008211
4. Dhala A. Pulmonary arterial hypertension in systemic lupus erythematosus: current status and future direction. *Clin Dev Immunol.* (2012) 2012:854941. doi: 10.1155/2012/854941
5. Tselios K, Gladman DD, Urowitz MB. Systemic lupus erythematosus and pulmonary arterial hypertension: links, risks, and management strategies. *Open Access Rheumatol.* (2017) 9:1–9. doi: 10.2147/OARRR.S123549
6. Chung L, Liu J, Parsons L, Hassoun PM, McGoon M, Badesch DB, et al. Characterization of connective tissue disease-associated pulmonary arterial hypertension from REVEAL: identifying systemic sclerosis as a unique phenotype. *Chest* (2010) 138:1383–94. doi: 10.1378/chest.10-0260
7. Perros F, Dorfmüller P, Montani D, Hammad H, Waelput W, Girerd B, et al. Pulmonary lymphoid neogenesis in idiopathic pulmonary arterial hypertension. *Am J Respir Crit Care Med.* (2012) 185:311–21. doi: 10.1164/rccm.201105-0927OC
8. Cool CD, Kennedy D, Voelkel NF, Tuder RM. Pathogenesis and evolution of plexiform lesions in pulmonary hypertension associated with scleroderma and human immunodeficiency virus infection. *Hum Pathol.* (1997) 28:434–42. doi: 10.1016/S0046-8177(97)90032-0
9. Neyt K, Perros F, GeurtsvanKessel CH, Hammad H, Lambrecht BN. Tertiary lymphoid organs in infection and autoimmunity. *Trends Immunol.* (2012) 33:297–305. doi: 10.1016/j.it.2012.04.006

10. Steinmetz OM, Velden J, Kneissler U, Marx M, Klein A, Helmchen U, et al. Analysis and classification of B-cell infiltrates in lupus and ANCA-associated nephritis. *Kidney Int.* (2008) 74:448–57. doi: 10.1038/ki.2008.191
11. Chang A, Henderson SG, Brandt D, Liu N, Guttikonda R, Hsieh C, et al. *In situ* B cell-mediated immune responses and tubulointerstitial inflammation in human lupus nephritis. *J Immunol.* (2011) 186:1849–60. doi: 10.4049/jimmunol.1001983
12. van de Pavert SA, Mebius RE. New insights into the development of lymphoid tissues. *Nat Rev Immunol.* (2010) 10:664–74. doi: 10.1038/nri2832
13. GeurtsvanKessel CH, Willart MA, Bergen IM, van Rijt LS, Muskens F, Elewaut D, et al. Dendritic cells are crucial for maintenance of tertiary lymphoid structures in the lung of influenza virus-infected mice. *J Exp Med.* (2009) 206:2339–49. doi: 10.1084/jem.20090410
14. McDonald KG, McDonough JS, Dieckgraefe BK, Newberry RD. Dendritic cells produce CXCL13 and participate in the development of murine small intestine lymphoid tissues. *Am J Pathol.* (2010) 176:2367–77. doi: 10.2353/ajpath.2010.090723
15. Kool M, van Loo G, Waelput W, De Prijck S, Muskens F, Sze M, et al.Kool M, et al. The ubiquitin-editing protein A20 prevents dendritic cell activation, recognition of apoptotic cells, and systemic autoimmunity. *Immunity* (2011) 35:82–96. doi: 10.1016/j.immuni.2011.05.013
16. Mattei F, Schiavoni G, Belardelli F, Tough DF. IL-15 is expressed by dendritic cells in response to type I IFN, double-stranded RNA, or lipopolysaccharide and promotes dendritic cell activation. *J Immunol.* (2001) 167:1179–87. doi: 10.4049/jimmunol.167.3.1179
17. Gasparini C, Foxwell BM, Feldmann M. RelB/p50 regulates CCL19 production, but fails to promote human DC maturation. *Eur J Immunol.* (2009) 39:2215–23. doi: 10.1002/eji.200939209
18. Doyle HA, Yang ML, Raycroft MT, Gee RJ, Mamula MJ. Autoantigens: novel forms and presentation to the immune system. *Autoimmunity* (2014) 47:220–33. doi: 10.3109/08916934.2013.850495
19. Wang W, Yan H, Zhu W, Cui Y, Chen J, Wang X, et al. Impairment of monocyte-derived dendritic cells in idiopathic pulmonary arterial hypertension. *J Clin Immunol.* (2009) 29:705–13. doi: 10.1007/s10875-009-9322-8
20. Jin O, Kavikondala S, Sun L, Fu R, Mok MY, Chan A, et al. Systemic lupus erythematosus patients have increased number of circulating plasmacytoid dendritic cells, but decreased myeloid dendritic cells with deficient CD83 expression. *Lupus* (2008) 17:654–62. doi: 10.1177/0961203308089410
21. Khan SA, Nowatzky J, Jiménez-Branda S, Greenberg JD, Clancy R, Buyon J, et al. Active systemic lupus erythematosus is associated with decreased blood conventional dendritic cells. *Exp Mol Pathol.* (2013) 95:121–3. doi: 10.1016/j.yexmp.2013.06.003
22. Migita K, Miyashita T, Maeda Y, Kimura H, Nakamura M, Yatsuhashi H, et al. Reduced blood BDCA-2+ (lymphoid) and CD11c+ (myeloid) dendritic cells in systemic lupus erythematosus. *Clin Exp Immunol.* (2005) 142:84–91. doi: 10.1111/j.1365-2249.2005.02897.x
23. Blomberg S, Eloranta ML, Magnusson M, Alm GV, Rönnblom L. Expression of the markers BDCA-2 and BDCA-4 and production of interferon-alpha by plasmacytoid dendritic cells in systemic lupus erythematosus. *Arthritis Rheum.* (2003) 48:2524–32. doi: 10.1002/art.11225
24. Carvalheiro T, Horta S, van Roon JAG, Santiago M, Salvador MJ, Trindade H, et al. Increased frequencies of circulating CXCL10-, CXCL8- and CCL4-producing monocytes and Siglec-3-expressing myeloid dendritic cells in systemic sclerosis patients. *Inflamm Res.* (2018) 67:169–77. doi: 10.1007/s00011-017-1106-7
25. van Bon L, Popa C, Huijbens R, Vonk M, York M, Simms R, et al. Distinct evolution of TLR-mediated dendritic cell cytokine secretion in patients with limited and diffuse cutaneous systemic sclerosis. *Ann Rheum Dis.* (2010) 69:1539–47. doi: 10.1136/ard.2009.128207
26. Broen JC, Bossini-Castillo L, van Bon L, Vonk MC, Knaapen H, Beretta L, et al. A rare polymorphism in the gene for Toll-like receptor 2 is associated with systemic sclerosis phenotype and increases the production of inflammatory mediators. *Arthritis Rheum.* (2012) 64:264–71. doi: 10.1002/art.33325
27. Marsh LM, Jandl K, Grünig G, Foris V, Bashir M, Ghanim B, et al. The inflammatory cell landscape in the lungs of patients with idiopathic pulmonary arterial hypertension. *Eur Respir J.* (2018) 51:1701214. doi: 10.1183/13993003.01214-2017
28. Roura-Mir C, Catálfamo M, Cheng TY, Marqusee E, Besra GS, Jaraquemada D, et al. CD1a and CD1c activate intrathyroidal T cells during Graves' disease and Hashimoto's thyroiditis. *J Immunol.* (2005) 174:3773–80. doi: 10.4049/jimmunol.174.6.3773
29. Ah Kioon MD, Tripodo C, Fernandez D, Kirou KA, Spiera RF, Crow MK, et al. Plasmacytoid dendritic cells promote systemic sclerosis with a key role for TLR8. *Sci Transl Med.* (2018) 10: eaam8458. doi: 10.1126/scitranslmed.aam8458
30. van Bon L, Affandi AJ, Broen J, Christmann RB, Marijnissen RJ, Stawski L, et al. Proteome-wide analysis and CXCL4 as a biomarker in systemic sclerosis. *N Engl J Med.* (2014) 370:433–43. doi: 10.1056/NEJMoa1114576
31. Farkas L, Beiske K, Lund-Johansen F, Brandtzaeg P, Jahnsen FL. Plasmacytoid dendritic cells (natural interferon- alpha/beta-producing cells) accumulate in cutaneous lupus erythematosus lesions. *Am J Pathol.* (2001) 159:237–43. doi: 10.1016/S0002-9440(10)61689-6
32. Raychaudhuri B, Bonfield TL, Malur A, Hague K, Kavuru MS, Arroliga AC, et al. Circulating monocytes from patients with primary pulmonary hypertension are hyporesponsive. *Clin Immunol.* (2002) 104:191–8. doi: 10.1006/clim.2002.5253
33. Pendergrass SA, Hayes E, Farina G, Lemaire R, Farber HW, Whitfield ML, et al. Limited systemic sclerosis patients with pulmonary arterial hypertension show biomarkers of inflammation and vascular injury. *PLoS ONE* (2010) 5:e12106. doi: 10.1371/journal.pone.0012106
34. Lescoat A, Lecureur V, Roussel M, Sunnaram BL, Ballerie A, Coiffier G, et al. CD16-positive circulating monocytes and fibrotic manifestations of systemic sclerosis. *Clin Rheumatol.* (2017) 36:1649–54. doi: 10.1007/s10067-017-3597-6
35. Hautefort A, Girerd B, Montani D, Cohen-Kaminsky S, Price L, Lambrecht BN, et al. T-helper 17 cell polarization in pulmonary arterial hypertension. *Chest* (2015) 147:1610-20. doi: 10.1378/chest.14-1678
36. Savai R, Pullamsetti SS, Kolbe J, Bieniek E, Voswinckel R, Fink L, et al. Immune and inflammatory cell involvement in the pathology of idiopathic pulmonary arterial hypertension. *Am J Respir Crit Care Med.* (2012) 186:897–908. doi: 10.1164/rccm.201202-0335OC
37. Nacionales DC, Kelly KM, Lee PY, Zhuang H, Li Y, Weinstein JS, et al. Type I interferon production by tertiary lymphoid tissue developing in response to 2,6,10,14-tetramethyl-pentadecane (pristane). *Am J Pathol.* (2006) 168:1227–40. doi: 10.2353/ajpath.2006.050125
38. Halle S, Dujardin HC, Bakocevic N, Fleige H, Danzer H, Willenzon S, et al. Induced bronchus-associated lymphoid tissue serves as a general priming site for T cells and is maintained by dendritic cells. *J Exp Med.* (2009) 206:2593–601. doi: 10.1084/jem.20091472
39. Fleige H, Bosnjak B, Permanyer M, Ristenpart J, Bubke A, Willenzon S, et al. Manifold roles of CCR7 and its ligands in the induction and maintenance of bronchus-associated lymphoid tissue. *Cell Rep.* (2018) 23:783–95. doi: 10.1016/j.celrep.2018.03.072
40. Guilliams M, Ginhoux F, Jakubzick C, Naik SH, Onai N, Schraml BU, et al.Guilliams M, et al. Dendritic cells, monocytes and macrophages: a unified nomenclature based on ontogeny. *Nat Rev Immunol.* (2014) 14:571–8. doi: 10.1038/nri3712
41. Collin M, Bigley V. Human dendritic cell subsets: an update. *Immunology* (2018) 154:3–20. doi: 10.1111/imm.12888
42. Guilliams M, Dutertre CA, Scott CL, McGovern N, Sichien D, Chakarov S, et al. Unsupervised high-dimensional analysis aligns dendritic cells across tissues and species. *Immunity* (2016) 45:669–84. doi: 10.1016/j.immuni.2016.08.015
43. Villani AC, Satija R, Reynolds G, Sarkizova S, Shekhar K, Fletcher J, et al. Single-cell RNA-seq reveals new types of human blood dendritic cells, monocytes, and progenitors. *Science* (2017) 356:eaah4573. doi: 10.1126/science.aah4573
44. Alcántara-Hernández M, Leylek R, Wagar LE, Engleman EG, Keler T, Marinkovich MP, et al. High-dimensional phenotypic mapping of human dendritic cells reveals interindividual variation and tissue specialization. *Immunity* (2017) 47:1037–1050 e6. doi: 10.1016/j.immuni.2017.11.001
45. Larsen KO, Yndestad A, Sjaastad I, Løberg EM, Goverud IL, Halvorsen B, et al. Lack of CCR7 induces pulmonary hypertension involving perivascular

leukocyte infiltration and inflammation. *Am J Physiol Lung Cell Mol Physiol.* (2011) 301:L50–9. doi: 10.1152/ajplung.00048.2010

46. Soon E, Holmes AM, Treacy CM, Doughty NJ, Southgate L, Machado RD, et al. Elevated levels of inflammatory cytokines predict survival in idiopathic and familial pulmonary arterial hypertension. *Circulation* (2010) 122:920–7. doi: 10.1161/CIRCULATIONAHA.109.933762
47. Steiner MK, Syrkina OL, Kolliputi N, Mark EJ, Hales CA, Waxman AB. Interleukin-6 overexpression induces pulmonary hypertension. *Circ Res.* (2009) 104:236–44:28p following 244. doi: 10.1161/CIRCRESAHA.108.182014
48. Savale L, Tu L, Rideau D, Izziki M, Maitre B, Adnot S, et al. Impact of interleukin-6 on hypoxia-induced pulmonary hypertension and lung inflammation in mice. *Respir Res.* (2009) 10:6. doi: 10.1186/1465-9921-10-6
49. Hernández-Sánchez J, Harlow L, Church C, Gaine S, Knightbridge E, Bunclark K, et al. Clinical trial protocol for TRANSFORM-UK: a therapeutic open-label study of tocilizumab in the treatment of pulmonary arterial hypertension. *Pulm Circ.* (2018) 8:2045893217735820. doi: 10.1177/2045893217735820
50. Liu X, Mayes MD, Tan FK, Wu M, Reveille JD, Harper BE, et al. Correlation of interferon-inducible chemokine plasma levels with disease severity in systemic sclerosis. *Arthritis Rheum.* (2013) 65:226–35. doi: 10.1002/art.37742
51. Eloranta ML, Franck-Larsson K, Lövgren T, Kalamajski S, Rönnblom A, Rubin K, et al. Type I interferon system activation and association with disease manifestations in systemic sclerosis. *Ann Rheum Dis.* (2010) 69:1396–402. doi: 10.1136/ard.2009.121400
52. Yang T, Li ZN, Chen G, Gu Q, Ni XH, Zhao ZH, et al. Increased levels of plasma CXC-Chemokine Ligand 10:12 and 16 are associated with right ventricular function in patients with idiopathic pulmonary arterial hypertension. *Heart Lung* (2014) 43:322–7. doi: 10.1016/j.hrtlng.2014.04.016
53. Ziegler-Heitbrock L. Blood monocytes and their subsets: established features and open questions. *Front Immunol.* (2015) 6:423. doi: 10.3389/fimmu.2015.00423
54. Wong KL, Yeap WH, Tai JJ, Ong SM, Dang TM, Wong SC. The three human monocyte subsets: implications for health and disease. *Immunol Res.* (2012) 53:41–57. doi: 10.1007/s12026-012-8297-3
55. Rossol M, Kraus S, Pierer M, Baerwald C, Wagner U. The CD14(bright) CD16+ monocyte subset is expanded in rheumatoid arthritis and promotes expansion of the Th17 cell population. *Arthritis Rheum.* (2012) 64:671–7. doi: 10.1002/art.33418
56. Wong KL, Tai JJ, Wong WC, Han H, Sem X, Yeap WH, et al. Gene expression profiling reveals the defining features of the classical, intermediate, and nonclassical human monocyte subsets. *Blood* (2011) 118:e16–31. doi: 10.1182/blood-2010-12-326355
57. Dorfmüller P, Zarka V, Durand-Gasselin I, Monti G, Balabanian K, Garcia G, et al. Chemokine RANTES in severe pulmonary arterial hypertension. *Am J Respir Crit Care Med.* (2002) 165:534–9. doi: 10.1164/ajrccm.165.4.2012112
58. Itoh T, Nagaya N, Ishibashi-Ueda H, Kyotani S, Oya H, Sakamaki F, et al. Increased plasma monocyte chemoattractant protein-1 level in idiopathic pulmonary arterial hypertension. *Respirology* (2006) 11:158–63. doi: 10.1111/j.1440-1843.2006.00821.x
59. Yamamoto T, Eckes B, Hartmann K, Krieg T. Expression of monocyte chemoattractant protein-1 in the lesional skin of systemic sclerosis. *J Dermatol Sci.* (2001) 26:133–9. doi: 10.1016/S0923-1811(00)00169-9
60. Distler O, Pap T, Kowal-Bielecka O, Meyringer R, Guiducci S, Landthaler M, et al. Overexpression of monocyte chemoattractant protein 1 in systemic sclerosis: role of platelet-derived growth factor and effects on monocyte chemotaxis and collagen synthesis. *Arthritis Rheum.* (2001) 44:2665–78. doi: 10.1002/1529-0131(200111)44:11<2665::AID-ART446>3.0.CO;2-S
61. Cella G, Vianello F, Cozzi F, Marotta H, Tona F, Saggiorato G, et al. Effect of bosentan on plasma markers of endothelial cell activity in patients with secondary pulmonary hypertension related to connective tissue diseases. *J Rheumatol.* (2009) 36:760–7. doi: 10.3899/jrheum.080542
62. van Hamburg JP, Tas SW. Molecular mechanisms underpinning T helper 17 cell heterogeneity and functions in rheumatoid arthritis. *J Autoimmun.* (2018) 87:69–81. doi: 10.1016/j.jaut.2017.12.006
63. Hashimoto-Kataoka T, Hosen N, Sonobe T, Arita Y, Yasui T, Masaki T, et al. Interleukin-6/interleukin-21 signaling axis is critical in the pathogenesis of pulmonary arterial hypertension. *Proc Natl Acad Sci USA* (2015) 112:E2677–86. doi: 10.1073/pnas.1424774112
64. Yang X, Yang J, Xing X, Wan L, Li M. Increased frequency of Th17 cells in systemic sclerosis is related to disease activity and collagen overproduction. *Arthritis Res Ther.* (2014) 16:R4. doi: 10.1186/ar4430
65. Kurasawa K, Hirose K, Sano H, Endo H, Shinkai H, Nawata Y, et al. Increased interleukin-17 production in patients with systemic sclerosis. *Arthritis Rheum.* (2000) 43:2455–63. doi: 10.1002/1529-0131(200011)43:11<2455::AID-ANR12>3.0.CO;2-K
66. Yang J, Chu Y, Yang X, Gao D, Zhu L, Yang X, et al. Th17 and natural Treg cell population dynamics in systemic lupus erythematosus. *Arthritis Rheum.* (2009) 60:1472–83. doi: 10.1002/art.24499
67. Xing X, Yang J, Yang X, Wei Y, Zhu L, Gao D, et al. IL-17A induces endothelial inflammation in systemic sclerosis via the ERK signaling pathway. *PLoS ONE* (2013) 8:e85032. doi: 10.1371/journal.pone.0085032
68. Hsu E, Shi H, Jordan RM, Lyons-Weiler J, Pilewski JM, Feghali-Bostwick CA. Lung tissues in patients with systemic sclerosis have gene expression patterns unique to pulmonary fibrosis and pulmonary hypertension. *Arthritis Rheum.* (2011) 63:783–94. doi: 10.1002/art.30159
69. Awasthi A, Riol-Blanco L, Jäger A, Korn T, Pot C, Galileos G, et al. Cutting edge: IL-23 receptor gfp reporter mice reveal distinct populations of IL-17-producing cells. *J Immunol.* (2009) 182:5904–8. doi: 10.4049/jimmunol.0900732
70. Gaublomme JT, Yosef N, Lee Y, Gertner RS, Yang LV, Wu C, et al. al. Single-cell genomics unveils critical regulators of Th17 cell pathogenicity. *Cell* (2015) 163:1400–12. doi: 10.1016/j.cell.2015.11.009
71. Rolla G, Fusaro E, Nicola S, Bucca C, Peroni C, Parisi S, et al. Th-17 cytokines and interstitial lung involvement in systemic sclerosis. *J Breath Res.* (2016) 10:046013. doi: 10.1088/1752-7155/10/4/046013
72. Huang WC, Ke MW, Cheng CC, Chiou SH, Wann SR, Shu CW, et al. Therapeutic benefits of induced pluripotent stem cells in monocrotaline-induced pulmonary arterial hypertension. *PLoS ONE* (2016) 11:e0142476. doi: 10.1371/journal.pone.0142476
73. Eid RE, Rao DA, Zhou J, Lo SF, Ranjbaran H, Gallo A, et al. Interleukin-17 and interferon-gamma are produced concomitantly by human coronary artery-infiltrating T cells and act synergistically on vascular smooth muscle cells. *Circulation* (2009) 119:1424–32. doi: 10.1161/CIRCULATIONAHA.108.827618
74. Maston LD, Jones DT, Giermakowska W, Resta TC, Ramiro-Diaz J, Howard TA, et al. Interleukin-6 trans-signaling contributes to chronic hypoxia-induced pulmonary hypertension. *Pulm Circ.* (2018) 8:2045894018780734. doi: 10.1177/2045894018780734
75. Le Hiress M, Tu L, Ricard N, Phan C, Thuillet R, Fadel E, et al. Proinflammatory signature of the dysfunctional endothelium in pulmonary hypertension. role of the macrophage migration inhibitory factor/CD74 complex. *Am J Respir Crit Care Med.* (2015) 192:983–97. doi: 10.1164/rccm.201402-0322OC
76. Hunter CA, Jones SA. IL-6 as a keystone cytokine in health and disease. *Nat Immunol.* (2015) 16:448–57. doi: 10.1038/ni.3153
77. Radstake TR, van Bon L, Broen J, Hussiani A, Hesselstrand R, Wuttge DM, et al. The pronounced Th17 profile in systemic sclerosis (SSc) together with intracellular expression of TGFbeta and IFNgamma distinguishes SSc phenotypes. *PLoS ONE* (2009) 4:e5903. doi: 10.1371/journal.pone.0005903
78. Stadhouders R, Lubberts E, Hendriks RW. A cellular and molecular view of T helper 17 cell plasticity in autoimmunity. *J Autoimmun.* (2018) 87:1–15. doi: 10.1016/j.jaut.2017.12.007
79. Rabinovitch M. Molecular pathogenesis of pulmonary arterial hypertension. *J Clin Invest.* (2012) 122:4306–13. doi: 10.1172/JCI60658
80. Gaowa S, Zhou W, Yu L, Zhou X, Liao K, Yang K, et al. Effect of Th17 and Treg axis disorder on outcomes of pulmonary arterial hypertension in connective tissue diseases. *Mediators Inflamm.* (2014) 2014:247372. doi: 10.1155/2014/247372
81. de Bourcy CFA, Dekker CL, Davis MM, Nicolls MR, Quake SR. Dynamics of the human antibody repertoire after B cell depletion in systemic sclerosis. *Sci Immunol.* (2017) 2:eaan8289. doi: 10.1126/sciimmunol.aan8289
82. Ulrich S, Taraseviciene-Stewart L, Huber LC, Speich R, Voelkel N. Peripheral blood B lymphocytes derived from patients with idiopathic pulmonary arterial hypertension express a different RNA pattern compared

with healthy controls: a cross sectional study. *Respir Res.* (2008) 9:20. doi: 10.1186/1465-9921-9-20

83. Blum LK, Cao RRL, Sweatt AJ, Bill M, Lahey LJ, Hsi AC, et al. Circulating plasmablasts are elevated and produce pathogenic anti-endothelial cell autoantibodies in idiopathic pulmonary arterial hypertension. *Eur J Immunol.* (2018) 48:874–84. doi: 10.1002/eji.201747460
84. Linterman MA, Rigby RJ, Wong RK, Yu D, Brink R, Cannons JL, et al. Follicular helper T cells are required for systemic autoimmunity. *J Exp Med.* (2009) 206:561–76. doi: 10.1084/jem.20081886
85. Vinuesa CG, Cook MC, Angelucci C, Athanasopoulos V, Rui L, Hill KM, et al. A RING-type ubiquitin ligase family member required to repress follicular helper T cells and autoimmunity. *Nature* (2005) 435:452–8. doi: 10.1038/nature03555
86. Taylor DK, Mittereder N, Kuta E, Delaney T, Burwell T, Dacosta K, et al. T follicular helper-like cells contribute to skin fibrosis. *Sci Transl Med.* (2018) 10:aaf5307. doi: 10.1126/scitranslmed.aaf5307
87. Zhu C, Ma J, Liu Y, Tong J, Tian J, Chen J, et al. Increased frequency of follicular helper T cells in patients with autoimmune thyroid disease. *J Clin Endocrinol Metab.* (2012) 97:943–50. doi: 10.1210/jc.2011-2003
88. Zhang X, Lindwall E, Gauthier C, Lyman J, Spencer N, Alarakhia A, et al. Circulating CXCR5+CD4+helper T cells in systemic lupus erythematosus patients share phenotypic properties with germinal center follicular helper T cells and promote antibody production. *Lupus* (2015) 24:909–17. doi: 10.1177/0961203314567750
89. Armengol MP, Juan M, Lucas-Martín A, Fernández-Figueras MT, Jaraquemada D, Gallart T, et al. Thyroid autoimmune disease: demonstration of thyroid antigen-specific B cells and recombination-activating gene expression in chemokine-containing active intrathyroidal germinal centers. *Am J Pathol.* (2001) 159:861–73. doi: 10.1016/S0002-9440(10)61762-2
90. Dib H, Tamby MC, Bussone G, Regent A, Berezné A, Lafine C, et al. Targets of anti-endothelial cell antibodies in pulmonary hypertension and scleroderma. *Eur Respir J.* (2012) 39:1405–14. doi: 10.1183/09031936.001 81410
91. Tamby MC, Chanseaud Y, Humbert M, Fermanian J, Guilpain P, Garcia-de-la-Peña-Lefebvre P, et al. Anti-endothelial cell antibodies in idiopathic and systemic sclerosis associated pulmonary arterial hypertension. *Thorax* (2005) 60:765–72. doi: 10.1136/thx.2004.029082
92. Arends SJ, Damoiseaux J, Duijvestijn A, Debrus-Palmans L, Boomars K, Broers B, et al. Prevalence of anti-endothelial cell antibodies in idiopathic pulmonary arterial hypertension. *Eur Respir J.* (2010) 35:923–5. doi: 10.1183/09031936.00164209
93. Arends SJ, Damoiseaux JG, Duijvestijn AM, Debrus-Palmans L, Vroomen M, Boomars KA, et al. Immunoglobulin G anti-endothelial cell antibodies: inducers of endothelial cell apoptosis in pulmonary arterial hypertension? *Clin Exp Immunol.* (2013) 174:433–40. doi: 10.1111/cei.12166
94. Arends SJ, Damoiseaux JG, Duijvestijn AM, Debrus-Palmans L, Boomars KA, Brunner-La Rocca HP, et al. Functional implications of IgG anti-endothelial cell antibodies in pulmonary arterial hypertension. *Autoimmunity* (2013) 46:463–70. doi: 10.3109/08916934.2013.812080
95. Bussone G, Tamby MC, Calzas C, Kherbeck N, Sahbatou Y, Sanson C, et al. IgG from patients with pulmonary arterial hypertension and/or systemic sclerosis binds to vascular smooth muscle cells and induces cell contraction. *Ann Rheum Dis.* (2012) 71:596–605. doi: 10.1136/annrheumdis-2011-200195
96. Becker MO, Kill A, Kutsche M, Guenther J, Rose A, Tabeling C, et al. Vascular receptor autoantibodies in pulmonary arterial hypertension associated with systemic sclerosis. *Am J Respir Crit Care Med.* (2014) 190:808–17. doi: 10.1164/rccm.201403-0442OC
97. Fang M, Huang Y, Zhang Y, Ning Z, Zhu L, Li X. Interleukin-6–572C/G polymorphism is associated with serum interleukin-6 levels and risk of idiopathic pulmonary arterial hypertension. *J Am Soc Hypertens* (2017) 11:171–77. doi: 10.1016/j.jash.2017.01.011
98. Phillips JA, Poling JS, Phillips CA, Stanton KC, Austin ED, Cogan JD, et al. Synergistic heterozygosity for TGFbeta1 SNPs and BMPR2 mutations modulates the age at diagnosis and penetrance of familial pulmonary arterial hypertension. *Genet Med.* (2008) 10:359–65. doi: 10.1097/GIM.0b013e318172dcdf
99. Dieudé P, Guedj M, Wipff J, Ruiz B, Riemekasten G, Matucci-Cerinic M, et al. Association of the TNFAIP3 rs5029939 variant with systemic sclerosis in the European Caucasian population. *Ann Rheum Dis.* (2010) 69:1958–64. doi: 10.1136/ard.2009.127928
100. Coornaert B, Carpentier I, Beyaert R. A20: central gatekeeper in inflammation and immunity. *J Biol Chem.* (2009) 284:8217–21. doi: 10.1074/jbc.R800032200
101. Price LC, Caramori G, Perros F, Meng C, Gambaryan N, Dorfmuller P, et al. Nuclear factor kappa-B is activated in the pulmonary vessels of patients with end-stage idiopathic pulmonary arterial hypertension. *PLoS ONE* (2013) 8:e75415. doi: 10.1371/journal.pone.0075415

4

Beyond cDC1: Emerging Roles of DC Crosstalk in Cancer Immunity

Rajkumar Noubade, Sonia Majri-Morrison and Kristin V. Tarbell*

Department of Inflammation and Oncology, Amgen Research, Amgen Inc., South San Francisco, CA, United States

***Correspondence:**
Rajkumar Noubade
rnoubade@amgen.com

Dendritic cells (DCs) efficiently process and present antigens to T cells, and by integrating environmental signals, link innate and adaptive immunity. DCs also control the balance between tolerance and immunity, and are required for T-cell mediated anti-tumor immunity. One subset of classical DCs, cDC1, are particularly important for eliciting CD8 T cells that can kill tumor cells. cDC1s are superior in antigen cross-presentation, a process of presenting exogenous antigens on MHC class I to activate $CD8^+$ T cells. Tumor-associated cDC1s can transport tumor antigen to the draining lymph node and cross-present tumor antigens, resulting in priming and activation of cytotoxic T cells. Although cross-presenting cDC1s are critical for eliciting anti-tumor T cell responses, the role and importance of other DC subsets in anti-tumor immunity is not as well-characterized. Recent literature in other contexts suggests that critical crosstalk between DC subsets can significantly alter biological outcomes, and these DC interactions likely also contribute significantly to tumor-specific immune responses. Therefore, antigen presentation by cDC1s may be necessary but not sufficient for maximal immune responses against cancer. Here, we discuss recent advances in the understanding of DC subset interactions to maximize anti-tumor immunity, and propose that such interactions should be considered for the development of better DC-targeted immunotherapies.

Keywords: dendritic cells, cDC1, cDC2, crosstalk, cancer immunity

INTRODUCTION

The interaction between various myeloid and lymphoid cell populations is crucial to initiate and orchestrate a robust anti-tumor response. By processing tumor associated antigens (TAAs) and migrating to draining lymph nodes (dLN), where T cell priming occurs, dendritic cells (DCs) are considered the most potent professional antigen presenting cells (APCs) to elicit adaptive anti-tumor immunity (1). In addition to presenting antigens, DCs use soluble molecules such as cytokines and chemokines as well as direct cell-cell contacts to prime and activate TAA-specific T cells. DCs were discovered by Ralph Steinman and Zanvil Cohn in 1973 as an APC population, distinct from macrophages, that initiate adaptive immune responses (2). As a result of more recent deep-phenotyping, DCs are now recognized to be a heterogenous population comprising several subsets distinguished by their development, phenotypic differences, localization, and functional specialization (2–6). This functional specialization of each subset allows DCs to initiate distinct immune responses in different immunological contexts (7). Here, we review literature supporting the hypothesis that, although one DC subset, conventional DC1(cDC1), has been shown to be crucial for anti-tumor immunity, multiple DC subsets, and interactions with other cells are needed for maximal responses.

DC Subsets Are Functionally Specialized

DCs are broadly classified as classical (or conventional) DCs (cDCs) and plasmacytoid DCs (pDCs), each with specialized functions. cDCs, specialized in antigen presentation to naïve T cells can be further segregated into cDC1s and cDC2s, excelling in MHC class I- and class II-mediated antigen-presentation, respectively (3, 6, 8–10). cDCs are found both as lymphoid and non-lymphoid tissue cells, the latter of which can migrate via the lymph to dLN to present tissue-derived antigens (3, 11). cDC1s, present at lower frequency compared to cDC2s, are identified by the expression of XCR1 (12), and in humans, also by the expression of CD141 (BDCA3) (5, 13, 14). cDC1s possess specialized mechanisms to mediate efficient antigen recognition, antigen transport to appropriate endosomal compartments and subsequent processing for the presentation to CD8 T cells in a process known as cross-presentation (15–18). cDC1s can also activate CD4 T cells through MHC class II antigen presentation and can polarize activated CD4 T cells toward a Th1 phenotype through the secretion of IL-12 (19).

cDC2s are specialized in MHC class II-mediated antigen presentation and are the most efficient APCs for activation and expansion of CD4 T cells (5, 13, 20). They are the most frequent DC population present in blood, lymphoid organs and tissues and promote a wide range of immune responses including Th1, Th2, and Th17 in specific contexts (13, 19, 21–25). Human cDC2s can be identified by their preferential expression of CD1c (BDCA1) and CD172a (SIRPα) (26). cDC2s are more heterogenous than cDC1s, and express various receptors that enable them to respond to broad spectrum of microbial products (22, 26–28). A subset of Notch2-dependent cDC2s specializes in IL-23 production and contributes to innate defense and adaptive immune responses (27, 29).

pDCs, distinguished by their ability to produce large amounts of type I IFN upon viral infection (30–33) are identified, in humans, by the expression of surface markers CD303 (BDCA-2), CD304 (BDCA-4/Neuropilin) and CD123 (5, 13). They are present mainly in lymphoid organs and can migrate to the LN through blood circulation (5, 34). Mature pDCs can also act as APCs and have distinct regulation of MHC class II surface expression that results in sustained membrane peptide-MHC complex and antigen presentation (30). A heterogeneity of pDCs is also described in terms of their ability to produce type I IFN and/or antigen presentation (35, 36).

Another related but developmentally distinct population, derived from monocytes, termed monocyte DCs (moDC) upregulates certain functional properties of DCs in some contexts and express tumor necrosis factor (TNF)- α and intracellular nitric oxide synthase (iNOS) (37). More commonly, the term moDCs refers to monocyte isolated from human peripheral blood mononuclear cells (PBMC) that are *in vitro* differentiated in the presence of granulocyte-macrophage colony-stimulating factor (GM-CSF) and interleukin (IL)-4 into cells sharing several phenotypic and functional features of DCs (26, 38, 39). moDCs are the most common *in vitro* model of DCs, yet are quite heterogeneous in both mouse and human, with unclear relationship to *in vivo* cell populations (40–42).

All DC subsets, including cDCs and pDCs, are found in the tumor microenvironment (TME) (30, 43–47) and among the cDCs, the cDC2s outnumber cDC1s, with cDC1s being the rarest APCs within the TME (43, 48). The role of pDCs in tumor immunity remains elusive and contradictory. Similarly, the precise role of cDC2s in anti-tumor immunity has been difficult to delineate due to lack of proper genetic tools. On the contrary, mounting evidence suggests cDC1s to be the critical antigen presenting DC subset for the generation of anti-tumor immunity. Here we summarize data supporting the importance of cDC1s in anti-tumor immunity, and then review the recent literature that documents DC crosstalk being necessary for effective immune responses, in other contexts such as anti-viral immune responses, and apply these principles to tumor immunity.

cDC1s Are Necessary for Anti-tumor Immunity

Since MHC class I molecules are expressed by every cell in the body (not just infected cells and cancer cells), to avoid bystander killing of healthy cells by CTLs, extracellular antigens do not enter the MHC class I-loading machinery (15, 18). Therefore, to generate an immune response, cancer cell antigens need special processing in APCs to be presented to naïve CD8 T cells. Moreover, naïve CD8 T cells primarily circulate through secondary lymphoid organs (15). Hence, cancer antigens must be brought to secondary lymphoid organs to be presented to naïve CD8 T cells. cDC1s fulfill both functions by patrolling tumor tissues, and by capturing, processing and presenting tumor-antigens on their surface through MHC class I molecules via antigen cross-presentation. cDC1s then migrate to dLN and deliver peptide/MHC class I signal to CD8 T cells which leads to their activation and the initiation of an immune response against tumor cells (15, 18).

Although other cell types have been reported to cross-present antigens (11, 49), this specialized function is mostly attributed to the cDC1 subset, owing to their unique adaptations of subcellular molecular machinery and vesicular trafficking (15, 18). Such adaptations include efficient antigen uptake of dying cells, delivery of cell-associated antigen to early endosomes, (15, 50–52), efficient phagosome-to-cytosol export of an ingested antigen possibly aided by ER-derived translocons and ER-associated degradation (ERAD) components such as Sec61, Derlin, p97 ATPase, Sec22 (15, 53–55), lower expression of lysosomal proteases (50) and antagonizing their degradative functions via NOX2-mediated ROS generation (56–60). The end result of such lower proteolysis, and therefore, increased antigen retention in cDC1s, is eventually an enhanced ability to carry the antigen all the way from peripheral tissues where the antigen is captured, to the dLN, where priming and activation of CD8 T cells occurs (56). The importance of cDC1s' ability to cross-present antigen in its immune functions is recently demonstrated using Wdfy4-deficient mice, which selectively lack cross-presentation (61).

Beyond their role in antigen cross-presentation, cDC1s are the major source of IL-12 production and thus influence anti-tumor immunity by activating NK cells and driving CD4 T cell responses toward Th1 responses (19, 62–64).

The critical role of cDC1s in anti-tumor immunity has been shown using mice deficient in basic leucine zipper transcription factor ATF-like 3 (Batf3), a transcription factor required for cDC1 differentiation (65). Batf3 knockout mice lack cDC1 cells but not other APCs and display impaired anti-tumor immunity in several models (43, 65–68). Expansion and activation of cDC1s using fms-related tyrosine kinase 3 ligand (Flt3L) and poly I:C leads to significant enhancement of antitumor responses (45). Immunotherapies such as PD1/PD-L1 blockade or CD137 agonists are ineffective in Batf3-deficient mice, highlighting the crucial role cDC1s in tumor immunity (68, 69). Furthermore, tumor-resident cDC1s are required for trafficking of adoptively transferred CD8 T cells into tumors through their ability to produce CXCL9 and CXCL10 (67, 70). DC-specific deletion of Sec22b leads not only to impaired cross-presentation of TAAs and reduced anti-tumor immune responses but also abolishes the efficacy of anti-PD1 therapy (53). In humans, the presence of cDC1s within the TME is associated with better prognosis and response to immunotherapy. Analysis of the cancer genome atlas (TCGA) dataset shows that a higher ratio of a cDC1 gene signature to a signature of all other myeloid cells (including monocyte/macrophage, and not just other DC subsets) is associated with better prognosis across human tumors (44, 71). Abundance of CD8 T cells positively correlates with cDC1 markers in pancreatic tumors (70). Taken together, these data show that cross-presenting cDC1s are crucial and necessary for the generation of an effective anti-tumor immunity.

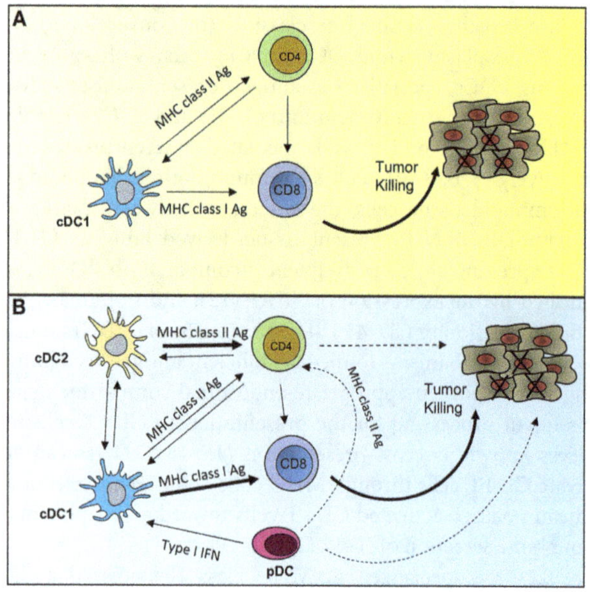

FIGURE 1 | Potential scenarios of DC crosstalk in anti-tumor immunity. **(A)** Describes a scenario where an effective anti-tumor immune response would rely solely on cDC1 functions. cDC1s can activate both CD8 T cells and CD4 T cells through MHC class I- and MHC class II-mediated antigen presentation, respectively. Activated CD4 T cells provide licensing signal to cDC1s, which relay that help to CD8 T cells. Helped CD8 T cells have enhanced cytotoxic properties to efficiently kill tumor cells. **(B)** Describes multi-cellular interactions to achieve full-strength CTL responses against tumor. In this scenario, cDC1s predominantly activate CD8 T cells and cDC2s predominantly activate CD4 T cells. Activated CD4 T cells, in addition to providing help to maximize CTL responses can directly exhibit anti-tumor responses. Activated pDCs can modulate the TME mainly via type I IFN production, but can also activate CD4 T cells via MHC class II-mediated antigen presentation. Solid line indicates strong experimental evidence in tumor setting and dashed line indicates data in non-tumor setting. Thick line indicates predominant function.

cDC1 Are Not Sufficient for Maximal Anti-tumor Immunity: Potential Roles of Other DC Subsets

Tumor immunology is built upon the tenet that cytotoxic CD8 T cells (CTLs) eliminate tumor cells (72) and the prevailing dogma is that cDC1s are the most potent APCs for the CTL response against tumor. Because of the strong evidence for the importance of cDC1 in tumor immunity, as presented in the previous section, in one scenario it is possible that cDC1s are the sole DC subset sufficient for optimal anti-tumor CTL generation through antigen presentation via MHC class I as well as MHC class II (**Figure 1A**). A major driver of the current dogma is the studies conducted in mice genetically manipulated to lack cDC1 such as Batf3-deficient or Zbtb46-Cre mice. However, these tools are imperfect. For example, Batf3 is expressed in cDC2 and effector CD4 T cells (65, 73) and Zbtb46 is also expressed in DC2s as well as in endothelial cells (74–76), raising the possibility of contributions from additional DC subsets and other cell types. Hence, it is not clear whether the cDC1 subset alone is sufficient to provide the maximal immunity against tumor. Recent evidence in non-tumor settings has demonstrated that cDC1s require significant contributions from other DC subsets and are not sufficient for an optimal CTL response (77–79), pointing toward a role for the other cells in shaping a robust and durable anti-tumor immunity.

Therefore, we describe a second scenario that includes possible roles of other DC subsets for a more robust anti-tumor immunity, directly and indirectly (**Figure 1B**). This scenario incorporates recent findings of spatiotemporal segregation of cDC1 and cDC2 activation within dLN to activate CD8 and CD4 T cells, respectively, during antiviral response. This robust CTL response requires interactions between multiple DC subsets, including cDCs and pDCs in a two-step priming process (77–79). Even though these responses are context dependent and are observed in anti-viral response, the general principals remain the same in anti-tumor immune response. Accordingly, in this scenario, the tumor-derived cDC1 primes CD8 T cells while tumor-derived cDC2 activates CD4 T cells in the first step of the CTL priming process and then in the second step, the activated CD4 T cells licenses a LN-resident cDC1 to relay the help for CTLs. Contributions of activated CD4 T cells to anti-tumor immunity can be more than just providing the help to CTLs, but also include activation of NK cells and macrophages through IFN-γ, modulation of tumor stroma and angiogenesis or direct cytolytic effects (80–83).

Additionally, during the two-step priming process, pDCs are recruited to cDC1-CD8 T cell priming sites, providing critical licensing signal to cDC1s through type 1 IFN. In this regard, lack of type 1 IFN receptor in cDC1s impairs their ability to reject tumors (84, 85). Furthermore, pDCs are usually weak APCs in the absence of activating signals but direct antigen presentation and T cell stimulation by pDCs has been described (30, 86). In fact, adoptive transfer of tumor-antigen-loaded pDCs induced potent anti-tumor T cell responses in melanoma patients (87), suggesting the possibility of anti-tumor immunity directly through APC functions by pDCs.

In the following sections, we mainly focus on this latter scenario of non-synchronous activation events by cDC1s and cDC2s and the reorganization of pDCs to the sites of CTL priming to describe the crosstalk between DC subsets and propose an integrated model of multi-DC subsets, multi-cell type interactions in achieving full-strength CTL responses in anti-tumor immunity.

Crosstalk Between DC Subsets

One of the goals of cancer immunotherapy is to promote tumor-antigen specific T cell responses. The current data supports the notion that cDC1s are well-suited for this purpose and that they are usually necessary for the generation of an anti-tumor response. However, as discussed below, they may not be sufficient for full-strength anti-tumor cytotoxic T cell responses and interactions with other DC subsets contribute to this process. In the following sections, we will review the interactions between each DC subsets separately.

cDC-pDC Crosstalk

cDCs and pDCs are co-localized in many immune contexts, e.g., non-inflamed LNs, skin biopsies from lupus erythematosus patients, thyroid glands from autoimmune thyroiditis patients and spleens of cancer patients (88–90). Such close-proximity of pDCs and cDCs suggests possible functional coordination. Indeed, local production of type I IFN by pDCs induces stimulatory molecules on cDCs driving their maturation during an effective immune response (79). Intravital two-photon microscopic analysis of DC subsets within dLN during vaccinia virus infection showed active, CCR5-mediated recruitment of pDCs to the site of CD8 T cell priming by virus-infected cDC1. The activated CD8 T cells also orchestrate, via XCL1, recruitment of resident, non-infected XCR1$^+$cDC1s. pDCs produce type I IFN to induce upregulation of costimulatory molecules including CD40, CD80, and CD86 on non-infected resident-cDC1s (79), driving their maturation and antigen-presentation functions leading to robust CTL response. pDC help for CTL response, either through type I IFN or other costimulatory molecules such as CD40L has been described in other viral infection models (91–93). Depletion of pDCs results in impaired CTL responses in many viral infections, e.g., VSV infection (94), LCMV infection (95), and cutaneous herpes simplex virus (HSV) (92). In the LCMV infection model, pDC-mediated CD4 T cell activation was essential in providing help and generation of anti-viral CTL response (95). These observations underscore the pivotal role of the crosstalk between DC subsets in maximizing immune response against cell-associated antigens.

Similarly, in the context of anti-tumor immune responses, cooperation between pDCs and cDC1s and the resulting synergistic effects dependent on soluble factors such as type I IFN and/or cell-cell contact between the two DC subsets are described (11, 47). The potent anti-tumor T cell responses induced in melanoma patients by adoptive transfer of tumor-antigen-loaded pDCs (87) could be either a result of direct priming by pDCs or via interactions with other cells, including cDCs. However, tumor infiltrating pDCs exhibit an abnormal or hypofunctional state, most likely due to immuno-suppressive effects of the TME such as TGFβ (96). The presence of pDCs in tumors is associated with poor prognosis in cancers such as breast and ovarian cancers (97, 98). pDCs are generally thought to contribute to tolerance induction and tumor promotion in this setting, most likely due to Treg induction and expression of immunosuppressive factors such as indoleamine 2,3-dioxygenase (IDO) (98, 99). Thus, the role of pDCs in shaping adaptive tumor immunity remains elusive. It likely depends on their activation status and involves cooperativity with other cells but how pDCs are activated needs further investigation.

cDC1-cDC2 Crosstalk

The two cDC subsets communicate not only through soluble mediators such as IL-12 but also through a third cell viz., activated CD4 T cell. Even though both cDC subsets are adept in priming naïve T cells, cDC2s are more proficient in activating CD4 T cells than CD8 T cells while cDC1s are potent activators of CD8 T cells but present antigen to CD4 T cells less efficiently, both *in vitro* and *in vivo* (8, 20, 43). However, recent literature demonstrates that robust and maximal induction of cytotoxic CD8 T cell responses against cell-associated antigens not only requires interactions with cDC1s, but also interactions involving cDC2s (77, 100). Intravital microscopy demonstrated that, in the dLN, the two cDC subsets exhibit differential localization wherein cDC1s are largely segregated to the T cell zone in deep paracortical regions and cDC2s are more peripherally distributed (78, 100–103) and that CD8 T cells cluster with cDC1s and CD4 T cells cluster with cDC2s during step one of two-step T cell priming event in anti-viral immunity (78, 100, 104), suggesting parallel activation of the two T cell subsets by two different cDCs in an asynchronous manner. Such differential localization of the cDC subsets into non-overlapping T cell regions is also reported in the spleen (105).

The peripheral DC subsets also exhibit different kinetics during their migration to dLN (106), with an implication that cDC2s might access CD4 T cells earlier. The CD4 T is cell activated in the first step of the priming process, then gets recruited to LN-resident, XCR1+ cDC1 during the second step of the priming process and delivers help signals to that cDC1. The receiver-cDC1 then transmits the help signal to CD8 T cell activated in the first step, resulting in a robust expansion of highly effective CTLs. In this regard, it is well-established that, in the absence of CD4 T cell help, CD8 T cell responses are weaker and insufficient to generate long-lasting memory (107–109). The CD4 T cell help includes molecules such as CD40L expressed on CD4 T cells, that induces expression of costimulatory molecules including CD70, CD80, CD86, and cytokines such as IL-12, IL-15 by cDC1 (66, 110–112). The molecular nature of CD4 T cell help in shaping the CTL response is recently reviewed (104) and will not be discussed here in detail. Signaling though type

I IFN is critical for proper functioning of cDC1s (85) and cDC2s are one of the important sources of this cytokine, as shown by depletion of pDCs using anti-pDCA antibodies in Batf3-deficient mice (84).

cDC1s and cDC2s may also collaborate for optimal Th1 induction. In the context of leishmania infection, targeting antigen to either cDC1 or cDC2 can elicit IFNγ-producing T cells, but interestingly, the cDC2s require IL-12 produced by the cDC1s to induce Th1 responses, whereas the cDC1s induce Th1 responses via CD70, independent of IL-12 (19). Therefore, each DC subset provides different signals that can contribute to effector T cell responses. Among the activated CD4 T cells, Th1 cells excel in providing the help to cDC1s to prime and expand CTLs through of production large amounts of IFNγ (113), thus fostering an important crosstalk between the two cDCs.

The majority of the experimental data described above originates from studies in anti-viral immunity. However, where and how naïve cancer cell-specific CD4 T cells get activated in a tumor setting is less clear. Lessons learnt on the importance of MHC class II-restricted CD4 T cell responses in autoimmune pathogenesis may shed light on this question in anti-tumor responses as well, since the anti-tumor response is essentially a self-specific response (114). The highest genetic risk for autoimmunity is conferred by HLA class II genes, with odds ratios >6, suggesting that CD4 T cell responses are necessary for immunity against self. In the context of autoimmunity, although some priming in the target tissue may occur (115–117), most studies suggest that self-specific CD4 T cells are first primed in the dLN, suggesting that a similar phenomenon might be happening in the generation of an anti-tumor immune response.

Evidence for the Importance of Tumor-Derived cDC2s and Activation of CD4 T Cells in the Draining Lymph Node

A large body of literature shows that naïve CD8 T cell activation for the generation of anti-tumor immunity occurs in dLN and is mediated by DCs (118–121). Interestingly, requirement of CD4 T cell help for optimal CD8 T cell effector functions in the context of tumor immunity is also well-documented, including the ability of CTLs to infiltrate the tumors (8, 119, 122–127). Non-helped CD8 T cells exhibit dysfunctional state with high expression of exhaustion markers in metastatic lung tumor model (127). In this regard, it is also well-established that the TME contains both cDC1 and cDC2 subsets (43–46). But importantly, both cDC1s and cDC2s scavenge tumor antigens (44) and migrate to dLN in a CCR7-dependent manner (46). Under right conditions, cDC2s can induce CD4 T cell activation in response to cell-associated antigen (51). Consistent with this, tumor-derived and dLN-derived cDC2s stimulate CD4 T cells more efficiently, *ex vivo*, in Lewis lung carcinoma model expressing ova as a model antigen (43). Furthermore, in this experimental setting, while cDC1 efficiently primed CD8 T cells, cDC2s are the most efficient activators of CD4 T cells. In addition, vaccination with the activated cDC2s reduced tumor growth, similar to that observed with cDC1s (43). Delivery of tumor antigen to cDC2 using dendritic cell immunoreceptor 2 (Dcir2) leads to significant anti-tumor effects in a mouse melanoma model (128). In a lung adenocarcinoma mouse model engineered to express MHC class II-restricted cytosolic antigen, activated cDC2 are observed both in the tumor and dLN and antigen-specific naïve CD4 T are activated in the dLN (129). In breast cancer patients gene signature of cDC2s positively correlates with better survival, similar to that observed with cDC1s, (130) and MHC class II expression predicts response to anti-PD1/PD-L1 therapy in melanoma patients (131). Collectively, tumor-derived cDC2s are likely to contribute to CD4 T cell activation in the dLN.

Integrated Model of DC Crosstalk in Tumor Draining Lymph Node

The spatiotemporal nature of DC crosstalk suggests two distinct DC-mediated events for maximal CD8 T cell responses: one after the initial antigen capture and another after the antigen is transferred to dLN-resident cDC1 cells (8). This sequential CTL activation is demonstrated by the exclusive clustering of migratory cDC1s with CD8 T cells early on during the initiation of an antiviral immune response. Subsequent clustering of activated CD8 T cells with the LN-resident cDC1s acts as a platform for signal relay from pDCs and activated CD4 T cells (79). According to this "consecutive interaction" model (79, 112), the generation of maximal CTL response and therapeutic anti-tumor immunity requires a multicellular orchestration of events in the tumor dLN (**Figure 2**) wherein migratory cDC1s capture the antigen in tumors, migrate to the dLN and form the initial priming site to activate CD8 T cells. The activated CD8 T cells produce CCL3/CCL4 and XCL1 to mediate recruitment of $CCR5^+$pDCs and $XCR1^+$LN-resident cDC1s, respectively. The migratory cDC1s handoff antigen to resident cDC1s in a yet-to-be-described mechanism (44, 106). In parallel, migratory cDC2s that have captured the antigen also move from the tumor to dLN and activate CD4 T cells. The pDCs induce the maturation of newly recruited, LN-resident cDC1s and the activated CD4 T cells licenses them for superior CTL responses. The overall effect of such orchestration and functional-cooperativity of pathways between different DC subsets is the amplification of CTL responses against a given antigen, without potentially missing out on the critical help necessary for CTLs to function at their peak. In fact, vaccine-mediated induction of such coordinated efforts of multiple DC subsets is known to trigger sustained and potent CTL responses while inhibiting immunosuppressive pathways in preclinical models (132). *Ex vivo* analyses of individual DC subsets might fail to identify such cellular orchestration to appreciate the relative contribution of each interaction between the different DC subsets in the generation of potent immune response.

DC Crosstalk in Tumors *in situ*

Accumulating evidence suggest that cross-priming by tumor-resident cDC1 *in situ* is also an important phenomenon in the generation of an anti-tumor immune response. Local T cell priming and activation within tumors were observed in mice that lacked LN, or when T cell recirculation was blocked (133–135). Furthermore, intratumoral cDCs are required for the tumor regression achieved with adoptively transferred T

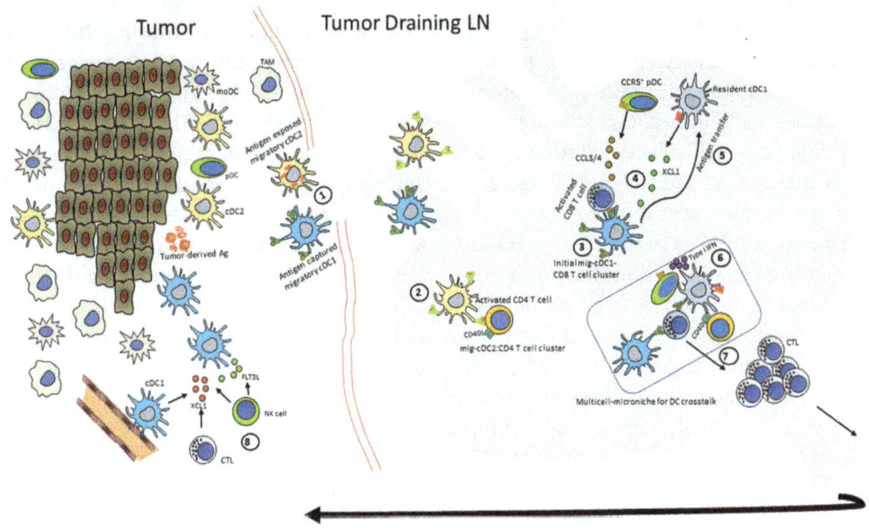

FIGURE 2 | An integrated model of DC crosstalk for anti-tumor immunity. Outline of the multicellular orchestration of events that can contribute to a robust anti-tumor response. (Note: not all events happen in every context, and the order may also differ). (1) Intratumoral migratory-cDC1 and -cDC2s scavenge tumor-derived antigens and migrate to tumor dLN. (2) migratory-cDC2s (mig-cDC2) present MHC class II-restricted tumor antigen to CD4 T cells and induce expression of molecules such as CD40L (3) Migratory-cDC1s (mig-cDC1) prime and activate naïve CD8 T cells; (4) these activated CD8 T cells produce XCL1 and CCL3/4 to draw in XCR1+LN-resident-cDC1s and CCR5+ pDCs to the site of initial priming. (5) Mig-cDC1s can hand-off antigen to the newly recruited, LN-resident-cDC1. (6) pDCs produce type I IFN to mature cDCs. (7) The licensed CTL with enhanced effector functions undergoes clonal expansion and moves to the tumor to induce tumor cell killing. (8) The activated CD8 T cells and NK cells can mediate further increase in cDC1 numbers by producing XCL1 and FLT3L.

cells in an experimental setting where migration of T cells to dLN was prevented (44). Moreover, tumor-resident cDC1s are the predominant sources of CXCL9 and CXCL10 and mediate recruitment effector T cells into the tumor (67). Similar to the events described for the dLN in the previous section, activated CD8 T cells could potentially orchestrate events *in situ* in the tumor where LN-like structures known as tertiary lymphoid structures (TLS) are present. A hallmark of TLS is the presence of high endothelial venules (HEVs) and expression of CCL19 and CCL21, the ligands for CCR7 (136, 137). DCs migrate in a CCR7-dependent manner (43, 45, 46, 138, 139). Moreover, well-organized TLSs contain B cell and T cells areas with mature DC subsets including cDCs and pDCs. Such organization makes TLS an ideal place to sustain proximity and the crosstalk between various subsets, and orchestrating local events required for maximal tumor immunity (135, 136). In fact, tumor-associated TLSs are functional structures capable of recruiting antigen-specific T cells and facilitating their activation through interactions with DCs (140). Interestingly, TLSs have been observed in several human tumors and their presence, particularly the ones containing high amounts of DCs and Th1 cells within the TLS, is associated with better prognosis (137, 141, 142) and increased TLS density is associated with strong infiltration of effector and memory CD8 T cells within the tumors (141), reflecting the importance of crosstalk between DC subsets and, CD4 help in increased CTL trafficking. Lung cancer patients with intratumoral CD8 T cells but no TLS had poor survival, indicating the necessity of their *in situ* education within the TLS for better effector functions (141, 143). In a metastatic lung tumor model, administration of TLR9 activator leads to CD8 T cell infiltration concurrent with TLS formation. The presence of TLS in this model was completely dependent on CD4 help (127). Taken together, these data suggest that TLSs promote DC crosstalk and anti-tumor immunity. Thus, induction of TLS provides another opportunity to promote communication between DC subsets to augment the magnitude of protective immunity, particularly against neoantigens that arise during the later phases of tumor progression (121). Moreover, induction of simultaneous trafficking and activation of cDCs and pDCs, using a vaccination strategy that combined DC subset-specific adjuvants (e.g., CpG-ODN and GM-CSF) leads to local accumulation of CD8 T cells and superior anti-tumor responses (132) suggesting that, even in the absence of TLS, evoking appropriate DC-crosstalk within the tumor tissue has the potential to boost superior CTL responses than targeting a single DC subset.

Influence of DC Crosstalk With Other Cells in the TME on Anti-tumor Immunity

DCs can also engage with other immune cell types in the TME and lymphoid organs. Such interactions can enhance or dampen DC functions and anti-tumor immunity, depending on the cell types involved. For example, DCs interact with Treg cells, resulting in the suppression of CD8 T cell-mediated anti-tumor immunity (144). Two-photon laser-scanning microscopy analysis showed that Treg cells engage in prolonged physical interactions with DCs, six times longer than that of DC-CD8 T cell interaction in tumor. This extended physical contact between Treg cells and DCs results in upregulation of the immunosuppressive molecules such as IDO and lower maturation molecules on DC surface (144).

Interactions with other immune cell types such as natural killer (NK) cells with DCs can boost the immune response against tumors. It has long been established that, through the secretion of IL-12, cDC1s can license NK cells to kill tumor cells (145–147). However, recent studies have shown that NK cells can also influence DC functions in the context of tumors. In fact, NK cells produce XCL1 to recruit XCR^{+}cDC1s to the TME (148). In addition, NK cells are one source of Flt3L within the tumor and dictate intratumoral accumulation of cDC1 cells by supporting DC survival, proliferation or development (71). Stimulation of NK cells with DC-derived factors such as IL-12, IL-15/IL-15Rα complex or contact–dependent interactions of OX40-OX40L augment NK cell functions to eliminate tumor cells (149–151). TCGA analysis suggests that NK cell/XCL1/cDC1 axis is associated with better survival in many cancer indications (148).

DCs also interact with NKT cells, the unconventional T lymphocytes expressing a semi-invariant T cell receptor (TCR) that recognize glycolipids presented by CD1d. (152). Although CD1d can be expressed by many hematopoietic cell types, DCs constitutively express CD1d and are the most potent APCs for exogenous glycolipids (153–155). The NKT cell ligand α-galactosylceramide (α-GalCer) acts as a potent *in vivo* adjuvant for DCs, resulting in increased expression of MHC class II and other costimulatory molecules (155). In addition, α-GalCer presented by DCs strongly activates NKT cells through CD40/CD40L interaction to induce IFN-γ production (156). Administration of α-GalCer was efficacious in preclinical tumor models (157) but not in patients (158), most likely due to soluble α-GalCer-induced anergy of NKT cell (159). Administration of α-GalCer, either soluble or loaded in DCs, is currently being explored to enhance anti-tumor immunity (160). Endogenous glycolipids are known to activate NKT cells (161) and CD1d expression is observed on tumor cells (162). In fact, the level of CD1d expression on tumor cells dictates NKT-mediated cytotoxicity (163).

Tumor-associated macrophages, in most carcinomas, are linked to poor prognosis primarily due to their immunosuppressive phenotype (164, 165). Macrophages produce IL-10 and in turn prevent IL-12 secretion of by DCs, resulting in dampened tumor-specific CD8 T cell activation (166). Among mononuclear phagocytes, monocyte-derived cells (including macrophages) are found at higher frequencies in tumors compared to DCs, and a higher monocyte-macrophage signature is associated with worse clinical prognosis (130, 167). These cells maintain a phenotype similar to *in vitro* M2 macrophages and contribute to the suppressive tumor microenvironment primarily via expression of anti-inflammatory mediators such as IL-10, TGF-β and IDO. Many of these signals dampen the ability of cDCs to present antigen in an immunogenic manner (164). However, in other contexts, macrophages can be inflammatory and effective APCs for eliciting T cell responses (168, 169). Thus, with the addition of the right signals, tumor macrophages have the potential to contribute to anti-tumor immunity.

Additionally, even though B cells have been described to play varied and often contrasting roles in the contexts of tumor immunity, emerging evidence suggests that B cells may also contribute to tumor immunity, both via antibody-mediated effects and by acting as APCs (170–172). Specifically, in terms of the crosstalk, DCs engage with B cells to promote their growth and differentiation, resulting in the production of antibodies. pDCs, through type I IFN production, can increase TLR7 expression and other activation markers on B cells (173). pDCs are specifically capable of inducing differentiation of activated B cells into Ig-secreting plasma cells through the secretion of type I IFN and IL-6 (174). Additionally, DCs dramatically enhance the secretion of IgG and IgA through the ligation of CD40 (175). B cells isolated from TLS-containing lung cancers showed significant antibody response against many TAAs (143, 176).

Finally, DC crosstalk with cancer cells has tremendous impact on the immune surveillance of the tumors. Cancer cells express several immunosuppressive factors such as PGE2, β-catenin and cytokines such as IL-10. PGE2 renders cDC1s unresponsive to XCL1 and CCL5 by downregulating *XCR1* and *CCR5* expression (148). β-catenin expression in cancer cells causes ATF3-mediated suppression of CCL4, the ligand for CCR5, leading to defective recruitment of cDC1 to the TME, and adversely affecting CD8 T cell priming against TAAs (177). Interestingly, PGE2 also induces the expression of β-catenin not only in tumor cells but also in stromal cells such as cancer associated fibroblasts (CAFs). CAFs respond to tumor-derived TNFα and IL-1β to secrete thymic stromal lymphopoietin (TSLP). TSLP is a strong driver of cDCs to activate Th2 CD4 T cells that are considered pro-tumorigenic (178). CAFs also produce stromal cell-derived factor 1 (SDF1) which drives cDCs toward tolerogenic DCs secreting IDO in a STAT3-dependent manner and promoting the recruitment and differentiation of Treg cells in tumors (179). However, co-targeting fibroblasts in combination with DC-based vaccine enhances the anti-tumor immune responses (180), suggesting that DC/stromal cell interactions can be manipulated to improve immunotherapies. Overall, with the property of bridging the innate and adaptive immune cells, DCs have a pivotal role in orchestrating an anti-tumor immune response by engaging interactions with many cell types within the TME.

Potential Therapeutic Applications of Tumor DC-Crosstalk

The field of cancer immunotherapy, energized by the effect of T cell checkpoint inhibitors (CPI) in some patients, is beginning to focus on ways to treat "cold" tumors that lack T cells which can be activated with an anti-PD1 or other CPI. There is a large unmet medical need to increase the proportion of patients who respond to immunotherapy. Enhancing innate immunity, and DC function in particular, is one way to make tumors "warmer" that has tremendous potential. To date, most cell-based DC cancer therapies have utilized moDCs and have shown limited efficacy (121, 181, 182). With our current knowledge of both the importance of cross-presenting cDC1s for tumor immunity and the plasticity of monocyte-derived cells, moDCs are likely not the best cell type to use for inducing optimal clinical outcomes against cancer. Most studies show that moDCs have limited capacity for both cross-presentation and migration to draining LN compared to Batf3-dependent cells (43, 183). In addition, most monocyte-derived cells in the TME are immunosuppressive, and even if *ex vivo* moDCs can be activated to sustain cDC1-like properties, these are not likely maintained in the TME (121, 181). Therefore, moDC-based vaccines may not be the answer, and a new generation of DC-focused cancer immunotherapies are needed.

Increasing cDC1 function is one important goal, but as described here, some of this can occur indirectly via the cooperative interactions with other cells. In addition, both cDCs and pDCs have the potential to directly activate T cells that can kill cancer cells if exposed to the right activating signals (**Figure 1B**). Therefore, targeting maturation signals specifically to just cDC1s may not be the optimal therapy, and delivering signals that can enhance the function of all DC subsets may enhance efficacy and durability. For example, although tumor pDCs often correlate with poor prognosis, they are the most efficient producers of type 1 IFN and have the capacity for sustained MHC class II expression; these functions together may inflame the tumor and elicit strong T cell help that in turn could be sustained by newly matured cDC1s. Therefore, identifying signals that target and activate all DC subsets, and the cells that crosstalk with them will help provide novel insights into the cellular and molecular nature of tumor-specific CTL priming. The goal is to design therapies that build a site of sustained, immunostimulatory tumor-antigen presentation and increase the magnitude of anti-tumor immunity, so we can successfully treat a broader set of patients.

AUTHOR CONTRIBUTIONS

RN, SM-M, and KT designed and wrote the manuscript.

ACKNOWLEDGMENTS

We thank Carlos Briseno, Michael Gonzalez, and Jackson G. Egen for critical reading of the manuscript and helpful discussions.

REFERENCES

1. Worbs T, Hammerschmidt SI, Forster R. Dendritic cell migration in health and disease. *Nat Rev Immunol.* (2017) 17:30–48. doi: 10.1038/nri.2016.116
2. Steinman RM, Cohn ZA. Identification of a novel cell type in peripheral lymphoid organs of mice. I. Morphology, quantitation, tissue distribution. *J Exp Med.* (1973) 137:1142–62. doi: 10.1084/jem.137.5.1142
3. Merad M, Sathe P, Helft J, Miller J, Mortha A. The dendritic cell lineage: ontogeny and function of dendritic cells and their subsets in the steady state and the inflamed setting. *Ann Rev Immunol.* (2013) 31:563–604. doi: 10.1146/annurev-immunol-020711-074950
4. Cosenza H, Leserman LD, Rowley DA. The third cell type required for the immune response of spleen cells *in vitro*. *J Immunol.* (1971) 107:414–21.
5. Anderson DA, 3rd, Murphy KM, Briseno CG. Development, diversity, and function of dendritic cells in mouse and human. *Cold Spring Harb Perspect Biol.* (2018) 10:a028613. doi: 10.1101/cshperspect.a028613
6. Guilliams M, Ginhoux F, Jakubzick C, Naik SH, Onai N, Schraml BU, et al. Dendritic cells, monocytes and macrophages: a unified nomenclature based on ontogeny. *Nat Rev Immunol.* (2014) 14:571–8. doi: 10.1038/nri3712
7. Dress RJ, Wong AY, Ginhoux F. Homeostatic control of dendritic cell numbers and differentiation. *Immunol Cell Biol.* (2018) 96:463–76. doi: 10.1111/imcb.12028
8. Theisen D, Murphy K. The role of cDC1s *in vivo*: CD8 T cell priming through cross-presentation. *F1000Res.* (2017) 6:98. doi: 10.12688/f1000research.9997.1
9. Devi KS, Anandasabapathy N. The origin of DCs and capacity for immunologic tolerance in central and peripheral tissues. *Seminars Immunopathol.* (2017) 39:137–52. doi: 10.1007/s00281-016-0602-0
10. Murphy TL, Grajales-Reyes GE, Wu X, Tussiwand R, Briseno CG, Iwata A, et al. Transcriptional control of dendritic cell development. *Ann Rev Immunol.* (2016) 34:93–119. doi: 10.1146/annurev-immunol-032713-120204
11. Nierkens S, Tel J, Janssen E, Adema GJ. Antigen cross-presentation by dendritic cell subsets: one general or all sergeants? *Trends Immunol.* (2013) 34:361–70. doi: 10.1016/j.it.2013.02.007
12. Scott CL, Soen B, Martens L, Skrypek N, Saelens W, Taminau J, et al. The transcription factor Zeb2 regulates development of conventional and plasmacytoid DCs by repressing Id2. *J Exp Med.* (2016) 213:897–911. doi: 10.1084/jem.20151715
13. Collin M, Bigley V. Human dendritic cell subsets: an update. *Immunology.* (2018) 154:3–20. doi: 10.1111/imm.12888
14. Poulin LF, Salio M, Griessinger E, Anjos-Afonso F, Craciun L, Chen JL, et al. Characterization of human DNGR-1+ BDCA3+ leukocytes as putative equivalents of mouse CD8alpha+ dendritic cells. *J Exp Med.* (2010) 207:1261–71. doi: 10.1084/jem.20092618
15. Cruz FM, Colbert JD, Merino E, Kriegsman BA, Rock KL. The biology and underlying mechanisms of cross-presentation of exogenous antigens on MHC-I molecules. *Ann Rev Immunol.* (2017) 35:149–76. doi: 10.1146/annurev-immunol-041015-055254
16. Haniffa M, Shin A, Bigley V, McGovern N, Teo P, See P, et al. Human tissues contain CD141hi cross-presenting dendritic cells with functional homology to mouse CD103+ nonlymphoid dendritic cells. *Immunity.* (2012) 37:60–73. doi: 10.1016/j.immuni.2012.04.012
17. Bachem A, Guttler S, Hartung E, Ebstein F, Schaefer M, Tannert A, et al. Superior antigen cross-presentation and XCR1 expression define human CD11c+CD141+ cells as homologues of mouse CD8+ dendritic cells. *J Exp Med.* (2010) 207:1273–81. doi: 10.1084/jem.20100348
18. Blander JM. Regulation of the cell biology of antigen cross-presentation. *Ann Rev Immunol.* (2018) 36:717–53. doi: 10.1146/annurev-immunol-041015-055523
19. Soares H, Waechter H, Glaichenhaus N, Mougneau E, Yagita H, Mizenina O, et al. A subset of dendritic cells induces CD4+ T cells to produce IFN-gamma by an IL-12-independent but CD70-dependent mechanism *in vivo*. *J Exp Med.* (2007) 204:1095–106. doi: 10.1084/jem.20070176
20. Dudziak D, Kamphorst AO, Heidkamp GF, Buchholz VR, Trumpfheller C, Yamazaki S, et al. Differential antigen processing by dendritic cell subsets *in vivo*. *Science.* (2007) 315:107–11. doi: 10.1126/science.1136080
21. Guilliams M, van de Laar L. A Hitchhiker's Guide to Myeloid Cell Subsets: practical implementation of a novel mononuclear phagocyte classification system. *Front Immunol.* (2015) 6:406. doi: 10.3389/fimmu.2015.00406
22. Tussiwand R, Everts B, Grajales-Reyes GE, Kretzer NM, Iwata A, Bagaitkar J, et al. Klf4 expression in conventional dendritic cells is required for T helper 2 cell responses. *Immunity.* (2015) 42:916–28. doi: 10.1016/j.immuni.2015.04.017

23. Gao Y, Nish SA, Jiang R, Hou L, Licona-Limon P, Weinstein JS, et al. Control of T helper 2 responses by transcription factor IRF4-dependent dendritic cells. *Immunity.* (2013) 39:722–32. doi: 10.1016/j.immuni.2013.08.028
24. Schlitzer A, McGovern N, Teo P, Zelante T, Atarashi K, Low D, et al. IRF4 transcription factor-dependent CD11b+ dendritic cells in human and mouse control mucosal IL-17 cytokine responses. *Immunity.* (2013) 38:970–83. doi: 10.1016/j.immuni.2013.04.011
25. Persson EK, Uronen-Hansson H, Semmrich M, Rivollier A, Hagerbrand K, Marsal J, et al. IRF4 transcription-factor-dependent CD103(+)CD11b(+) dendritic cells drive mucosal T helper 17 cell differentiation. *Immunity.* (2013) 38:958–69. doi: 10.1016/j.immuni.2013.03.009
26. Alcantara-Hernandez M, Leylek R, Wagar LE, Engleman EG, Keler T, Marinkovich MP, et al. High-dimensional phenotypic mapping of human dendritic cells reveals interindividual variation and tissue specialization. *Immunity.* (2017) 47:1037–50 e6. doi: 10.1016/j.immuni.2017.11.001
27. Satpathy AT, Briseno CG, Lee JS, Ng D, Manieri NA, Kc W, et al. Notch2-dependent classical dendritic cells orchestrate intestinal immunity to attaching-and-effacing bacterial pathogens. *Nat Immunol.* (2013) 14:937–48. doi: 10.1038/ni.2679
28. Villani AC, Satija R, Reynolds G, Sarkizova S, Shekhar K, Fletcher J, et al. Single-cell RNA-seq reveals new types of human blood dendritic cells, monocytes, and progenitors. *Science.* (2017) 356:eaah4573. doi: 10.1126/science.aah4573
29. Lewis KL, Caton ML, Bogunovic M, Greter M, Grajkowska LT, Ng D, et al. Notch2 receptor signaling controls functional differentiation of dendritic cells in the spleen and intestine. *Immunity.* (2011) 35:780–91. doi: 10.1016/j.immuni.2011.08.013
30. Colonna M, Trinchieri G, Liu YJ. Plasmacytoid dendritic cells in immunity. *Nat Immunol.* (2004) 5:1219–26. doi: 10.1038/ni1141
31. Grouard G, Rissoan MC, Filgueira L, Durand I, Banchereau J, Liu YJ. The enigmatic plasmacytoid T cells develop into dendritic cells with interleukin (IL)-3 and CD40-ligand. *J Exp Med.* (1997) 185:1101–11. doi: 10.1084/jem.185.6.1101
32. Cella M, Jarrossay D, Facchetti F, Alebardi O, Nakajima H, Lanzavecchia A, et al. Plasmacytoid monocytes migrate to inflamed lymph nodes and produce large amounts of type I interferon. *Nat Med.* (1999) 5:919–23. doi: 10.1038/11360
33. Siegal FP, Kadowaki N, Shodell M, Fitzgerald-Bocarsly PA, Shah K, Ho S, et al. The nature of the principal type 1 interferon-producing cells in human blood. *Science.* (1999) 284:1835–7. doi: 10.1126/science.284.5421.1835
34. Cisse B, Caton ML, Lehner M, Maeda T, Scheu S, Locksley R, et al. Transcription factor E2-2 is an essential and specific regulator of plasmacytoid dendritic cell development. *Cell.* (2008) 135:37–48. doi: 10.1016/j.cell.2008.09.016
35. Alculumbre SG, Saint-Andre V, Di Domizio J, Vargas P, Sirven P, Bost P, et al. Diversification of human plasmacytoid predendritic cells in response to a single stimulus. *Nat Immunol.* (2018) 19:63–75. doi: 10.1038/s41590-017-0012-z
36. Rodrigues PF, Alberti-Servera L, Eremin A, Grajales-Reyes GE, Ivanek R, Tussiwand R. Distinct progenitor lineages contribute to the heterogeneity of plasmacytoid dendritic cells. *Nat Immunol.* (2018) 19:711–22. doi: 10.1038/s41590-018-0136-9
37. Serbina NV, Salazar-Mather TP, Biron CA, Kuziel WA, Pamer EG. TNF/iNOS-producing dendritic cells mediate innate immune defense against bacterial infection. *Immunity.* (2003) 19:59–70. doi: 10.1016/S1074-7613(03)00171-7
38. Sallusto F, Lanzavecchia A. Efficient presentation of soluble antigen by cultured human dendritic cells is maintained by granulocyte/macrophage colony-stimulating factor plus interleukin 4 and downregulated by tumor necrosis factor alpha. *J Exp Med.* (1994) 179:1109–18. doi: 10.1084/jem.179.4.1109
39. Steinman RM, Banchereau J. Taking dendritic cells into medicine. *Nature.* (2007) 449:419–26. doi: 10.1038/nature06175
40. Helft J, Bottcher J, Chakravarty P, Zelenay S, Huotari J, Schraml BU, et al. GM-CSF mouse bone marrow cultures comprise a heterogeneous population of CD11c(+)MHCII(+) macrophages and dendritic cells. *Immunity.* (2015) 42:1197–211. doi: 10.1016/j.immuni.2015.05.018
41. Sander J, Schmidt SV, Cirovic B, McGovern N, Papantonopoulou O, Hardt AL, et al. Cellular differentiation of human monocytes is regulated by time-dependent interleukin-4 signaling and the transcriptional regulator NCOR2. *Immunity.* (2017) 47:1051–66 e12. doi: 10.1016/j.immuni.2017.11.024
42. Wu X, Briseno CG, Durai V, Albring JC, Haldar M, Bagadia P, et al. Mafb lineage tracing to distinguish macrophages from other immune lineages reveals dual identity of Langerhans cells. *J Exp Med.* (2016) 213:2553–65. doi: 10.1084/jem.20160600
43. Laoui D, Keirsse J, Morias Y, Van Overmeire E, Geeraerts X, Elkrim Y, et al. The tumour microenvironment harbours ontogenically distinct dendritic cell populations with opposing effects on tumour immunity. *Nat Commun.* 2016;7:13720. doi: 10.1038/ncomms13720
44. Broz ML, Binnewies M, Boldajipour B, Nelson AE, Pollack JL, Erle DJ, et al. Dissecting the tumor myeloid compartment reveals rare activating antigen-presenting cells critical for T cell immunity. *Cancer Cell.* 2014;26(6):938. doi: 10.1016/j.ccell.2014.11.010
45. Salmon H, Idoyaga J, Rahman A, Leboeuf M, Remark R, Jordan S, et al. Expansion and activation of CD103(+) dendritic cell progenitors at the tumor site enhances tumor responses to therapeutic PD-L1 and BRAF inhibition. *Immunity.* (2016) 44:924–38. doi: 10.1016/j.immuni.2016.03.012
46. Roberts EW, Broz ML, Binnewies M, Headley MB, Nelson AE, Wolf DM, et al. Critical role for CD103(+)/CD141(+) dendritic cells bearing CCR7 for tumor antigen trafficking and priming of T cell immunity in melanoma. *Cancer Cell.* (2016) 30:324–36. doi: 10.1016/j.ccell.2016.06.003
47. Lou Y, Liu C, Kim GJ, Liu YJ, Hwu P, Wang G. Plasmacytoid dendritic cells synergize with myeloid dendritic cells in the induction of antigen-specific antitumor immune responses. *J Immunol.* (2007) 178:1534–41. doi: 10.4049/jimmunol.178.3.1534
48. Lavin Y, Kobayashi S, Leader A, Amir ED, Elefant N, Bigenwald C, et al. Innate immune landscape in early lung adenocarcinoma by paired single-cell analyses. *Cell.* (2017) 169:750–65 e17. doi: 10.1016/j.cell.2017.04.014
49. Tang-Huau TL, Gueguen P, Goudot C, Durand M, Bohec M, Baulande S, et al. Human *in vivo*-generated monocyte-derived dendritic cells and macrophages cross-present antigens through a vacuolar pathway. *Nat Commun.* 2018;9(1):2570. doi: 10.1038/s41467-018-04985-0
50. Cohn L, Chatterjee B, Esselborn F, Smed-Sorensen A, Nakamura N, Chalouni C, et al. Antigen delivery to early endosomes eliminates the superiority of human blood BDCA3+ dendritic cells at cross presentation. *J Exp Med.* (2013) 210:1049–63. doi: 10.1084/jem.20121251
51. Kretzer NM, Theisen DJ, Tussiwand R, Briseno CG, Grajales-Reyes GE, Wu X, et al. RAB43 facilitates cross-presentation of cell-associated antigens by CD8alpha+ dendritic cells. *J Exp Med.* (2016) 213:2871–83. doi: 10.1084/jem.20160597
52. Chatterjee B, Smed-Sorensen A, Cohn L, Chalouni C, Vandlen R, Lee BC, et al. Internalization and endosomal degradation of receptor-bound antigens regulate the efficiency of cross presentation by human dendritic cells. *Blood.* (2012) 120:2011–20. doi: 10.1182/blood-2012-01-402370
53. Alloatti A, Rookhuizen DC, Joannas L, Carpier JM, Iborra S, Magalhaes JG, et al. Critical role for Sec22b-dependent antigen cross-presentation in antitumor immunity. *J Exp Med.* (2017) 214:2231–41. doi: 10.1084/jem.20170229
54. Wu SJ, Niknafs YS, Kim SH, Oravecz-Wilson K, Zajac C, Toubai T, et al. A critical analysis of the role of SNARE protein SEC22B in antigen cross-presentation. *Cell Rep.* (2017) 19:2645–56. doi: 10.1016/j.celrep.2017.06.013
55. Cebrian I, Visentin G, Blanchard N, Jouve M, Bobard A, Moita C, et al. Sec22b regulates phagosomal maturation and antigen crosspresentation by dendritic cells. *Cell.* (2011) 147:1355–68. doi: 10.1016/j.cell.2011.11.021
56. Savina A, Jancic C, Hugues S, Guermonprez P, Vargas P, Moura IC, et al. NOX2 controls phagosomal pH to regulate antigen processing during crosspresentation by dendritic cells. *Cell.* (2006) 126:205–18. doi: 10.1016/j.cell.2006.05.035
57. Mantegazza AR, Savina A, Vermeulen M, Perez L, Geffner J, Hermine O, et al. NADPH oxidase controls phagosomal pH and antigen cross-presentation in human dendritic cells. *Blood.* (2008) 112:4712–22. doi: 10.1182/blood-2008-01-134791
58. Savina A, Peres A, Cebrian I, Carmo N, Moita C, Hacohen N, et al. The small GTPase Rac2 controls phagosomal alkalinization and antigen

crosspresentation selectively in CD8(+) dendritic cells. *Immunity.* (2009) 30:544–55. doi: 10.1016/j.immuni.2009.01.013
59. Jancic C, Savina A, Wasmeier C, Tolmachova T, El-Benna J, Dang PM, et al. Rab27a regulates phagosomal pH and NADPH oxidase recruitment to dendritic cell phagosomes. *Nat Cell Biol.* (2007) 9:367–78. doi: 10.1038/ncb1552
60. Ding Y, Guo Z, Liu Y, Li X, Zhang Q, Xu X, et al. The lectin Siglec-G inhibits dendritic cell cross-presentation by impairing MHC class I-peptide complex formation. *Nat Immunol.* (2016) 17:1167–75. doi: 10.1038/ni.3535
61. Theisen DJ, Davidson JTt, Briseno CG, Gargaro M, Lauron EJ, Wang Q, et al. WDFY4 is required for cross-presentation in response to viral and tumor antigens. *Science.* (2018) 362:694–9. doi: 10.1126/science.aat5030
62. Mashayekhi M, Sandau MM, Dunay IR, Frickel EM, Khan A, Goldszmid RS, et al. CD8α^+ dendritic cells are the critical source of interleukin-12 that controls acute infection by *Toxoplasma gondii* tachyzoites. *Immunity.* (2011) 35:249–59. doi: 10.1016/j.immuni.2011.08.008
63. Martinez-Lopez M, Iborra S, Conde-Garrosa R, Sancho D. Batf3-dependent CD103+ dendritic cells are major producers of IL-12 that drive local Th1 immunity against Leishmania major infection in mice. *Eur J Immunol.* (2015) 45:119–29. doi: 10.1002/eji.201444651
64. Everts B, Tussiwand R, Dreesen L, Fairfax KC, Huang SC, Smith AM, et al. Migratory CD103+ dendritic cells suppress helminth-driven type 2 immunity through constitutive expression of IL-12. *J Exp Med.* (2016) 213:35–51. doi: 10.1084/jem.20150235
65. Hildner K, Edelson BT, Purtha WE, Diamond M, Matsushita H, Kohyama M, et al. Batf3 deficiency reveals a critical role for CD8alpha+ dendritic cells in cytotoxic T cell immunity. *Science.* (2008) 322:1097–100. doi: 10.1126/science.1164206
66. Byrne KT, Vonderheide RH. CD40 Stimulation obviates innate sensors and drives T cell immunity in cancer. *Cell Rep.* (2016) 15:2719–32. doi: 10.1016/j.celrep.2016.05.058
67. Spranger S, Dai D, Horton B, Gajewski TF. Tumor-residing Batf3 dendritic cells are required for effector T cell trafficking and adoptive T cell therapy. *Cancer Cell.* (2017) 31:711–23 e4. doi: 10.1016/j.ccell.2017.04.003
68. Meyer MA, Baer JM, Knolhoff BL, Nywening TM, Panni RZ, Su X, et al. Breast and pancreatic cancer interrupt IRF8-dependent dendritic cell development to overcome immune surveillance. *Nat Commun.* (2018) 9:1250. doi: 10.1038/s41467-018-03600-6
69. Sanchez-Paulete AR, Cueto FJ, Martinez-Lopez M, Labiano S, Morales-Kastresana A, Rodriguez-Ruiz ME, et al. Cancer Immunotherapy with immunomodulatory anti-CD137 and anti-PD-1 monoclonal antibodies requires BATF3-dependent dendritic cells. *Cancer Discov.* (2016) 6:71–9. doi: 10.1158/2159-8290.CD-15-0510
70. Li J, Byrne KT, Yan F, Yamazoe T, Chen Z, Baslan T, et al. Tumor cell-intrinsic factors underlie heterogeneity of immune cell infiltration and response to immunotherapy. *Immunity.* (2018) 49:178–93 e7. doi: 10.1016/j.immuni.2018.06.006
71. Barry KC, Hsu J, Broz ML, Cueto FJ, Binnewies M, Combes AJ, et al. A natural killer-dendritic cell axis defines checkpoint therapy-responsive tumor microenvironments. *Nat Med.* (2018) 24:1178–91. doi: 10.1158/2326-6074.CRICIMTEATIAACR18-PR04
72. Vonderheide RH. The immune revolution: a case for priming, not checkpoint. *Cancer Cell.* (2018) 33:563–9. doi: 10.1016/j.ccell.2018.03.008
73. Lee W, Kim HS, Hwang SS, Lee GR. The transcription factor Batf3 inhibits the differentiation of regulatory T cells in the periphery. *Exp Mol Med.* (2017) 49:e393. doi: 10.1038/emm.2017.157
74. Meredith MM, Liu K, Darrasse-Jeze G, Kamphorst AO, Schreiber HA, Guermonprez P, et al. Expression of the zinc finger transcription factor zDC (Zbtb46, Btbd4) defines the classical dendritic cell lineage. *J Exp Med.* (2012) 209:1153–65. doi: 10.1084/jem.20112675
75. Robbins SH, Walzer T, Dembele D, Thibault C, Defays A, Bessou G, et al. Novel insights into the relationships between dendritic cell subsets in human and mouse revealed by genome-wide expression profiling. *Genome Biol.* (2008) 9:R17. doi: 10.1186/gb-2008-9-1-r17
76. Satpathy AT, Kc W, Albring JC, Edelson BT, Kretzer NM, Bhattacharya D, et al. Zbtb46 expression distinguishes classical dendritic cells and their committed progenitors from other immune lineages. *J Exp Med.* (2012) 209:1135–52. doi: 10.1084/jem.20120030
77. Eickhoff S, Brewitz A, Gerner MY, Klauschen F, Komander K, Hemmi H, et al. Robust anti-viral immunity requires multiple distinct T cell-dendritic cell interactions. *Cell.* (2015) 162:1322–37. doi: 10.1016/j.cell.2015.08.004
78. Hor JL, Whitney PG, Zaid A, Brooks AG, Heath WR, Mueller SN. Spatiotemporally distinct interactions with dendritic cell subsets facilitates $CD4^+$ and $CD8^+$ T cell activation to localized viral infection. *Immunity.* (2015) 43:554–65. doi: 10.1016/j.immuni.2015.07.020
79. Brewitz A, Eickhoff S, Dahling S, Quast T, Bedoui S, Kroczek RA, et al. $CD8^+$ T cells orchestrate pDC-$XCR1^+$ dendritic cell spatial and functional cooperativity to optimize priming. *Immunity.* (2017) 46:205–19. doi: 10.1016/j.immuni.2017.01.003
80. Quezada SA, Simpson TR, Peggs KS, Merghoub T, Vider J, Fan X, et al. Tumor-reactive $CD4^+$ T cells develop cytotoxic activity and eradicate large established melanoma after transfer into lymphopenic hosts. *J Exp Med.* (2010) 207:637–50. doi: 10.1084/jem.20091918
81. Qin Z, Blankenstein T. CD4+ T cell–mediated tumor rejection involves inhibition of angiogenesis that is dependent on IFN gamma receptor expression by nonhematopoietic cells. *Immunity.* (2000) 12:677–86. doi: 10.1016/S1074-7613(00)80218-6
82. Kim HJ, Cantor H. CD4 T-cell subsets and tumor immunity: the helpful and the not-so-helpful. *Cancer Immunol Res.* (2014) 2:91–8. doi: 10.1158/2326-6066.CIR-13-0216
83. Kennedy R, Celis E. Multiple roles for CD4+ T cells in anti-tumor immune responses. *Immunol Rev.* (2008) 222:129–44. doi: 10.1111/j.1600-065X.2008.00616.x
84. Fuertes MB, Kacha AK, Kline J, Woo SR, Kranz DM, Murphy KM, et al. Host type I IFN signals are required for antitumor CD8+ T cell responses through CD8{alpha}+ dendritic cells. *J Exp Med.* (2011) 208:2005–16. doi: 10.1084/jem.20101159
85. Diamond MS, Kinder M, Matsushita H, Mashayekhi M, Dunn GP, Archambault JM, et al. Type I interferon is selectively required by dendritic cells for immune rejection of tumors. *J Exp Med.* (2011) 208:1989–2003. doi: 10.1084/jem.20101158
86. Fonteneau JF, Gilliet M, Larsson M, Dasilva I, Munz C, Liu YJ, et al. Activation of influenza virus-specific CD4+ and CD8+ T cells: a new role for plasmacytoid dendritic cells in adaptive immunity. *Blood.* (2003) 101:3520–6. doi: 10.1182/blood-2002-10-3063
87. Tel J, Aarntzen EH, Baba T, Schreibelt G, Schulte BM, Benitez-Ribas D, et al. Natural human plasmacytoid dendritic cells induce antigen-specific T-cell responses in melanoma patients. *Cancer Res.* (2013) 73:1063–75. doi: 10.1158/0008-5472.CAN-12-2583
88. Perez-Cabezas B, Naranjo-Gomez M, Ruiz-Riol M, Bastos-Amador P, Fernandez MA, Carmona F, et al. TLR-activated conventional DCs promote gamma-secretase-mediated conditioning of plasmacytoid DCs. *J Leukoc Biol.* (2012) 92:133–43. doi: 10.1189/jlb.0911452
89. Nascimbeni M, Perie L, Chorro L, Diocou S, Kreitmann L, Louis S, et al. Plasmacytoid dendritic cells accumulate in spleens from chronically HIV-infected patients but barely participate in interferon-alpha expression. *Blood.* (2009) 113:6112–9. doi: 10.1182/blood-2008-07-170803
90. Vermi W, Lonardi S, Morassi M, Rossini C, Tardanico R, Venturini M, et al. Cutaneous distribution of plasmacytoid dendritic cells in lupus erythematosus. Selective tropism at the site of epithelial apoptotic damage. *Immunobiology.* (2009) 214:877–86. doi: 10.1016/j.imbio.2009.06.013
91. Rogers GL, Shirley JL, Zolotukhin I, Kumar SRP, Sherman A, Perrin GQ, et al. Plasmacytoid and conventional dendritic cells cooperate in crosspriming AAV capsid-specific $CD8^+$ T cells. *Blood.* (2017) 129:3184–95. doi: 10.1182/blood-2016-11-751040
92. Yoneyama H, Matsuno K, Toda E, Nishiwaki T, Matsuo N, Nakano A, et al. Plasmacytoid DCs help lymph node DCs to induce anti-HSV CTLs. *J Exp Med.* (2005) 202:425–35. doi: 10.1084/jem.20041961
93. Asselin-Paturel C, Boonstra A, Dalod M, Durand I, Yessaad N, Dezutter-Dambuyant C, et al. Mouse type I IFN-producing cells are immature APCs with plasmacytoid morphology. *Nat Immunol.* (2001) 2:1144–50. doi: 10.1038/ni736
94. Swiecki M, Gilfillan S, Vermi W, Wang Y, Colonna M. Plasmacytoid dendritic cell ablation impacts early interferon responses and

antiviral NK and CD8+ T cell accrual. *Immunity.* (2010) 33:955–66. doi: 10.1016/j.immuni.2010.11.020
95. Cervantes-Barragan L, Lewis KL, Firner S, Thiel V, Hugues S, Reith W, et al. Plasmacytoid dendritic cells control T-cell response to chronic viral infection. *Proc Natl Acad Sci USA.* (2012) 109:3012–7. doi: 10.1073/pnas.1117359109
96. Terra M, Oberkampf M, Fayolle C, Rosenbaum P, Guillerey C, Dadaglio G, et al. Tumor-derived TGFbeta alters the ability of plasmacytoid dendritic cells to respond to innate immune signaling. *Cancer Res.* (2018) 78:3014–26. doi: 10.1158/0008-5472.CAN-17-2719
97. Treilleux I, Blay JY, Bendriss-Vermare N, Ray-Coquard I, Bachelot T, Guastalla JP, et al. Dendritic cell infiltration and prognosis of early stage breast cancer. *Clinical Cancer Res.* (2004) 10:7466–74. doi: 10.1158/1078-0432.CCR-04-0684
98. Conrad C, Gregorio J, Wang YH, Ito T, Meller S, Hanabuchi S, et al. Plasmacytoid dendritic cells promote immunosuppression in ovarian cancer via ICOS costimulation of Foxp3+ T-regulatory cells. *Cancer Res.* (2012) 72:5240–9. doi: 10.1158/0008-5472.CAN-12-2271
99. Mellor AL, Munn DH. IDO expression by dendritic cells: tolerance and tryptophan catabolism. *Nat Rev Immunol.* (2004) 4:762–74. doi: 10.1038/nri1457
100. Kitano M, Yamazaki C, Takumi A, Ikeno T, Hemmi H, Takahashi N, et al. Imaging of the cross-presenting dendritic cell subsets in the skin-draining lymph node. *Proc Natl Acad Sci USA.* (2016) 113:1044–9. doi: 10.1073/pnas.1513607113
101. Gerner MY, Torabi-Parizi P, Germain RN. Strategically localized dendritic cells promote rapid T cell responses to lymph-borne particulate antigens. *Immunity.* (2015) 42:172–85. doi: 10.1016/j.immuni.2014.12.024
102. Gerner MY, Kastenmuller W, Ifrim I, Kabat J, Germain RN. Histo-cytometry: a method for highly multiplex quantitative tissue imaging analysis applied to dendritic cell subset microanatomy in lymph nodes. *Immunity.* (2012) 37:364–76. doi: 10.1016/j.immuni.2012.07.011
103. Gerner MY, Casey KA, Kastenmuller W, Germain RN. Dendritic cell and antigen dispersal landscapes regulate T cell immunity. *J Exp Med.* (2017) 214:3105–22. doi: 10.1084/jem.20170335
104. Borst J, Ahrends T, Babala N, Melief CJM, Kastenmuller W. CD4+ T cell help in cancer immunology and immunotherapy. *Nat Rev Immunol.* (2018) 18:635–47. doi: 10.1038/s41577-018-0044-0
105. Calabro S, Liu D, Gallman A, Nascimento MS, Yu Z, Zhang TT, et al. Differential intrasplenic migration of dendritic cell subsets tailors adaptive immunity. *Cell Rep.* (2016) 16:2472–85. doi: 10.1016/j.celrep.2016.07.076
106. Allan RS, Waithman J, Bedoui S, Jones CM, Villadangos JA, Zhan Y, et al. Migratory dendritic cells transfer antigen to a lymph node-resident dendritic cell population for efficient CTL priming. *Immunity.* (2006) 25:153–62. doi: 10.1016/j.immuni.2006.04.017
107. Amigorena S. Helping the help for CD8+ T cell responses. *Cell.* (2015) 162:1210–2. doi: 10.1016/j.cell.2015.08.051
108. Janssen EM, Lemmens EE, Wolfe T, Christen U, von Herrath MG, Schoenberger SP. CD4+ T cells are required for secondary expansion and memory in CD8+ T lymphocytes. *Nature.* (2003) 421:852–6. doi: 10.1038/nature01441
109. Shedlock DJ, Shen H. Requirement for CD4 T cell help in generating functional CD8 T cell memory. *Science.* (2003) 300:337–9. doi: 10.1126/science.1082305
110. Bennett SR, Carbone FR, Karamalis F, Flavell RA, Miller JF, Heath WR. Help for cytotoxic-T-cell responses is mediated by CD40 signalling. *Nature.* (1998) 393:478–80. doi: 10.1038/30996
111. Schoenberger SP, Toes RE, van der Voort EI, Offringa R, Melief CJ. T-cell help for cytotoxic T lymphocytes is mediated by CD40-CD40L interactions. *Nature.* (1998) 393:480–3. doi: 10.1038/31002
112. Ridge JP, Di Rosa F, Matzinger P. A conditioned dendritic cell can be a temporal bridge between a CD4+ T-helper and a T-killer cell. *Nature.* (1998) 393:474–8. doi: 10.1038/30989
113. Nishimura T, Iwakabe K, Sekimoto M, Ohmi Y, Yahata T, Nakui M, et al. Distinct role of antigen-specific T helper type 1 (Th1) and Th2 cells in tumor eradication *in vivo*. *J Exp Med.* (1999) 190:617–27. doi: 10.1084/jem.190.5.617
114. Tarbell KV, Egen JG. Breaking self-tolerance during autoimmunity and cancer immunity: myeloid cells and type I IFN response regulation. *J Leukoc Biol.* (2018) 103:1117–29. doi: 10.1002/JLB.3MIR1017-400R
115. Gagnerault MC, Luan JJ, Lotton C, Lepault F. Pancreatic lymph nodes are required for priming of beta cell reactive T cells in NOD mice. *J Exp Med.* (2002) 196:369–77. doi: 10.1084/jem.20011353
116. Hoglund P, Mintern J, Waltzinger C, Heath W, Benoist C, Mathis D. Initiation of autoimmune diabetes by developmentally regulated presentation of islet cell antigens in the pancreatic lymph nodes. *J Exp Med.* (1999) 189:331–9. doi: 10.1084/jem.189.2.331
117. Unanue ER. Perspectives on anti-CD47 antibody treatment for experimental cancer. *Proc Natl Acad Sci USA.* (2013) 110:10886–7. doi: 10.1073/pnas.1308463110
118. Engelhardt JJ, Boldajipour B, Beemiller P, Pandurangi P, Sorensen C, Werb Z, et al. Marginating dendritic cells of the tumor microenvironment cross-present tumor antigens and stably engage tumor-specific T cells. *Cancer Cell.* (2012) 21:402–17. doi: 10.1016/j.ccr.2012.01.008
119. Gerner MY, Casey KA, Mescher MF. Defective MHC class II presentation by dendritic cells limits CD4 T cell help for antitumor CD8 T cell responses. *J Immunol.* (2008) 181:155–64. doi: 10.4049/jimmunol.181.1.155
120. Anderson MJ, Shafer-Weaver K, Greenberg NM, Hurwitz AA. Tolerization of tumor-specific T cells despite efficient initial priming in a primary murine model of prostate cancer. *J Immunol.* (2007) 178:1268–76. doi: 10.4049/jimmunol.178.3.1268
121. Gardner A, Ruffell B. Dendritic cells and cancer immunity. *Trends Immunol.* (2016) 37:855–65. doi: 10.1016/j.it.2016.09.006
122. Zhu Z, Cuss SM, Singh V, Gurusamy D, Shoe JL, Leighty R, et al. CD4+ T cell help selectively enhances high-avidity tumor antigen-specific CD8+ T cells. *J Immunol.* (2015) 195:3482–9. doi: 10.4049/jimmunol.1401571
123. Bos R, Sherman LA. CD4+ T-cell help in the tumor milieu is required for recruitment and cytolytic function of CD8+ T lymphocytes. *Cancer Res.* (2010) 70:8368–77. doi: 10.1158/0008-5472.CAN-10-1322
124. Schietinger A, Philip M, Liu RB, Schreiber K, Schreiber H. Bystander killing of cancer requires the cooperation of CD4+ and CD8+ T cells during the effector phase. *J Exp Med.* (2010) 207:2469–77. doi: 10.1084/jem.20092450
125. Marzo AL, Kinnear BF, Lake RA, Frelinger JJ, Collins EJ, Robinson BW, et al. Tumor-specific CD4+ T cells have a major "post-licensing" role in CTL mediated anti-tumor immunity. *J Immunol.* (2000) 165:6047–55. doi: 10.4049/jimmunol.165.11.6047
126. Ahrends T, Spanjaard A, Pilzecker B, Babala N, Bovens A, Xiao Y, et al. CD4+ T cell help confers a cytotoxic T cell effector program including coinhibitory receptor downregulation and increased tissue invasiveness. *Immunity.* (2017) 47:848–61 e5. doi: 10.1016/j.immuni.2017.10.009
127. Gallotta M, Assi H, Degagne E, Kannan SK, Coffman RL, Guiducci C. Inhaled TLR9 agonist renders lung tumors permissive to PD-1 blockade by promoting optimal CD4+ and CD8+ T-cell Interplay. *Cancer Res.* (2018) 78:4943–56. doi: 10.1158/0008-5472.CAN-18-0729
128. Neubert K, Lehmann CH, Heger L, Baranska A, Staedtler AM, Buchholz VR, et al. Antigen delivery to CD11c+CD8- dendritic cells induces protective immune responses against experimental melanoma in mice *in vivo*. *J Immunol.* (2014) 192:5830–8. doi: 10.4049/jimmunol.1300975
129. Alonso R, Flament H, Lemoine S, Sedlik C, Bottasso E, Peguillet I, et al. Induction of anergic or regulatory tumor-specific CD4+ T cells in the tumor-draining lymph node. *Nat Commun.* (2018) 9:2113. doi: 10.1038/s41467-018-04524-x
130. Michea P, Noel F, Zakine E, Czerwinska U, Sirven P, Abouzid O, et al. Adjustment of dendritic cells to the breast-cancer microenvironment is subset specific. *Nat Immunol.* (2018) 19:885–97. doi: 10.1038/s41590-018-0145-8
131. Johnson DB, Estrada MV, Salgado R, Sanchez V, Doxie DB, Opalenik SR, et al. Melanoma-specific MHC-II expression represents a tumour-autonomous phenotype and predicts response to anti-PD-1/PD-L1 therapy. *Nat Commun.* 2016;7:10582. doi: 10.1038/ncomms10582

132. Ali OA, Emerich D, Dranoff G, Mooney DJ. *In situ* regulation of DC subsets and T cells mediates tumor regression in mice. *Sci Transl Med.* (2009) 1:8ra19. doi: 10.1126/scitranslmed.3000359
133. Thompson ED, Enriquez HL, Fu YX, Engelhard VH. Tumor masses support naive T cell infiltration, activation, and differentiation into effectors. *J Exp Med.* (2010) 207:1791–804. doi: 10.1084/jem.20092454
134. Ma Y, Adjemian S, Mattarollo SR, Yamazaki T, Aymeric L, Yang H, et al. Anticancer chemotherapy-induced intratumoral recruitment and differentiation of antigen-presenting cells. *Immunity.* (2013) 38:729–41. doi: 10.1016/j.immuni.2013.03.003
135. Yu P, Lee Y, Liu W, Chin RK, Wang J, Wang Y, et al. Priming of naive T cells inside tumors leads to eradication of established tumors. *Nat Immunol.* (2004) 5:141–9. doi: 10.1038/ni1029
136. Pitzalis C, Jones GW, Bombardieri M, Jones SA. Ectopic lymphoid-like structures in infection, cancer and autoimmunity. *Nat Rev Immunol.* (2014) 14:447–62. doi: 10.1038/nri3700
137. Dieu-Nosjean MC, Goc J, Giraldo NA, Sautes-Fridman C, Fridman WH. Tertiary lymphoid structures in cancer and beyond. *Trends Immunol.* (2014) 35:571–80. doi: 10.1016/j.it.2014.09.006
138. Gunn MD, Kyuwa S, Tam C, Kakiuchi T, Matsuzawa A, Williams LT, et al. Mice lacking expression of secondary lymphoid organ chemokine have defects in lymphocyte homing and dendritic cell localization. *J Exp Med.* (1999) 189:451–60. doi: 10.1084/jem.189.3.451
139. Forster R, Schubel A, Breitfeld D, Kremmer E, Renner-Muller I, Wolf E, et al. CCR7 coordinates the primary immune response by establishing functional microenvironments in secondary lymphoid organs. *Cell.* (1999) 99:23–33. doi: 10.1016/S0092-8674(00)80059-8
140. Joshi NS, Akama-Garren EH, Lu Y, Lee DY, Chang GP, Li A, et al. Regulatory T cells in tumor-associated tertiary lymphoid structures suppress anti-tumor T cell responses. *Immunity.* (2015) 43:579–90. doi: 10.1016/j.immuni.2015.08.006
141. Goc J, Germain C, Vo-Bourgais TK, Lupo A, Klein C, Knockaert S, et al. Dendritic cells in tumor-associated tertiary lymphoid structures signal a Th1 cytotoxic immune contexture and license the positive prognostic value of infiltrating CD8$^+$ T cells. *Cancer Res.* (2014) 74:705–15. doi: 10.1158/0008-5472.CAN-13-1342
142. Dieu-Nosjean MC, Antoine M, Danel C, Heudes D, Wislez M, Poulot V, et al. Long-term survival for patients with non-small-cell lung cancer with intratumoral lymphoid structures. *J Clin Oncol.* (2008) 26:4410–7. doi: 10.1200/JCO.2007.15.0284
143. Remark R, Becker C, Gomez JE, Damotte D, Dieu-Nosjean MC, Sautes-Fridman C, et al. The non-small cell lung cancer immune contexture. A major determinant of tumor characteristics and patient outcome. *Am J Respir Crit Care Med.* (2015) 191:377–90. doi: 10.1164/rccm.201409-1671PP
144. Jang JE, Hajdu CH, Liot C, Miller G, Dustin ML, Bar-Sagi D. Crosstalk between regulatory T cells and tumor-associated dendritic cells negates anti-tumor immunity in pancreatic cancer. *Cell Rep.* (2017) 20:558–71. doi: 10.1016/j.celrep.2017.06.062
145. Fernandez NC, Lozier A, Flament C, Ricciardi-Castagnoli P, Bellet D, Suter M, et al. Dendritic cells directly trigger NK cell functions: cross-talk relevant in innate anti-tumor immune responses *in vivo*. *Nat Med.* (1999) 5:405–11. doi: 10.1038/7403
146. Borg C, Jalil A, Laderach D, Maruyama K, Wakasugi H, Charrier S, et al. NK cell activation by dendritic cells (DCs) requires the formation of a synapse leading to IL-12 polarization in DCs. *Blood.* (2004) 104:3267–75. doi: 10.1182/blood-2004-01-0380
147. Morvan MG, Lanier LL. NK cells and cancer: you can teach innate cells new tricks. *Nat Rev Cancer.* (2016) 16:7–19. doi: 10.1038/nrc.2015.5
148. Bottcher JP, Bonavita E, Chakravarty P, Blees H, Cabeza-Cabrerizo M, Sammicheli S, et al. NK cells stimulate recruitment of cDC1 into the tumor microenvironment promoting cancer immune control. *Cell.* (2018) 172:1022–37 e14. doi: 10.1016/j.cell.2018.01.004
149. Ferlazzo G, Pack M, Thomas D, Paludan C, Schmid D, Strowig T, et al. Distinct roles of IL-12 and IL-15 in human natural killer cell activation by dendritic cells from secondary lymphoid organs. *Proc Natl Acad Sci USA.* (2004) 101:16606–11. doi: 10.1073/pnas.0407522101
150. Lucas M, Schachterle W, Oberle K, Aichele P, Diefenbach A. Dendritic cells prime natural killer cells by trans-presenting interleukin 15. *Immunity.* (2007) 26:503–17. doi: 10.1016/j.immuni.2007.03.006
151. Liu C, Lou Y, Lizee G, Qin H, Liu S, Rabinovich B, et al. Plasmacytoid dendritic cells induce NK cell-dependent, tumor antigen-specific T cell cross-priming and tumor regression in mice. *J Clin Invest.* (2008) 118:1165–75. doi: 10.1172/JCI33583
152. Godfrey DI, Uldrich AP, McCluskey J, Rossjohn J, Moody DB. The burgeoning family of unconventional T cells. *Nat Immunol.* (2015) 16:1114–23. doi: 10.1038/ni.3298
153. Fujii S, Shimizu K, Kronenberg M, Steinman RM. Prolonged IFN-gamma-producing NKT response induced with alpha-galactosylceramide-loaded DCs. *Nat Immunol.* (2002) 3:867–74. doi: 10.1038/ni827
154. Fujii S, Liu K, Smith C, Bonito AJ, Steinman RM. The linkage of innate to adaptive immunity via maturing dendritic cells *in vivo* requires CD40 ligation in addition to antigen presentation and CD80/86 costimulation. *J Exp Med.* (2004) 199:1607–18. doi: 10.1084/jem.20040317
155. Fujii S, Shimizu K, Smith C, Bonifaz L, Steinman RM. Activation of natural killer T cells by alpha-galactosylceramide rapidly induces the full maturation of dendritic cells *in vivo* and thereby acts as an adjuvant for combined CD4 and CD8 T cell immunity to a coadministered protein. *J Exp Med.* (2003) 198:267–79. doi: 10.1084/jem.20030324
156. Kitamura H, Iwakabe K, Yahata T, Nishimura S, Ohta A, Ohmi Y, et al. The natural killer T (NKT) cell ligand alpha-galactosylceramide demonstrates its immunopotentiating effect by inducing interleukin (IL)-12 production by dendritic cells and IL-12 receptor expression on NKT cells. *J Exp Med.* (1999) 189:1121–8. doi: 10.1084/jem.189.7.1121
157. Kobayashi E, Motoki K, Uchida T, Fukushima H, Koezuka Y. KRN7000, a novel immunomodulator, and its antitumor activities. *Oncol Res.* (1995) 7:529–34.
158. Giaccone G. Clinical impact of novel treatment strategies. *Oncogene.* (2002) 21:6970–81. doi: 10.1038/sj.onc.1205565
159. Parekh VV, Wilson MT, Olivares-Villagomez D, Singh AK, Wu L, Wang CR, et al. Glycolipid antigen induces long-term natural killer T cell anergy in mice. *J Clin Invest.* (2005) 115:2572–83. doi: 10.1172/JCI24762
160. King LA, Lameris R, de Gruijl TD, van der Vliet HJ. CD1d-Invariant natural killer T cell-based cancer immunotherapy: alpha-galactosylceramide and beyond. *Front Immunol.* (2018) 9:1519. doi: 10.3389/fimmu.2018.01519
161. Mattner J, Debord KL, Ismail N, Goff RD, Cantu C, III, Zhou D, et al. Exogenous and endogenous glycolipid antigens activate NKT cells during microbial infections. *Nature.* (2005) 434:525–9. doi: 10.1038/nature03408
162. Nair S, Dhodapkar MV. Natural killer T cells in cancer immunotherapy. *Front Immunol.* (2017) 8:1178. doi: 10.3389/fimmu.2017.01178
163. Haraguchi K, Takahashi T, Nakahara F, Matsumoto A, Kurokawa M, Ogawa S, et al. CD1d expression level in tumor cells is an important determinant for anti-tumor immunity by natural killer T cells. *Leuk Lymphoma.* (2006) 47:2218–23. doi: 10.1080/10428190600682688
164. Bingle L, Brown NJ, Lewis CE. The role of tumour-associated macrophages in tumour progression: implications for new anticancer therapies. *J Pathol.* (2002) 196:254–65. doi: 10.1002/path.1027
165. Ries CH, Cannarile MA, Hoves S, Benz J, Wartha K, Runza V, et al. Targeting tumor-associated macrophages with anti-CSF-1R antibody reveals a strategy for cancer therapy. *Cancer Cell.* (2014) 25:846–59. doi: 10.1016/j.ccr.2014.05.016
166. Ruffell B, Chang-Strachan D, Chan V, Rosenbusch A, Ho CM, Pryer N, et al. Macrophage IL-10 blocks CD8+ T cell-dependent responses to chemotherapy by suppressing IL-12 expression in intratumoral dendritic cells. *Cancer Cell.* (2014) 26:623–37. doi: 10.1016/j.ccell.2014.09.006
167. Franklin RA, Liao W, Sarkar A, Kim MV, Bivona MR, Liu K, et al. The cellular and molecular origin of tumor-associated macrophages. *Science.* (2014) 344:921–5. doi: 10.1126/science.1252510
168. Pozzi LA, Maciaszek JW, Rock KL. Both dendritic cells and macrophages can stimulate naive CD8 T cells *in vivo* to proliferate, develop effector function, and differentiate into memory cells. *J Immunol.* (2005) 175:2071–81. doi: 10.4049/jimmunol.175.4.2071

169. Unanue ER. Antigen-presenting function of the macrophage. *Ann Rev Immunol.* (1984) 2:395–428. doi: 10.1146/annurev.iy.02.040184.002143
170. Joseph CG, Darrah E, Shah AA, Skora AD, Casciola-Rosen LA, Wigley FM, et al. Association of the autoimmune disease scleroderma with an immunologic response to cancer. *Science.* (2014) 343:152–7. doi: 10.1126/science.1246886
171. Tsou P, Katayama H, Ostrin EJ, Hanash SM. The Emerging Role of B Cells in Tumor Immunity. *Cancer Res.* (2016) 76:5597–601. doi: 10.1158/0008-5472.CAN-16-0431
172. Yuen GJ, Demissie E, Pillai S. B lymphocytes and cancer: a love-hate relationship. *Trends Cancer.* (2016) 2:747–57. doi: 10.1016/j.trecan.2016.10.010
173. Bekeredjian-Ding IB, Wagner M, Hornung V, Giese T, Schnurr M, Endres S, et al. Plasmacytoid dendritic cells control TLR7 sensitivity of naive B cells via type I IFN. *J Immunol.* (2005) 174:4043–50. doi: 10.4049/jimmunol.174.7.4043
174. Jego G, Palucka AK, Blanck JP, Chalouni C, Pascual V, Banchereau J. Plasmacytoid dendritic cells induce plasma cell differentiation through type I interferon and interleukin 6. *Immunity.* (2003) 19:225–34. doi: 10.1016/S1074-7613(03)00208-5
175. Dubois B, Vanbervliet B, Fayette J, Massacrier C, Van Kooten C, Briere F, et al. Dendritic cells enhance growth and differentiation of CD40-activated B lymphocytes. *J Exp Med.* (1997) 185:941–51. doi: 10.1084/jem.185.5.941
176. Germain C, Gnjatic S, Tamzalit F, Knockaert S, Remark R, Goc J, et al. Presence of B cells in tertiary lymphoid structures is associated with a protective immunity in patients with lung cancer. *Am J Respir Crit Care Med.* (2014) 189:832–44. doi: 10.1164/rccm.201309-1611OC
177. Spranger S, Bao R, Gajewski TF. Melanoma-intrinsic beta-catenin signalling prevents anti-tumour immunity. *Nature.* (2015) 523:231–5. doi: 10.1038/nature14404
178. Liu YJ, Soumelis V, Watanabe N, Ito T, Wang YH, Malefyt Rde W, et al. TSLP: an epithelial cell cytokine that regulates T cell differentiation by conditioning dendritic cell maturation. *Ann Rev Immunol.* (2007) 25:193–219. doi: 10.1146/annurev.immunol.25.022106.141718
179. Cheng JT, Deng YN, Yi HM, Wang GY, Fu BS, Chen WJ, et al. Hepatic carcinoma-associated fibroblasts induce IDO-producing regulatory dendritic cells through IL-6-mediated STAT3 activation. *Oncogenesis.* (2016) 5:e198. doi: 10.1038/oncsis.2016.7
180. Ohshio Y, Teramoto K, Hanaoka J, Tezuka N, Itoh Y, Asai T, et al. Cancer-associated fibroblast-targeted strategy enhances antitumor immune responses in dendritic cell-based vaccine. *Cancer Sci.* (2015) 106:134–42. doi: 10.1111/cas.12584
181. Palucka K, Banchereau J. Dendritic-cell-based therapeutic cancer vaccines. *Immunity.* (2013) 39:38–48. doi: 10.1016/j.immuni.2013.07.004
182. Constantino J, Gomes C, Falcao A, Cruz MT, Neves BM. Antitumor dendritic cell-based vaccines: lessons from 20 years of clinical trials and future perspectives. *Transl Res.* (2016) 168:74–95. doi: 10.1016/j.trsl.2015.07.008
183. Adema GJ, de Vries IJ, Punt CJ, Figdor CG. Migration of dendritic cell based cancer vaccines: *in vivo* veritas? *Curr Opin Immunol.* (2005) 17:170–4. doi: 10.1016/j.coi.2005.01.004

5

Flagellin/NLRC4 Pathway Rescues NLRP3-Inflammasome Defect in Dendritic Cells from HIV-Infected Patients: Perspective for New Adjuvant in Immunocompromised Individuals

Edione Cristina dos Reis[1*], *Vinícius Nunes Cordeiro Leal*[1], *Jaíne Lima da Silva Soares*[1], *Fernanda Pereira Fernandes*[1], *Dhêmerson Souza de Lima*[1], *Bruna Cunha de Alencar*[2] and *Alessandra Pontillo*[1]

[1] *Laboratory of Immunogenetics, Department of Immunology, Institute of Biomedical Sciences/ICB, University of São Paulo/USP, São Paulo, Brazil,* [2] *Laboratory of Immune System Cell Biology, Department of Immunology, Institute of Biomedical Sciences/ICB, University of São Paulo/USP, São Paulo, Brazil*

***Correspondence:**
Edione Cristina dos Reis
edionereis@usp.br

Introduction: NLRP3 inflammasome plays a key role in dendritic cells (DC) activation in response to vaccine adjuvants, however we previously showed that it is not properly activated in DC from HIV-infected patients (HIV-DC), explaining, at least in part, the poor response to immunization of these patients. Taking in account that several cytoplasmic receptors are able to activate inflammasome, and that bacterial components are considered as a novel and efficient adjuvant, we postulated that bacterial flagellin (FLG), a natural ligand of NAIP/NLRC4 inflammasome, could rescue the activation of the complex in HIV-DC.

Objective: Demonstrate that FLG is able to activate monocyte-derived dendritic cells from HIV-infected individuals better than LPS, and to what extent the entity of inflammasome activation differs between DC from HIV-infected patients and healthy donors.

Methods: Monocyte-derived dendritic cells from HIV-infected patients (HIV-DC) and healthy donors (HD-DC) were stimulated with FLG, and inflammasome as well as DC activation (phenotypic profile, cytokine production, autologous lymphocytes activation) were compared. Chemical and genetic inhibitors were used to depict the relative contribution of NLRC4 and NLRP3 in HIV/HD-DC response to FLG.

Results: FLG properly activates HD-DC and HIV-DC. FLG induces higher inflammasome activation than LPS in HIV-DC. FLG acts through NLRC4 and NLRP3 in HD-DC, but at a lesser extent in HIV-DC due to intrinsic NLRP3 defect.

Conclusions: FLG by-passes NLRP3 defect in HIV-DC, through the activation of NAIP/NLRC4 inflammasome, indicating possible future use of the bacterial component as an efficient adjuvant in immunocompromised individuals.

Keywords: dendritic cell, inflammasome, HIV, flagellin, NLRC4, adjuvant

INTRODUCTION

Dendritic cells (DC) are a specialized professional antigen presenting cells (APC) with unique capability to initiate and maintain primary immune responses when pulsed with antigens (1–3). Following recognition of pathogen- or damage-associated molecular patterns (PAMPs or DAMPs, respectively) by innate pattern recognition receptors (PRRs), DC activate and turn into a potent APC. The final differentiation of activated DC is characterized by plasma membrane up-regulation of MHC-II and co-stimulatory molecules (i.e., CD86, CD80), and the production of cytokines important for T CD4$^+$ lymphocytes activation at the immunologic synapsis (i.e., IL-12 and IL-18; and/or IL-1ß; or IL-4). The result of DC activation drives the polarization of T CD4$^+$ lymphocytes, and therefore of the immune response (4).

Successful vaccine preparations have to properly activate DC to induce a long-term memory protective immunity. Together with pathogen' antigens, adjuvants strongly contribute to the effectiveness of a vaccine. Their action is mediated by DC PRRs, such as Toll-like receptors (TLRs) and NACHT and LRR containing receptors (NLRs), through the activation of intracellular pathways leading to the production of cytokines important for T cell activation (5). Alum (aluminum hydroxide), a commonly used adjuvant, activates murine DC through the induction of the NLR-containing a PYD domain 3 (NLRP3) and the consequent mounting of the cytoplasmic complex, known as inflammasome, which results in caspase-1 activation and IL-1ß and IL-18 production. The absence of NLRP3 results in the loss of adjuvant responsivity (6), emphasizing the central role of inflammasome in the activation of DC and in the induction of an efficient immune response.

Accordingly, recent findings have reported that individuals with a low response to vaccines, such infants (7) or cancer patients (8) present a substantial alteration in inflammasome expression and/or activity.

Immune response to many current vaccines is known to be impaired and/or less effective in chronically HIV-infected individuals (9). This impairment has been associated to both a reduced frequency of DC (10, 11), together with phenotypic and functional alterations of these cells (12). As HIV-infected patients present well-documented DC impairment, it has been proposed that a poor response to vaccination could be caused by a diminished and/or defective response to common adjuvants (13).

We have previously demonstrated that NLRP3 inflammasome is not correctly activated by bacterial lipopolysaccharide (LPS) in monocyte-derived dendritic cells (MDDC) from HIV-infected patients (HIV-DC) (14), possibly as a result of the HIV-associated chronic inflammation and the consequent immune system exhaustion (15). As NLRP3 inflammasome is involved in the activation of DC by vaccine adjuvants (6, 16), the defect observed in NLRP3 inflammasome possibly contributes to the less extend immunization response in HIV-infected individuals.

To counteract the low immune response, new vaccination strategies have been proposed, such as the use of PRRs agonists, such as LPS or flagellin (FLG), as largely reviewed in (17).

FLG is the main component of a bacterial flagellum, and it is recognized extracellularly by TLR5 inducing a Myd88 signaling and promoting the transcription of NF-κB-related genes (18, 19); and by the intracellular receptors, NLR-containing a BIR domain (NAIP) and NLR-containing a CARD domain (NLRC)-4. NAIP directly binds FLG, while NLRC4 recognizes the NAIP:FLG complex and mounts the NAIP/NLRC4 inflammasome, resulting in IL-1ß and IL-18 production (20–22).

FLG has already been used as an adjuvant in a number of clinical trials of healthy individuals (23, 24), however to our knowledge none or poor data are available about its ability to activate MDDC in both healthy or immuno-compromised individuals via NAIP/NLRC4 inflammasome.

Taking in account the key role of the inflammasome in proper DC activation, and the impairment of NLRP3 activation observed in HIV-DC, we hypothesize that FLG could represent an alternative adjuvant for HIV-infected patients, by activating inflammasome in DC through NAIP and NLRC4 receptors, and in this way by-passing the NLRP3 defect. Therefore, the aim of this study was to demonstrate that FLG is able to activate MDDC from HIV-infected individuals better than LPS, and to what extent the entity of inflammasome activation differs between HIV-DC and HD-DC.

MATERIALS AND METHODS

HIV-Infected Patients

Twenty-seven HIV-infected adults patients (16 males/11 females; 51.9 ± 11.7 years), proceeding from the metropolitan area of São Paulo (SP, Brazil), seropositive for at least 5 years (26.9 ± 16.9 years), in antiretroviral therapy (ART), with blood CD4$^+$ T cells count >500 cells/μl, without clinical AIDS or other chronic diseases (i.e., neoplasias, cardiovascular disease, autoimmune disease, kidney disease, obesity) or infectious diseases (i.e., human T-lymphotropic virus/HTLV, hepatitis B or hepatitis C virus), were recruited from January 2016 to May 2018 at the "Serviço de Extensão ao Atendimento de Pacientes HIV/AIDS" (SEAP) of the Faculty of Medicine, University of São Paulo (São Paulo, SP, Brazil). Fifty milliliter of the peripheral blood was collected in heparin tubes. All volunteers assigned the informed consent approved by the Institutional Ethical Committee. Patients' main characteristics are summarized in **Table 1**.

Healthy Donors (HD)

Twenty-seven adults (15 males/12 females; 45.5 ± 13.4 years), proceeding from the metropolitan area of São Paulo (SP, Brazil), without clinical HIV or other chronic or infectious diseases, were recruited at the Blood Bank Service of the Hospital "Oswaldo Cruz" (São Paulo, SP, Brazil). Fifty milliliter of the peripheral blood was collected in heparin tubes. All volunteers assigned the informed consent approved by the Hospital Ethical Committee. HD demographic data were included in **Table 1**. Of note, any significant difference exists in gender ratio (Fisher test $p > 0.05$) or age mean value (t- test $p > 0.05$) between HD and HIV-infected patients.

TABLE 1 | Main characteristics of healthy donors and HIV-infected patients.

	HD (n = 27)	HIV (n = 27)
Gender (M/F), n	15/12	16/11
Age (years), mean ± SD	45.5 ± 13.4	51.9 ± 11.7
Time from diagnosis (years), mean ± SD		26.9 ± 16.9
PVL* (log RNA copies/μL), mean ± SD		1.77 ± 0.37
PVL^0 (log RNA copies/μL), mean ± SD		4.00 ± 1.02
PVL^1 (log RNA copies/μL), mean ± SD		2.25 ± 0.77
$CD4^+$ T* (cells/μL), mean ± SD		768.9 ± 283.1
$CD4^+$ T^0 (cells/μL), mean ± SD		377.5 ± 389.9
$CD4^+$ T^1 (cells/μL), mean ± SD		679.0 ± 252.7

Gender and age are reported for healthy donors (HD) and HIV-infected patients (HIV). Time from HIV-1 diagnosis as well as plasma viral load (PVL) and $CD4^+$ T cells counts at the time of blood collection (*), before (^{0}) and after (^{1}) the start of anti-retroviral therapy (ART) were included for HIV-infected patients. The detection limit of PVL was 1.70 log HIV-1 RNA copies/ml. M, males; F, females; n, number of individuals; SD, standard deviation.

Human Monocyte-Derived Dendritic Cells (MDDC)

Mononuclear cells were isolated from 50 mL of peripheral blood by Ficoll-Hypaque (GE Healthcare) density gradient, and monocytes were separated from lymphocytes by plastic adherence. Briefly, 4 × 10^6 mononuclear cells/well were incubated in 24-wells culture plates (Corning-Costar). After 2 h, non-adherent cells (mainly lymphocytes) were removed and cryopreserved at −80°C for co-culture assays, while adherent cells (mainly monocytes) were cultured with 50 ng/mL GM-CSF (Peprotech) and 50 ng/mL IL-4 (Peprotech) in RPMI-1640 (Gibco, Thermo Fisher Scientific) supplemented with 10% of fetal bovine serum (FBS; Gibco) at 37°C in 5% CO_2 for 5 days (25). Monocytes-to-DC differentiation was confirmed by flow cytometry analysis of CD14 and CD11c surface markers (**Supplementary File 1**).

MDDC (HIV-DC or HD-DC) were stimulated with purified 5 μg/mL FLG from S. *typhimurium* (FLA-ST, Invivogen) or 1 μg/mL LPS from E. *coli* (Sigma-Aldrich, Merck) for 3, 8, 18, and 24 h and 1 mM ATP was added for more 15 min (26). In some experiments, MDDC were pre-incubated with 10 μg/mL MCC-950 (Invivogen), a specific NLRP3 inhibitor (27), or 10 μM parthenolide (PTD; Sigma-Aldrich, Merck), a NF-κB and caspases inhibitor (28); or with 1,000 UI/mL IFN-α-2b (Schering-Plough) for 18 h (29, 30). Cell supernatants were collected for cytokines measurement. MDDC were used for cytometric assays or RNA isolation and genes expression analysis.

To assess MDDC ability to activate $CD4^+$ T lymphocytes, 0.4 × 10^5 MDDC were distributed in 96-well U-bottom suspension culture plates with 4.0 × 10^5 autologous lymphocytes (cryopreserved non-adherent peripheral blood mononuclear cells) (co-culture MDDC/lymphocytes ratio: 1/10) in duplicates and cultured in the presence of unspecific (not antigen-specific) stimuli for 96 or 120 h to measure IFN-γ production and lymphocytes proliferation, respectively. Lymphocytes alone were used as a negative control (Neg).

MDDC Phenotype Analysis

2 × 10^5 DC/mL were incubated in Phosphate Buffer Saline (PBS; Sigma-Aldrich, Merck) with the optimal dilution of anti-CD14 PE (MEM15; Exbio), anti-CD11c (3.9; Biolegend), anti-HLA-DR V500 (G46-6; BD Biosciences), anti-CD86 PE-cy7 (2331/FUN-1, B), and anti-CD40 Horizon 450 (5C3; BD Biosciences) antibodies for 20 min at 4°C. Cells were then washed twice with PBS and resuspended in 200 μL of 4% Formaldehyde-PBS. The Live/Dead Fixable Cell Stain Kit (Life Technology, Thermo Fisher Scientific) was added to the assay according to the manufacturer's instructions. A minimum of 50,000 events was acquired on a LSRFortessa™ X-20 flow cytometer (BD Biosciences) using the FACS Diva software (BD Biosciences). Data were analyzed using the FlowJo software (Tree Star). The gates strategy for one representative experiment was reported in **Supplementary File 2**.

$CD4^+$ T Lymphocytes Activation Assay

$CD4^+$ T lymphocytes activation was measured by the meaning of intracellular staining of IFN-γ. Briefly, autologous co-cultures of MDDC and lymphocytes were treated with lymphocyte mitogens Ionomycin (1 μg/mL; Sigma-Aldrich, Merck) and Phorbol Myristate Acetate (10 ng/mL; Sigma-Aldrich, Merck) for 96 h (31). Twenty microgram per milliliter Brefeldin A (Sigma-Aldrich, Merck) was added 6 h before the end of co-culture to block Golgi secretory pathway. Cells were then labeled for surface marker anti-CD3 APC (MEM-57) and anti-CD4 PE (RPAT4) (BD Biosciences), permeabilized with Cytofix/Cytoperm solution (BD Biosciences), and finally stained for anti-IFN-γ V450 (B27; BD Biosciences). The Live/Dead Fixable Cell Stain Kit was added to the assay according to the manufacturer's instructions. Cells were then washed twice with PBS and resuspended in 200 μL of 4% Formaldehyde-PBS to proceed to flow cytometry analysis as above-mentioned.

$CD4^+$ T Lymphocytes Proliferation Assay

The CFSE Cell Division Tracker Kit (Biolegend) was used for flow cytometry analysis of *in vitro* $CD4^+$ T cells proliferation assay according to manufacturers' protocol. Briefly, autologous lymphocytes were pre-treated with 0.1 μM CFSE before being added to MDDC cultures in the presence of the lymphocyte mitogen Concanavalin A (5 μg/mL; Sigma Aldrich, Merck) for 120 h (32). At the end of assay, cells were then labeled for anti-CD3 APC (MEM-57) and anti-CD4 PE (RPAT4) (BD Biosciences). The Live/Dead Fixable Cell Stain Kit was added to the assay according to the manufacturer's instructions. Cells were then washed twice with PBS and resuspended in 200 μL of 4% Formaldehyde-PBS to proceed to flow cytometry analysis as above-mentioned.

Cytokines Measurement in Culture Supernatants

IL-1β, IL-18, TNF-α, and IL-12p70 were measured in MDDC culture supernatants by ELISA according to the manufacturers' protocols (Biolegend for IL-1β; IL-18, TNF; eBioscience for IL12p70). Data were reported as pg/mL.

Caspase-1 Activity Assay

The detection of caspase-1 activity in MDDC was measured with the FAM FLICA Caspase-1 Assay Kit (Immunochemistry Technologies) and flow cytometry according to the manufacturer's protocol. Briefly, 10 μL 30x FLICA was added to 2 × 10^5 MDDC in 300 mL and cells incubated for 1 h at 37°C 5% CO_2. The Live/Dead Fixable Cell Stain Kit was used. Cells were then washed twice with PBS and resuspended in 200 μL of 4% Formaldehyde-PBS to proceed to flow cytometer analysis as above-mentioned. Live MDDC were gated based on their forward (FSC) and side light scatter (SSC). Histograms for one representative experiment was reported in **Supplementary File 3**.

Inflammasome Genes Expression Analysis

Total RNA was isolated from 2 × 10^5 MDDC using the RNAqueous-Micro kit (Ambion, Thermo Fisher Scientific) according to manufacturer's protocol and quantified using Nanodrop N-1000 (Agilent). 0.5 μg of total RNA was converted into cDNA using Superscript III RT kit and random primers (Invitrogen, Thermo Fisher Scientific). *NLRP1* (hs00248187), *NLRP3* (hs00366465), *NAIP* (hs03037952), *NLRC4* (hs00368367), *CASP1* (hs00354836), *IL1B* (hs01555410), *IL18* (hs01038788), *CARD8* (hs01088221), *BRCC3* (hs02386484), and *NEDD8* (hs01921826) genes were amplified using TaqMan® gene-specific assays (Applied Biosystems, Thermo Fisher Scientific) and qPCR on the QuantStudio 3.0 Real-Time PCR equipment (Applied Biosystems, Thermo Fisher Scientific). The QuantStudio 3.0 software was used to obtain cycle threshold values (Ct) for relative gene expression analysis according to Fold Change (FC) method (33). Raw expression data (Ct) were normalized with the expression of the housekeeping gene glyceraldehyde-3-phosphate dehydrogenase/*GAPDH* (hs02758991; TaqMan® assay) (ΔCt), and the FC was calculated comparing stimulated and unstimulated (UN) conditions ($FC = 2^{-\Delta\Delta Ct}$; $\Delta\Delta Ct = \Delta Ct_{stimulated} - \Delta Ct_{UN}$). Alternatively, the basal (constitutive) gene expression was calculated as $2^{-\Delta Ct}$.

miR-223 Expression Analysis

Total RNA was isolated from 2 × 10^5 MDDC by mirVana™ miRNA Isolation Kit (Ambion, Thermo Fisher Scientific) according to the manufacturer's instructions. 0.5 μg of total RNA were converted into cDNA using kit TaqMan™ MicroRNA Reverse Transcription and miRNA-specific primers (Applied Biosystems, Thermo Fisher Scientific). miR-223 was amplified using TaqMan® miR-specific assays (*TM:002098*; Applied Biosystems, Thermo Fisher Scientific) and qPCR on the QuantStudio 3.0 Real-Time PCR equipment. The QuantStudio 3.0 software was used to obtain cycle threshold values (Ct) for relative gene expression analysis according to Fold Change (FC) method (33). Raw expression data (Ct) were normalized with the expression of and non-coding small RNA control U6 (*TM:001973*; TaqMan® assay) (ΔCt), and the FC was calculated comparing stimulated and unstimulated (UN) conditions ($FC=2^{-\Delta\Delta Ct}$; $\Delta\Delta Ct= \Delta Ct_{stimulated} - \Delta Ct_{UN}$). Alternatively, the basal (constitutive) gene expression was calculated as $2^{-\Delta Ct}$.

Detection of "Specks" Formation

Detection of inflammasome "specks" formation was performed by confocal microscopy and immunofluorescence, as previously described (34). Briefly, 2 × 10^5 MDDC were cultured in 16-wells chamber slides (Thermo Fisher Scientific) and stimulated with 5 μg/mL FLG or 1 μg/mL LPS for 24 h at 37°C 5% CO_2 with or without 1 mM ATP. Cells were then fixed and permeabilized with Cytofix/Cytoperm reagent (BD Biosciences) for 30 min at 37°C 5% CO_2, and incubated with primary antibody for NLRP3 (1:100 mouse anti-human NLRP3, Abcam) and/or NLRC4 (1:200 rabbit anti-human NLRC4; Biolegend) overnight at room temperature. Fluorescent secondary antibodies (Alexa 488-conjugated goat-anti-mouse IgG1, or Alexa 647-conjugated goat-anti-rabbit IgG1; Biolegend) were then added for 1 h. Finally, cells were washed and fixed to image acquisition at DMi8 confocal laser scanning microscope (Leica). 4′,6-Diamidine-2′-phenylindole dihydrochloride (DAPI; Sigma-Aldrich, Merck) was used for nuclear counterstaining. ImageJ software and related plugins (National Institutes of Health) were used for image processing. The counting of NLRP3+ and NLRC4+ specks in MDDC was performed manually by observing specks formation within the cells (34), and through the ImageJ software by calculating the corrected total cellular fluorescence (CTCF) for each marker as integrated density–(area of selected cell × mean fluorescence of background readings) (35).

NLRC4 and *NLRP3* Silencing

Pre-validated shRNA for human *NLRC4* and *NLRP3* was obtained from MISSION® shRNA Plasmid DNA (Sigma-Aldrich, Merck). The shRNAs for NLRP3 and NLRC4 used in the study are listed in **Supplementary File 4**. 2 × 10^5 MDDC were transduced using with the same amounts of lentiviral particles encoding non-targeting control or gene-specific shRNA in the presence of SIV3+ VLP for 48 h. Thereafter, cells were treated with 5 μg/mL FLG or 1 μg/mL LPS for 24 h. The shRNA knockdown efficiency of the target protein in lentivirus-transduced cells was assessed by gene expression (**Supplementary File 5**). The concentrations of IL-1β in cell culture supernatants was measured by ELISA.

Data Analysis

All data were collected and analyzed from at least three independent experiments. Normality test was applied to the data, and parametric or non-parametric analysis was used accordingly to compare two or more data sets as specified for each graph. The level of significance was $p < 0.05$. Calculations were performed using the statistical software package GraphPad Prism 7.0.

Biosecurity and Institutional Safety Procedures

All research was performed following the guidelines of biosecurity and safety of Institute of Biomedical Science (ICB/USP).

RESULTS

Flagellin Similarly Activates MDDC From HIV-Infected Patients and Healthy Donors

MDDC were treated with 5 μg/mL FLG for 24 h and phenotypic profile, TNF and IL-12 secretion as well as $CD4^+$ T lymphocytes activation in co-culture experiments were assessed based on previously published protocols (31, 32).

FLG activates MDDC, both HIV-DC and HD-DC, as indicated by the increase of co-stimulatory molecules, cytokines release and $CD4^+$ T lymphocytes activation (**Figure 1**).

As expected, FLG induced the up-regulation of HLA-DR (95.83 ± 0.68 % positive cells) compared to untreated cells (UN: 77.5 ± 4.4 % positive cells) and the significant increase of CD40 (FLG: 39.8 ± 3.7 %, vs. UN: 7.8 ± 2.0 % positive cells; $p = 3 \times 10^{-5}$) in HD-DC, but not of CD86, which appeared to be decreased in HD-DC+FLG compared to untreated cells (FLG: 62.8 ± 4.3 %, vs. UN: 91.1 ± 2.9 % positive cells; $p = 0.001$) (**Figure 1A**). However, this result could be due to a previously reported positive feedback mechanism and not to a negative effect of FLG (36). A significant augment of HLA-DR (FLG: 83.5 ± 6.1 %, vs. UN: 49.2 ± 9.5 % positive cells; $p = 0.006$) and CD40 (FLG: 48.7 ± 5.4 %, vs. UN: 17.4 ± 1.7 % positive cells; $p = 0.020$) was observed in HIV-DC challenged with FLG. The expression of CD86 did not change in treated or untreated cells (**Figure 1A**).

It is interesting to emphasize that the entity of surface markers expression did not significantly differ between HIV-DC and HD-DC in both untreated or treated conditions (**Figure 1A**). Even if we observed lower viability in HIV-DC compared to HD-DC, this difference did not result statistically significant ($p > 0.999$).

FLG induced the secretion of a good and similar amount of TNF in HD-DC and HIV-DC ($p < 0.05$) (**Figure 1B**). On the other hand, the production of IL-12 differs between HD-DC and HIV-DC ($p = 0.029$): while HD-DC produced significant level of IL-12 in response to the molecular pattern (FLG: 212.7 ± 53.1 pg/mL, vs. UN: 50.5 ± 2.9 pg/mL; $p = 7 \times 10^{-4}$), the induction of cytokine appeared to be less pronounced in HIV-DC (FLG: 63.9 ± 6.9 pg/mL, vs. UN: 38.2 ± 12.1 pg/mL; $p > 0.05$) (**Figure 1C**).

Altogether these data indicate that FLG is able to activate HIV-DC in a similar way to that seen for HD-DC.

To test whether FLG-treated MDDC are able to induce a properly adaptive immunity response, a MDDC/lymphocytes co-culture assay was performed using autologous cells as previously described (31, 32). Lymphocytes alone were used as a negative control (Neg) (**Figures 1D,E**).

A significant increment of IFN-γ^+ $CD4^+$ T cells was observed in healthy donors (FLG: 12.9 ± 5.5 % vs. UN: 1.3 ± 0.4 % positive cells; $p = 0.022$) as well as in HIV-infected individuals (FLG: 9.6 ± 1.8 % vs. UN: 0.1 ± 0.1 % positive cells; $p = 0.014$). Of note, the percentage of IFN-γ^+ $CD4^+$ T cells after FLG treatment was similar in healthy donor and patients ($p > 0.999$). Negative control resulted similar to untreated co-cultures ($p > 0.05$) (**Figure 1D**), emphasizing that the increasing percentage of positive cells is not an artifact.

Moreover, FLG-treated MDDC were able to induce a significant proliferation of $CD4^+$ T lymphocytes in healthy donors (FLG: 51.0 ± 12.1 %, vs. UN: 3.7 ± 0.9 % positive cells; $p = 0.026$) and patients (FLG: 24.3 ± 2.8 %, vs. UN: 3.5 ± 0.8 % positive cells; $p = 0.038$), even if in a lesser extent in patients compared to HD ($p = 0.004$). Negative control presented a proliferation rate similar to untreated co-cultures ($p > 0.05$) (**Figure 1E**).

It is interesting to underline that the limited percentage of positive cells in this type of assay is in accord with previously published data for autologous MDDC and T cells co-culture both in healthy donors (32) and even in HIV-infected patients (31) treated with unspecific stimuli (mitogens). Moreover, despite its limited entity, the activation of lymphocytes is consequence of MDDC stimulation as in the absence of MDDC (negative control) mitogens cannot activate T cells (**Figures 1D,E**).

Taking in account the activation status of FLG-treated HIV-DC (**Figures 1A–C**) together with their ability to induce lymphocytes activation (**Figures 1D,E**), we clearly demonstrated that FLG is able to activate HIV-DC similarly to what observed for HD-DC. It is interesting to emphasize that, on the contrary, we have previously shown that HIV-DC did not properly respond to bacterial LPS (14).

Flagellin, but Not LPS, Induces Comparable Inflammasome Activation in MDDC From HIV-Infected Patients and Healthy Donors

We then investigated the ability of flagellin to stimulate inflammasome in MDDC by the meaning of inflammasome cytokines production and caspase-1 activity. LPS alone or in combination with ATP was added to the assay as a positive control for inflammasome or NLRP3 inflammasome activation, respectively (26) (**Figure 2**). A time-course assay treating MDDC with 5 μg/mL FLG or 1 μg/mL LPS was performed to determine the best experimental time for IL-1ß detection in this model, (**Supplementary File 6**), and selected 24 h for all the experiments.

FLG induced a significant IL-1ß release in HD-DC (155.3 ± 20.7 pg/mL), compared to unstimulated cells (4.0 ± 1.9 pg/mL; $p < 0.0001$) and similarly to LPS (132.4 ± 9.9 pg/mL; $p < 0.0001$). The treatment with LPS+ATP resulted in a significant increase of IL-1ß release compared to LPS ($p = 0.002$), indicating a proper response of NLRP3 inflammasome in HD-DC (**Figure 2A**).

In HIV-DC, the entity of IL-1ß production resulted lower than in HD-DC but significantly augmented compared to resting cells (FLG: 121.3 ± 34.3 pg/mL, vs. UN: 18.3 ± 9.3 pg/mL; $p = 2 \times 10^{-4}$) and also to LPS-treated cells (84.4 ± 17.5 pg/mL; $p = 0.002$). However, ATP did not alter LPS-induced IL-1ß production ($p > 0.05$) (**Figure 2A**), confirming the previously observed dysregulation of NLRP3 inflammasome in MDDC from HIV-infected patients (14).

In a similar way, FLG also induced significantly IL-18 release in HD-DC (FLG: 91.1 ± 19.3 pg/mL, vs. UN: 12.8 ± 6.1 pg/mL; $p = 0.018$) and at lower extent in HIV-DC (FLG: 50.5 ± 5.6 pg/mL, vs. UN: 2.9 ± 1.5 pg/mL; $p = 0.009$). HD-DC better respond to LPS and LPS+ATP than HIV-DC also in term of IL-18. There

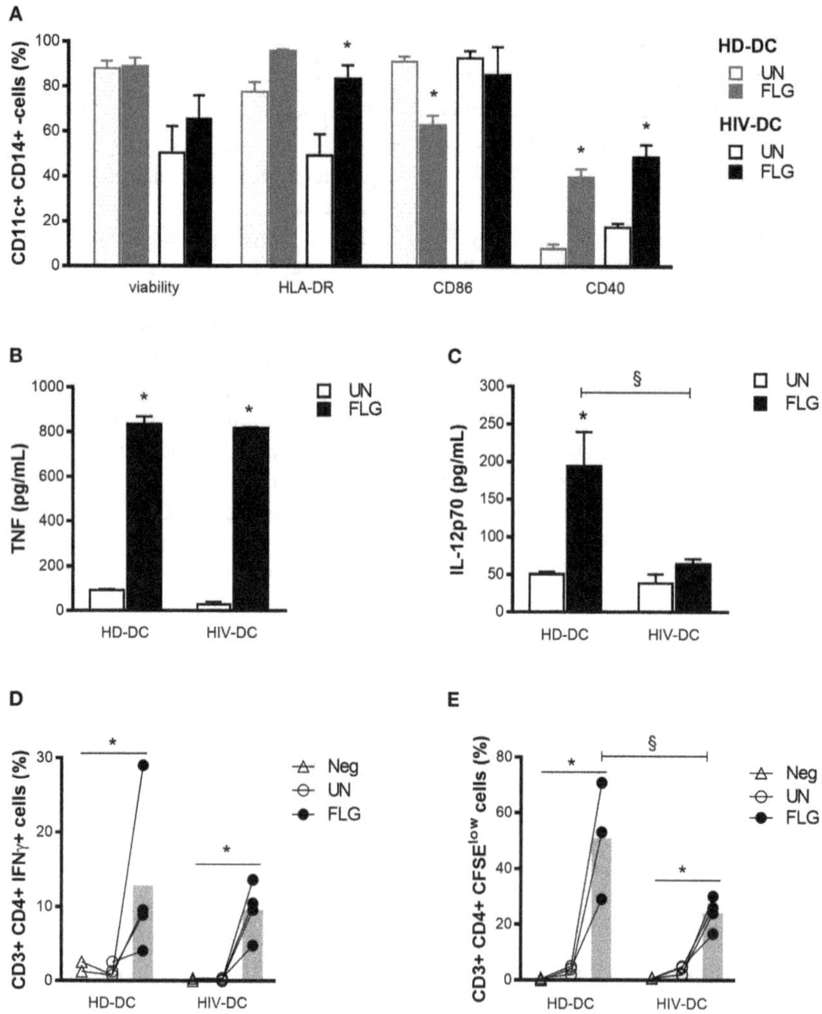

FIGURE 1 | Flagellin similarly activates HIV-DC and HD-DC. 2×10^5 MDDC from healthy donors (HD-DC; $n = 5$) and HIV-infected patients (HIV-DC; $n = 5$) were stimulated with 5 μg/ml flagellin (FLG) for 24 hours. Viability, expression of characteristic DC surface markers **(A)** as well as TNF **(B)** and IL-12p70 **(C)** secretion were analyzed and compared between untreated (UN) and stimulated (FLG) conditions as well between HD-DC and HIV-DC groups 0.4×10^5 FLG-treated MDDC were cultured with 4×10^5 autologous lymphocytes (MDDC/lymphocytes ratio: 1/0) for 96 hours to detect IFN-γ production in $CD4^+$ T lymphocytes (percentage of $CD3^+$ $CD4^+$ T IFN-γ^+ cells) **(D)**, or 120 hours to measure $CD4^+$ T lymphocytes proliferation (percentage of $CD3^+$ $CD4^+$ T $CSFE^{low}$ cells) **(E)**. Lymphocytes alone were used as a negative control (Neg). Data are reported as mean ± standard error. Multiple *t*-test **(A)** and Two-Way ANOVA test **(B–E)** were applied to compare conditions within a group (HIV-DC or HD-DC; $^*p < 0.05$) and between groups (HIV-DC vs. HD-DC; $^§p < 0.05$).

were no statistical differences in the production of IL-18 between HD- and HIV-DC (**Figure 2B**).

Inflammasome cytokines release revealed that FLG is able to induce complex activation in MDDC from healthy as well as HIV-infected individuals. Accordingly, FLG increased caspase-1 activity in HD-DC (FLG: 6.8 ± 2.0 %, vs. UN: 0.3 ± 0.0 % positive cells) and in HIV-DC (FLG: 6.9 ± 0.7 %, vs. UN: 3.5 ± 0.5 % positive cells). HIV-DC presented a constitutively activated caspase-1, however a lower activation in response to LPS+ATP compared to HD-DC, once more emphasizing the specific dysregulation of NLRP3 pathway (**Figure 2C**). Even if these differences did not reach statistical significance ($p = 0.07$), we underline that caspase-1 activity accompanies above-mentioned cytokines data, and that this is the first study showing a tendency in caspase-1 activation defect in MDDC from HIV-infected individuals. Although other studies have reported statistically significant differences in caspase-1 activity in healthy donors and HIV-infected patients, those results referred to lymphoid compartment or peripheral blood mononuclear cells, while little is known in myeloid cells (37–40).

Flagellin Induces Inflammasome Activation by Stimulated NAIP/NLRC4 and NLRP3 Receptors in HD-DC, but Not in HIV-DC

Once assessed that FLG is able to induce inflammasome activation in MDDC, we therefore tried to depict the pathways involved in complex formation and to detect any differences between HD-DC and HIV-DC.

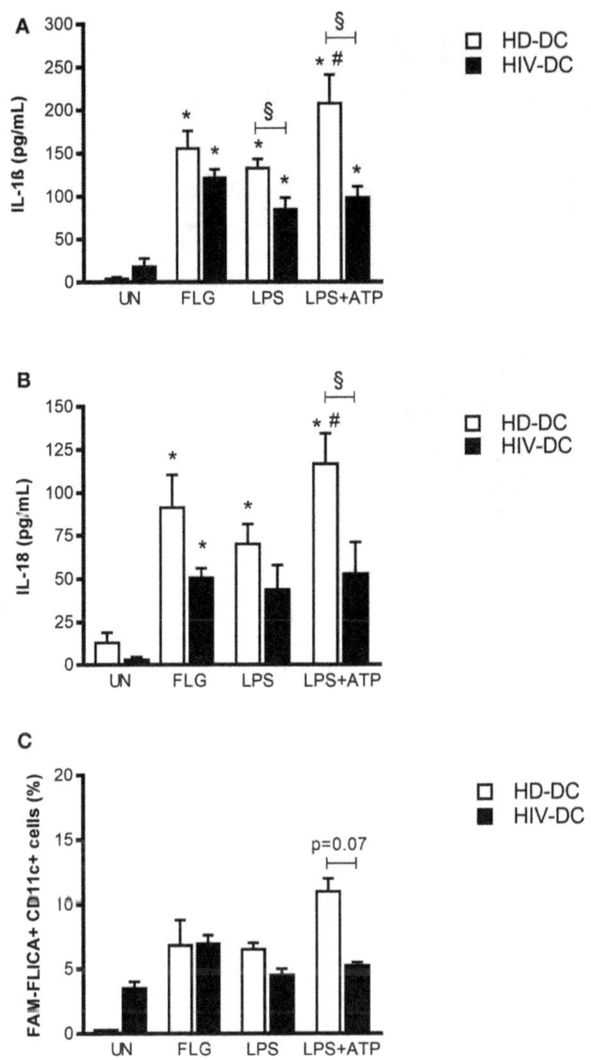

FIGURE 2 | Flagellin induces better inflammasome activation in HIV-DC than LPS. 2 × 10^5 MDDC from healthy donors (HD-DC; $n = 20$) or HIV-infected patients (HIV-DC; $n = 20$) were stimulated with 5 μg/mL flagellin (FLG) for 24 hours. 1 μg/mL LPS for 24 hours, or 1 μg/mL LPS for 24 hours plus 1 mM ATP for more 15 minutes were used as positive control for the activation of inflammasome and NLRP3 inflammasome, respectively. Culture supernatants were used to measure IL-1β **(A)** and IL-18 **(B)** concentration (pg/mL). Cells were harvested for analysis of caspase-1 activity by FAM-FLICA assay and flow cytometry. Percentage of FAM-FLICA+CD11c$^+$ cells were reported for FLG-treated (FLG) and untreated (UN) MDDC **(C)**. Data are represented as mean ± standard error. Two-Way ANOVA test was applied to compare conditions within a group (HIV-DC or HD-DC; *$p < 0.05$; LPS+ATP vs. LPS: #$p < 0.05$) and between groups (HIV-DC vs. HD-DC; $^{§}p < 0.05$).

Gene expression analysis revealed that HIV-DC presents a significant higher constitutive expression of *IL1B* and *IL18* compared to HD-DC. *NLRP3* also resulted increased even if not in a statistically significant way, while the level of *NAIP* and *NLRC4* was similar between MDDC (**Figure 3A**).

When the effect of flagellin was evaluated in genes modulation, we observed a revealed a different expression profile in HD-DC and HIV-DC at all the analyzed time-points (3, 8, 18, and 24 h) (**Figure 3B**).

In particular, we focused our attention on the two receptors *NLRP3* and *NLRC4*. While, as expected, FLG induces NLRC4 gene modulation in HD-DC and HIV-DC (**Figure 3C**), NLRP3 appeared to be defective in HIV-DC, as FLG was able to induce NLRP3 expression in HD, but not in HIV-DC (**Figure 3D**), according to our previously published data (14).

The dysregulation observed for NLRP3 could be due to an imbalance of inhibitor and activator signals. NLRP3 is tightly regulated by endogenous proteins CARD8 (41), BRCC3 (42) and NEDD8 (43), and by miR-223 (44). Interestingly, the basal expression of *CARD8* and *BRCC3*, as well as of miR-223, resulted significantly augmented in HIV-DC compared to HD-DC (**Figure 3E**), suggesting a possible cause of low responsiveness of NLRP3. Moreover, taking in account that IFN-I also contributes to the negative regulation of NLRP3 (29, 30) and that HIV-infected patients are known to present high level of circulating IFN-I (45–47), we shown that the treatment of HD-DC with IFN-a significantly reduced IL-1ß release specifically in LPS+ATP treated cells up to cytokine level observed in HIV-DC (**Figure 3F**), emphasizing the inhibitory role of IFN-I on NLRP3 and suggesting that this could be another cause of a specific NLRP3 defect in HIV-DC.

According to our initial hypothesis, flagellin appears to be able to by-pass this defect of NLRP3 in HIV-DC, and at the same time our results have shown the involvement of both NLRC4 and NLRP3 receptors in HD-DC response to flagellin.

This hypothesis of a "two-receptors" mechanism is supported also by inflammasome "specks" detection through immunofluorescence staining of NLRP3 and NLRC4 (**Figure 4**). NLRC4+ specks were evidenced in confocal imagines of FLG-treated HD-DC (**Figure 4A**) and HIV-DC (**Figure 4B**). NLRP3+ specks resulted more in FLG-treated HD-DC (**Figure 4A**) than in HIV-DC (**Figure 4B**). In general NLRC4 and NLRP3 staining localized in the same cells. By the use of CTCF index, we showed that FLG significantly induced both NLRC4+ and NLRP3+ specks in HD-DC (FLG vs. UN: $p < 0.0001$) (**Figure 4C**). On the other hands, in HIV-DC FLG induced preferentially NLRC4+ specks (CTCF FLG vs. UN: $p = 0.0001$) and at lesser extent NLRP3+ specks ($p > 0.05$) (**Figure 4D**). These findings demonstrated that in healthy donor cells, FLG not only activates inflammasome through the expected NAIP/NLRC4 pathway but also through the NLRP3 one.

To better investigate the involvement of NAIP/NLRC4 and NLRP3 in response to FLG in our model, we evaluated the IL-1ß production in FLG-treated MDDC previously incubated with 10 μM MCC-950, a specific NLRP3 inhibitor (27), or with 10 μM parthenolide/PTD, a large spectrum inflammasome inhibitor (28) (**Figures 5A,B**).

MCC-950 and PTD significantly inhibited IL-1ß production in FLG-treated HD-DC (78 and 90% of inhibition, respectively; $p < 0.05$), as well as LPS+ATP-treated cells (78 and 90% of inhibition, respectively; $p < 0.05$), and partially LPS-induced inflammasome activation (78 and 90% of inhibition, respectively; $p < 0.05$) (**Figure 5A**), due to the contribution of other pathway in inflammasome activation by LPS (48).

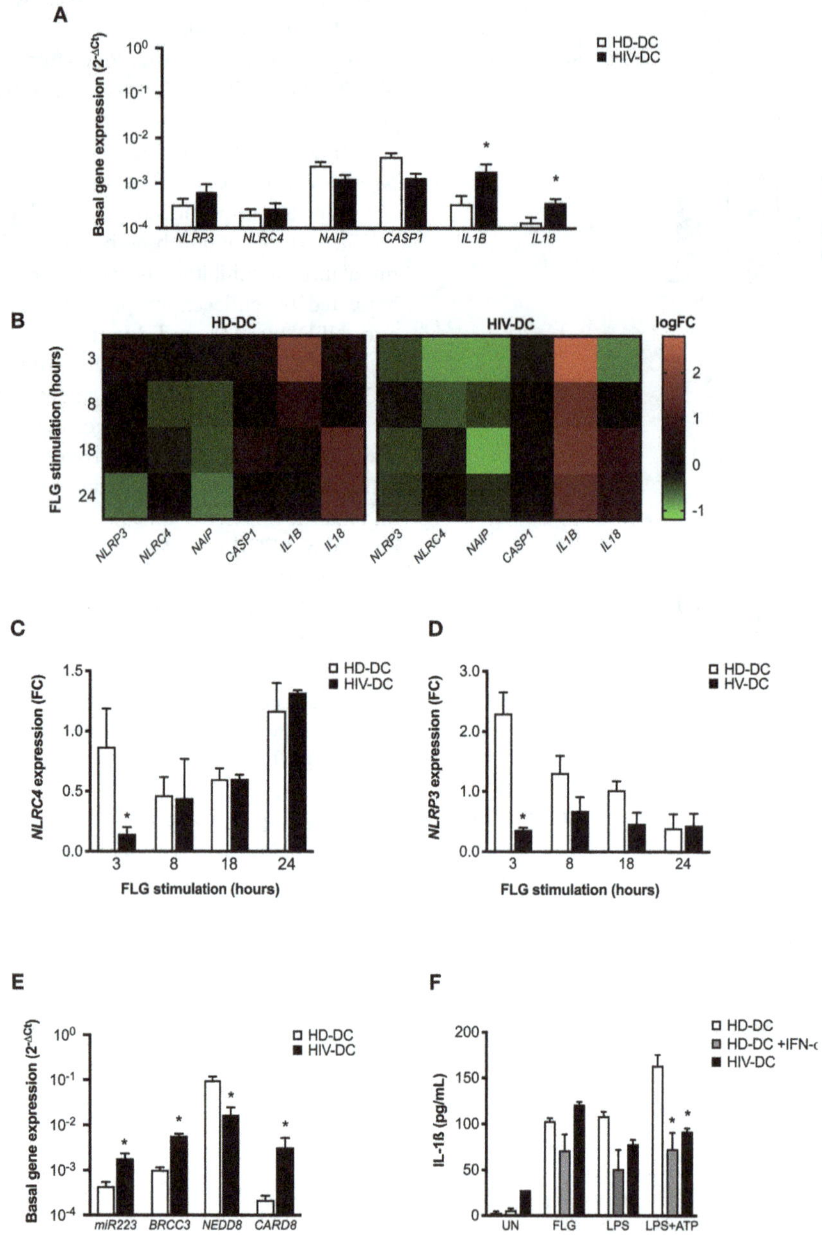

FIGURE 3 | NLRC4 and NLRP3 are differentially involved in flagellin activation in HD-DC and HIV-DC. 2 × 10^5 MDDC from healthy donors (HD-DC; $n = 5$) or HIV-infected patients (HIV-DC; $n = 5$) were stimulated with 5 μg/ml flagellin (FLG) for 3, 8, 18, and 24 hours. Cells were harvested for total RNA isolation and evaluation of relative gene expression by qPCR **(A–E)**. **(A)** Basal gene expression of *NLRP3, NAIP, NLRC4, CASP1, IL18,* and *IL1B* was expressed as $2^{-\Delta Ct}$. **(B)** FLG-induced expression of *NLRP1, NLRP3, NLRC4, NAIP, CASP1, IL1B,* and *IL18* genes was calculated as $2^{-\Delta\Delta Ct}$ (fold-change, FC) and reported as logFC in a heat-map graph for HD-DC and HIV-DC. **(C)** FC values for *NLRC4* are compared between HD-DC and HIV-DC at all the time-points. **(D)** FC values for *NLRP3* are compared between HD-DC and HIV-DC at all the time-points. **(E)** Basal gene expression of *miR223, BRCC3, NEDD8,* and *CARD8* was expressed as $2^{-\Delta Ct}$. **(F)** 2 × 10^5 MDDC from healthy donors (HD-DC; $n = 3$) were pre-treated with 1,000 UI/mL of IFN-α-2b (Schering-Plough) for 18 h and then with 5 μg/ml flagellin (FLG) or LPS 1 μg/mL LPS for 24 hours, or 1 μg/mL LPS for 24 hours plus 1 mM ATP for more 15 minutes. IL-1ß concentration was measured in culture supernatants of HD-DC with and without IFN-α-2b pre-treatment and compared with HIV-DC ($n = 3$) stimulated with FLG. Data are represented as mean ± standard error. Multiple *t*-test was applied to compare HD- and HIV-DC in **(A,C–E)**. Kruskall-Wallis test was applied to compare HD-DC, HD-DC + IFN-α-2b, and HIV-DC sets in **(F)** (*$p < 0.05$).

On the other side, MCC-950 was not able to significantly reduce cytokine release in HIV-DC stimulated with FLG (48% of inhibition; $p > 0.05$), LPS (48% of inhibition; $p > 0.05$) or LPS+ATP (48% of inhibition; $p > 0.05$) (**Figure 5B**). Accordingly, in the presence of MCC-950 a reduction not significantly of NLRP3+ specks was observed in HIV-DC (**Supplementary File 7**). PTD similarly inhibited IL-1β production in both FLG-treated HIV-DC (84% of inhibition $p = 0.002$), LPS or LPS+ATP-treated HIV-DC (84% of inhibition; $p = 0.002$), as expected due to

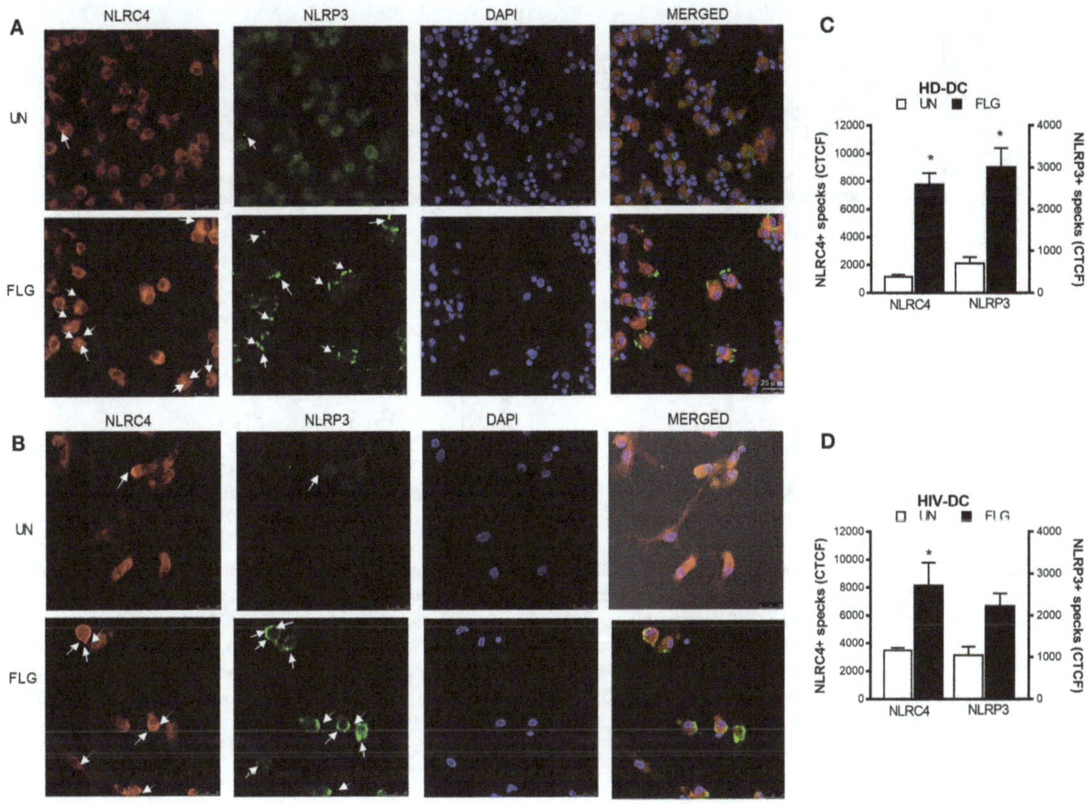

FIGURE 4 | Flagellin induces NLRC4+ and NLRP3+ specks formation in MDDC. 2 × 10^5 MDDC from healthy donors (HD-DC; $n = 3$) or HIV-infected patients (HIV-DC; $n = 3$) were cultured in 16-wells chamber slides and stimulated with 5 µg/mL FLG or 1 µg/mL LPS for 24 hours at 37°C 5% CO_2 with or without 1 mM ATP for more 15 minutes. Mouse anti-human NLRP3 and rabbit anti-human NLRC4 antibodies and fluorescent secondary antibodies (Alexa 488-conjugated goat-anti-mouse IgG1; Alexa 647-conjugated goat-anti-rabbit IgG1) were used to label NLRP3+ and NLRC4+ specks, respectively. DAPI was used to counterstain nuclei. Images acquisition was performed using a DMi8 confocal laser scanning microscope. A representative experiment (magnification: 63x) was reported for HD-DC **(A)** and HIV-DC **(B)**. Arrows indicated NLRC4+ or NLRP3+ specks. **(C,D)** CTCF index for NLRP3+ and NLRC4+ specks in untreated (UN) and FLG-treated (FLG) MDDC. Data are represented as mean ± standard error. Mann-Whitney test was applied to compare UN and FLG conditions in **(C,D)** ($^*p < 0.05$).

the caspase-1 and NF-kB dependency for FLG-induced response (49), as well as for LPS-mediated one (48). These data confirm the greater involvement of NLRP3 in response to FLG in healthy donors compared to HIV-infected individuals.

Then we compared the differences in IL-1ß release in FLG-treated MDDC following *NLRC4* or *NLRP3* shRNA knockdown (**Figures 5C,D**). In *NLRC4* shRNA-transduced MDDC, FLG induced a lower level of IL-1ß production compared to untreated cells both in HD-DC (**Figure 5C**) and in HIV-DC (**Figure 5D**). In *NLRP3* siRNA-transducted MDDC, FLG induced a lower level of IL-1ß compared to untreated cells in HD-DC (**Figure 5C**), however this effect was not observed in HIV-DC (**Figure 5D**). These data are in accord with above-reported effect of chemical NLRP3 inhibitor MCC-950 (**Figures 5A,B**).

Altogether these findings allow us to suggest that FLG activates the inflammasome in human MDDC through the induction of NAIP/NLRC4 and NLRP3 receptors; the contribution of NLRP3 in FLG-signaling is less pronounced in HIV-DC due to the well-known "exhausted" profile of these cells (50).

DISCUSSION

A number of microbial components have been proposed as alternative adjuvants to augment the immune responses of poorly immunogenic vaccines and/or of not fully immunocompetent individuals. Emerging evidence pointed out the possible use of bacterial flagellin in this context, firstly in mice [as extensively revised in Hajam et al. (17)], but also in a human clinical trial of prophylactic vaccine (23). Studies in mice show the stimulatory capacity of flagellin to induce both humoral and cellular immune responses when implied together with pathogen' antigens as adjuvant (51, 52) or in cancer immunotherapy (53).

Taking in account that, even in ART treatment, HIV-infected individuals continue to experience immune dysfunction, leading, among others side effects, to a deficient vaccine response (9), the necessity of new vaccine strategy in this population appear to be urgent.

Using the *in vitro* model of peripheral blood monocytes-derived-dendritic cells developed for HIV-infected patient's immunotherapy by Lu and collaborators (54), we demonstrated

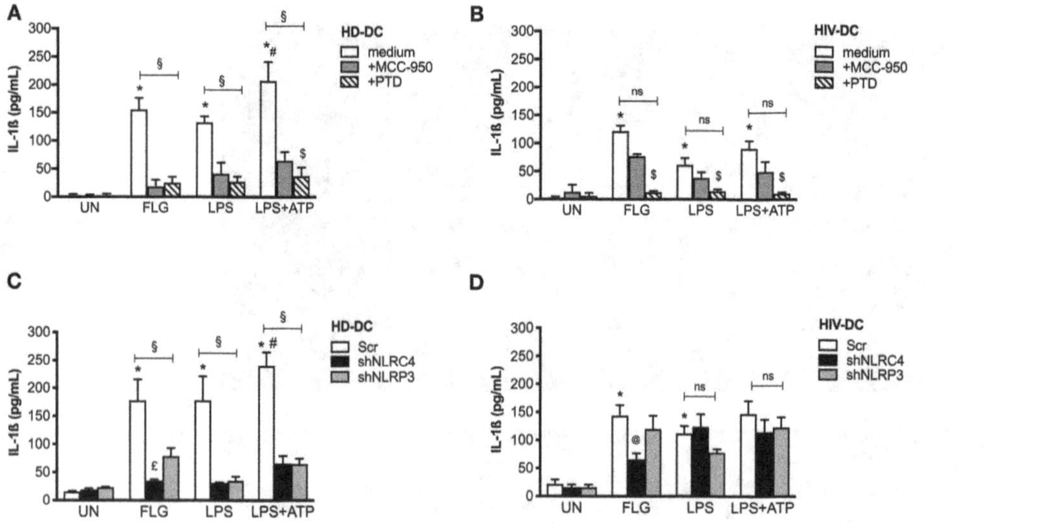

FIGURE 5 | Flagellin significantly induces NLRC4 but not NLRP3 in HIV-DC. 2 × 10^5 MDDC from healthy donors (HD-DC; $n = 5$) **(A)** and HIV-infected patients (HIV-DC; $n = 5$) **(B)** were pretreated with 10 µM MCC-950 or 10 µM parthenolide (PTD), and then stimulated with 5 µg/ml FLG for 24 hours or 1 µg/mL LPS for 24 hours with or without 1 mM ATP for more 15 minutes. IL-1ß concentration was measured in culture supernatants. 2 × 10^5 MDDC from healthy donors (HD-DC; $n = 3$) **(C)** and HIV-infected patients (HIV-DC; $n = 3$) **(D)** were transduced with empty vector (scramble: Scr), shNLRC4 or shNLRP3, and then stimulated with 5 µg/ml FLG for 24 hours, or 1 µg/mL LPS for 24 hours with or without 1 mM ATP for more 15 minutes. IL-1ß concentration was measured in culture supernatants. Kruskal-Wallis test with multi comparison post-test was applied (treated vs. UN: $^*p < 0.05$; LPS+ATP vs. LPS $^{\#}p < 0.05$; within each group: $^{\S}p < 0.05$; +MCC-950 vs. +PTD: $^{\$}p < 0.05$; shNLRC4 vs. shNLRP3: £$p < 0.05$; shNLRC4 vs. Scr: @p<0.05).

that flagellin is able to activate MDDC from HIV-infected patients as well as from healthy donors. Previous studies have evidenced the ability of flagellin to activate primary human monocytes, or human pro-monocytic cell line U38 (55), however here we demonstrated that flagellin is able to activate human MDDC considering both the MDDC profile as well as the MDDC-mediated lymphocytes activation (**Figure 1**), with the exception of IL-12 production which results lower in HIV-DC compared to HD-DC, but in accord with previously published data (56).

Flagellin is sensed by two main innate immune receptors, TLR5 (18) and NAIP/NLRC4 (57–59). While it has been shown that flagellin induces NAIP/NLRC4 inflammasome activation in primary human macrophages and monocytes (49, 60, 61), little is known about its role in human DC. Despite it has been previously reported that flagellin stimulates IL-1β production in human MDDC (62), any evidence about NLRC4 or NLRP3 pathway in IL-1ß induction have been shown nor hypothesized. Besides the description of these two receptors within inflammasome activation by flagellin, our study also demonstrated for the first time the different contribution of the two receptors in HIV-DC response to flagellin.

As expected, flagellin induces the inflammasome activation through NAIP/NLRC4 both in HD-DC as well as HIV-DC (**Figure 2**), suggesting that this pathway is still effective in HIV-infected patients, contrary to what seen for NLRP3 (14). Actually, HIV-DC presents a basal increased expression of NLRP3 inhibitory molecules, namely CARD8 (41), BRCC3 (42) and miR-223 (44), compatible with specific inhibition of this receptor (**Figure 3E**).

While the low rate of NLRP3 response in HIV-DC has been attributed to the chronic inflammation of HIV-infected patients, consequent of HIV-1 persistence, endogenous viruses reactivation (i.e., herpes simplex virus), immune system exhaustion, increased intestinal permeability and microbial translocation (mainly LPS) and antiretroviral drugs cytotoxicity (15, 63) and taking in account that flagellate bacteria also could be present in gut microbiota, it remains obscure why the NAIP/NLRC4 pathway continues "ready-to-go." The administration of continues doses of LPS was found to be tolerogenic in mice (64), however any data are available about flagellin. We speculated that the increased IFN-a production in HIV-infected individuals (even if at lower levels in ART-treated patients) could be a possible cause of specific NLRP3 inhibition due to the known effect of the anti-viral mediator as NLRP3 negative regulators (30). It is important to underline that our cohort of ART-treated HIV-infected individuals presented a mean value of plasma IFN-a of about 50 pg/mL, 5-fold more than healthy individuals (about 10 pg/mL) (data not shown). Moreover, when HD-DC were treated with IFN-a their NLRP3 response is diminished similarly to what observed in HIV-DC (**Figure 3F**), supporting our hypothesis. Another possible explication concerns the higher constitutive recruitment of adaptor molecule ASC (Apoptosis speck like with a CARD) in inflammasome complex in HIV-infected patients compared to healthy controls as recently observed by Ahmad and colleagues (65) in PBMC. In this case, inflammasome receptors, which need ASC to mount the complex (i.e., NLRP3), could be disadvantaged in respect to sensors that directly recruit caspase-1, such as NLRC4.

Beyond the main purpose of this article, and for the first time to our knowledge, we demonstrated that NLRP3 also contribute to flagellin response in human MDDC, as revealed by NLRP3+ specks formation in FLG-treated cells (**Figure 4**) and by specific (chemical and genetic) inhibition of this receptor (**Figure 5**). Our findings are in lines with previous reports about NLRC4 and NLRP3 co-localization into a unique complex in HEK293 cells (66) and in mice bone marrow-derived macrophages during *Salmonella* infection (67).

Therefore, flagellin induces the two pathways in HD-DC, whereas it preferentially activates NLRC4 pathway in HIV-DC due to the defect in NLRP3 in these cells. Despite the immunofluorescence visualization of both NLRP3+ and NLRC4+ specks, our data are not sufficient to determine whether the two receptors are truly co-localized in the same inflammasome complex, and further investigations will be needed to finally prove it.

In conclusion, our data support the use of flagellin in the design of future vaccines effective also in immunocompromised individuals, such as HIV-infected patients. According to our findings, flagellin activates human MDDC from healthy and HIV-infected individuals through the NAIP/NLRC4 inflammasome, with the participation of NLRP3 at least in healthy donors cells. Flagellin was able to by-pass the NLRP3 defect in HIV-DC, contributing to inflammasome activation and consequently full MDDC maturation in HIV-infected patients.

AUTHOR CONTRIBUTIONS

EdR, BdA, and AP: conceived and designed experiments. EdR: performed MDDC experiments. VL: collection of samples. DdL: performed the immunofluorescence experiments. FF and JdS: ELISA. EdR, DdL, and AP: statistical analysis. EdR, DdL, VL, FF, and AP: discussion of results. EdR and AP: wrote the article. BdA: designed and discussed silencing experiments.

FUNDING

This project was supported by the Fundação de Amparo à Pesquisa do Estado de São Paulo (FAPESP) (research grant 2015/23395-6 and 2015/50660-7 to AP; 2014/23225-0 to BdA). ECR (2015/17373-0), VL (2017/10824-1) and FF (2018/04361-1) receive FAPESP post-graduation fellowships; JdS had received a CAPES master' degree fellowships; DdL receives a Ph.D. fellowship from the Fundação de Amparo à Pesquisa do Estado Amazonas (FAPEAM). AP receives a CNPq Researcher Fellowship. The funders had no role in this study design, data collection and analysis, decision to publish, or preparation of the manuscript.

ACKNOWLEDGMENTS

We are very grateful to the Oswaldo Cruz Hospital Blood Bank Service and the Serviço de Extensão ao Atendimento de Pacientes HIV/AIDS (SEAP) of the FMUSP (SP, Brazil) for the recruitment of healthy donors and HIV-infected patients, respectively. We acknowledge Prof. Niels Olsen Câmara for slide chambers and qPCR reagents; Dr. Telma Miyuki Oshiro for anti-human NLRP3 antibody, and IL-12p70 ELISA reagents; Prof. Karina Ramalho Bortoluci, Dr. Paula Ordonhez Rigato, and Prof. Silvia Boscardin for helpful suggestions and discussion. We acknowledge Prof. Eliana Faquim and the technician Alexsander Souza for the microscope facility of the Laboratory of Cellular Biology at the Butantan Institute (São Paulo, SP, Brazil) by the use of a DMi8 confocal laser scanning microscope; the Laboratory of Immune Cell Biology (Department of Immunology, ICB, USP) for technical support in silencing experiments.

REFERENCES

1. Steinman RM. The dendritic cell system and its role in immunogenicity. *Annu Rev Immunol.* (1991) 9:271–96. doi: 10.1146/annurev.iy.09.040191.001415
2. Banchereau J, Steinman RM. Dendritic cells and the control of immunity. *Nature.* (1998) 392:245–52. doi: 10.1038/32588
3. Wu L, Dakic A. Development of dendritic cell system. *Cell Mol Immunol.* (2004) 1:112–8.
4. Steinman RM. Dendritic cells: understanding immunogenicity. *Eur J Immunol.* (2007) (37Suppl. 1):S53–60. doi: 10.1002/eji.200737400
5. Maisonneuve C, Bertholet S, Philpott DJ, De Gregorio E. Unleashing the potential of NOD- and Toll-like agonists as vaccine adjuvants. *Proc Natl Acad Sci USA.* (2014) 111:12294. doi: 10.1073/pnas.1400478111
6. Li H, Willingham SB, Ting JPY, Re F. Cutting edge: inflammasome activation by alum and alum's adjuvant effect are mediated by NLRP3. *J Immunol.* (2008) 181:17. doi: 10.4049/jimmunol.181.1.17
7. Surendran N, Nicolosi T, Pichichero M. Infants with low vaccine antibody responses have altered innate cytokine response. *Vaccine.* (2016) 34:5700–3. doi: 10.1016/j.vaccine.2016.09.050
8. Van Deventer HW, Burgents JE, Wu QP, Woodford RMT, Brickey WJ, Allen IC, et al. The inflammasome component Nlrp3 impairs antitumor vaccine by enhancing the accumulation of tumor-associated myeloid-derived suppressor cells. *Cancer Res.* (2010) 70:10161–9. doi: 10.1158/0008-5472.CAN-10-1921
9. Geretti AM, Doyle T. Immunization for HIV-positive individuals. *Curr Opin Infect Dis.* (2010) 23:32–8. doi: 10.1097/QCO.0b013e328334fec4
10. Donaghy H, Gazzard B, Gotch F, Patterson S. Dysfunction and infection of freshly isolated blood myeloid and plasmacytoid dendritic

cells in patients infected with HIV-1. *Blood.* (2003) 101:4505–11. doi: 10.1182/blood-2002-10-3189
11. Sabado RL, O'brien M, Subedi A, Qin L, Hu N, Taylor E, et al. Evidence of dysregulation of dendritic cells in primary HIV infection. *Blood.* (2010) 116:3839–52. doi: 10.1182/blood-2010-03-273763
12. Cardone M, Ikeda KN, Varano B, Gessani S, Conti L. HIV-1-induced impairment of dendritic cell cross talk with γδ T lymphocytes. *J Virol.* (2015) 89:4798–808. doi: 10.1128/JVI.03681-14
13. Liu J, Ostrowski M. Development of targeted adjuvants for HIV-1 vaccines. *AIDS Res Ther.* (2017) 14:43. doi: 10.1186/s12981-017-0165-8
14. Pontillo A, Silva LT, Oshiro TM, Finazzo C, Crovella S, Duarte AJ. HIV-1 induces NALP3-inflammasome expression and interleukin-1beta secretion in dendritic cells from healthy individuals but not from HIV-positive patients. *AIDS.* (2012) 26:11–8. doi: 10.1097/QAD.0b013e32834d697f
15. Deeks SG, Tracy R, Douek DC. Systemic effects of inflammation on health during chronic HIV infection. *Immunity.* (2013) 39:633–45. doi: 10.1016/j.immuni.2013.10.001
16. Kool M, Pétrilli V, De Smedt T, Rolaz A, Hammad H, Van Nimwegen M, et al. Cutting edge: alum adjuvant stimulates inflammatory dendritic cells through activation of the NALP3 inflammasome. *J Immunol.* (2008) 181:3755–9. doi: 10.4049/jimmunol.181.6.3755
17. Hajam IA, Dar PA, Shahnawaz I, Jaume JC, Lee JH. Bacterial flagellin-a potent immunomodulatory agent. *Exp Mol Med.* (2017) 49:e373. doi: 10.1038/emm.2017.172
18. Hayashi F, Smith KD, Ozinsky A, Hawn TR, Yi EC, Goodlett DR, et al. The innate immune response to bacterial flagellin is mediated by Toll-like receptor 5. *Nature.* (2001) 410:1099–103. doi: 10.1038/35074106
19. Yoon SI, Kurnasov O, Natarajan V, Hong M, Gudkov AV, Osterman AL, et al. Structural basis of TLR5-flagellin recognition and signaling. *Science.* (2012) 335:859–64. doi: 10.1126/science.1215584
20. Diebolder CA, Halff EF, Koster AJ, Huizinga EG, Koning RI. Cryoelectron tomography of the NAIP5/NLRC4 inflammasome: implications for NLR activation. *Structure.* (2015) 23:2349–57. doi: 10.1016/j.str.2015.10.001
21. Hu Z, Zhou Q, Zhang C, Fan S, Cheng W, Zhao Y, et al. Structural and biochemical basis for induced self-propagation of NLRC4. *Science.* (2015) 350:399–404. doi: 10.1126/science.aac5489
22. Zhang L, Chen S, Ruan J, Wu J, Tong AB, Yin Q, et al. Cryo-EM structure of the activated NAIP2-NLRC4 inflammasome reveals nucleated polymerization. *Science.* (2015) 350:404–9. doi: 10.1126/science.aac5789
23. Treanor JJ, Taylor DN, Tussey L, Hay C, Nolan C, Fitzgerald T, et al. Safety and immunogenicity of a recombinant hemagglutinin influenza-flagellin fusion vaccine (VAX125) in healthy young adults. *Vaccine.* (2010) 28:8268–74. doi: 10.1016/j.vaccine.2010.10.009
24. Turley CB, Rupp RE, Johnson C, Taylor DN, Wolfson J, Tussey L, et al. Safety and immunogenicity of a recombinant M2e-flagellin influenza vaccine (STF2.4xM2e) in healthy adults. *Vaccine.* (2011). 29:5145–52. doi: 10.1016/j.vaccine.2011.05.041
25. Sallusto F, Palermo B, Lenig D, Miettinen M, Matikainen S, Julkunen I, et al. Distinct patterns and kinetics of chemokine production regulate dendritic cell function. *Eur J Immunol.* (1999) 29:1617–25. doi: 10.1002/(SICI)1521-4141(199905)29:05<1617::AID-IMMU1617>3.0.CO;2-3
26. Gattorno M, Tassi S, Carta S, Delfino L, Ferlito F, Pelagatti MA, et al. Pattern of interleukin-1beta secretion in response to lipopolysaccharide and ATP before and after interleukin-1 blockade in patients with CIAS1 mutations. *Arthritis Rheum.* (2007) 56:3138–48. doi: 10.1002/art.22842
27. Coll RC, Robertson AA, Chae JJ, Higgins SC, Munoz-Planillo R, Inserra MC, et al. A small-molecule inhibitor of the NLRP3 inflammasome for the treatment of inflammatory diseases. *Nat Med.* (2015) 21:248–55. doi: 10.1038/nm.3806
28. Juliana C, Fernandes-Alnemri T, Wu J, Datta P, Solorzano L, Yu JW, et al. Anti-inflammatory compounds parthenolide and Bay 11-7082 are direct inhibitors of the inflammasome. *J Biol Chem.* (2010) 285:9792–802. doi: 10.1074/jbc.M109.082305
29. Guarda G, Braun M, Staehli F, Tardivel A, Mattmann C, Forster I, et al. Type I interferon inhibits interleukin-1 production and inflammasome activation. *Immunity.* (2011) 34:213–23. doi: 10.1016/j.immuni.2011.02.006
30. Simmons DP, Wearsch PA, Canaday DH, Meyerson HJ, Liu YC, Wang Y, et al. Type I IFN drives a distinctive dendritic cell maturation phenotype that allows continued class II MHC synthesis and antigen processing. *J Immunol.* (2012) 188:3116–26. doi: 10.4049/jimmunol.1101313
31. Da Silva LT, Da Silva WC, De Almeida A, Da Silva Reis D, Santillo BT, Rigato PO, et al. Characterization of monocyte-derived dendritic cells used in immunotherapy for HIV-1-infected individuals. *Immunotherapy.* (2018) 10:871–85. doi: 10.2217/imt-2017-0165
32. Shinde P, Fernandes S, Melinkeri S, Kale V, Limaye L. Compromised functionality of monocyte-derived dendritic cells in multiple myeloma patients may limit their use in cancer immunotherapy. *Sci Rep.* (2018) 8:5705. doi: 10.1038/s41598-018-23943-w
33. Schmittgen TD, Livak KJ. Analyzing real-time PCR data by the comparative C(T) method. *Nat Protoc.* (2008) 3:1101–8. doi: 10.1038/nprot.2008.73
34. Stutz A, Horvath GL, Monks BG, Latz E. ASC speck formation as a readout for inflammasome activation. *Methods Mol Biol.* (2013) 1040:91–101. doi: 10.1007/978-1-62703-523-1_8
35. Mccloy RA, Rogers S, Caldon CE, Lorca T, Castro A, Burgess A. Partial inhibition of Cdk1 in G 2 phase overrides the SAC and decouples mitotic events. *Cell Cycle.* (2014) 13:1400–12. doi: 10.4161/cc.28401
36. Baravalle G, Park H, Mcsweeney M, Ohmura-Hoshino M, Matsuki Y, Ishido S, et al. Ubiquitination of CD86 is a key mechanism in regulating antigen presentation by dendritic cells. *J Immunol.* (2011). 187:2966–73. doi: 10.4049/jimmunol.1101643
37. Doitsh G, Galloway NLK, Geng X, Yang Z, Monroe KM, Zepeda O, et al. Cell death by pyroptosis drives CD4 T-cell depletion in HIV-1 infection. *Nature.* (2013) 505:509. doi: 10.1038/nature12940
38. Walsh JG, Reinke SN, Mamik MK, Mckenzie BA, Maingat F, Branton WG, et al. Rapid inflammasome activation in microglia contributes to brain disease in HIV/AIDS. *Retrovirology.* (2014) 11:35. doi: 10.1186/1742-4690-11-35
39. Bandera A, Masetti M, Fabbiani M, Biasin M, Muscatello A, Squillace N, et al. The NLRP3 inflammasome is upregulated in HIV-infected antiretroviral therapy-treated individuals with defective immune recovery. *Front Immunol.* (2018) 9:214. doi: 10.3389/fimmu.2018.00214
40. Feria MG, Taborda NA. HIV replication is associated to inflammasomes activation, IL-1beta, IL-18 and caspase-1 expression in GALT and peripheral Blood. *PLoS ONE.* (2018) 13:e0192845. doi: 10.1371/journal.pone.0192845
41. Ito S, Hara Y, Kubota T. CARD8 is a negative regulator for NLRP3 inflammasome, but mutant NLRP3 in cryopyrin-associated periodic syndromes escapes the restriction. *Arthritis Res Ther.* (2014) 16:R52. doi: 10.1186/ar4483
42. Py BF, Kim MS, Vakifahmetoglu-Norberg H, Yuan J. Deubiquitination of NLRP3 by BRCC3 critically regulates inflammasome activity. *Mol Cell.* (2013) 49:331–8. doi: 10.1016/j.molcel.2012.11.009
43. Segovia JA, Tsai S-Y, Chang T-H, Shil NK, Weintraub ST, Short JD, et al. Nedd8 regulates inflammasome-dependent caspase-1 activation. *Mol Cell Biol.* (2015) 35:582–97. doi: 10.1128/MCB.00775-14
44. Yang Z, Zhong L, Xian R, Yuan B. MicroRNA-223 regulates inflammation and brain injury via feedback to NLRP3 inflammasome after intracerebral hemorrhage. *Mol Immunol.* (2015) 65:267–76. doi: 10.1016/j.molimm.2014.12.018
45. Von Sydow M, Sonnerborg A, Gaines H, Strannegard O. Interferon-alpha and tumor necrosis factor-alpha in serum of patients in various stages of HIV-1 infection. *AIDS Res Hum Retrovirus.* (1991) 7:375–80. doi: 10.1089/aid.1991.7.375
46. Khatissian E, Tovey MG, Cumont MC, Monceaux V, Lebon P, Montagnier L, et al. The relationship between the interferon alpha response and viral burden in primary SIV infection. *AIDS Res Hum Retrovirus.* (1996) 12:1273–8. doi: 10.1089/aid.1996.12.1273
47. Stylianou E, Aukrust P, Bendtzen K, Muller F, Froland SS. Interferons and interferon (IFN)-inducible protein 10 during highly active anti-retroviral therapy (HAART)-possible immunosuppressive role of IFN-alpha in HIV infection. *Clin Exp Immunol.* (2000) 119:479–85. doi: 10.1046/j.1365-2249.2000.01144.x
48. Kayagaki N, Wong MT, Stowe IB, Ramani SR, Gonzalez LC, Akashi-Takamura S, et al. Noncanonical inflammasome activation by intracellular LPS independent of TLR4. *Science.* (2013) 341:1246–9. doi: 10.1126/science.1240248

49. Kortmann J, Brubaker SW, Monack DM. Cutting edge: inflammasome activation in primary human macrophages is dependent on flagellin. *J Immunol.* (2015) 195:815–9. doi: 10.4049/jimmunol.1403100
50. Blanchet FP, Moris A, Nikolic DS, Lehmann M, Cardinaud S, Stalder R, et al. Human immunodeficiency virus-1 inhibition of immunoamphisomes in dendritic cells impairs early innate and adaptive immune responses. *Immunity.* (2010) 32:654–69. doi: 10.1016/j.immuni.2010.04.011
51. Mcsorley SJ, Ehst BD, Yu Y, Gewirtz AT. Bacterial flagellin is an effective adjuvant for CD4+ T cells *in vivo. J Immunol.* (2002) 169:3914–9. doi: 10.4049/jimmunol.169.7.3914
52. Didierlaurent A, Ferrero I, Otten LA, Dubois B, Reinhardt M, Carlsen H, et al. Flagellin promotes myeloid differentiation factor 88-dependent development of Th2-type response. *J Immunol.* (2004) 172:6922–30. doi: 10.4049/jimmunol.172.11.6922
53. Zheng JH, Nguyen VH, Jiang SN, Park SH, Tan W, Hong SH, et al. Two-step enhanced cancer immunotherapy with engineered Salmonella typhimurium secreting heterologous flagellin. *Sci Transl Med.* (2017) 9:9537. doi: 10.1126/scitranslmed.aak9537
54. Lu W, Arraes LC, Ferreira WT, Andrieu JM. Therapeutic dendritic-cell vaccine for chronic HIV-1 infection. *Nat Med.* (2004) 10:1359–65. doi: 10.1038/nm1147
55. Ciacci-Woolwine F, Blomfield IC, Richardson SH, Mizel SB. Salmonella flagellin induces tumor necrosis factor alpha in a human promonocytic cell line. *Infect Immun.* (1998) 66:1127–34.
56. Buisson S, Benlahrech A, Gazzard B, Gotch F, Kelleher P, Patterson S. Monocyte-derived dendritic cells from HIV type 1-infected individuals show reduced ability to stimulate T cells and have altered production of interleukin (IL)-12 and IL-10. *J Infect Dis.* (2009) 199:1862–71. doi: 10.1086/599122
57. Franchi L, Amer A, Body-Malapel M, Kanneganti TD, Ozoren N, Jagirdar R, et al. Cytosolic flagellin requires Ipaf for activation of caspase-1 and interleukin 1beta in salmonella-infected macrophages. *Nat Immunol.* (2006) 7:576–82. doi: 10.1038/ni1346
58. Miao EA, Alpuche-Aranda CM, Dors M, Clark AE, Bader MW, Miller SI, et al. Cytoplasmic flagellin activates caspase-1 and secretion of interleukin 1beta via Ipaf. *Nat Immunol.* (2006) 7:569–75. doi: 10.1038/ni1344
59. Kofoed EM, Vance RE. Innate immune recognition of bacterial ligands by NAIPs determines inflammasome specificity. *Nature.* (2011) 477:592–5. doi: 10.1038/nature10394
60. Canna SW, De Jesus AA, Gouni S, Brooks SR, Marrero B, Liu Y, et al. An activating NLRC4 inflammasome mutation causes autoinflammation with recurrent macrophage activation syndrome. *Nat Genet.* (2014) 46:1140–6. doi: 10.1038/ng.3089
61. Reyes Ruiz VM, Ramirez J, Naseer N, Palacio NM, Siddarthan IJ, Yan BM, et al. Broad detection of bacterial type III secretion system and flagellin proteins by the human NAIP/NLRC4 inflammasome. *Proc Natl Acad Sci USA.* (2017) 114:13242. doi: 10.1073/pnas.1710433114
62. Means TK, Hayashi F, Smith KD, Aderem A, Luster AD. The toll-like receptor 5 stimulus bacterial flagellin induces maturation and chemokine production in human dendritic cells. *J Immunol.* (2003) 170:5165. doi: 10.4049/jimmunol.170.10.5165
63. Maartens G, Celum C, Lewin SR. HIV infection: epidemiology, pathogenesis, treatment, and prevention. *Lancet.* (2014) 384:258–71. doi: 10.1016/S0140-6736(14)60164-1
64. Geisel J, Kahl F, Müller M, Wagner H, Kirschning CJ, Autenrieth IB, et al. IL-6 and maturation govern TLR2 and TLR4 induced TLR agonist tolerance and cross-tolerance in dendritic cells. *J Immunol.* (2007) 179:5811. doi: 10.4049/jimmunol.179.9.5811
65. Ahmad F, Mishra N, Ahrenstorf G, Franklin BS, Latz E, Schmidt RE, et al. Evidence of inflammasome activation and formation of monocyte-derived ASC specks in HIV-1 positive patients. *AIDS.* (2018) 32:299–307. doi: 10.1097/QAD.0000000000001693
66. Man SM, Hopkins LJ, Nugent E, Cox S, Glück IM, Tourlomousis P, et al. Inflammasome activation causes dual recruitment of NLRC4 and NLRP3 to the same macromolecular complex. *Proc Natl Acad Sci USA.* (2014) 111:7403–8. doi: 10.1073/pnas.1402911111
67. Qu Y, Misaghi S, Newton K, Maltzman A, Izrael-Tomasevic A, Arnott D, et al. NLRP3 recruitment by NLRC4 during *Salmonella* infection. *J Exp Med.* (2016) 213:877–85. doi: 10.1084/jem.20132234

6

Molecular Aspects of Dendritic Cell Activation in Leishmaniasis: An Immunobiological View

Rafael Tibúrcio [1,2], Sara Nunes [1,2], Ivanéia Nunes [1,2], Mariana Rosa Ampuero [1,2], Icaro Bonyek Silva [1,2], Reinan Lima [1,2], Natalia Machado Tavares [1,2,3] and Cláudia Brodskyn [1,2,3]**

[1] Gonçalo Moniz Institute, Oswaldo Cruz Foundation, Salvador, Brazil, [2] Federal University of Bahia, Salvador, Brazil, [3] Instituto Nacional de Ciência e Tecnologia (INCT) iii Instituto de Investigação em Imunologia, São Paulo, Brazil

***Correspondence:**
Natalia Machado Tavares
natalia.tavares@bahia.fiocruz.br
Cláudia Brodskyn
brodskyn@bahia.fiocruz.br

Dendritic cells (DC) are a diverse group of leukocytes responsible for bridging innate and adaptive immunity. Despite their functional versatility, DCs exist primarily in two basic functional states: immature and mature. A large body of evidence suggests that upon interactions with pathogens, DCs undergo intricate cellular processes that culminate in their activation, which is paramount to the orchestration of effective immune responses against *Leishmania* parasites. Herein we offer a concise review of the emerging hallmarks of DCs activation in leishmaniasis as well as a comprehensive discussion of the following underlying molecular events: DC-*Leishmania* interaction, antigen uptake, costimulatory molecule expression, parasite ability to affect DC migration, antigen presentation, metabolic reprogramming, and epigenetic alterations.

Keywords: dendritic cell activation, *leishmania*- dendritic cell interaction, parasite uptake, dendritic cells migration, metabolism of infection, epigenetic modifications

INTRODUCTION

Important Considerations in Leishmaniasis

Leishmaniasis comprises a collection of neglected protozoan infections caused by unicellular organisms belonging to the genus *Leishmania* spp. According to the current World Health Organization estimation, 12 million people are affected by leishmaniasis and 350 million are at risk of infection worldwide (1-3).

The pathology of this disease results in a wide spectrum of clinical manifestations not only associated with the biological aspects of *Leishmania* species and strains, but also with host immune responses. Interestingly, it has been recently suggested that the clinical progression of the disease is influenced by several other factors, ranging from the host's nutritional status to the presence of RNA viruses in the *Leishmania* species (4–7).

These manifestations are dichotomically divided into Visceral (VL) and Tegumentary Leishmaniasis (TL). The former is characterized by the dissemination of parasites to visceral organs, while the latter branch includes Localized Cutaneous Leishmaniasis (LCL), a frequent form of TL in which ulcerated skin lesions are common. It has been abundantly reported that a modest fraction of LCL cases can evolve into mucosal lesions, which is termed as Mucocutaneous Leishmaniasis (MCL). Additionally, TL can also present as a variety of clinical manifestations, such as Disseminated Cutaneous Leishmaniasis (DCL), which comprises multiple nodular ulcerated lesions, whereas Diffuse Leishmaniasis (DL) is characterized by scattered non-ulcerated lesions (5, 8, 9).

Leishmania transmission occurs when infected sandflies inoculate the promastigote forms of the parasite into the host skin. Additionally, the arthropod vector also introjects various parasite-associated compounds, along with other molecules found in salivary secretions, which collectively exert immunomodulatory effects on the host defense (10). The early events of infection are characterized by the engagement of different phagocytic cells (e.g., tissue-resident macrophages, dermal DCs, and neutrophils) in the recognition and uptake of parasites (8). Emerging pieces of evidence indicate that neutrophils are one of the first cell types to interact with *Leishmania* parasites (11). Subsequently, depending chiefly on the *Leishmania* species, infected neutrophils become apoptotic and can be phagocytized by macrophages (12). Accordingly, parasite transmission to these cells becomes facilitated, leading to the subsequent differentiation of promastigotes into intracellular replicative amastigotes that occurs in the interior of macrophages phagolysosomes. Additionally, the literature upholds that dendritic cells (DCs) are also key elements in the early interaction with *Leishmania* parasites, thusly these are thought to be a decisive in the outcome of infection (13). Indeed, the complex interactions occurring between DCs and parasites may lead to long-term *Leishmania* replication, or to the establishment of an effective immune response against this pathogen.

The Immunobiology of Dendritic Cells

DCs are competent antigen presenting cells (APC) that take center stage in both the induction of immunological responses and the generation of tolerance (14). In the context of inflammation and infection, DCs are responsible for orchestrating the connection between the innate and adaptive axis of immunity. Interestingly, despite the significant importance of DCs in several immunological processes, these cells do not comprise a homogeneous population, and are further classified into distinct subtypes according to origin, differential expression of surface proteins, cell localization, and immunological function (15).

Dendritic Cell Origin

It has been long hypothesized that DCs stem from a bone-marrow resident population of hematopoietic stem cells (HSC), which eventually give rise to both granulocyte-macrophage progenitors (GMP), and multi-lymphoid progenitors (MLP), the precursors of all DC subsets (16). Subsequent stages in DC ontogeny involve precursors, such as CD14+ monocytes, circulating blood myeloid DCs (mDCs), or plasmacytoid DCs, from which all myeloid and lymphoid DCs are derived. It is noteworthy that mDC precursors comprise a heterogeneous lineage of cells predetermined to develop into CD1+ or CD141+ DCs. Additionally, human mDCs express conventional myeloid markers, including CD11c, CD11b, CD13, and CD33 (17). In mice, these cell populations are often referred to as conventional DCs. Interestingly, it has been well-elucidated that in humans, both CD14+DCs and inflammatory DCs are derived from classical monocytes, which justifies the fact that these cells present greater similarity to monocytes and macrophages than other DC subsets (18).

Dendritic Cell Subtypes

Myeloid/Conventional Dendritic Cells

Typically, myeloid DCs are classified into two subtypes: cDC1 and cDC2. The human cDC1 subset is identified by the expression of CD141 (BDCA-3), while the murine equivalent is subdivided into a splenic CD8α-bearing population and another CD141+ DC subset residing in non-lymphoid tissues (19–21). Human and mouse cDC1 express Clec9A (C-type lectin domain family 9-member A) and XCR1 (a chemokine receptor), which provide specificity for their biological activities in combating invasive microorganisms and tumors (22). In regard to the expression of transcription factors, cDC1s are characterized as producing both BAFT3 (Basic leucine zipper transcription factor) and IRF8 (Interferon regulatory factor 8). It has been long suggested that cDC1s have the capacity to effectively induce the activation of CD8+ T cells via the process of antigen cross-presentation, as well as produce copious amounts of IL-12p70 (23, 24).

cDC2s express both common myeloid markers, such as CD11b, CD11c, CD13, and CD33, in addition to other antigens more recently identified in these cells: CD1c, CD2, FceR1, and SIRPA (15). cDC2s comprise a large portion of the human conventional DCs found in blood and tissues. The immunological function of cDC2s is granted by a myriad of immune receptors, including Toll-like receptors (TLRs) 2,4,5,7 and 8, C-type lectins, including Dectin-1 and−2 as well as Nod- and RIG-like receptors (**Figure 1** and **Table 1**) (15).

Plasmacytoid Dendritic Cells

Plasmacytoid DCs (pDCs) comprise a group of Type I interferon (IFN)-producing cells whose distinguishing feature is their participation in the response against viral infection. Interestingly, human pDCs were first identified as a population of cells found in the peripheral blood and tonsils. With respect to morphology, blood pDCs are mainly recognized by their resemblance to lymphocytes, whereas IL-3/CD40L-cultured pDCs possess a microscopic appearance similar to mDCs (22, 25). Typically, human pDCs are characterized by the unique expression of both cell-surface receptors and transcription factors. Of note, the distinctly expressed receptors include both conventional and other recently identified markers. The former includes CD123 (IL-3R), CD303 (BDCA-2), and CD304 (BDCA-4), while the later includes FceR1, DR6 (CD358), and CD300A. As previously mentioned, these cells also exhibit distinctive TF expression, including E2-2, IRF8, and IRF4 (26, 27). It is particularly interesting to note that, in contrast to cDCs, human pDCs do not express any conventional myeloid markers, e.g., CD11b, CD11c, CD13, and CD33 (15). Murine pDCs express siglecH (Sialic acid-binding immunoglobulin-type lectin), bst2 and Ly6C. SiglecH is a surface receptor responsible for binding glycans presenting sialic acids residues. Interestingly, Blasius et al demonstrated that siglecH regulates type I IFN production in a DAP12-dependent manner (28). Bst2, an integral membrane protein associated with lipid rafts, has also been associated with IFN-mediated responses against viral infection (29). Additionally, several reports have demonstrated that both murine and human pDCs rely on TLR7 and TLR9 expression for IFN-α production

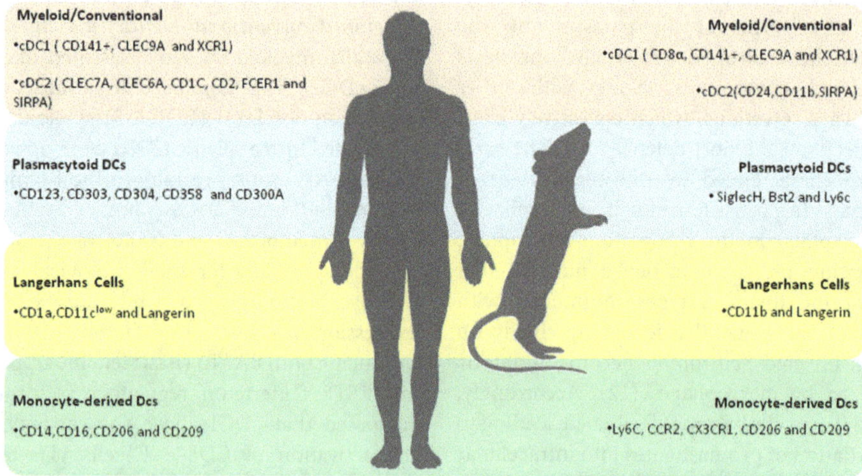

FIGURE 1 | Overview of human and murine DC subtypes–Summary of the molecular markers that characterize each human and murine DC subtypes.

and immunity against viruses (30). Interestingly, mounting evidence have demonstrated that pDCs also play a role in the establishment of peripheral tolerance by delivering antigens to the lymph nodes (**Figure 1** and **Table 1**) (31–33).

Langerhans Cells

A distinct lineage of epidermis-resident DCs, known as Langerhans cells (LC), mainly characterized by the expression of C-type lectin Langerin and CD1a, grant organisms immunity against several skin pathogens, such as fungi and bacteria (34). Uniquely, LCs possess Langerin-replete organelles, known as Birbeck granules. Although their main function has not been well-elucidated, the depletion of these granules has not been determined to mitigate the process of antigen presentation (**Figure 1** and **Table 1**) (35).

Monocyte-Derived Dendritic Cells

Monocytes constitute a very plastic group of mononuclear phagocytic cells long thought to be the source of macrophages and DCs. Several reports suggest that monocytes possess both pro- and anti-inflammatory functional specializations which are, in turn, chiefly regulated by tissue environments (36). Human monocytes comprise two subsets of peripheral blood circulating cells mainly characterized by the expression of CD14 and CD16, whereas murine monocytes can be identified by the presence of Ly6C, CCR2, and CX3CR1 (22). Of note, in the presence of inflammation, blood-circulating monocytes invade tissues, subsequently differentiating into monocyte-derived Dendritic cells (moDCs). It has been long established that *in vitro* moDCs are obtained by stimulating monocytes with GM-CSF and IL-4 (37). These cells possess a broad functional repertoire, including lymphocyte activation and the production of cytokines, such as IL-6, TNF-α, IL-12, IL-23, and IL-1 (15). Inflammatory DCs (iDCs) express both CD14 and CD16, in addition to CD206, CD209 (DC-SIGN), and CD163. Importantly, a novel tumor necrosis factor (TNF)-and inducible nitric oxide synthase (iNOS)-producing DCs (TIP-DCs) subset has been reported to exert a pivotal role in the course of several infectious diseases, including experimental leishmaniasis (**Figure 1** and **Table 1**) (38).

Adaptative Immunity Gatekeepers: The Role of DCs and T Cells Activation

In an immature state, DCs are typically located in peripheral tissues and express low levels of major histocompatibility complex II (MHC II) and costimulatory molecules. These cells possess highly efficient cellular machinery for antigen recognition and capture (39). In response to signals associated with infection and inflammation, such as the presence of pathogens and other damaging elements, DCs undergo intricate molecular processes that culminate in the acquisition of a mature functional state, whose main characteristic is the ability to induce both naïve $CD4^+$ T cell activation and proliferation via antigen presentation (40). Most importantly, the signaling process that induces DC maturation involves the recognition of pathogen-associated molecular patterns (PAMPs) by way of a sophisticated surface and intracellular molecular detection system consisting of pattern recognition receptors (PRRs) and downstream signaling (41).

After interaction with antigen-bearing DCs, naïve $CD4^+$ T cells are capable of differentiating into two main functional phenotypes: T helper 1 (Th1) and T helper 2 (Th2) profiles. It should be noted that this dichotomy is a rather simplistic representation of the Th cell repertoire. In recent decades, several studies have identified other Th subtypes, including Th17 (whose hallmark is the production of IL-17 in response to viruses, bacteria and fungi), Th9 (a producer of IL-9 and IL-10, and also a key element in humoral interplay with B cells), Th follicular (characterized by the production of IL-4 and IL-2 (also related to supporting B cell-mediated immunity), and T regulatory (Tregs), involved in the promotion of self-tolerance (42). Since T regs exert a prevalent immunological role in the regulation of other immune cells, their populations

TABLE 1 | Summary of the hallmarks of *Leishmania* induced DC activation.

Leishmania-prompted effects in DC activation	DC subsets	Parasite species	Experimental model	Functional aftermath	References
TLR9 activation	BMDCs	*L. infantum*	C57BL/6	Increases Neutrophil chemoattraction and IL-12 production	Sacramento et al. (53)
		L. major		Enhances IFN-γ production and cytotoxicity in NK cells	Liese et al. (54)
TLR2/TLR4 activation	BMDCs	*L major*	BALB/c	Upregulation of CD80, CD86, and MHC-II expression	Komai-Koma et al. (49)
TLR2 activation	BMDCs	*L. braziliensis*	C57BL/6	Decreases DC activation and IL-12 production	Vargas-Inchaustegui et al. (50)
Engagement of MyD88 signaling pathway	BMDCs	*L. braziliensis*	C57BL/6	Enhances IL-12 production	Vargas-Inchaustegui et al. (50)
A2B receptor activation	BMDCs	*L amazonensis*	C57BL/6J	Decreases of CD40 expression and IL-12 production	Figueiredo et al. (64)
Increased expression of HIF1 α	Murine splenic DCs	*Leishmania donovani*		Decreases production of IL-12, parasite survival, limited generation of Th1 cells	Hammami et al. (111)
Up-regulation of MHC class II, CD40, CD54, CD80, and CD86	Epidermal Langerhans cells-like DC	*L. major* amastigotes	C57BL/6	Increase production of IL-12	Von Stebut et al. (78)
Did not change the expression of CD80, CD54, and MHC II molecules	BMDCs	*L. mexicana* amastigotes	C57BL/6	Did not alter the production of IL-12	Bennett et al. (79)
Lower levels of MHCII, CD86, and CD40 expression	BMDCs	*L. amazonensis*	C57BL/6	Declined T-cell proliferation	Figueiredo et al. (65)
Low levels of CD40 expression	BMDCs	*L. donovani*	BALB/c	T regulatory cells expansion and disease intensification	Martin et al. (71)
Fail in producing IL-12 through a CD40-dependent manner	BMDCs	*L. amazonensis*	BALB/c	Increase in IL-4 levels	Qi et al. (74)
Down-regulation of CD80 and up-regulation of CD86	Human moDCs	*L. amazonensis*	*in vitro*	Increase in IL-6 during DC differentiation	Favali et al. (75)
Alterations in DC migration		*L. major*		Inhibition of DCs motility	Steigerwald et al. (98); Ponte-Sucre et al. (100)

BMDC, bone marrow -derived dendritic cell; IFN-γ, interferon gamma; IL-12, interleukine-12; NK, natural killer cells; TLR, toll-like receptors; HIF1α, hypoxia-inducible factor 1 α.

heterogeneity and functional specializations are of particular interest. Commonly, T regs are dichotomically classified as "natural" ($CD4^+CD25^+Foxp3^+$ T cells) or inducible T regs (a group that includes the IL-10-secreting Treg1 cells, the Th3 population that produces both TGF-b and IL-10, and $foxp3^+$ Tregs). A more detailed description of the diversity and functions of T regulatory cells can be found elsewhere (43).

DC as Modulators of the Adaptive Immune Response in Leishmaniasis

The biological features of pathogens and activation PRRs as well as the underlying signaling processes, are determinant in the specific cytokines secreted by activated DCs, which in turn are one of the key element in the polarization of Th cell subtypes (44).

In general, Th1 cells produce pro-inflammatory cytokines, such as Interferon Gamma (IFN-γ), which lead to Tumor Necrosis Factor Alpha (TNF-α) production by innate immune cells, promoting a resistance profile against *Leishmania*. The hallmark of IFN-γ leishmanicidal activity relies on the classical activation of infected macrophages, leading to increased production of nitric oxide (NO) and reactive oxygen species (ROS), which subsequently culminate in intracellular *Leishmania* elimination (13). By contrast, the Th2 profile is characterized by the production of IL-4, IL-5, and IL-13, which are mostly associated with enhanced arginase activity accompanied by the alternative activation of macrophages, parasite survival and proliferation, and pronounced susceptibility (13). Additionally, in recent decades, the contributions of the Th17 subtype on the progression of leishmaniasis has become a growing concern. The hallmark of the Th17 profile is the production of IL-17, and the subsequent recruitment of neutrophils to the site of inflammation. As reviewed elsewhere, the joint actions of this subtype paradoxically play a dual role in leishmaniasis, since these cells are not only responsible for the elimination of parasites, but also for the exacerbation of the inflammatory process and tissue damage (45). Crosstalk between *Leishmania* and DCs via the stimulation of various cellular apparatuses and the engagement of multiple signaling processes culminates in phenotypic and functional alterations in DCs. Such modifications are imperative for proper cytokine production and the activation of Th cells, which induce immune events that can result in parasite control (46).

DENDRITIC CELL-*LEISHMANIA* INTERACTION

Leishmanial Signals Prompt DCs Activation

One of the biological functions of DCs is to recognize molecular patterns associated with pathogens (PAMPs). To this end, DCs employ PRRs that interact with a variety of PAMPs expressed by distinct species of *Leishmania*. The activation of DCs can be substantially modulated by these interactions, which greatly influence the immune response against *Leishmania* (46).

The DC Recognition Apparatus: the Role of PRRs in Leishmania-DC Interplay

Toll-like receptors (TLRs) are germline-encoded immune receptors that play a pivotal role in the immunosurveillance function of DCs. These receptors are subdivided into 10 families in humans (TLR1 to TLR10) and 12 families in mice (TLR1 to TLR9, and TLR11 to TLR13) (47), and are expressed on either the cell membrane surface or in intracellular compartments. TLRs possess leucine-rich repeats that serve as molecular docking sites for ligand-receptor interactions. Upon ligand-mediated activation, TLRs undergo an intricate dimerization process that activates a variety of biochemical pathways, culminating in the transcription of several inflammatory genes. Of note, it has been proposed that TLRs may be central elements in the establishment of immune homeostasis, as these cells participate in the delicate balance between pro-inflammatory and anti-inflammatory responses (48). However, despite their relevance in the recognition of several pathogens and the induction of immune responses, only TLR2, TLR4, and TLR9 have been described in the mediation of DC-*Leishmania* interaction.

It has been demonstrated that the neutralization of TLR2 and TLR4 decreases the expression of molecules involved in the process of antigen presentation during *L. major* infection, which suggests that both receptors may be key players in the establishment of effective responses against *Leishmania* (49). Interestingly, a study documented that TLR2 deficiency increases DC activation, leading to IL-12 production during *L. braziliensis* infection. On the other hand, a deficiency of MyD88 results in lower levels of DC activation and IL-12 production, both essential elements in mounting protective immunity against *L. braziliensis* (50).

TLR2 also recognizes Lipophosphoglycan (LPG), a surface molecule conserved in all *Leishmania* species that is considered an important virulence factor, especially due to its role in the modulation of immune cell activation (51). When LPG of *L. mexicana* is recognized by the TLR2 of moDCs, the expression of MHC-II and CD86 as well as the secretion of IL-12p70, are enhanced. Subsequently, the interaction of DCs with NKT cells culminates in higher IFN-γ production. This cellular interaction could possibly contribute to the protective state observed during the acute phase of *L. mexicana* infection (52).

TLR9 has been described as important in DC activation as well as in the production of neutrophil chemoattractant during *L. infantum* infection in C57BL/6 mice (53). Additionally, TLR9 is also required for the induction of IL-12 production in mouse bone marrow-derived DCs (BMDCs) infected with *L. major*, leading to both IFN-γ expression and cytotoxicity enhancement in NK cells (54). Collectively, these findings contribute to the understanding of how the intracellular TLRs in DCs mediate the stimulation of other immune cells that promote parasite eradication.

Different *Leishmania* species can mitigate the signaling pathways of CTLRs to promote parasite proliferation and survival. Iborra et al. showed that *L. major* releases a soluble protein ligand of Mincle (Macrophage inducible Ca^{2+}-dependent lectin receptor) that targets an inhibitory ITAM signaling pathway, resulting in the impairment of DC activation and migration (55). In a similar vein, Zimara et al. experimentally demonstrated the importance of CTLRs in mounting an adaptive immune response against *L. major*. These researchers observed an increased expansion of Dectin-1^+ DCs following *L. major* inoculation in C57BL/6 and BALB/c mice as well as in the peripheral blood of CL patients. Additionally, experiments with BMDM stimulated with a Dectin-1 agonist revealed both high levels of DC maturation and the expansion of CD 4 T cells (56). Collectively, these findings serve to indicate the significance of both CTRL signaling and the physical interactions between these cells and pathogens in the promotion of an effective immune response.

Mechanisms of Leishmania Uptake

In addition to their importance as major mediators of the innate and adaptive branches of immunity, DCs are also recognized for their highly efficient phagocytic activity (57). These cells actively collect antigens in their surroundings, and couple subsequent antigen processing with epitope exhibition via antigen presentation platforms–the major histocompatibility complex molecules (58).

Typically, the mechanisms of capturing pathogens involve specific receptor-ligand interactions as well as the mobilization of cytoskeleton elements that promotes the internalization of parasites (59). Several studies have proposed that the uptake of *Leishmania* by DCs occurs in a parasite life form-dependent manner, since DCs preferentially phagocytose IgG -coated amastigotes. In fact, amastigotes internalization involves the participation of FcγRI and FcγRIII (60). It has been suggested that GP63, a protease found on leishmanial membranes, mediates the conversion of C3b into its inactive form, iC3b. Subsequently, iC3b binds to CR3, resulting in the adherence of leishmania to the surface membrane of DCs (60).

Argueta-Donohué et al. demonstrated that DC-SIGN (Dendritic Cell-Specific Intercellular adhesion molecule-3-Grabbing Non-integrin), a surface receptor mainly found in DCs, mediates a more efficient internalization rates of *L. mexicana* promastigotes after 3 h of *in vitro* infection (52). Moreover, these authors also confirmed that the experimental neutralization of DC-SIGN significantly reduces the rates of infection in moDCs. These intriguing findings illustrate the fundamental role of DC-SIGN in several instances of *Leishmania*-DC interplay, ranging from the initiation of parasite phagocytosis to discrimination between *Leishmania* life cycle stages (52). Additionally, mounting evidence indicates that DC-SIGN also recognizes *L. pifanoi* surface molecules, contributing to the subsequent uptake of parasite amastigotes (61). Furthermore, *L. major* and *L. donovani*- infected moDCs exhibit reduced surface expression of DC-SIGN in contrast to uninfected cells, with this immunomodulation being accentuated in cells stimulated with excreted-secreted antigens (ESA) of both *Leishmania* species (62). Together, these studies suggest that the consequences of the DC-SIGN-mediated crosstalk between *Leishmania* and host DCs may have profound biological consequences in *Leishmania* infection.

The Effects of Purinergic Receptors on DC Activation During Leishmania Infection

Purinergic receptors play a significant role in the recognition of damage-associated molecular pattern (DAMPs), including the detection of extracellular Adenosine Triphosphate (ATP), a potent pro-inflammatory trigger of immune responses (63). In pathophysiological contexts, ATP is converted into Adenosine (ADO) via the action of the ectonucleotidases CD39 and CD73, and the accumulation of ADO in the extracellular milieu results in the activation of its A2 receptor. This phenomenon has been observed during *L. amazonensis* infection, which was accompanied by the suppression of DC functions via decreased rates of CD40 expression and IL-12 production. Additionally, the activation of the A2b receptor of DCs decreases the capacity of these cells to stimulate T cell proliferation and the production of IFN-γ, leading to an insufficient protective immune response, a peculiarity of *L. amazonensis* infection (64). While increases in CD39 and CD73 expression are also observed in *L. braziliensis* and *L. major* infection, A2b receptor activation has not been detected. Interestingly, it has been proposed that the main evasion mechanism employed by these two species is reduced expression of the molecules involved in antigen presentation, which includes the exploitation of the IL-10 receptor (IL-10R). Notwithstanding, this evasion mechanism employed by *L. braziliensis* and *L. major* is followed by the upregulation of CD40, which may suggest that it does not prevent T cell activation (65).

Together, these findings provide evidence that early interactions between DCs and *Leishmania* can have profound effects on disease outcome. Several of the mechanisms of immune evasion employed by *Leishmania* include the mitigation of DC immunobiological functioning via the exploitation of different receptors and the disruption of downstream signaling pathways. In addition, recent data indicate that the impairment of DC activation is directly associated with the enhancement of parasite survival and persistence in hosts.

CO-STIMULATORY MOLECULES AND ANTIGEN PRESENTATION

Following the recognition and internalization of pathogens, DCs migrate to secondary lymphoid organs to present processed antigens to naïve T cells (66). Subsequently, the adaptive immune response becomes initiated via the presentation of small peptides through either MHC class I or class II molecules. Basically, the former class mediates the recognition of endogenous peptides by cytotoxic CD8+ T cells, while the latter is involved in the presentation of exogenous peptides to CD4+ T helper cells. Notably, the process of antigen fragmentation is of paramount importance to allow for proper antigen presentation, since MHCII molecules only present peptides with a specific number of amino acids (67). Alternatively, DCs are also capable of mobilizing MHC I molecules in order to display exogenously derived-antigens, a process known as cross-presentation (68). Additionally, co-stimulatory molecules (such as CD40, CD80, and CD86) are essential to effective antigen presentation, by providing secondary signals for T cell expansion and differentiation (69).

Several species of *Leishmania* employ distinct strategies to regulate the expression of co-stimulatory molecules, which dampens the process of antigen presentation (70). Accordingly, the modulation of co-stimulatory molecules can be associated not only with enhanced parasites survival and growth, but also with subsequent disease outcome.

Figueiredo et al. experimentally demonstrated that *L. amazonensis* induced lower levels of MHCII, CD86 and CD40 expression in BMDCs (bone marrow -derived DCs) from C57BL/6 mice, resulting in a decline in T-cell proliferation (65). Furthermore, the adoptive transfer of BMDCs expressing low levels of CD40 was associated not only with T regulatory cell expansion, but also with an increase in *L. donovani* burden in BALB/c mice (71). It has been also shown that CD40 and its ligand are important for the development of resistance against *L. major* infection (72, 73). Hai Qi et al. reported that *L. amazonensis* amastigotes mitigated IL-12 production in a CD40-dependent manner in a BALB/c infection model, which was followed by an increase in levels of IL-4 (74). Subsequently, amastigote-infected DCs were observed to be able to activate pathogenic CD4+ T cells, which could potentially lead to exacerbated *Leishmania* proliferation and the progression of pathogenesis (72). Thus, emerging evidence suggests that reduced CD40 expression could possibly facilitate *Leishmania* infection.

The importance of CD80 and CD86 expression has been highlighted in the establishment of early immune responses. For instance, the infection of human moDCs with *L. amazonensis* downregulates the expression of CD80 and upregulates the expression of CD86, which is followed by a decrease in IL-6 production during DC differentiation (75). Although CD86 possibly takes center stage in this context, the equivalent expression of other costimulatory molecules can lead to the early production of IFN-γ or IL-4 during infection by *L. major* depending on the experimental model (76). Together, these results reinforce the contribution of these molecules in the production of different cytokines by properly stimulated T cells.

Several species of *Leishmania* can modulate antigen processing and the expression of MHC II molecules (77). DCs infected with *L. major* amastigotes not only upregulate the expression of several molecules involved in antigen presentation,

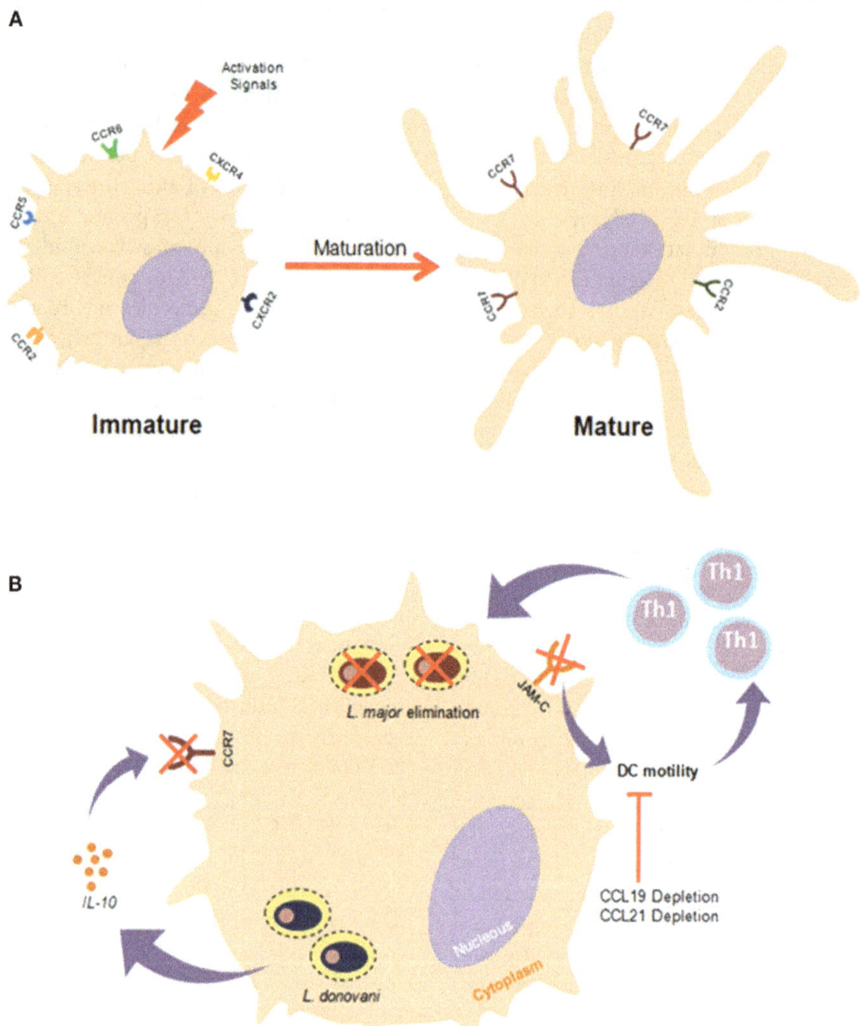

FIGURE 2 | Effects of *Leishmania* parasites in DC migration. **(A)** Immature DCs exhibit particular membrane surface markers such as CCR2,CCR5,CXCR4, and CXCR2. Once stimulated by effective activation signals, DCs undergo a maturation process that culminate in the upregulation CCR7 expression as well as enhanced mobilility. **(B)** The establishment of effective immune responses against *Leishmania* depends substantially on the migration of DCs to lymph nodes where these cells activate T lymphocytes. *Leishmania* impairs the highly coordinated process of DC migration as an evasion strategy to prevent the leishmanicidal effects of the adaptative immunity. *L. donovani* mitigates the functionality of CCR7 in an IL-10 dependent manner, thus hampering DC migration. Furthermore, it has been documented that the experimental blockage of junctional adhesion molecule-C (JAM-C) enhances DC migration and immunity against *L. major*.

such as MHC class II, CD40, CD54, CD80, and CD86, but also exhibit elevated rates of IL-12 production. It should be noted that only the amastigote forms of these parasites were capable of inducing this increase in *L. major*-infected DCs (78). Conversely, *L. mexicana* amastigotes do not promote increased expression of CD80, CD54, and MHC II molecules in BMDCs, suggesting that these discrepancies in the immune response by DCs occur in a species-specific manner (79).

Interestingly, a recent study by Resende et al. reported a dichotomic response between *L. infantum*-infected and non-infected DCs. In this study, the authors observed that uninfected DCs expressed higher levels of IL-12p40 and other co-stimulatory molecules, which enabled DCs to elicit appropriate $CD4^+$ T cell immunoprotective responses, whereas infected DCs expressed lower levels of co-stimulatory molecules and high IL-10 production (80). This finding suggests that *L.infantum*-infected DCs and their uninfected counterparts exert antagonistic roles in the activation and polarization of T cells, mechanistically revealing a novel evasion strategy employed by this species. Along the same lines, a study carried out by Carvalho et al demonstrated that, in contrast to *L-braziliensis*-infected DCs, only uninfected DCs upregulate the expression of MHC II, CD80, and CD86. Interestingly, it was also observed that despite enhancing the expression of such molecules, *L-braziliensis*-infected DCs produced higher levels of TNF-α in response to stimulation with LPS. These findings corroborate the hypothesis that uninfected and *Leishmania*-infected DCs can act conjointly, yet distinctly, to promote immune responses against the parasite, since uninfected DCs can lead to enhanced T cell activation, while the production of TNF-α by infected DCs may

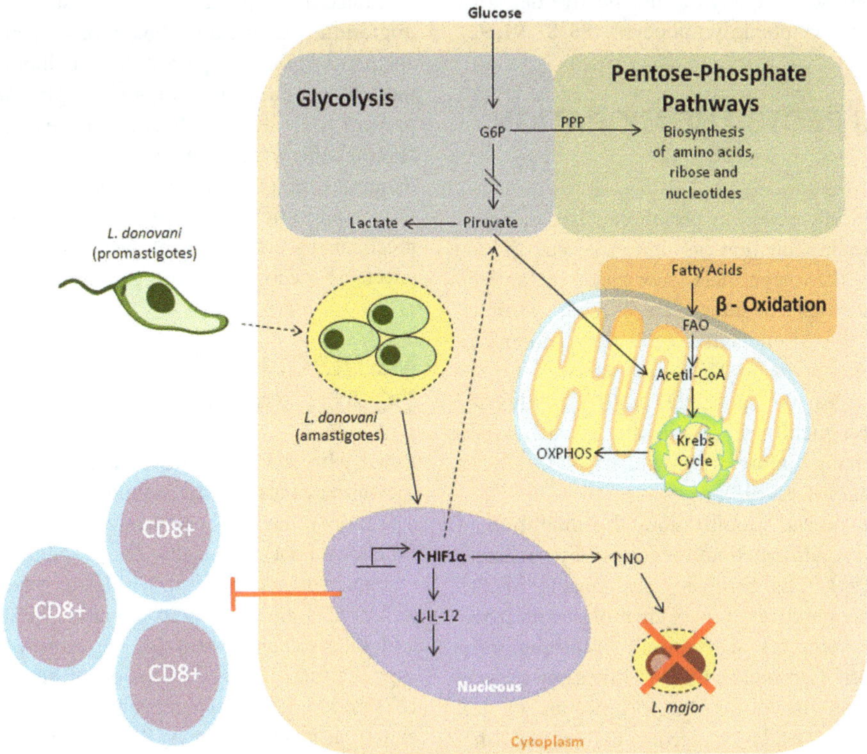

FIGURE 3 | Overview of the major metabolic pathways in Dendritic cells. Cellular metabolic processes provide DCs with the necessary energy to sustain their immunological functions. In a resting state, DCs rely on oxidative phosphorylation to meet their bioenergetic requirements. When faced with pathogens, DCs undergo metabolic reprogramming skewed toward aerobic glycolysis for ATP generation, and the establishment of pro-inflammatory responses. Of note, different reports seem to suggest that HIF1a play a dual role in metabolic reprogramming in leishmaniasis. It has been shown that *L. donovani* infection enhances the stabilization of HIF1a, which in turn leads to decreased IL-12 production. Conversely, It has been demonstrated that HIF1a increases nitric oxide production, which subsequently results in *L. major* elimination.

contribute to the control of parasite proliferation at the site of infection (81).

Paradoxically, DCs are also able to present exogenous antigens through MHC-I, with significant consequences on the activation of CD8 T cells (82). It has been reported that this phenomenon, also known as cross-presentation, is of great importance to the expansion of antigen-specific cytotoxic CD8 T cells, which are responsible for eliciting an effective immune responses against *Leishmania*. Accordingly, in this context, DC figure as the most potent inducers of IFN-γ production by CD8+ T lymphocytes. Brewig et al. demonstrated that, in experimental leishmaniasis, the priming of $CD4^+$ and $CD8^+$ T cell relies essentially on the activity of distinct DC subtypes (83). Indeed, it was reported that the depletion of $Langerin^+$ DCs was associated with the reduced proliferation of *L. major*-specific CD8+ T cells. As a consequence, the amount of primed CD8 T cells found at the site of infection and in lymph nodes was significantly reduced (83). In a similar vein, a study conducted by Ashok et al revealed the importance of cross-priming DCs in the effective constraint of *L. major* infection. It was shown that $Batf3^{-/-}$ mice (which lack $CD8^+/CD103^+$ DCs) exhibited increased susceptibility *to L. major* (84). Furthermore, a study by Lemos et al explored the function of $CD8^+$ DCs in antigen presentation during *L. major* infection in a murine model that restricted the expression of MHC-II to $CD8a^+/CD11b^+$ DCs. Notably, it was observed that $CD8a^+/CD11b^+$ DCs could efficiently restrain *L. major* infection by eliciting the effective constraint of parasites by CD4 T cells (85).

Numerous studies have revealed that the underlying mechanisms of antigen processing depend not only on the constitutive proteasome or the immunoproteosome, but also on the involvement of alternative molecular machineries of cytosolic degradation, such as tripeptidyl peptidase II (TPPII) and nardilysin (86–88). TPPII is a known eukaryotic peptidase related to several cellular processes, such as antigen processing, apoptosis and cell division. However, it should be noted that TPPII activation occurs mainly when proteasome function becomes compromised (89).

Although little is known about the detailed mechanisms of cytosolic endopeptidases, such as Nardilysin, their role seems to be indispensable in the generation of some specific epitopes (90). The importance of alternative antigen processing machinery should be further investigated in the context of leishmaniasis.

Although the participation of $CD8^+$ T cells in *Leishmania* infection is still controversial, growing evidence indicates that protective responses rely substantially on the effective dendritic cell-mediated activation of cytotoxic lymphocytes (86, 87, 91, 92).

LEISHMANIA AFFECTS THE MIGRATION OF DCS

Immature DCs strategically reside in peripheral tissues, where they exercise their main function as immune guards. As discussed previously, these sentinels specialize in antigen uptake via their apparatus to internalize foreign particles. In peripheral tissues, PAMP-mediated activation confers an immunostimulatory phenotype to DCs, characterized by the upregulation of molecules also associated with an enhanced migratory ability. Subsequently, DCs migrate toward lymph nodes, where they exchange information with naïve T cells via the antigen presentation process (93).

In order to ensure precise mobilization, the migration of DCs needs to be highly coordinated and regulated by particular recruitment signals (94). The primary mechanisms of DC migration involve the cooperative action of chemokines and their receptors. Chemokine receptors are typically transmembrane proteins associated with G-proteins whose activation triggers signaling pathways responsible for the promotion of cell mobilization (95). Some evidence seems to suggest that DC subtypes exhibit diverse chemokine receptors, conferring subtype-specific migration dynamics. Commonly, immature DCs express CCR2, CCR5, CCR6, CXCR2, and CXCR4 in a predominant fashion. Upon pathogen-mediated activation, DCs undergo a maturation processes that culminates in the crucial upregulation of CCR7 (**Figure 2A**) (96).

By way of evolution, protozoan parasites developed strategies to mitigate DC functioning by inhibiting access to T cells, thusly restricting the establishment of efficient adaptive immune responses. In the context of flagellate protozoan infection, successful DC migration to draining lymph nodes (dLNs) is substantially dependent on both CCR2 and CCR7 expression (97). Several studies have reported that *Leishmania* can induce a reduction in rates of DC migration (98, 99). *In vitro* studies have elucidated the roles of both soluble products and membrane constituents, such as *L. major* LPG, in the inhibition of DC motility (98, 100). The underlying molecular mechanisms of *Leishmania*-induced mitigation of DC motility remain elusive. A recent study suggested that *L. major* exploits the junction adhesion molecule C (JAM-C) to reduce DC migration rates, and demonstrated that the experimental blockage of this molecule enhanced the immunological response against this parasite (101). An investigation in an animal model exhibited an *L. major*-susceptible phenotype, suggesting that the depletion of CCR2 culminated in poor DC migration and a skewed Th2 immune response (102). Furthermore, infection with *L. donovani*, a viscerotropic species, promotes an inhibition in the expression of CCR7 mediated by IL-10 production, which ensures that DCs will not be able to reach splenic regions, thereby contributing to the progression of visceral leishmaniasis (**Figure 2B**) (103). Another *in vivo* study associated CCL19/CCL21 deficiency with a reduction in both DC mobility and resistance to *L. donovani* infection (103).

Collectively, the current data suggest that efficacious DC migration is essential to the establishment of effective responses against *Leishmania* parasites. The literature clearly indicates that these parasites employ a plenitude of strategies to prevent DCs from activating T cells during the course of several clinical forms of leishmaniasis. Deciphering the complex dynamics surrounding the *Leishmania*-mediated impairment of DC mobilization will provide new insights into the evasion mechanisms employed by these parasites and elucidate their effects on the immunopathogenesis of leishmaniasis.

METABOLIC REPROGRAMMING DURING DC ACTIVATION

Faced with infection and inflammation, DCs must cope with increasing catabolic and anabolic demands via the redirection of a plethora of metabolic pathways to support their major immune functions (104). Typically, the metabolism of inactive DCs is characterized by the central roles of oxidative phosphorylation (OXPHOS) and fatty acid oxidation (FAO), for energy supply and biomolecule synthesis, respectively (105). New evidence suggests that, after the initiation of PAMP-mediated activation, DCs undergo metabolic reprogramming, relying substantially on anaerobic glycolysis for ATP production, a process characterized by the conversion of pyruvate into lactate. Despite being ineffective in the generation of ATP, glycolysis can be coupled with several anabolic pathways, such as fatty acid synthesis and the pentose phosphate pathway, allowing for the biosynthesis of other macromolecules, namely lipids and nucleotides, respectively (106, 107). In this scenario, DCs exhibit low rates of oxidative phosphorylation. These deviations in the metabolic repertoire of DCs are prominent regulators of immune responses, as metabolic enzymes and their products can influence the establishment of inflammation (108).

In this inflammatory milieu, immune cells are poorly supplied with oxygen and nutrients for their metabolic processes, leading to the activation of hypoxia-inducible transcription factor 1α (HIF-1α) (109). Recently, HIF-1α was recognized as a major player in the induction of glycolysis, since it promotes the transcription of several enzymes involved in glucose metabolism (110). Nevertheless, its expression was shown to favor *L. donovani* infection in a model of chronic visceral leishmaniasis, as increased HIF-1a expression in murine splenic DCs was correlated with decreased IL-12 production, allowing parasite survival through limited Th1 cell expansion (111). In consonance with these observations, Hammani et al. demonstrated the importance of the IRF-5/HIF1α transcription factor axis in the impairment of DCs to promote the expansion of $CD8^+$ T cells (112). Conversely, *in vitro* experiments showed that HIF1α enhanced both *Leishmania major* elimination and levels of NO production in macrophages (**Figure 3**) (113). Together, while these observations suggest that HIF1α downregulates some DC functions against *Leishmania*, this effect may be cell-specific. Moreover, a recent study highlighted the contribution of two energetic sensors, Sirtuin 1 (SIRT1) and AMP-activated protein kinase (AMPK), to *L. infantum* survival and replication in macrophages (114).

Given the relevance of the metabolic processes of DCs in supporting the immunobiological functioning of these cells, it is unsurprising that an increasing number of studies have contemplated this interesting topic in recent years. Nevertheless, few studies have attempted to investigate the role of DC immunometabolism in *Leishmania* infection. Currently, the molecular players involved in metabolic reprogramming and the mechanistic basis of immunometabolism continue to remain elusive in the context of leishmaniasis.

EFFECTS OF EPIGENETIC MODIFICATIONS ON DC DEVELOPMENT AND COURSE OF INFECTION

Interactions between host cells and parasites prompt several alterations in a range of biological processes occurring in DCs, including epigenetic alteration via modified gene expression. This phenomenon is not dependent on DNA sequence modifications and includes DNA methylation, histone modifications, chromatin remodeling and regulation by non-coding RNAs (115–117).

The activation of transcription factors is one of the major regulatory elements occurring in epigenetic alterations (118, 119). PU.1 transcription factor has been described as an essential TF for the development and functioning of DCs, as evidenced by the expression of FLT3, granulocyte-macrophage colony-stimulating factor receptor (GM-CSFR) and macrophage colony stimulating factor receptor (M-GSFR) (119, 120). It has been demonstrated that PU.1 is also involved in the regulation of basal expression of DC-SIGN, which in turn influences the repertoire of antigen uptake in DCs (121). PU.1 can also regulate the promoter region of genes CD80 and CD86 in murine bone marrow–derived DCs, leading to the overexpression of these co-stimulatory molecules, thereby enhancing DC migration and the activation of T cells (122).

In face of tissue damage or infection, several modifications in the histones alter chromatin conformation, leading to changes in the expression profile of critical genes in specific DC subsets (123, 124). Tserel et al. showed by GWAS (Genome-wide Association Study) that histone modifications can influence the processes of differentiation, phagocytosis and antigen presentation in moDCs through the upregulation of surface marker expression and chemokine production. Similar findings have been reported in macrophages, reinforcing the similarity of epigenetic mechanisms in the development of both cell types (125).

The importance of epigenetic changes in DCs infected by *Leishmania* remains unclear. However, *L. donovani* infection in macrophages was shown to lead to changes in the methylation of CpGs sites via parasite exosome secretion, which may enhance parasite replication and survival (126). Furthermore, *L. amazonensis* infection promoted epigenetic modifications at the IL-10 *locus* in murine macrophages, which activated ERK1/2 pathways and promoted parasite survival (127). In addition, this parasite species can upregulate histone deacetylases (HDACs), which enhances iNOS promoters in macrophages, thusly favoring infection (128).

Taken together, in addition to playing a crucial role in the development of DCs, these findings seem to suggest that interactions between *Leishmania* and immune cells can trigger epigenetic modifications that may alter the course of the infection. However, much remains to be elucidated with regard to this topic.

CONCLUSION REMARKS

DCs are relevant immunological agents in the concatenation of innate and adaptative branches of immunity. Here, we have attempted to integrate recent advances in molecular aspects of the immunobiological functioning of DCs with the current state of understanding regarding the pathogenic mechanisms of leishmaniasis. Although a large body of evidence supports the central role of DC activation in the establishment of responses against *Leishmania* parasites, the overwhelming complexity of *Leishmania*-DC interactions impedes the attainment of a comprehensive understanding of the molecular processes involved in DC activation. Further clarification is required to unravel the interplay between different DC subtypes and different species and life cycle stages of *Leishmania* as well as how parasites subvert particular aspects of DC activation in the effort to successfully establish infection. Finally, an enhanced understanding of the fundamental molecular events underlying DC activation will lead to the expansion of our current base of knowledge surrounding leishmaniasis as well as offer new therapeutic targets.

AUTHOR CONTRIBUTIONS

RT and SN designed the review and wrote the manuscript. IN, MR, IS, and RL assembled the review and wrote the manuscript. NM and CB supervised the work, designed the review, and wrote the manuscript.

REFERENCES

1. Alvar J, Vélez ID, Bern C, Herrero M, Desjeux P, Cano J, et al. Leishmaniasis worldwide and global estimates of its incidence. *PLoS ONE* (2012) 7:e35671. doi: 10.1371/journal.pone.0035671
2. Desjeux P. Leishmaniasis: current situation and new perspectives. *Comp Immunol Microbiol Infect Dis.* (2004) 27:305–318. doi: 10.1016/j.cimid.2004.03.004
3. WHO. *Who Technical Report Series Control of the Leishmaniases* (2016).

4. Kaye P, Scott P. Leishmaniasis: complexity at the host-pathogen interface. *Nat Rev Microbiol.* (2011) 9:604–15. doi: 10.1038/nrmicro2608
5. Amato VS, Tuon FF, Bacha HA, Neto VA, Nicodemo AC. Mucosal leishmaniasis. current scenario and prospects for treatment. *Acta Trop.* (2008) 105:1–9. doi: 10.1016/j.actatropica.2007.08.003
6. Ives A, Ronet C, Prevel F, Ruzzante G, Fuertes-marraco S, Schutz F, Zangger H, et al. *Leishmania* RNA virus controls the severity of mucocutaneous leishmaniasis. *Learn Instr.* (2011) 331:775–8. doi: 10.1126/science.1199326
7. Gatto M, Abreu MM de, Tasca KI, Simão JC, Fortaleza CMCB, Pereira PCM, et al. Biochemical and nutritional evaluation of patients with visceral leishmaniasis before and after treatment with leishmanicidal drugs. *Rev Soc Bras Med Trop.* (2013) 46:735–40. doi: 10.1590/0037-8682-0198-2013
8. Scott P, Novais FO. Cutaneous leishmaniasis: immune responses in protection and pathogenesis. *Nat Publ Gr.* (2016) 16:581–92. doi: 10.1038/nri.2016.72
9. De Oliveira CI, Brodskyn CI. The immunobiology of leishmania braziliensis infection. *Front Immunol.* (2012) 3:145. doi: 10.3389/fimmu.2012.00145
10. Oliveira F, de Carvalho AM, de Oliveira CI. Sand-fly saliva-leishmania-man: the trigger trio. *Front Immunol.* (2013) 4:375. doi: 10.3389/fimmu.2013.00375
11. Ribeiro-Gomes FL, Sacks D. The influence of early neutrophil-leishmania interactions on the host immune response to infection. *Front Cell Infect Microbiol.* (2012) 2:59. doi: 10.3389/fcimb.2012.00059
12. Laskay T, Zandbergen G, Solbach W. Neutrophil granulocytes – trojan horses for *Leishmania major* and other intracellular microbes ? (2003) 11:210–4. doi: 10.1016/S0966-842X(03)00075-1
13. Liu D, Uzonna JE. The early interaction of leishmania with macrophages and dendritic cells and its influence on the host immune response. *Front Cell Infect Microbiol.* (2012) 2:83. doi: 10.3389/fcimb.2012.00083
14. Steinman RM. Dendritic cells: understanding immunogenicity. *Eur J Immunol.* (2007) 37:53–60. doi: 10.1002/eji.200737400
15. Collin M, Bigley V. Human dendritic cell subsets: an update. *Immunology* (2018) 154:3–20. doi: 10.1111/imm.12888
16. Doulatov S, Notta F, Eppert K, Nguyen LT, Ohashi PS, Dick JE. Revised map of the human progenitor hierarchy shows the origin of macrophages and dendritic cells in early lymphoid development. *Nat Immunol.* (2010) 11:585–93. doi: 10.1038/ni.1889
17. Collin M, Mcgovern N. Human dendritic cell subsets. (2013) 140:22–30. doi: 10.1111/imm.12117
18. Sprangers S, Vries TJD, Everts V. Monocyte heterogeneity: consequences for monocyte-derived immune cells. *J Immunol Res.* (2016) 2016:1475435. doi: 10.1155/2016/1475435
19. Bachem A, Güttler S, Hartung E, Ebstein F, Schaefer M, Tannert A, et al. Superior antigen cross-presentation and XCR1 expression define human CD11c $^{+}$ CD141 $^{+}$ cells as homologues of mouse cd8 $^{+}$ dendritic cells. *J Exp Med.* (2010) 207:1273–81. doi: 10.1084/jem.20100348
20. Crozat K, Guiton R, Contreras V, Feuillet V, Dutertre C-A, Ventre E, et al. The XC chemokine receptor 1 is a conserved selective marker of mammalian cells homologous to mouse CD8α $^{+}$ dendritic cells. *J Exp Med.* (2010) 207:1283–92. doi: 10.1084/jem.20100223
21. Haniffa M, Shin A, Bigley V, McGovern N, Teo P, See P, et al. Human tissues contain CD141 hi cross-presenting dendritic cells with functional homology to mouse CD103 + nonlymphoid dendritic cells. *Immunity* (2012) 37:60–73. doi: 10.1016/j.immuni.2012.04.012
22. Reynolds G, Haniffa M. Human and mouse mononuclear phagocyte networks: a tale of two species? *Front Immunol.* (2015) 6:330. doi: 10.3389/fimmu.2015.00330
23. den Haan JMM, Lehar SM, Bevan MJ. Cd8 $^{+}$ but not Cd8 $^{-}$ dendritic cells cross-prime cytotoxic t cells *in vivo*. *J Exp Med.* (2000) 192:1685–96. doi: 10.1084/jem.192.12.1685
24. Bedoui S, Whitney PG, Waithman J, Eidsmo L, Wakim L, Caminschi I, et al. Cross-presentation of viral and self antigens by skin-derived CD103+ dendritic cells. *Hisp Sacra* (2012) 64:661–719. doi: 10.1038/ni.1724
25. Reizis B, Bunin A, Ghosh HS, Lewis KL, Sisirak V. Plasmacytoid dendritic cells : recent progress and open questions. *Annu Rev Immunol.* (2011) 29:163–83. doi: 10.1146/annurev-immunol-031210-101345
26. Cisse B, Caton ML, Lehner M, Maeda T, Scheu S, Locksley R, et al. Transcription factor E2-2 is an essential and specific regulator of plasmacytoid dendritic cell development. *Cell* (2008) 135:37–48. doi: 10.1016/j.cell.2008.09.016
27. Ghosh HS, Cisse B, Bunin A, Lewis KL, Reizis B. Continuous expression of the transcription factor E2-2 maintains the cell fate of mature plasmacytoid dendritic cells. *Immunity* (2010) 33:905–16. doi: 10.1016/j.immuni.2010.11.023
28. Blasius AL, Cella M, Maldonado J, Takai T, Colonna M. Brief report siglec-H is an IPC-specific receptor that modulates type I IFN secretion through DAP12. (2017) 107:2474–7. doi: 10.1182/blood-2005-09-3746.supported
29. Douglas JL, Gustin JK, Viswanathan K, Mansouri M, Moses AV, Früh K. The great escape: viral strategies to counter BST-2/ tetherin. *PLoS Pathog.* (2010) 6:e1000913. doi: 10.1371/journal.ppat.1000913
30. Fuchsberger M, Hochrein H, O'Keeffe M. Activation of plasmacytoid dendritic cells. *Immunol Cell Biol.* (2005) 83:571–7. doi: 10.1111/j.1440-1711.2005.01392.x
31. Ochando JC, Homma C, Yang Y, Hidalgo A, Garin A, Tacke F, et al. Alloantigen-presenting plasmacytoid dendritic cells mediate tolerance to vascularized grafts. *Nat Immunol.* (2006) 7:652–62. doi: 10.1038/ni1333
32. de Heer HJ, Hammad H, Soullié T, Hijdra D, Vos N, Willart MAM, et al. Essential role of lung plasmacytoid dendritic cells in preventing asthmatic reactions to harmless inhaled antigen. *J Exp Med.* (2004) 200:89–98. doi: 10.1084/jem.20040035
33. Kohli K, Janssen A, Förster R. Plasmacytoid dendritic cells induce tolerance predominantly by cargoing antigen to lymph nodes. *Eur J Immunol.* (2016) 46:2659–68. doi: 10.1002/eji.201646359
34. Ginhoux F, Merad M. Ontogeny and homeostasis of langerhans cells. *Immunol Cell Biol.* (2010) 88:387–92. doi: 10.1038/icb.2010.38
35. Birbeck MS, Breathnach AS, Everall JD. An electron microscope study of basal melanocytes and high-level clear cells (langerhans cells) in vitiligo**from the chester beatty research institute, Royal Cancer Hospital, London, S.W. 3, and the Departments of Anatomy, and Dermatology, St. Mary's Hos. *J Invest Dermatol.* (1961) 37:51–64. doi: 10.1038/jid.1961.80
36. Jakubzick CV, Randolph GJ, Henson PM. Monocyte differentiation and antigen-presenting functions. *Nat Rev Immunol.* (2017) 17:349–62. doi: 10.1038/nri.2017.28
37. Auffray C, Sieweke MH, Geissmann F. Blood Monocytes : development, heterogeneity, and relationship with dendritic cells. *Annu Rev Immunol.* (2009) 27:669–92. doi: 10.1146/annurev.immunol.021908.132557
38. Schmid M, Wege AK, Ritter U. Characteristics of "Tip-DCs and MDSCs" and their potential role in leishmaniasis. *Front Microbiol.* (2012) 3:74. doi: 10.3389/fmicb.2012.00074
39. Hammer GE, Ma A. Molecular control of steady-state dendritic cell maturation and immune homeostasis. *Annu Rev Immunol.* (2013) 31:743–91. doi: 10.1146/annurev-immunol-020711-074929
40. Haniffa M, Bigley V, Collin M. Human mononuclear phagocyte system reunited. *Semin Cell Dev Biol.* (2015) 41:59–69. doi: 10.1016/j.semcdb.2015.05.004
41. Dalod M, Chelbi R, Malissen B, Lawrence T. Dendritic cell maturation: functional specialization through signaling specificity and transcriptional programming. *EMBO J.* (2014) 33:1104–16. doi: 10.1002/embj.201488027
42. Pennock ND, White JT, Cross EW, Cheney EE, Tamburini BA, Kedl RM. T cell responses: naive to memory and everything in between. *AJP Adv Physiol Educ.* (2013) 37:273–83. doi: 10.1152/advan.00066.2013
43. Peterson RA. Regulatory T-cells: diverse phenotypes integral to immune homeostasis and suppression. *Toxicol Pathol.* (2012) 40:186–204. doi: 10.1177/0192623311430693
44. Kapsenberg ML. Dendritic-cell control of pathogen-driven T-cell polarization. *Nat Rev Immunol.* (2003) 3:984–93. doi: 10.1038/nri1246
45. Gonçalves-de-Albuquerque SC, Pessoa-e-Silva R, Trajano-Silva LAM, de Goes TC, de Morais RCS, Oliveira CNC, et al. The equivocal role of Th17 cells and neutrophils on immunopathogenesis of leishmaniasis. *Front Immunol.* (2017) 8:1437. doi: 10.3389/fimmu.2017.01437
46. Soong L. Modulation of dendritic cell function by leishmania parasites. *J Immunol.* (2008) 180:4355–60. doi: 10.4049/jimmunol.180.7.4355
47. Kawasaki T, Kawai T. Toll-like receptor signaling pathways. *Front Immunol.* (2014) 5:461. doi: 10.3389/fimmu.2014.00461

48. Chauhan P, Shukla D, Chattopadhyay D, Saha B. Redundant and regulatory roles for toll-like receptors in leishmania infection. *Clin Exp Immunol.* (2017) 190:167–86. doi: 10.1111/cei.13014
49. Komai-Koma M, Li D, Wang E, Vaughan D, Xu D. Anti-Toll-like receptor 2 and 4 antibodies suppress inflammatory response in mice. *Immunology* (2014) 143:354–62. doi: 10.1111/imm.12312
50. Vargas-Inchaustegui DA, Tai W, Xin L, Hogg AE, Corry DB, Soong L. Distinct roles for MyD88 and toll-like receptor 2 during leishmania braziliensis infection in mice. *Infect Immun.* (2009) 77:2948–56. doi: 10.1128/IAI.00154-09
51. Becker I, Salaiza N, Aguirre M, Delgado J, Carrillo-Carrasco N, Kobeh LG, et al. *Leishmania lipophosphoglycan* (LPG) activates NK cells through toll-LIKE receptor-2. *Mol Biochem Parasitol.* (2003) 130:65–74. doi: 10.1016/S0166-6851(03)00160-9
52. Argueta-Donohué J, Wilkins-Rodríguez AA, Aguirre-García M, Gutiérrez-Kobeh L. Differential phagocytosis of leishmania mexicana promastigotes and amastigotes by monocyte-derived dendritic cells. *Microbiol Immunol.* (2016) 60:369–81. doi: 10.1111/1348-0421.12325
53. Sacramento L, Trevelin SC, Nascimento MS, Lima-Jùnior DS, Costa DL, Almeida RP, et al. Toll-like receptor 9 signaling in dendritic cells regulates neutrophil recruitment to inflammatory foci following leishmania infantum infection. *Infect Immun.* (2015) 83:4604–16. doi: 10.1128/IAI.00975-15
54. Liese J, Schleicher U, Bogdan C. TLR9 signaling is essential for the innate NK cell response in murine cutaneous leishmaniasis. *Eur J Immunol.* (2007) 37:3424–34. doi: 10.1002/eji.200737182
55. Iborra S, Cueto FJ, Soto M, Lowell CA, Sancho D, Cueto FJ, et al. *Leishmania* uses mincle to target an inhibitory ITAM signaling pathway in dendritic cells that dampens adaptive immunity to infection. *Adaptive Imm.* (2016) 45:788–801. doi: 10.1016/j.immuni.2016.09.012
56. Zimara N, Chanyalew M, Aseffa A, van Zandbergen G, Lepenies B, Schmid M, et al. Dectin-1 positive dendritic cells expand after infection with *Leishmania major* parasites and represent promising targets for vaccine development. *Front Immunol.* (2018) 9:263. doi: 10.3389/fimmu.2018.00263
57. Savina A. Phagocytosis and antigen presentation in dendritic cells. (2007) 219:143–56. doi: 10.1111/j.1600-065X.2007.00552.x
58. Gordon S. Phagocytosis: an immunobiologic process. *Immunity* (2016) 44:463–75. doi: 10.1016/j.immuni.2016.02.026
59. Jaumouillé V, Grinstein S. Molecular mechanisms of phagosome formation. *Microbiol Spectr.* (2016) 4:1–18. doi: 10.1128/microbiolspec.MCHD-0013-2015
60. Woelbing F, Kostka SL, Moelle K, Belkaid Y, Sunderkoetter C, Verbeek S, et al. Uptake of *Leishmania major* by dendritic cells is mediated by Fcγ receptors and facilitates acquisition of protective immunity. *J Exp Med.* (2006) 203:177–88. doi: 10.1084/jem.20052288
61. Colmenares M, Puig-Kröger A, Pello OM, Corbí AL, Rivas L. Dendritic cell (DC)-specific intercellular adhesion molecule 3 (ICAM-3)-grabbing nonintegrin (DC-SIGN, CD209), a C-type surface lectin in human DCs, is a receptor for leishmania amastigotes. *J Biol Chem.* (2002) 277:36766–9. doi: 10.1074/jbc.M205270200
62. Revest M, Donaghy L, Cabillic F, Guiguen C, Gangneux JP. Comparison of the immunomodulatory effects of *L. donovani* and *L. major* excreted-secreted antigens, particulate and soluble extracts and viable parasites on human dendritic cells. *Vaccine* (2008) 26:6119–23. doi: 10.1016/j.vaccine.2008.09.005
63. Cronstein BN. Adenosine and inflammation. *Immunol Endocr Metab Agents Med Chem.* (2007) 7:280–5. doi: 10.2174/187152207781369841
64. Figueiredo AB, Souza-Testasicca MC, Mineo TWP, Afonso LCC. *Leishmania amazonensis*-induced cAMP triggered by adenosine A2Breceptor is important to inhibit dendritic cell activation and evade immune response in infected mice. *Front Immunol.* (2017) 8:849. doi: 10.3389/fimmu.2017.00849
65. Figueiredo AB, Serafim TD, Marques-da-Silva EA, Meyer-Fernandes JR, Afonso LCC. *Leishmania amazonensis* impairs DC function by inhibiting CD40 expression via A 2B adenosine receptor activation. *Eur J Immunol.* (2012) 42:1203–15. doi: 10.1002/eji.201141926
66. Banchereau J, Steinman RM. Dendritic cells and the control of immunity. *Nature* (1998) 392:245–52. doi: 10.1038/32588
67. Rock KL, Reits E, Neefjes J. Present yourself! By MHC Class I and MHC class II molecules. *Trends Immunol.* (2016) 37:724–37. doi: 10.1016/j.it.2016.08.010
68. Fonteneau JF, Kavanagh DG, Lirvall M, Sanders C, Timothy L, Bhardwaj N, et al. Characterization of the MHC class I cross-presentation pathway for cell-associated antigens by human dendritic cells characterization of the MHC class I cross-presentation pathway for cell-associated antigens by human dendritic cells. *Am Soc Hematol.* (2003) 102:4448–55. doi: 10.1182/blood-2003-06-1801
69. Kalinski P, Hilkens CMU, Wierenga EA, Kapsenberg ML. T-cell priming by type-1 and type-2 polarized dendritic cells: the concept of a third signal. *Immunol Today* (1999) 20:561–7. doi: 10.1016/S0167-5699(99)01547-9
70. Ghosh M, Bandyopadhyay S. Interaction of leishmania parasites with dendritic cells and its functional consequences. *Immunobiology* (2004) 209:173–7. doi: 10.1016/j.imbio.2004.02.007
71. Martin S, Agarwal R, Murugaiyan G, Saha B. CD40 expression levels modulate regulatory T cells in leishmania donovani infection. *J Immunol.* (2010) 185:551–9. doi: 10.4049/jimmunol.0902206
72. Campbell KA, Ovendale PJ, Kennedy MK, Fanslow WC, Reed SG, Maliszewski CR. CD40 ligand is required for protective cell-mediated immunity to *Leishmania major*. *Immunity* (1996) 4:283–9. doi: 10.1016/S1074-7613(00)80436-7
73. Kamanaka M, Yu P, Yasui T, Yoshida K, Kawabe T, Horii T. Protective role of CD40 in *Leishmania major* infection at two distinct phases of cell-mediated immunity CD40–CD40L interaction also plays a critical role in cell- mediated immune responses. *Immunity* (1996) 4:275–81.
74. Qi H, Popov V, Soong L. *Leishmania amazonensis*-dendritic cell interactions *in vitro* and the priming of parasite-specific CD4+ T cells *in vivo*. *J Immunol.* (2001) 167:4534–42. doi: 10.4049/jimmunol.167.8.4534
75. Favali C, Tavares N, Clarencio J, Barral A, Barral-Netto M, Brodskyn C. *Leishmania amazonensis* infection impairs differentiation and function of human dendritic cells. *J Leukoc Biol.* (2007) 82:1401–6. doi: 10.1189/jlb.0307187
76. Elloso MM, Scott P. Expression and contribution of B7-1 (CD80) and B7-2 (CD86) in the early immune response to *Leishmania major* infection. *J Immunol.* (1999) 162. 6708–15.
77. Feijó D, Tibúrcio R, Ampuero M, Brodskyn C, Tavares N. Dendritic cells and leishmania infection : adding layers of complexity to a complex disease. (2016) 2016:3967436. doi: 10.1155/2016/3967436
78. von Stebut E, Belkaid Y, Jakob T, Sacks DL, Udey MC. Uptake of *Leishmania major* amastigotes results in activation and interleukin 12 release from murine skin–derived dendritic cells: implications for the initiation of *Anti-Leishmania* immunity. *J Exp Med.* (1998) 188:1547–52. doi: 10.1084/jem.188.8.1547
79. Bennett CL, Misslitz A, Colledge L, Aebischer T, Clare Blackburn C. Silent infection of bone marrow-derived dendritic cells by leishmania mexicana amastigotes. *Eur J Immunol.* (2001) 31:876–83. doi: 10.1002/1521-4141(200103)31:3<876::AID-IMMU876>3.0.CO;2-I
80. Resende M, Moreira D, Augusto J, Cunha J, Neves B, Cruz MT, et al. Leishmania-infected MHC Class II high dendritic cells polarize CD4+ T cells toward a nonprotective T-bet+ IFN- + IL-10+ phenotype. *J Immunol.* (2013) 191:262–73. doi: 10.4049/jimmunol.1203518
81. Carvalho LP, Pearce EJ, Scott P. Functional dichotomy of dendritic cells following interaction with leishmania braziliensis: infected cells produce high levels of TNF- whereas bystander dendritic cells are activated to promote T cell responses. *J Immunol.* (2008) 181:6473–80. doi: 10.4049/jimmunol.181.9.6473
82. Embgenbroich M, Burgdorf S. Current concepts of antigen cross-presentation. *Front Immunol.* (2018) 9:1643. doi: 10.3389/fimmu.2018.01643
83. Brewig N, Kissenpfennig A, Malissen B, Veit A, Bickert T, Fleischer B, et al. Priming of CD8+ and CD4+ T cells in experimental leishmaniasis is initiated by different dendritic cell subtypes. *J Immunol.* (2009) 182:774–83. doi: 10.4049/jimmunol.182.2.774

84. Ashok D, Schuster S, Ronet C, Rosa M, Mack V, Lavanchy C, et al. Cross-presenting dendritic cells are required for control of *Leishmania major* infection. *Eur J Immunol.* (2014) 44:1422–32. doi: 10.1002/eji.201344242
85. Lemos MP, Esquivel F, Scott P, Laufer TM. MHC class II expression restricted to CD8{alpha}+ and CD11b+ dendritic cells is sufficient for control of *Leishmania major. J Exp Med.* (2004) 199:725–30. doi: 10.1084/jem.20 030795
86. Belkaid Y, Von Stebut E, Mendez S, Lira R, Caler E, Bertholet S, et al. CD8+ T cells are required for primary immunity in C57BL/6 mice following low-dose, intradermal challenge with *Leishmania major. J Immunol.* (2002) 168:3992–4000. doi: 10.4049/jimmunol.168.8.3992
87. Brosch S, Tenzer S, Akkad N, Lorenz B, Schild H, Stebut EV. Priming of leishmania-reactive CD8 T cells *in vivo* does not require LMP7-containing immunoproteasomes. *J Invest Dermatol.* (2012) 132:1302–5. doi: 10.1038/jid.2011.454
88. von Stebut E, Tenzer S. Cutaneous leishmaniasis: distinct functions of dendritic cells and macrophages in the interaction of the host immune system with *Leishmania major. Int J Med Microbiol.* (2017) 308:206–14. doi: 10.1016/j.ijmm.2017.11.002
89. Rockel B, Kopec KO, Lupas AN, Baumeister W. Structure and function of tripeptidyl peptidase II, a giant cytosolic protease. *Biochim Biophys Acta Proteins Proteomics* (2012) 1824:237–45. doi: 10.1016/j.bbapap.2011.07.002
90. Kessler JH, Khan S, Seifert U, Le Gall S, Chow KM, Paschen A, et al. Antigen processing by nardilysin and thimet oligopeptidase generates cytotoxic T cell epitopes. *Nat Immunol.* (2011) 12:45–53. doi: 10.1038/ni.1974
91. Maji M, Mazumder S, Bhattacharya S, Choudhury ST, Sabur A, Shadab M, et al. A Lipid Based antigen delivery system efficiently facilitates MHC class-I antigen presentation in dendritic cells to stimulate CD8+T cells. *Sci Rep.* (2016) 6:27206. doi: 10.1038/srep27206
92. Hernández-Ruiz J, Salaiza-Suazo N, Carrada G, Escoto S, Ruiz-Remigio A, Rosenstein Y, et al. CD8 cells of patients with diffuse cutaneous leishmaniasis display functional exhaustion: the latter is reversed, *in vitro*, by TLR2 agonists. *PLoS Negl Trop Dis.* (2010) 4:871. doi: 10.1371/journal.pntd.0000871
93. Randolph GJ, Ochando J, Partida-Sánchez S. Migration of dendritic cell subsets and their precursors. *Annu Rev Immunol.* (2008) 26:293–316. doi: 10.1146/annurev.immunol.26.021607.090254
94. Tiberio L, Del Prete A, Schioppa T, Sozio F, Bosisio D, Sozzani S. Chemokine and chemotactic signals in dendritic cell migration review-article. *Cell Mol Immunol.* (2018) 15:346–52. doi: 10.1038/s41423-018-0005-3
95. Hughes CE, Nibbs RJB. A guide to chemokines and their receptors. *FEBS J.* (2018) 285:2944–71. doi: 10.1111/febs.14466
96. Ohl L, Mohaupt M, Czeloth N, Hintzen G, Kiafard Z, Zwirner J, et al. CCR7 governs skin dendritic cell migration under inflammatory and steady-state conditions. *Immunity* (2004) 21:279–88. doi: 10.1016/j.immuni.2004.06.014
97. Teixeira MJ, Teixeira CR, Andrade BB, Barral-Netto M, Barral A. Chemokines in host-parasite interactions in leishmaniasis. *Trends Parasitol.* (2006) 22:32–40. doi: 10.1016/j.pt.2005.11.010
98. Steigerwald M, Moll H. *Leishmania major* modulates chemokine and chemokine receptor expression by dendritic cells and affects their migratory capacity *Leishmania major* modulates chemokine and chemokine receptor expression by dendritic cells and affects their migratory capacity. *Infect Immun.* (2005) 73:2564–7. doi: 10.1128/iai.73.4.2564
99. Hermida MDR, Doria PG, Taguchi AMP, Mengel JO, dos-Santos WLC. *Leishmania amazonensis* infection impairs dendritic cell migration from the inflammatory site to the draining lymph node. *BMC Infect Dis.* (2014) 14:450. doi: 10.1186/1471-2334-14-450
100. Ponte-Sucre A, Heise D, Moll H. *Leishmania major* lipophosphoglycan modulates the phenotype and inhibits migration of murine langerhans cells. *Immunology* (2001) 104:462–7. doi: 10.1046/j.1365-2567.2001.01333.x
101. Ballet R, Emre Y, Jemelin S, Charmoy M, Tacchini-Cottier F, Imhof BA. Blocking junctional adhesion molecule C enhances dendritic cell migration and boosts the immune responses against *Leishmania major. PLoS Pathog.* (2014) 10:e1004550. doi: 10.1371/journal.ppat.1004550
102. Sato N, Ahuja SK, Quinones M, Kostecki V, Reddick RL, Melby PC, et al. CC chemokine receptor (CCR)2 is required for langerhans cell migration and localization of T helper cell type 1 (Th1)-inducing dendritic cells. absence of CCR2 shifts the *Leishmania major*-resistant phenotype to a susceptible state dominated by Th2 cytokin. *J Exp Med.* (2000) 192:205–18. doi: 10.1084/jem.192.2.205
103. Ato M, Maroof A, Zubairi S, Nakano H, Kakiuchi T, Kaye PM. Loss of dendritic cell migration and impaired resistance to leishmania donovani infection in mice deficient in CCL19 and CCL21. *J Immunol.* (2006) 176:5486–93. doi: 10.4049/jimmunol.176.9.5486
104. Kelly B, O'Neill LAJ. Metabolic reprogramming in macrophages and dendritic cells in innate immunity. *Cell Res.* (2015) 25:771–84. doi: 10.1038/cr.2015.68
105. Pearce EJ, Everts B. Dendritic cell metabolism. *Nat Rev Immunol.* (2015) 15:18–29. doi: 10.1038/nri3771
106. Krawczyk CM, Holowka T, Sun J, Blagih J, Amiel E, DeBerardinis RJ, et al. Toll-like receptor-induced changes in glycolytic metabolism regulate dendritic cell activation. *Blood* (2010) 115:4742–9. doi: 10.1182/blood-2009-10-249540
107. Everts B, Amiel E, Huang SCC, Smith AM, Chang CH, Lam WY, et al. TLR-driven early glycolytic reprogramming via the kinases TBK1-IKKε supports the anabolic demands of dendritic cell activation. *Nat Immunol.* (2014) 15:323–32. doi: 10.1038/ni.2833
108. Gaber T, Strehl C, Buttgereit F. Metabolic regulation of inflammation. *Nat Rev Rheumatol.* (2017) 13:267–79. doi: 10.1038/nrrheum.2017.37
109. Krzywinska E, Stockmann C. Hypoxia, metabolism and immune cell function. *Biomedicines* (2018) 6:56. doi: 10.3390/biomedicines6020056
110. Corcoran SE, Neill LAJO, Corcoran SE, Neill LAJO. HIF1 a and metabolic reprogramming in inflammation find the latest version : HIF1 α and metabolic reprogramming in inflammation. (2016) 126:3699–707. doi: 10.1172/JCI84431
111. Hammami A, Abidin BM, Heinonen KM, Stäger S. HIF-1α hampers dendritic cell function and Th1 generation during chronic Visceral leishmaniasis. *Sci Rep.* (2018) 8:3500. doi: 10.1038/s41598-018-21891-z
112. Hammami A, Charpentier T, Smans M, Stäger S. IRF-5-mediated inflammation limits $CD8^{+}$ T cell expansion by inducing HIF-1α and Impairing dendritic cell functions during leishmania infection. *PLoS Pathog.* (2015) 11:e1004938. doi: 10.1371/journal.ppat.1004938
113. Schatz V, Strüssmann Y, Mahnke A, Schley G, Waldner M, Ritter U, et al. Myeloid cell–derived HIF-1α promotes control of *Leishmania major. J Immunol.* (2016) 197:4034–41. doi: 10.4049/jimmunol.1601080
114. Moreira ML, Costa-Pereira C, Alves MLR, Marteleto BH, Ribeiro VM, Peruhype-Magalhães V, et al. Vaccination against canine leishmaniosis increases the phagocytic activity, nitric oxide production and expression of cell activation/migration molecules in neutrophils and monocytes. *Vet Parasitol.* (2016) 220:33–45. doi: 10.1016/j.vetpar.2016.02.009
115. Wen H, Schaller MA, Dou Y, Hogaboam CM, Kunkel SL. Dendritic cells at the interface of innate and acquired immunity : the role for epigenetic changes. *J Leukoc Biol.* (2008) 83:439–46. doi: 10.1189/jlb.0607357
116. Lin Q, Chauvistré H, Costa IG, Gusmao EG, Mitzka S, Hanzelmann S, et al. Epigenetic program and transcription factor circuitry of dendritic cell development. *Nucleic Acid Res.* (2018) 43:9680–93. doi: 10.1093/nar/gkv1056
117. Tian Y, Meng L, Zhang Y. Epigenetic regulation of dendritic cell development and function. *Cancer J.* (2017) 23:302–7. doi: 10.1097/PPO.0000000000000280
118. Cirillo LA, Lin FR, Cuesta I, Friedman D, Jarnik M, Zaret KS. Opening of compacted chromatin by early developmental transcription factors HNF3 (FoxA) and GATA-4. *Mol Cell* (2002) 9:279–89. doi: 10.1016/S1097-2765(02)00459-8
119. Satpathy AT, Murphy KM. Transcription factor networks in dendritic cell development. *Semin Immunol.* (2011) 23:388–97. doi: 10.1016/j.smim.2011.08.009
120. Carotta S, Dakic A, D'Amico A, Pang SHM, Greig KT, Nutt SL, et al. The transcription factor PU.1 controls dendritic cell development and Flt3 cytokine receptor expression in a dose-dependent manner. *Immunity* (2010) 32:628–41. doi: 10.1016/j.immuni.2010.05.005
121. Dominguez-Soto A, Puig-Kröger A, Vega MA, Corbí AL. PU 1 regulates the tissue-specific expression of dendritic cell-specific intercellular adhesion molecule (ICAM)−3-grabbing nonintegrin*. *J Biol Chem.* (2005) 280:33123–31. doi: 10.1074/jbc.M503401200

122. Kanada S, Nishiyama C, Nakano N, Suzuki R, Maeda K, Hara M, et al. Critical role of transcription factor PU. 1 in the expression of CD80 and CD86 on dendritic cells. *Blood* (2018) 117:2211–23. doi: 10.1182/blood-2010-06-291898
123. Wang Z, Zang C, Rosenfeld JA, Schones DE, Cuddapah S, Cui K, et al. Combinatorial patterns of histone acetylations and methylations in the human genome. *Nat Genet.* (2009) 40:897–903. doi: 10.1038/ng.154.Combinatorial
124. Bornstein C, Winter D, Barnett-Itzhaki Z, David E, Kadri S, Garber M, et al. A negative feedback loop of transcription factors specifies alternative dendritic cell chromatin states. *Mol Cell* (2014) 56:749–62. doi: 10.1016/j.molcel.2014.10.014
125. Tserel L, Kolde R, Rebane A, Kisand K, Org TÃ, Peterson H, et al. Genome-wide promoter analysis of histone modifications in human monocyte-derived antigen presenting cells. *BMC Genomics* (2010) 11:642. doi: 10.1186/1471-2164-11-642
126. Marr AK, MacIsaac JL, Jiang R, Airo AM, Kobor MS, McMaster WR. *Leishmania donovani* infection causes distinct epigenetic DNA methylation changes in host macrophages. *PLoS Pathog.* (2014) 10:e1004419. doi: 10.1371/journal.ppat.1004419
127. Yang Z, Mosser DM, Zhang X. Activation of the MAPK, ERK, following *Leishmania amazonensis* infection of macrophages. *J Immunol.* (2007) 178:1077–85. doi: 10.4049/jimmunol.178.2.1077
128. Calegari-Silva TC, Vivarini ÁC, Pereira RMS, Dias-Teixeira KL, Rath CT, Pacheco ASS, et al. *Leishmania amazonensis* downregulates macrophage iNOS expression via histone deacetylase 1 (HDAC1): a novel parasite evasion mechanism. *Eur J Immunol Immunol.* (2018) 48:1188-98. doi: 10.1002/eji.201747257

7

Co- but not Sequential Infection of DCs Boosts their HIV-Specific CTL-Stimulatory Capacity

Manuela Schönfeld[1†], *Ulla Knackmuss*[1†], *Parul Chandorkar*[1], *Paul Hörtnagl*[2], *Thomas John Hope*[3], *Arnaud Moris*[4,5], *Rosa Bellmann-Weiler*[6], *Cornelia Lass-Flörl*[1], *Wilfried Posch*[1*] and *Doris Wilflingseder*[1*]

[1] Division of Hygiene and Medical Microbiology, Medical University of Innsbruck, Innsbruck, Austria, [2] Central Institute for Blood Transfusion and Immunological Department, Medical University of Innsbruck, Innsbruck, Austria, [3] Department of Cell and Molecular Biology, Feinberg School of Medicine, Northwestern University, Chicago, IL, United States, [4] Sorbonne Université, INSERM, CNRS, Center for Immunology and Microbial Infections - CIMI-Paris, Paris, France, [5] Institute for Integrative Biology of the Cell (I2BC), CEA, CNRS, Université Paris-Sud, Université Paris-Saclay, Gif-sur-Yvette, France, [6] Department of Internal Medicine II, Medical University of Innsbruck, Innsbruck, Austria

***Correspondence:**
Doris Wilflingseder
doris.wilflingseder@i-med.ac.at
Wilfried Posch
wilfried.posch@i-med.ac.at

† These authors have contributed equally to this work

Pathogenic bacteria and their microbial products activate dendritic cells (DCs) at mucosal surfaces during sexually transmitted infections (STIs) and therefore might also differently shape DC functions during co-infection with HIV-1. We recently illustrated that complement (C) coating of HIV-1 (HIV-C), as primarily found during the acute phase of infection before appearance of HIV-specific antibodies, by-passed SAMHD1-mediated restriction in DCs and therefore mediated an increased DC activation and antiviral capacity. To determine whether the superior antiviral effects of HIV-C-exposed DCs also apply during STIs, we developed a co-infection model in which DCs were infected with *Chlamydia spp.* simultaneously (HIV-C/Chlam-DCs or HIV/Chlam-DCs) or a sequential infection model, where DCs were exposed to *Chlamydia* for 3 or 24 h (Chlam-DCs) followed by HIV-1 infection. Co-infection of DCs with HIV-1 and *Chlamydia* significantly boosted the CTL-stimulatory capacity compared to HIV-1-loaded iDCs and this boost was independent on the opsonization pattern. This effect was lost in the sequential infection model, when opsonized HIV-1 was added delayed to *Chlamydia*-loaded DCs. The reduction in the CTL-stimulatory capacity of Chlam-DCs was not due to lower HIV-1 binding or infection compared to iDCs or HIV-C/Chlam-DCs, but due to altered fusion and internalization mechanisms within DCs. The CTL-stimulatory capacity of HIV-C in Chlam-DCs correlated with significantly reduced viral fusion compared to iDCs and HIV-C/Chlam-DCs and illustrated considerably increased numbers of HIV-C-containing vacuoles than iDCs. The data indicate that *Chlamydia* co-infection of DCs mediates a transient boost of their HIV-specific CTL-stimulatory and antiviral capacity, while in the sequential infection model this is reversed and associated with hazard to the host.

Keywords: HIV-1, STIs, dendritic cell, complement, CTL

INTRODUCTION

Dendritic cells (DCs) play a pivotal role in the defense against invading pathogens. DCs reside in the peripheral tissue, where they capture antigens and transport them to lymph nodes to present them to naive T cells. Hence, DCs play a key role in shaping the adaptive immune response. Of all new HIV-1 infections, 60–90 % are caused by sexual transmission (1, 2). Since HIV-1 transmission occurs at mucosal surfaces, DCs are amongst the first cells to encounter the virus (3). At the same time, HIV-1 spontaneously activates the classical complement (C) pathway (4), even in seminal fluid (5), through direct binding of C1q to the viral surface. Therefore, C-opsonized HIV (HIV-C) is accumulating at mucosal sites during early HIV-1 infection (6, 7).

We have previously shown that HIV-C interacts with complement receptors 3 (CR3) and 4 (CR4) on iDCs, whereas non-opsonized HIV binds DCs via gp120 to DC-SIGN (8) and via CD169 (Siglec-1) binding to virions. Furthermore, iDCs were efficiently infected with HIV-C compared to non- or antibody-opsonized HIV (7, 9). HIV-C was able to bypass SAMHD1 restriction in DCs, an intrinsic cellular defense mechanism, which usually inhibits HIV-1 replication in myeloid cells. Thus, complement opsonization of the virus counteracted viral defenses in DCs. DCs exposed to HIV-C had a significantly higher maturation and co-stimulatory capacity compared to DCs exposed to non-opsonized HIV (9).

In general, efficiency of HIV-1 transmission is low (10). However, it is known that viral and bacterial genital infections that cause inflammation or ulcers increase risk of infection and/or susceptibility to HIV transmission (10). Epidemiological studies also revealed a link between an increased incidence of STIs with increased efficiency to transmit the virus to an uninfected partner (11). Among the STIs most commonly associated with high genital HIV loads are *Gardnerella vaginalis* (12, 13) associated with bacterial vaginosis (BV), herpes simplex virus type 2 (HSV-2), *Chlamydia trachomatis, Neisseria gonorrheae,* and *Trichomonas vaginalis* (10). Dendritic cells incubated with mucosal fluid from women with BV were found to up-regulate maturation and activation markers like HLA-DR, CD40, and CD83, and to have an increased T cell-stimulatory capacity indicating an impact on mucosal immunity (14). To determine if model pathogenic bacteria could similarly pereturb the complement-mediated avoidance of antiviral effects when DCs are exposed to bacteria, we added *Chlamydia* and opsonized HIV-1 either simultaneously mimicking a co-infection (HIV-C/Chlam-DCs) or by delayed addition of HIV-C (Chlam-DCs). *Chlamydia (C.) trachomatis* are gram-negative obligate intracellular bacteria and a primary agent causing non-gonococcal urethritis (15). During infection of cells within the vaginal mucosa, *C. trachomatis* initiates disruption of the mucosal-epithelial layer allowing better tissue entry of HIV-1 (10). Immunological alterations due to the presence of *C. trachomatis* may further support the transmission of HIV to susceptible cells or impact the antigen-presenting capacity of DCs (10).

Given that infection of iDCs is modulated by the opsonization pattern of HIV-1, which also had an impact on outcomes of both humoral and cellular antiviral immune responses (9, 16, 17) and given that HIV-1 particles are opsonized *in vivo* (18) and *in vitro* (4, 5), we analyzed whether the presence of *Chlamydia* modulates DC properties and function during co-infection with HIV-C.

MATERIALS AND METHODS

Ethics Statement

This study was carried out in accordance with the recommendations of the Ethics Committee of the Medical University of Innsbruck. The protocol was approved by the Ethics Committee of the Medical University of Innsbruck. All subjects gave written informed consent in accordance with the Declaration of Helsinki.

Generation of Human Monocyte-Derived iDCs and mDCs

Monocytes were isolated from whole blood of healthy donors by using CD14 BD IMAG Beads (Becton-Dickinson), according to the manufacturer's instructions. Differentiation into iDCs was done using IL-4 (200 U/ml) and GM-CSF (1,000 U/ml) and the iDC phenotype was routinely confirmed on day 5 by flow cytometry using CD11b, CD11c, DC-SIGN, HLA-DR, and CD83 (9, 16, 19). Representative histogram plots of these markers on iDCs are illustrated in **Figure S1** (upper panel, red; isotype, blue). To generate LPS-DCs, day 5 iDCs were stimulated for 24 h with 100 ng/ml pure LPS-EB (Sigma) prior to HIV-1 infection.

Acute and chronic *Chlamydia* exposure was mimicked by stimulation of day 5 iDCs with infectious or heat-inactivated *Chlamydia* for either 24 h prior to (Chlam-DCs) or at the same time (HIV-C/Chlam-DCs or HIV/Chlam-DCs) as HIV-1 infection. For first experiments (DC maturation, binding, internalization) infectious as well as heat-inactivated bacteria were used. Since no differences were observed and since we intended to study PAMP-associated changes in DCs induced by *Chlamydia*, for all other analyses we used heat-inactivated bacteria. A representative histogram plot of CD83 expression on iDCs (red), DCs treated with heat-inactivated *Chlamydia* (dark green) or live *Chlamydia* (light green) is depicted in **Figure S1**, lower panel. Since isotype controls between the conditions did not differ, the iDC isotype control is shown (**Figure S1**, lower panel).

Bacteria

Chlamydia spp. propagated in human epithelial HL cells and aliquots of purified bacteria were stored in sucrose phosphate glutamic acid at −80°C until use (20). For quantification of infection, coverslips overlaid with HL-cell-monolayers were fixed in methanol and stained with FITC-conjugated anti-Chlamydia LPS monoclonal antibody (OXOID (Ely) Ltd., Ely, UK). Chlamydial inclusion bodies within cells were counted by fluorescence microscopy at a magnification of x100 with a Scope A1 microscope (Zeiss). For experiments using infectious, purified *Chlamydia* cells were infected at a multiplicity of infection/MOI of 10 as described earlier (20). An aliquot of tested, purified *Chlamydia spp.* was used for heat-inactivation at 70°C for 20 min.

Plasmids

The infectious R5-tropic HIV-1 proviral clone R9Bal was used for maturation, binding/internalization and DC infection studies. For HIV-1 fusion assays the R9Bal and vpr/β-lam expression constructs were used to generate chimeric R9Bal/β-lam proviral clones. Confocal microscopic analyses and HC/HT imaging analyses were performed by using chimeric R9Bal/mCherry virus preparations originating from R9Bal and vpr/m-Cherry expression plasmids (21).

Virus Production

HIV-1 proviral clones were produced by transfecting HEK293T cells. R9Bal/β-lam and R9Bal/mCherry virus stocks were prepared by co-transfection of HEK293T cells with the proviral R9Bal DNA and the vpr-β-lam or vpr-mCherry expression constructs (9). Freshly produced virus was obtained via ultracentrifugation (70,000 × g/90 min/4°C). Concentration of the ultracentrifuged virus was measured by p24 ELISA (22) and viral infectivity was confirmed by the determination of the $TCID_{50}$ using PHA/IL-2-stimulated PBLs. To monitor productive infection of DCs or DC/T cell co-cultures, p24 ELISA was used.

Opsonization of Viral Stocks

Viruses were opsonized by incubation with normal human serum (NHS) as a complement (C) source in a 1:10 dilution for 1 h at 37°C (HIV-C). As negative control, the viruses were incubated under the same conditions in medium, which reflects non-opsonized HIV-1 (HIV). After opsonization, viruses were thoroughly washed, pelleted by ultracentrifugation (25,000 × g/90 min/4°C) and re-suspended in RPMI medium. The opsonization pattern was determined by virus capture assay (VCA) as described (7). 96-well high-binding plates were coated using anti-human C3c, C3d, or IgG antibodies. Mouse IgG antibody was used as a control for background binding. Plates were then incubated overnight at 4°C with the differentially opsonized virus preparations (10 ng p24/well). After extensive washing, virus was lysed and p24 ELISA was performed.

Capture of HIV-1

Differentially matured DCs (1 × 10^5 cells/well/100 μl) were exposed to 25 ng p24/ml of R5 tropic non-opsonized (R9Bal) or complement-opsonized (R9Bal-C) HIV-1. After 6 h incubation at either 4°C for binding or 37°C for internalization, cells were washed 4 times to remove unbound virus. Cell pellets were lysed with 2% Igepal and viral amount was assessed by p24 ELISA.

Viral Fusion Assay

DCs were plated into 96-well plates (1 × 10^5 cells/well/100 μl) and infected with 250 ng p24/ml non-opsonized or opsonized R9Bal/β-lam. After 5 h incubation cells were washed and loaded for 1 h with CCF2-AM substrate solution according to the manufacturer's instructions (LiveBLAzer™ FRET-B/G Loading Kit with CCF2-AM, LifeTechnologies). Cells were washed again and developed for 16 h in CO_2-independent medium (Gibco) containing 10% FCS and 2.5 mM probenicid. Cleavage of CCF2 was analyzed by flow cytometry after fixation of DCs in 4% paraformaldehyde.

Microscopy

To visualize intracellular HIV-1 localization by confocal microscopy, iDCs, HIV-C or HIV/Chlam, Chlam- and LPS-DCs were plated onto Poly-L-lysine (Sigma)-coated coverslips and exposed to R9Bal/mCherry or –GFP (350 ng p24/ml) for 24 h. For HC/HT screening analyses, various matured DCs (50,000/well) were seeded in CellCarrier Ultra plates (Perkin Elmer) and infected over night with fluorescently labeled HIV-C (350 ng p24/ml). DCs were fixed with 4% paraformaldehyde, labeled using Hoechst 33342 (Cell Signaling Technologies), permeabilized (Permeabilization Wash Buffer, BioLegend), and stained with HLA-DR (BioLegend). Following staining, cells were washed and mounted (confocal microscopy) or re-suspended in D-PBS (HC/HT Screening). Confocal microscopy was performed on a Leica SP5 (Leica Microsystems) using a glycerol objective. Images were analyzed using LAS AF Lite (Leica Microsystems) and Fiji (ImageJ). For 3-D-rendered stacks, Imaris (Bitplane) was used. HC/HT analyses were performed using an Operetta CLS™ (Perkin Elmer) and co-localization of mCherry/HLA-DR or GFP/Siglec-1 automatically quantified using the Harmony™ Software and RMS Spot Analyses (Perkin Elmer). For these automated analyses, first fluorescence intensities were measured, since if HIV particles are in the cytoplasm, the fluorescence intensities are significantly lower compared to packed virus in endosomes. Lower intensities can then be excluded from the automatic screening process. Then co-localization of virus particles with HLA-DR, which is in endosomal compartments only, was measured.

DC Infection

Day 6 iDCs, HIV-C or HIV/Chlam-DCs, Chlam-DCs and LPS-DCs (1 × 10^5cells/well/100 μl) were infected in triplicate with 25 ng p24/ml of R9Bal or R9Bal-C. After 24 h incubation, DCs were thoroughly washed and cultured at 37°C and 5 % CO_2 for 15 days. For co-infection experiments, autologous $CD4^+$ T cells were added to washed DCs the day after HIV-infection. After several days post-infection, supernatants were taken and diluted 1:10 with 2% Igepal to lyse the virus. Productive infection was determined by measuring p24 concentrations in the supernatant.

Interferon-γ Elispot

SL9 clone 2, a HIV-specific $CD8^+$ CTL clone, was derived from an HIV-infected patient and recognizes the well-characterized immune-dominant epitope of Gag p17 SLYNTVATL (SL9) presented by HLA-A*02:01 (23, 24). The human immune response to the HLA-A*02:01-restricted Gag_{77-85} SLYNTVATL epitope is the most studied—SL9 is a highly immunogenic, help-independent HIV-1 epitope and a strong negative association was demonstrated between SL9-CTL levels and viral load (25). DCs were co-cultured overnight with SL9-CTLs (2,500–10,000 clones/well). As positive controls, DCs were incubated with 1 μg/ml of cognate peptide before washing and addition of the HIV-specific CTL clones overnight. IFN-γ production was monitored in an Elispot assay as described (24). All antibodies (Abs) used for the IFN-γ Elispot were purchased from Mabtech.

Multicolor FACS Analyses

Differentiation and maturation of DCs exposed to *Chlamydia* or LPS and HIV-1 were analyzed by using anti-human CD11c-AlexaFluor488, HLA-DR-PerCP/Cy5.5, DC-SIGN-PE (Biolegend), CD86-BV421, CD83-APC, CD169-PE (BD Biosciences) on a FACS Verse flow cytometer (BD Biosciences). Cell surface expression of receptors for HIV and HIV-C binding was determined by flow cytometry as described using anti-human CD11b-APC, CD4 PerCP/Cy5.5 and DC-SIGN-PE (BioLegend). Data was analyzed using FACS DIVA software (BD Biosciences) and R.

Statistical Analysis

Data were analyzed using GraphPad Prism software (GraphPad Software Inc.). Statistical analyses were performed using two-way ANOVA with Dunnett's posttest for multiple comparisons.

RESULTS

Reduced Maturation of DCs During Chlamydial Co-infection Compared to Sequential Infection

We initially evaluated whether exposure to *Chlamydia* induced maturation of DCs similarily to the positive control LPS. Therefore, we analyzed cell surface expression of the specific markers CD83, CD86 and HLA-DR after the different treatments. We found that long-term exposure (24 h) of iDCs to *Chlamydia* induced significant up-regulation of CD83, CD86, and HLA-DR compared to untreated iDCs (**Figure 1A**). However, expression levels of CD83, CD86, and HLA-DR on Chlam-DCs were lower compared to LPS-stimulated DCs (LPS-DCs) in all donors tested (**Figure 1A**, $n = 6$). Independent of DC stimulation, the expression levels of DC-SIGN and the complement receptors 3 and 4 (CR3, CD11b/CD18; CR4, CD11c/CD18) were only moderately changed and CD4 expression was slightly reduced under all maturation conditions as also shown by Chen et al. (26) (not shown). Exposure of such various matured DCs (Chlam-DCs, LPS-DCs) to HIV-C did not change the expression of up-regulated markers CD83 (**Figure 1B**, left panel), CD86 (**Figure 1B**, middle panel), and HLA-DR (**Figure 1B**, right panel). In contrast, a reduced maturation of DCs was observed upon co-infection with HIV-C and *Chlamydia* (HIV-C/Chlam-DCs) and this maturation was comparable to that when iDCs were exposed to HIV-C only (**Figure 1B**, CD83—left panel, CD86—middle panel, HLA-DR—right panel). Expression of all maturation and activation markers was significantly higher on HIV-C- and HIV-C/Chlam-DCs compared to iDCs. We demonstrated that stimulation of DCs with *Chlamydia* caused a lower DC maturation compared to LPS and this maturation was not increased due to additional HIV-C exposure.

Binding of HIV-C Depends on the DC Maturation Status

Since expression of activation markers was shown to be different on iDCs, Chlam- and LPS-DCs, we assessed whether this might lead to differential binding of HIV-C to DCs. To characterize binding of HIV-C co-cultures of various matured DCs and HIV-C were incubated for 6 h at 4°C (8). At 4°C, DCs just bind but do not internalize viral pathogens (8). HIV-C (25 ng p24/ml) was added to iDCs, Chlam- and LPS-DCs for 6 h at 4°C. Using the co-infection model, DCs were incubated with simultaneously added HIV-C and *Chlamydia* under above mentioned conditions. Cell-bound virus was determined after thorough washing and lysing of DCs by quantification of p24 protein. Similar amounts of HIV-C were attached to iDCs and HIV-C/Chlam-DCs, while Chlam- and LPS-DCs depicted a significantly increased binding of HIV-C (**Figure 2A**). A similar binding pattern was analyzed for non-opsonized HIV-1 (HIV, **Figure S2A**). Therefore, binding to DCs was independent of the opsonization pattern, but was modulated by DC maturation status.

DC Maturation Affects HIV-C Internalization

To also see if internalization of HIV-C in iDCs, HIV-C/Chlam-, Chlam-, and LPS-DCs differs, we incubated differentially stimulated cells for 6 h at 37°C. Virus was added as described above and bound/internalized HIV-C was determined by p24 ELISA after washing and lysing the cells. These analyses revealed that LPS-DCs show a ~5-fold higher internalization compared to iDCs and HIV-C/Chlam-DCs (**Figure 2B**). Internalization of HIV-C into LPS-DCs was significantly higher compared to its non-opsonized counterpart (**Figure S2B**, $p = 0.005$). Though the internalization of HIV-C in Chlam-DCs was lower compared to LPS-DCs, a significantly higher internalization of HIV-C compared to both iDCs ($p = 0.0030$) and HIV-C/Chlam-DCs ($p = 0.0071$) was identified (**Figure 2B**). The increase in HIV-1 internalization upon DC maturation was observed independent on whether the virus was opsonized (**Figure 2B**) or not (**Figure S2B**).

DC Maturation Affects HIV-C Fusion

To further evaluate the impact of iDC maturation by the different treatments on the interaction of cell and virions, we analyzed virion fusion using Vpr-β-lactamase (Vpr-blam)-containing HIV-C (**Figure 2C**) or HIV (**Figure S2C**). We found that fusion was not inhibited in HIV-C/Chlam-DCs relative to HIV-C-exposed iDC controls (**Figure 2C**). In contrast fusion was significantly decreased in Chlam-DCs and LPS-DCs (**Figure 2C**). It is notable that fusion was completely inhibited in the LPS-DCs independent of the opsonization pattern of the virus (**Figure 2C** and **Figure S2C**). iDCs and co-infection of DCs with *Chlamydia* were associated with the highest fusion with HIV-1, while sequential infection with *Chlamydia* displayed significantly lower fusion levels with a complete inhibition of fusion in LPS-DCs.

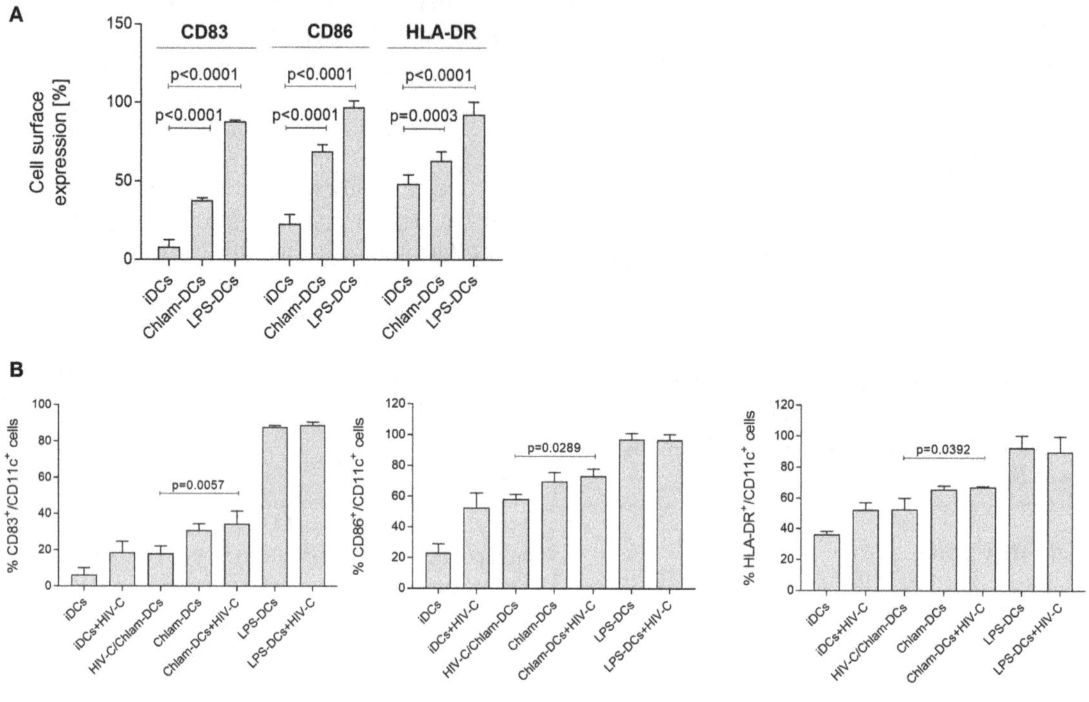

FIGURE 1 | *Chlamydia* induces maturation of DCs *in vitro*. **(A)** Representative flow cytometric analysis of CD83, CD86, and HLA-DR expression on $CD11c^+$ DCs upon stimulation with *Chlamydia* or LPS for 24 h. Percentages+/-SD of double positive ($CD83^+/CD11c^+$, $CD86^+/CD11c^+$, $HLA\text{-}DR^+/CD11c^+$) DCs are indicated for 6 independent donors. **(B)** CD83 (left), CD86 (middle) and HLA-DR (right panel) expression levels are not changed in co- or sequential infected cells. Levels of HIV-C/Chlam-DCs and HIV-C-DCs are similar, while delayed addition of HIV-C to Chlam-DCs represents the maturation and activation status of Chlam-DCs. LPS-DCs were used as positive controls. To simplify the graph, statistics are only depicted for differences between the co- and sequential infection model. Percentages+/-SD of double positive ($CD83^+/CD11c^+$, $CD86^+/CD11c^+$, $HLA\text{-}DR^+/CD11c^+$) DCs are indicated for 3 donors. Statistical analysis was performed using 2way ANOVA and Dunnett's multiple comparisons test.

Siglec-1 Does Not Play a Role With Respect to HIV-C Capture

Since Siglec-1 (CD169) was described—at least *in vitro* - to exert a prominent role with respect to capture and transfer of HIV-1 in LPS-stimulated mDCs (27–29), we analyzed co-localization of this molecule with GFP-tagged HIV or HIV-C in differently stimulated DCs. For this, we performed high content screening of differentially stimulated and infected DCs and analyzed the co-localization of GFP-tagged virus with PE-labeled Siglec-1. We automatically analyzed two fields á 100 cells for their co-localization of HIV-1 and Siglec-1 using the Harmony™ software (Perkin-Elmer) and mean values of spots co-localizing within 100 cells are depicted in **Figure S3**. These analyses revealed no significant differences but only slightly higher Siglec-1/HIV-C co-localization in Chlam-DCs compared to iDCs or HIV/Chlam-DCs and compared to background fluorescence of non-infected cells, which served as negative controls (**Figure S3**). As positive controls, mature DCs (Chlam-DCs or LPS-DCs) infected with non-opsonized HIV-1 (HIV) were used, which displayed significantly higher co-localization compared to HIV-C-infected DCs. the results suggest that a modulation of the interaction of HIV-1 and Siglec-1 is not playing a major role in viral capture.

HIV-C Localizes to HLA-DR-Containing Compartments in Chlam- and LPS-DCs

To gain additional insights into potential differences in the interaction of HIV-1 with iDCs matured by the different treatments, we evaluated the intracellular localization of HIV-C in iDCs, HIV/Chlam-, Chlam-, and LPS-DCs. To this end, we infected the respective different DC populations using fluorescently labeled HIV-C and analyzed viral particle distribution of internalized HIV-C by high-content/high-throughput (HC/HT) image analyses and confocal microscopy (**Figure 3**, **Figure S4**). For these analyses, cells were additionally labeled using a nuclear stain (**Figure 3**, **Figure S4**, Hoechst, blue) and HLA-DR as marker for endosomal compartments including virus containing compartments (VCCs) (**Figure 3**, **Figure S4**, green). The analyses revealed significantly lower levels of HIV-C-containing HLA-DR-containing compartments in iDCs compared to HIV-C/Chlam-, Chlam-, and LPS-DCs (**Figure 3**, left, histogram plot). Significantly higher HLA-DR-containing compartment levels were detected in LPS-DCs compared to both, HIV-C/Chlam- and Chlam-DCs (**Figure 3**, left, histogram plot). The accumulation of the virus in HLA-DR-containing compartments in LPS-DCs was confirmed using confocal microscopic analyses (**Figure 3**, right)—these revealed vacuolar and cytoplasmic distribution of HIV-C in iDCs (**Figure 3**, right,

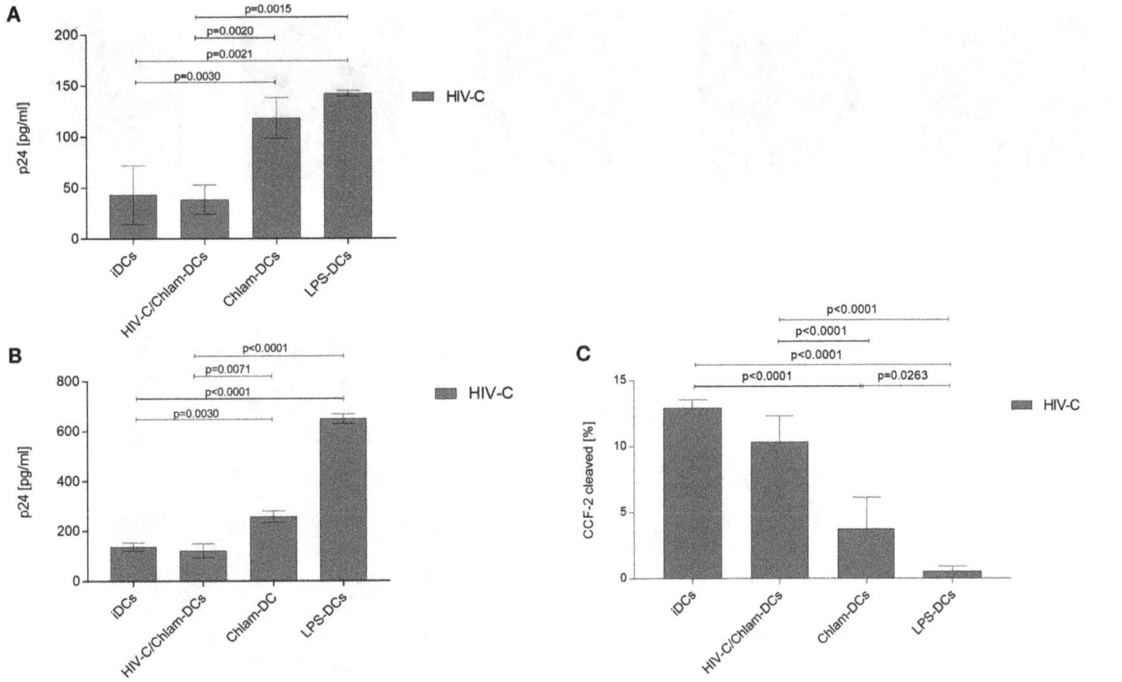

FIGURE 2 | Chlam- and LPS-DCs efficiently capture HIV-C. Binding at 4°C **(A)** and internalization at 37°C **(B)** were performed in triplicates using 25 ng/ml of R5-tropic opsonized HIV-1. Bar graphs show means ± SD from three independent experiments. p24 levels within the cell lysates were determined by ELISA. Prior to cell lysate preparation, cells were thoroughly washed to remove unbound virus. Statistical analysis shows 2-way ANOVA with Tukey's multiple comparisons test. **(C)** Fusion assays were performed after addition of HIV-C bearing the chimeric protein β-lactamase-Vpr to iDCs, Chlam-DCs, and LPS-DCs or after simultaneous HIV-C-VprBlam/Chlamydia stimulation of iDCs (HIV-C/Chlam-DCs). The amount of fused virus was determined by flow cytometric analyses of cleaved CCF2 in the cytoplasm. Percentages of cleaved CCF2-positive cells from three independent donors are depicted.

upper panel, **Figure S4**, left), while only HLA-DR-containing compartments, but no cytoplasmic HIV-1, were detected in LPS-DCs (**Figure 3**, right, lower panel, **Figure S4**, right). **Figure 3** shows volume projections of maximal pixel intensity of all layers analyzed and **Figure S4** the respective 3D-rendered z-stacks. Fusion and image analyses by HC/HT screening and confocal microscopy revealed a high cytoplasmic distribution of HIV-C in iDCs and under conditions of co-infection. The cytoplasmic distribution was reduced in sequentially infected DCs and completely abrogated in LPS-DCs. In contrast HIV-1-containing vacuoles were mainly detected in LPS-exposed DCs, to lower levels in *Chlamydia*-exposed DCs and only marginally in iDCs.

DC Infection Is Enhanced by *Chlamydia* Co- and Sequential Infection

We recently demonstrated that HIV-C overcomes restriction in iDCs resulting in significantly higher productive DC infection, improved antigen-presentation as well as humoral antiviral immune responses (30). We analyzed productive DC infection using HIV-C in co- (HIV+Chlam-) and sequential infection (Chlam-) DC models as well as LPS-DCs. iDCs were used as controls—again we found that non-opsonized HIV caused a significantly lower productive infection of iDCs (**Figure 4**, upper panel, dotted green line, HIV, vs. green line, HIV-C and **Figure S5**) compared to HIV-C despite similar binding and internalization (**Figure 4**, upper panel, and **Figure S1**). However, neither HIV (not shown) nor HIV-C (**Figure 4**, upper and lower panels) caused any productive infection in LPS-DCs. Within the co-infection model, both HIV-C (**Figure 4**, upper and lower panels) and HIV (**Figure S5**) exerted an enhanced productive DC infection compared to iDCs (**Figure S5**)—nevertheless, complement opsonization of HIV-1 still promoted a significantly increased DC infection compared to its non-opsonized counterpart (**Figure S5**). Although Chlam-DCs—representing the sequential infection—showed a high maturation and low viral fusion, they were infected to high levels with both HIV-C (**Figure 4**) and HIV (**Figure S5**). These data suggest that HIV-C facilitated productive infection in DCs during chlamydial co- and sequential infection as well as a different maturation status between LPS- and *Chlamydia*-matured DCs.

HIV-C/*Chlamydia* Co- but not Sequential Infection of DCs Is Associated With Reduced HIV Transfer

Lastly, we evaluated HIV-1 trans-infection from differently matured DCs to autologous, stimulated $CD4^+$ T cells as revealed by a co-culture with T cells. In these studies, we found that simultaneous stimulation of DCs with HIV-C and *Chlamydia*

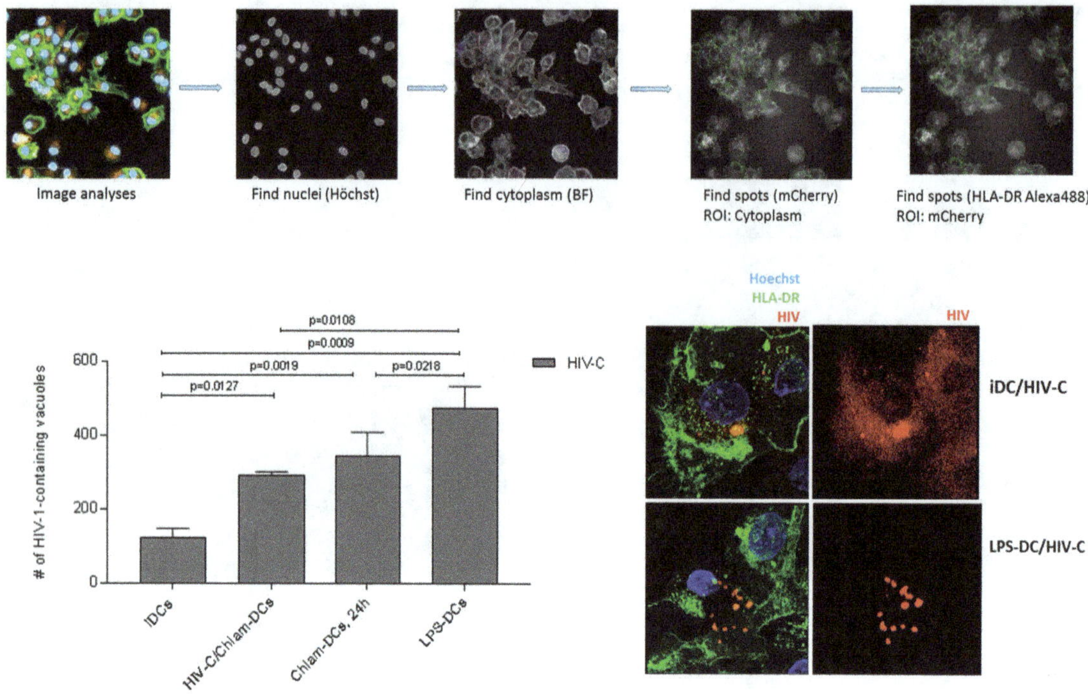

FIGURE 3 | HIV-C/Chlam-, Chlam-, and LPS-DCs show significantly higher levels of vacuolar HIV-C. Intracellular localization of HIV-C in LPS-DCs was investigated by HC/HT screening and confocal microscopic analyses. The path of image analyses is illustrated in the upper panel. Briefly, nuclei (Hoechst) and cytoplasm (Brightfield) of differentially matured and HIV-C-infected DCs were identified using the Harmony 4.6 software (Perkin Elmer). Within at least 50 to 100 scanned cells, mCherry-labeled HIV-spots co-localizing with Alexa488-labeled HLA-DR were identified. Quantitative analyses of HIV-C-containing HLA-DR-positive vacuoles are depicted in the lower left panel. Co-localization of HIV-C and HLA-DR in LPS-DCs was further confirmed using confocal microscopic analyses. iDCs show, besides some compartmentalized HIV, randomly distributed cytoplasmic HIV-C (red) while LPS-DCs display solely concentrated HIV-C within cellular compartments.

resulted in similar infection rates to $CD4^+$ T cells as HIV-C-exposed iDCs. Compared to Chlam- and LPS-DCs, these conditions illustrated significantly reduced trans-infection in co-culture experiments (**Figure 5**). As demonstrated previously for non-opsonized HIV (27, 31), LPS-matured DCs, too, transmitted significantly more virus when complement-opsonized compared to iDCs, HIV/Chlam- and Chlam-DCs (**Figure 5**). Therefore, levels of transmitted HIV-C in *Chlamydia*-matured DCs differ in co- and sequential infection models and transfer does not correlate with Siglec-1 co-localization in the HIV-C model (**Figure S3**).

Chlamydia Co-infection Promotes Significant Activation of HIV-Specific CTLs, While Reversing the Situation During Sequential Infection

Bypassing of restriction mechanisms in iDCs and enhanced productive infection using HIV-C rendered the cells capable to activate highly specific anti-HIV-cellular and humoral immune responses (9, 17). To determine the potential impact of *Chlamydia* on cellular HIV responses, we evaluated the ability of differently matured DCs (iDCs, HIV-C or HIV/Chlam-, Chlam-DCs, and LPS-DCs) exposed to HIV-C (**Figure 6**) or HIV (**Figure S6**) to stimulate HLA-matched HIV-specific CTLs. While in the co-infection model, when *Chlamydia* and HIV-C were added simultaneously, we detected a significantly higher CTL stimulatory capacity compared to HIV-C-exposed iDCs (**Figure 6**). Within the sequential infection model (Chlam-DCs, LPS-DCs) a significantly abrogated potential to stimulate HIV-specific $CD8^+$ T cells was observed (**Figure 6**). SLYNTVATL-exposed DCs were used as positive controls (**Figure 6**). The CTL-stimulatory power of DCs was also drastically augmented using co-infection of the cells with bacteria and non-opsonized HIV-1 (**Figure S6**). As already observed during our earlier work, HIV-loaded iDCs exerted a very weak CTL-stimulatory capacity (**Figure S6**) (9, 18). These observations illustrate that co-infection of DCs with *Chlamydia* and HIV-C or HIV is associated with induction of HIV-specific CTL responses, while sequential infection results in increased hazard with respect to the weak CTL-stimulatory capacity of DCs.

DISCUSSION

The studies presented here reveal that infection of the host with *Chlamydia* and HIV-1 have both potential positive and negative impact on HIV infection. Simultaneous infection of DCs with *Chlamydia* and HIV might be beneficial for the host as this triggers a higher HIV-specific CTL activation and lower transfer of HIV to autologous $CD4^+$ T cells. In

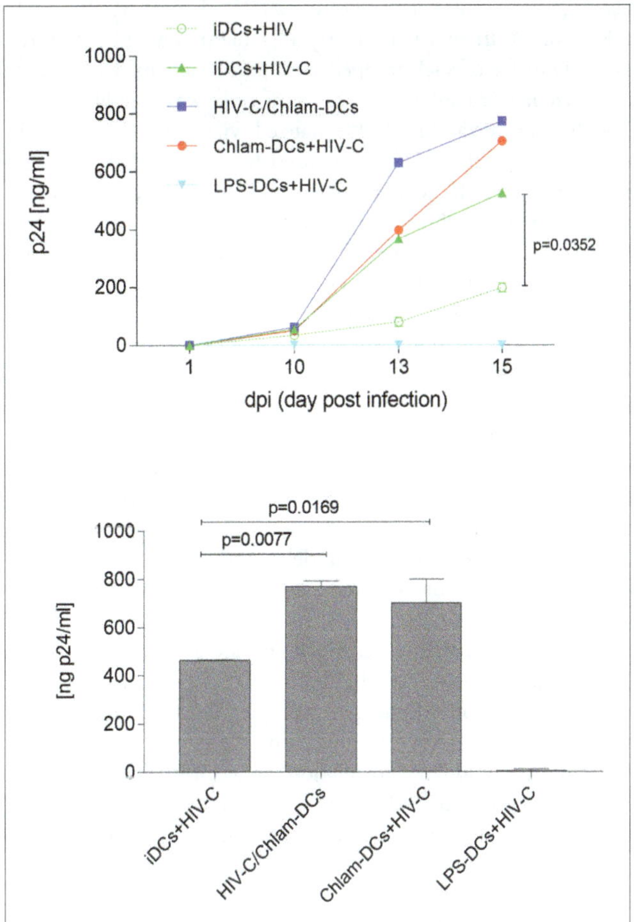

FIGURE 4 | Enhanced productive infection of Chlam-DCs mediated by HIV-C. DCs were infected with 25 ng p24/ml of HIV-C. The graph depicts an infection course of DCs—p24 levels (means ± SD) within the supernatant were analyzed on day 1 10 13 and 15 post-infection. Highest productive infection was measured in supernatants from HIV-C-infected HIV-C/Chlam- (blue) and Chlam-DCs (red) followed by HIV-C-exposed iDCs (green, solid line). Non-opsonized HIV caused the already described low-productive infection in DCs (green, dashed line) (9). No infection was detected in LPS-DCs independent of the opsonization pattern of the virus (turquoise). The upper panel shows the kinetics of one out of three representative assays including technical triplicates, while in the lower panel all three donors were combined and day 15 post infection is depicted.

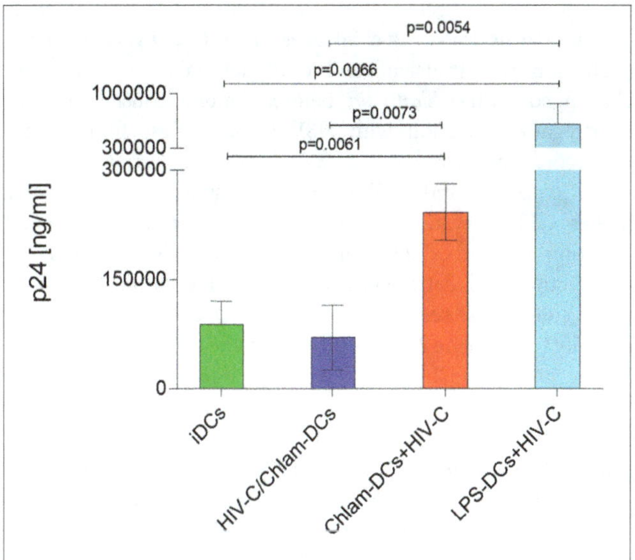

FIGURE 5 | HIV-C is efficiently transferred from Chlam- and LPS-DCs. In co-culture experiments differentially stimulated DCs (iDCs, green; HIV/Chlam-DCs, blue; Chlam-DCs, red; LPS-DCs, turquoise) were infected using HIV-C (25 ng p24/ml), thoroughly washed and autologous CD4$^+$ T cells were added. Significantly higher infectivity was measured in Chlam-DC- and LPS-DC co-cultures compared to iDC- and HIV-C/Chlam-DC-CD4$^+$ T cell co-cultures. p24 ELISAs of differently stimulated DC/T cell co-cultures performed in triplicates from two donors exposed to HIV-C are summarized and statistical analyses were performed using two-way ANOVA with Dunnett's posttest for multiple comparisons.

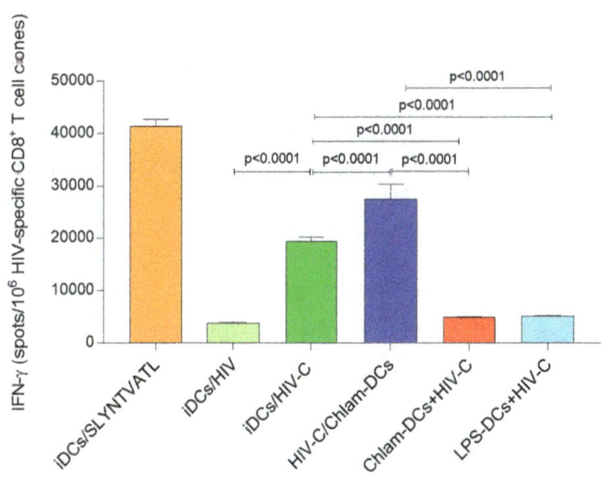

FIGURE 6 | Enhanced stimulation of HIV-specific T cell clones at simultaneous addition. IFNγ induction in CD8$^+$ T cell clones by HIV-C-exposed iDCs and HIV-C/Chlam-DCs was significantly stronger than that of non-opsonized HIV-loaded DCs (HIV-DCs; $p < 0.0001$ for CD8$^+$ T cell clones), or Chlam- and LPS-DCs exposed to HIV-C ($p < 0.0001$ for all). As positive controls specific peptide-loaded DCs for CD8$^+$ T cell clones were used (iDCs/SLYNTVATL). IFNγ Elispots of CD8$^+$ T cell clones were repeated using HLA-matched and differently stimulated DCs from three donors exposed to HIV-C, or HIV. Statistical analyses were performed using two-way ANOVA with Dunnett's posttest for multiple comparisons.

contrast, sequential infection of DCs with *Chlamydia* and HIV, which might be a common situation in the host, results in detrimental outcomes as it is associated with higher productive DC infection and viral transmission to susceptible CD4$^+$ T cells as well as poorer stimulation of HIV-1-specific CD8$^+$ T cell clones.

Upon simultaneous stimulation of DCs with *Chlamydia* and either complement-opsonized HIV-1 or untreated control HIV, a significantly improved CTL response was observed. This is in contrast to the requirement for complement-opsonization we previously reported in the absence of *Chlamydia* exposure to act as an endogenous adjuvant for DC-mediated CTL activation of iDC (16). We also find that HIV-exposed DCs co-infected simultaneously with *Chlamydia* exerted a superior CTL-stimulatory capacity of HIV-specific CD8$^+$ T cell clones compared to their HIV-iDC counterparts (9, 16, 18). As shown recently in a murine vaginal co-infection model (32), chlamydial pre-infection protected the mice from subsequent Herpes Simplex Virus (HSV)-2 challenges. This *Chlamydia*-mediated protection was transient and only detectable in mice pre-challenged with *Chlamydia* before, simultaneously with, or shortly after infection with HSV-2 (32). These findings are in accordance with our data, where co-infection of DCs with *Chlamydia* and HIV or HIV-C resulted in significantly higher CTL activation via DCs. In contrast, DC sequential infection for 3 h or 24 h with *Chlamydia* followed by HIV-C infection had detrimental outcomes (**Figures 4, 5**). Under these conditions, sequentially infected DCs only had a poor capacity to stimulate HIV-specific CTLs and allowed significantly higher productive HIV infection (*cis* infection). In contrast, no *cis*-infection was analyzed at all in DCs challenged for 3 or 24 h with LPS prior infection with HIV-C. The impact of pre-existing STIs on HIV immune responses was studied by Sheung et al. (33) in high risk Kenyan female sex workers. They found that mucosal *Neisseria gonorrhoeae* co-infection during HIV-1 acquisition was associated with substantially enhanced HIV-specific $CD8^+$ T cell responses (33). The enhanced CTL response was not seen in women with *Chlamydia* co-infection, which correlates well with our findings within the sequential infection model of DCs with *Chlamydia* and HIV-1, which exerted a weak HIV-specific CTL activation. However, to study the impact of simultaneous STI on HIV immune responses is logistically impossible in the human host.

LPS-DCs had the highest binding and internalization of HIV-C followed by Chlam-DCs, while iDCs and HIV-C/Chlam-DCs showed similar HIV-C up-take levels. As described earlier, maturation of DCs—as seen in LPS- or Chlam-DCs—enhances their virus capture and *trans* infection capacity while reducing viral fusion events (34). HIV-C/Chlam-DCs are not as mature as Chlam-DCs, when binding and internalization were measured. Therefore, HIV-C/Chlam-DCs more act like iDCs, which show less binding and internalization, but enhanced fusion. Consistent with this interpretation, the highest levels of fusion were measured in iDCs and HIV-C/Chlam-DCs, while Chlam- and LPS-DCs demonstrated considerably reduced fusion levels (34). Consistent with our fusion data, the accumulation of HIV-C in HLA-DR-containing compartments was highest in LPS-DCs and also Chlam-DCs showed significantly higher HIV-C-containing compartments compared to iDCs. In macrophages, virus containing compartments (VCCs) were described to resemble late endosomes or multi-vesicular body (MVB) compartments and to show enrichment of CD9, CD53, CD81, CD82, and MHC class II (35, 36). We previously illustrated co-localization of HIV-C with these markers (7). VCCs are non-acidic and often express surface-connected tubular conduits to the plasma membrane (35, 37, 38). VCC formation was demonstrated to greatly facilitate *trans*-infection of HIV-1 from macrophages to autologous $CD4^+$ T cells (39). Accumulation of viral particles within intracellular DC compartments was illustrated to share multiple features with macrophage VCCs (30, 40, 41). Concentration of non-opsonized HIV-1 particles in large sac-like and tetraspanin-rich/MHC II compartments within LPS-mDCs was shown by various imaging studies (27, 42, 43). We also show a similar distribution of HIV-C in MHC II (HLA-DR-) compartments particularly in Chlam- and LPS-matured DCs. Transfer of such trapped viral particles, which were non-opsonized, from mDCs to $CD4^+$ T cells was highly effective (44–46). Localization of internalized virus differs greatly in endocytically active iDCs compared to mDCs—mDCs storing intact HIV particles within large vesicles correlate with increased *trans*-infection abilities (34). We here demonstrate (47), that similar to non-opsonized HIV-1, mature DCs (i.e., LPS-DCs and Chlam-DCs) retained HIV-C particles in an infectious form and efficiently transmitted the virus particles to target $CD4^+$ T cells through *trans* infection. Despite co-infection with *Chlamydia*, DCs displayed significantly higher amounts of trapped virus particles compared to iDCs loaded with HIV-C. Such co-infected DCs exerted superior antiviral functions as increased HIV-specific CTL-stimulation and reduced transfer to $CD4^+$ T cells. These effects were likely a consequence of higher viral fusion of HIV-C during co-infection compared to LPS-DCs and the sequential infection model, where DCs were incubated with *Chlamydia* for a prolonged period prior to addition of HIV-C.

Siglec-1 was recently described to play a major role during HIV-1 capture and transfer in LPS-mDCs. Here, we also analyzed co-localization of GFP-tagged complement-opsonized HIV-1 and Siglec-1 in iDCs, HIV+Chlam-, Chlam-, and LPS-DCs. We did not find any correlation between co-localization of Siglec-1/HIV-C, the maturation status of DCs and transfer to susceptible T cells. These findings are consistent with recent *in vivo* studies by Martinez-Picado et al. where they demonstrated that Siglec-1 protein truncation did not have a measurable impact on HIV-1 acquisition or AIDS outcomes *in vivo* (48). The missing correlation of Siglec-1/HIV-C and transfer from differently matured DCs to target cells which was described *in vitro* for non-opsonized HIV-1 by recent studies (41, 49–51) might rely on the fact that C3 fragments covalently bind to the surface of HIV-1 (52) potentially hampering interactions of Siglec-1 with virus-incorporated host-cell-derived glycosphingolipid GM3. GM3 was shown to allow capture by DCs, monocytes and macrophages *in vitro* (51). In our analyses, we, too, found higher co-localization of non-opsonized HIV with Siglec-1, in particular in the sequential infection model, but also in LPS-mDCs. *In vivo*, HIV-1 was found to be opsonized with complement fragments or specific antibodies in all compartments tested so far (53–57). Therefore, the findings by Martinez-Picado et al. that Siglec-1 protein truncation did not correlate with HIV-1 acquisition or AIDS outcomes *in vivo* could be explained by covalent coating of the virus with C3. C3 bound to the viral particles would mediate interactions with complement receptors 3 and 4 (CR3, CD11b/CD18; CR4, CD11c/CD18) abundantly expressed by immature and mature DCs rather than allowing interactions of GM3 with Siglec-1. We earlier found that the covalently linked cloud of C3 fragments on the viral surface impaired interactions of the HIV envelope glycoproteins with C-type lectins expressed on iDCs (8).

The presented data shows that co- or sequential infection of DCs with *Chlamydia* alters the progression of subsequent HIV-1 infection with implications for HIV-1 processing into peptides for MHC presentation, transfer to target cells via *trans*-infection and CTL responses (58, 59). STIs are an important public health issue and in HIV-positive women, STIs are associated not only with gynecological complications but with increased risk of HIV transmission to HIV-negative partners and newborns (60). We find that infection of DCs with HIV-C (or HIV) and *Chlamydia* are associated with mechanisms but only if added simultaneously. The mechanisms are likely due to simultaneous stimulation of innate immune mechanisms on DCs. One such trigger might be activation of Toll-like receptors (TLRs), since *Chlamydia* was illustrated to activate TLR2/6 (61). Therefore, within the chlamydial/HIV-C co-infection model TLRs in concerted action with CR3/CR4 (HIV-C) or C-type lectins (HIV) could stimulate a more robust DC activation compared to HIV-C- or HIV-DCs alone. This would result in even higher stimulation of HIV-specific CTLs and reduction of viral infectivity in the co-infection model. Other host innate immune responses, which might contribute to the higher anti-HIV-1 activity of co-infected DCs comprise superior induction of pro-inflammatory cytokines and/or antimicrobial peptides (62–64). However, the sequential infection model, which probably occurs more often *in vivo* compared to simultaneous DC stimulation with both pathogens, was associated with harm to the host due to significantly enhanced *cis* and *trans* infection with HIV-1 and significantly reduced HIV-specific CTL-stimulation. In future studies, we want to elucidate the mechanisms in DCs involved in the observed differences in *Chlamydia*-mediated effects to characterize factors associated with protection, which might be applied as therapeutic interventions during STIs to lower the risk of HIV-1 transmission and infection.

AUTHOR CONTRIBUTIONS

MS, UK, and PC performed experiments, analyzed data, and read the manuscript, PH, TJH, AM, and RB-W contributed essential components, read and discussed the manuscript, CL-F helped in designing the study, provided financial support and read and discussed the manuscript, WP and DW designed the study, conducted experiments, analyzed data, and wrote the manuscript with input from all authors. All authors provided critical feedback and helped shape the research, analysis and manuscript.

ACKNOWLEDGMENTS

We would like to thank our technician Karolin Thurnes, Divison of Hygiene and Medical Microbiology, and Prof. Oliver Keppler, Max-von-Pettenkofer Institute, Munich, Germany, for supplying the HIV plasmids. We would like to thank the Austrian Science Fund (MCBO graduate program/W011010-21 and P24598 to DW, P25389 to WP) and the Oesterreichische Nationalbank Anniversary Fund (Project number: 17614 to WP) for supporting this work. Further, this publication was made possible with help from the HIV Vaccine Trials Network Mucosal Immunology Group Program, an NIH funded program (HVTN LC Grant UM1AI068618 to TJH and DW) and the Tyrolean Science Fund (to DW). AM is supported by ANRS, Sidaction and ANR fundings.

SUPPLEMENTARY MATERIAL

Figure S1 | Flow cytometric analyses of DC profiles of iDCs and differentially treated DCs. (Upper panel) Monocyte-derived iDCs are routinely checked for characteristic markers CD11b, CD11c, and DC-SIGN, which are homogenously expressed on day 5 iDCs. Characteristic maturation markers CD83 and HLA-DR are not expressed or do show a low expression on day 5 iDCs dependent on the donor. Representative histogram plots for the various markers are illustrated. (Lower panel) Day 5 iDCs were treated for further 2 days with live (light green) or heat-inactivated (dark green) Chlamydia or not (iDCs, red) and analyzed for expression of characteristic maturation markers. A representative histogram plot for CD83 is depicted.

Figure S2 | Chlam- and LPS-DCs efficiently capture HIV. Binding at 4°C **(A)** and internalization at 37°C **(B)** were performed in triplicates using 25 ng/ml of R5-tropic non-opsonized HIV-1. Bar graphs show means ± SD from three independent experiments. p24 levels within the cell lysates were determined by ELISA. Prior to cell lysate preparation, cells were thoroughly washed to remove unbound virus. Statistical analysis shows 2-way ANOVA with Tukey's multiple comparisons test. Six donors are summarized. **(C)** Fusion assays were performed by exposure of HIV/Chlam-DCs and LPS-DCs to HIV bearing the chimeric protein β-lactamase-vpr. The amount of fused virus was determined by flow cytometric analyses of cleaved CCF2 in the cytoplasm. Percentages of cleaved CCF2-positive cells from three independent donors are depicted.

Figure S3 | Siglec-1-independent transfer of HIV-C. Enhanced transfer of HIV-C from Chlam- and LPS-DCs was independent on Siglec-1 as analyzed by high content screening as depicted (upper panel). Only low spots of HIV-C/Siglec-1-co-localization were quantified in 2 fields of 100 cells each (lower panel, right). The co-localization was compared to non-infected differentially stimulated DCs, which represent background values (lower panel, left), and HIV-infected differentially stimulated DCs (lower panel, middle). 200 cells were analyzed in total.

Figure S4 | Localization of HIV-C in iDCs and LPS-DCs. For three-dimensional reconstructions, confocal z stacks of iDCs and LPS-DCs exposed to HIV-C were processed with Imaris software using surface reconstruction (Surpass, IMARIS 8.2). About 30 cells per condition were analyzed.

Figure S5 | Enhanced DC infection by HIV-C independent of stimulation. iDCs, HIV/Chlam- and Chlam-DCs exerted a significantly enhanced infection using HIV-C (gray) compared to HIV (white). Nevertheless, also productive DC infection of HIV/Chlam-DCs was significantly increased compared to the low-level infection of iDCs using non-opsonized HIV. Three independent donors were summarized in the graph and means ± SD are shown.

Figure S6 | Enhanced CTL stimulation by HIV+Chlam DCs. IFNγ induction in CD8+ T cell clones by DCs simultaneously exposed to HIV and Chlamydia was significantly higher than that iDCs, Chlam-, and LPS-DCs exposed to HIV (p < 0.0001 for all). Means ± SD of three independent experiments are illustrated.

REFERENCES

1. Doncel GF, Joseph T, Thurman AR. Role of semen in HIV-1 transmission: inhibitor or facilitator? *Am J Reproduc Immunol.* (2011) 65:292–301. doi: 10.1111/j.1600-0897.2010.00931.x
2. Royce RA, Seña A, Cates WJ, Cohen MS. Sexual Transmission of HIV. *N Engl J Med.* (1997) 336:1072–8. doi: 10.1056/NEJM199704103361507
3. Shen R, Richter HE, Smith PD. Early HIV-1 target cells in human vaginal and ectocervical mucosa. *Am J Reproduc Immunol.* (2011) 65:261–7. doi: 10.1111/j.1600-0897.2010.00939.x
4. Ebenbichler CF, Thielens NM, Vornhagen R, Marschang P, Arlaud GJ, Dierich MP. Human immunodeficiency virus type 1 activates the classical pathway of complement by direct C1 binding through specific sites in the transmembrane glycoprotein gp41. *J Exp Med.* (1991) 174:1417–24. doi: 10.1084/jem.174.6.1417
5. Bouhlal H, Chomont N, Haeffner-Cavaillon N, Kazatchkine MD, Belec L, Hocini H. Opsonization of HIV-1 by semen complement enhances infection of human epithelial cells. *J Immunol.* (2002) 169:3301–6. doi: 10.4049/jimmunol.169.6.3301
6. Stoiber H, Soederholm A, Wilflingseder D, Gusenbauer S, Hildgartner A, Dierich MP. Complement and antibodies: a dangerous liaison in HIV infection? *Vaccine.* 26(Suppl. 8):I79–85. doi: 10.1016/j.vaccine.2008.11.050
7. Wilflingseder D, Banki Z, Garcia E, Pruenster M, Pfister G, Muellauer B, et al. IgG opsonization of HIV impedes provirus formation in and infection of dendritic cells and subsequent long-term transfer to T cells. *J Immunol.* (2007) 178:7840–8. doi: 10.4049/jimmunol.178.12.7840
8. Pruenster M, Wilflingseder D, Bánki Z, Ammann CG, Muellauer B, Meyer M, et al. C-type lectin-independent interaction of complement opsonized HIV with monocyte-derived dendritic cells. *Eur J Immunol.* (2005) 35:2691–8. doi: 10.1002/eji.200425940
9. Posch W, Steger M, Knackmuss U, Blatzer M, Baldauf HM, Doppler W, et al. Complement-opsonized HIV-1 overcomes restriction in dendritic cells. *PLoS Pathog.* (2015) 11:e1005005. doi: 10.1371/journal.ppat.1005005
10. Galvin SR, Cohen MS. The role of sexually transmitted diseases in HIV transmission. *Nat Rev Microbiol.* (2004) 2:33–42. doi: 10.1038/nrmicro794
11. Fleming DT, Wasserheit JN. From epidemiological synergy to public health policy and practice: the contribution of other sexually transmitted diseases to sexual transmission of HIV infection. *Sexually Transmitted Infect.* (1999) 75:3–17. doi: 10.1136/sti.75.1.3
12. Hillier SL. Diagnostic microbiology of bacterial vaginosis. *Am J Obstetr Gynecol.* (1993) 169(2, Part 2):455–9. doi: 10.1016/0002-9378(93)90340-O
13. Sewankambo N, Gray RH, Wawer MJ, Paxton L, McNairn D, Wabwire-Mangen F, et al. HIV-1 infection associated with abnormal vaginal flora morphology and bacterial vaginosis. *Lancet.* (1997) 350:546–50. doi: 10.1016/S0140-6736(97)01063-5
14. St. John EP, Martinson J, Simoes JA, Landay AL, Spear GT. Dendritic cell activation and maturation induced by mucosal fluid from women with bacterial vaginosis. *Clin Immunol.* (2007) 125:95–102. doi: 10.1016/j.clim.2007.06.004
15. Bachmann NL, Polkinghorne A, Timms P. Chlamydia genomics: providing novel insights into chlamydial biology. *Trends Microbiol.* (2014) 22:464–72. doi: 10.1016/j.tim.2014.04.013
16. Banki Z, Posch W, Ejaz A, Oberhauser V, Willey S, Gassner C, et al. Complement as an endogenous adjuvant for dendritic cell-mediated induction of retrovirus-specific CTLs. *PLoS Pathog.* (2010) 6:e1000891. doi: 10.1371/journal.ppat.1000891
17. Wilflingseder D, Schroll A, Hackl H, Gallasch R, Frampton D, Lass-Florl C, et al. Immediate T-helper 17 polarization upon triggering CD11b/c on HIV-exposed dendritic cells. *J Infect Dis.* (2015) 212:44–56. doi: 10.1093/infdis/jiv014
18. Sullivan BL, Knopoff EJ, Saifuddin M, Takefman DM, Saarloos MN, Sha BE, et al. Susceptibility of HIV-1 Plasma Virus to Complement-mediated lysis. *Immunol J.* (1996) 157:1791–8.
19. Posch W, Cardinaud S, Hamimi C, Fletcher A, Muhlbacher A, Loacker K, et al. Antibodies attenuate the capacity of dendritic cells to stimulate HIV-specific cytotoxic T lymphocytes. *J Allergy Clin Immunol.* (2012) 130:1368–74 e2. doi: 10.1016/j.jaci.2012.08.025
20. Bellmann-Weiler R, Martinz V, Kurz K, Engl S, Feistritzer C, Fuchs D, et al. Divergent modulation of Chlamydia pneumoniae infection cycle in human monocytic and endothelial cells by iron, tryptophan availability and interferon gamma. *Immunobiology.* (2010) 215:842–8. doi: 10.1016/j.imbio.2010.05.021
21. Campbell EM, Perez O, Anderson JL, Hope TJ. Visualization of a proteasome-independent intermediate during restriction of HIV-1 by rhesus TRIM5alpha. *J Cell Biol.* (2008) 180:549–61. doi: 10.1083/jcb.200706154
22. Purtscher M, Trkola A, Gruber G, Buchacher A, Predl R, Steindl F, et al. A broadly neutralizing human monoclonal antibody against gp41 of human immunodeficiency virus type 1. *AIDS Res Hum Retroviruses.* (1994) 10:1651–8. doi: 10.1089/aid.1994.10.1651
23. Moris A, Nobile C, Buseyne F, Porrot F, Abastado JP, Schwartz O. DC-SIGN promotes exogenous MHC-I-restricted HIV-1 antigen presentation. *Blood.* (2004) 103:2648–54. doi: 10.1182/blood-2003-07-2532
24. Casartelli N, Guivel-Benhassine F, Bouziat R, Brandler S, Schwartz O, Moris A. The antiviral factor APOBEC3G improves CTL recognition of cultured HIV-infected T cells. *J Exp Med.* (2010) 207:39–49. doi: 10.1084/jem.20091933
25. Ogg GS, Jin X, Bonhoeffer S, Dunbar PR, Nowak MA, Monard S, et al. Quantitation of HIV-1-specific cytotoxic T lymphocytes and plasma load of viral RNA. *Science.* (1998) 279:2103–6. doi: 10.1126/science.279.5359.2103
26. Chen Q, Swaminathan S, Yang D, Dai L, Sui H, Yang J, et al. Interleukin-27 is a potent inhibitor of cis HIV-1 replication in monocyte-derived dendritic cells via a type I interferon-independent pathway. *PLoS ONE.* (2013) 8:e59194. doi: 10.1371/journal.pone.0059194
27. Rodriguez-Plata MT, Puigdomenech I, Izquierdo-Useros N, Puertas MC, Carrillo J, Erkizia I, et al. The infectious synapse formed between mature dendritic cells and CD4(+) T cells is independent of the presence of the HIV-1 envelope glycoprotein. *Retrovirology.* (2013) 10:42. doi: 10.1186/1742-4690-10-42
28. Izquierdo-Useros N, Lorizate M, Puertas MC, Rodriguez-Plata MT, Zangger N, Erikson E, et al. Siglec-1 is a novel dendritic cell receptor that mediates HIV-1 trans-infection through recognition of viral membrane gangliosides. *PLoS Biol.* (2012) 10:e1001448. doi: 10.1371/journal.pbio.1001448
29. Martinez-Picado J, McLaren PJ, Telenti A, Izquierdo-Useros N. Retroviruses as myeloid cell riders: what natural human siglec-1 "Knockouts" tell us about pathogenesis. *Front Immunol.* (2017) 8:1593. doi: 10.3389/fimmu.2017.01593
30. Izquierdo-Useros N, Lorizate M, McLaren PJ, Telenti A, Krausslich HG, Martinez-Picado J. HIV-1 capture and transmission by dendritic cells: the role of viral glycolipids and the cellular receptor Siglec-1. *PLoS Pathog.* (2014) 10:e1004146. doi: 10.1371/journal.ppat.1004146
31. Izquierdo-Useros N, Naranjo-Gomez M, Erkizia I, Puertas MC, Borras FE, Blanco J, et al. HIV and mature dendritic cells: trojan exosomes riding the Trojan horse? *PLoS Pathog.* (2010) 6:e1000740. doi: 10.1371/journal.ppat.1000740
32. Slade J, Hall JV, Kintner J, Schoborg RV. Chlamydial pre-infection protects from subsequent herpes simplex virus-2 challenge in a murine vaginal super-infection model. *PLoS ONE.* (2016) 11:e0146186. doi: 10.1371/journal.pone.0146186
33. Sheung A, Rebbapragada A, Shin LY, Dobson-Belaire W, Kimani J, Ngugi E, et al. Mucosal Neisseria gonorrhoeae coinfection during HIV acquisition is associated with enhanced systemic HIV-specific CD8 T-cell responses. *AIDS.* (2008) 22:1729–37. doi: 10.1097/QAD.0b013e32830baf5e
34. Cavrois M, Neidleman J, Kreisberg JF, Fenard D, Callebaut C, Greene WC. Human immunodeficiency virus fusion to dendritic cells declines as cells mature. *J Virol.* (2006) 80:1992–9. doi: 10.1128/JVI.80.4.1992-1999.2006
35. Deneka M, Pelchen-Matthews A, Byland R, Ruiz-Mateos E, Marsh M. In macrophages, HIV-1 assembles into an intracellular plasma membrane domain containing the tetraspanins CD81, CD9, and CD53. *J Cell Biol.* (2007) 177:329–41. doi: 10.1083/jcb.200609050
36. Pelchen-Matthews A, Kramer B, Marsh M. Infectious HIV-1 assembles in late endosomes in primary macrophages. *J Cell Biol.* (2003) 162:443–55. doi: 10.1083/jcb.200304008
37. Bennett AE, Narayan K, Shi D, Hartnell LM, Gousset K, He H, et al. Ion-abrasion scanning electron microscopy reveals surface-connected tubular conduits in HIV-infected macrophages. *PLoS Pathog.* (2009) 5:e1000591. doi: 10.1371/journal.ppat.1000591

38. Welsch S, Keppler OT, Habermann A, Allespach I, Krijnse-Locker J, Krausslich HG. HIV-1 buds predominantly at the plasma membrane of primary human macrophages. *PLoS Pathog.* (2007) 3:e36. doi: 10.1371/journal.ppat.0030036
39. Hammonds JE, Beeman N, Ding L, Takushi S, Francis AC, Wang JJ, et al. Siglec-1 initiates formation of the virus-containing compartment and enhances macrophage-to-T cell transmission of HIV-1. *PLoS Pathog.* (2017) 13:e1006181. doi: 10.1371/journal.ppat.1006181
40. Puryear WB, Akiyama H, Geer SD, Ramirez NP, Yu X, Reinhard BM, et al. Interferon-inducible mechanism of dendritic cell-mediated HIV-1 dissemination is dependent on Siglec-1/CD169. *PLoS Pathog.* (2013) 9:e1003291. doi: 10.1371/journal.ppat.1003291
41. Puryear WB, Gummuluru S. Role of glycosphingolipids in dendritic cell-mediated HIV-1 trans-infection. *Adv Exp Med Biol.* (2013) 762:131–53. doi: 10.1007/978-1-4614-4433-6_5
42. Yu HJ, Reuter MA, McDonald D. HIV traffics through a specialized, surface-accessible intracellular compartment during trans-infection of T cells by mature dendritic cells. *PLoS Pathog.* (2008) 4:e1000134. doi: 10.1371/journal.ppat.1000134
43. Garcia E, Pion M, Pelchen-Matthews A, Collinson L, Arrighi JF, Blot G, et al. HIV-1 trafficking to the dendritic cell-T-cell infectious synapse uses a pathway of tetraspanin sorting to the immunological synapse. *Traffic.* (2005) 6:488–501. doi: 10.1111/j.1600-0854.2005.00293.x
44. Izquierdo-Useros N, Esteban O, Rodriguez-Plata MT, Erkizia I, Prado JG, Blanco J, et al. Dynamic imaging of cell-free and cell-associated viral capture in mature dendritic cells. *Traffic.* (2011) 12:1702–13. doi: 10.1111/j.1600-0854.2011.01281.x
45. Sanders RW, de Jong EC, Baldwin CE, Schuitemaker JH, Kapsenberg ML, Berkhout B. Differential transmission of human immunodeficiency virus type 1 by distinct subsets of effector dendritic cells. *J Virol.* (2002) 76:7812–21. doi: 10.1128/JVI.76.15.7812-7821.2002
46. Wang JH, Janas AM, Olson WJ, Wu L. Functionally distinct transmission of human immunodeficiency virus type 1 mediated by immature and mature dendritic cells. *J Virol.* (2007) 81:8933–43. doi: 10.1128/JVI.00878-07
47. Granelli-Piperno A, Delgado E, Finkel V, Paxton W, Steinman RM. Immature dendritic cells selectively replicate macrophagetropic (M-tropic) human immunodeficiency virus type 1, while mature cells efficiently transmit both M- and T-tropic virus to T cells. *J Virol.* (1998) 72:2733–7.
48. Martinez-Picado J, McLaren PJ, Erkizia I, Martin MP, Benet S, Rotger M, et al. Identification of Siglec-1 null individuals infected with HIV-1. *Nat Commun.* (2016) 7:12412. doi: 10.1038/ncomms12412
49. Pino M, Erkizia I, Benet S, Erikson E, Fernandez-Figueras MT, Guerrero D, Dalmau J, et al. HIV-1 immune activation induces Siglec-1 expression and enhances viral trans-infection in blood and tissue myeloid cells. *Retrovirology.* (2015) 12:37. doi: 10.1186/s12977-015-0160-x
50. Izquierdo-Useros N, Naranjo-Gomez M, Archer J, Hatch SC, Erkizia I, Blanco J, et al. Capture and transfer of HIV-1 particles by mature dendritic cells converges with the exosome-dissemination pathway. *Blood.* (2009) 113:2732–41. doi: 10.1182/blood-2008-05-158642
51. Puryear WB, Yu X, Ramirez NP, Reinhard BM, Gummuluru S. HIV-1 incorporation of host-cell-derived glycosphingolipid GM3 allows for capture by mature dendritic cells. *Proc Natl Acad Sci USA.* (2012) 109:7475–80. doi: 10.1073/pnas.1201104109
52. Stoiber H, Ebenbichler C, Schneider R, Janatova J, Dierich MP. Interaction of several complement proteins with gp120 and gp41, the two envelope glycoproteins of HIV-1. *AIDS.* (1995) 9:19–26. doi: 10.1097/00002030-199501000-00003
53. Hess C, Klimkait T, Schlapbach L, Del Zenero V, Sadallah S, Horakova E, et al. Association of a pool of HIV-1 with erythrocytes *in vivo*: a cohort study. *Lancet.* (2002) 359:2230–4. doi: 10.1016/S0140-6736(02)09291-7
54. Burton GF, Masuda A, Heath SL, Smith BA, Tew JG, Szakal AK. Follicular dendritic cells (FDC) in retroviral infection: host/pathogen perspectives. *Immunol Rev.* (1997) 156:185–97. doi: 10.1111/j.1600-065X.1997.tb00968.x
55. Moir S, Malaspina A, Li Y, Chun TW, Lowe T, Adelsberger J, et al. B cells of HIV-1-infected patients bind virions through CD21-complement interactions and transmit infectious virus to activated T cells. *J Exp Med.* (2000) 192:637–46. doi: 10.1084/jem.192.5.637
56. Kacani L, Prodinger WM, Sprinzl GM, Schwendinger MG, Spruth M, Stoiber H, et al. Detachment of human immunodeficiency virus type 1 from germinal centers by blocking complement receptor type 2. *J Virol.* (2000) 74:7997–8002. doi: 10.1128/JVI.74.17.7997-8002.2000
57. Schifferli JA. Complement and immune complexes. *Res Immunol.* (1996) 147:109–10. doi: 10.1016/0923-2494(96)87183-5
58. McDonald D, Wu L, Bohks SM, KewalRamani VN, Unutmaz D, Hope TJ. Recruitment of HIV and its receptors to dendritic cell-T cell junctions. *Science.* (2003) 300:1295–7. doi: 10.1126/science.1084238
59. Turville SG, Santos JJ, Frank I, Cameron PU, Wilkinson J, Miranda-Saksena M, et al. Immunodeficiency virus uptake, turnover, and 2-phase transfer in human dendritic cells. *Blood.* (2004) 103:2170–9. doi: 10.1182/blood-2003-09-3129
60. Alcaide ML, Jones DL, Chitalu N, Weiss S. Chlamydia and Gonorrhea Infections in HIV-positive Women in Urban Lusaka, Zambia. *J Glob Infect Dis.* (2012) 4:141–4. doi: 10.4103/0974-777X.100566
61. Wang Y, Liu Q, Chen D, Guan J, Ma L, Zhong G, et al. Chlamydial lipoproteins stimulate toll-like receptors 1/2 mediated inflammatory responses through MyD88-dependent pathway. *Front Microbiol.* (2017) 8:78. doi: 10.3389/fmicb.2017.00078
62. Liechti GW, Kuru E, Hall E, Kalinda A, Brun YV, VanNieuwenhze M, et al. A new metabolic cell-wall labelling method reveals peptidoglycan in Chlamydia trachomatis. *Nature.* (2014) 506:507–10. doi: 10.1038/nature12892
63. Hickey DK, Patel MV, Fahey JV, Wira CR. Innate and adaptive immunity at mucosal surfaces of the female reproductive tract: stratification and integration of immune protection against the transmission of sexually transmitted infections. *J Reprod Immunol.* (2011) 88:185–94. doi: 10.1016/j.jri.2011.01.005
64. Wira CR, Patel MV, Ghosh M, Mukura L, Fahey JV. Innate immunity in the human female reproductive tract: endocrine regulation of endogenous antimicrobial protection against HIV and other sexually transmitted infections. *Am J Reprod Immunol.* (2011) 65:196–211. doi: 10.1111/j.1600-0897.2011.00970.x

8

Generation of an Oncolytic Herpes Simplex Virus 1 Expressing Human MelanA

Jan B. Boscheinen [1], Sabrina Thomann [1], David M. Knipe [2], Neal DeLuca [3], Beatrice Schuler-Thurner [4], Stefanie Gross [4], Jan Dörrie [4], Niels Schaft [4], Christian Bach [5], Anette Rohrhofer [6], Melanie Werner-Klein [7], Barbara Schmidt [1,6,8] and Philipp Schuster [8]*

[1] Institute of Clinical and Molecular Virology, Friedrich-Alexander-Universität Erlangen-Nürnberg, Erlangen, Germany, [2] Department of Microbiology and Immunobiology, Harvard Medical School, Boston, MA, United States, [3] Department of Microbiology and Molecular Genetics, University of Pittsburgh School of Medicine, Pittsburgh, PA, United States, [4] Department of Dermatology, Universitätsklinikum Erlangen, Friedrich-Alexander-Universität Erlangen-Nürnberg, Erlangen, Germany, [5] Lab for Immunogenetics, Universitätsklinikum Erlangen, Erlangen, Germany, [6] Institute of Clinical Microbiology and Hygiene, University Hospital Regensburg, Regensburg, Germany, [7] Chair of Immunology, Regensburg Center for Interventional Immunology (RCI), University of Regensburg, Regensburg, Germany, [8] Institute of Medical Microbiology and Hygiene, University of Regensburg, Regensburg, Germany

***Correspondence:**
Barbara Schmidt
barbara.schmidt@ukr.de

Robust anti-tumor immunity requires innate as well as adaptive immune responses. We have shown that plasmacytoid dendritic cells develop killer cell-like activity in melanoma cell cocultures after exposure to the infectious but replication-deficient herpes simplex virus 1 (HSV-1) *d*106S. To combine this innate effect with an enhanced adaptive immune response, the gene encoding human MelanA/MART-1 was inserted into HSV-1 *d*106S via homologous recombination to increase direct expression of this tumor antigen. Infection of Vero cells using this recombinant virus confirmed MelanA expression by Western blotting, flow cytometry, and immunofluorescence. HSV-1 *d*106S-MelanA induced expression of the transgene in fibroblast and melanoma cell lines not naturally expressing MelanA. Infection of a melanoma cell line with CRISPR-Cas9-mediated knockout of MelanA confirmed *de novo* expression of the transgene in the viral context. Dependent on MelanA expression, infected fibroblast and melanoma cell lines induced degranulation of HLA-matched MelanA-specific $CD8^+$ T cells, followed by killing of infected cells. To study infection of immune cells, we exposed peripheral blood mononuclear cells and *in vitro*-differentiated macrophages to the parental HSV-1 *d*106S, resulting in expression of the transgene GFP in $CD11c^+$ cells and macrophages. These data provide evidence that the application of MelanA-encoding HSV-1 *d*106S could enhance adaptive immune responses and re-direct MelanA-specific $CD8^+$ T cells to tumor lesions, which have escaped adaptive immune responses via downregulation of their tumor antigen. Hence, HSV-1 *d*106S-MelanA harbors the potential to induce innate immune responses in conjunction with adaptive anti-tumor responses by $CD8^+$ T cells, which should be evaluated in further studies.

Keywords: vaccine, oncolytic viruses, malignant melanoma, herpes virus, cytotoxic T cell response

INTRODUCTION

Based on the results of a large phase III trial (1), Talimogene laherparepvec (T-VEC) was recently approved as first oncolytic herpes virus 1 for the treatment of patients with stage IIIB, IIIC, or IVM1a malignant melanoma. This attenuated virus induces regression of injected or distant cutaneous, lymphatic, and visceral lesions (2). It preferentially replicates in tumor cells due to defects in the type I interferon pathway, which renders these cells more susceptible to virus replication (3). T-VEC encodes GM-CSF, which contributes to recruitment of antigen-presenting cells to the site of injection. Via lysis of melanoma cells and uptake into antigen-presenting cells, T-VEC enhances cross-presentation of tumor-associated antigens to T cells, which, in particular in combination with immune checkpoint inhibitors, induces strong anti-tumoral responses leading to significantly improved survival of the patients (4, 5).

T-VEC is one of several oncolytic herpes simplex viruses, which have made their way to the clinic. Amongst them are G207, HSV 1716, NV1020, and HF10, which have been used in phase I/II trials in glioma, glioblastoma, melanoma, neuroblastoma, breast, and pancreatic cancer (6). All these viruses are attenuated, but replication-competent. In addition to inactivation of the neurovirulence gene γ34.5 and the TAP-binding protein ICP47, the third generation oncolytic herpes virus Δ47 has mutated the ribonucleotide reductase ICP6, resulting in a more pronounced attenuation of the virus (7).

We have investigated the oncolytic effects of the HSV-1 *d*106S strain, which, in contrast to other oncolytic herpes viruses, is infectious but replication-deficient due to deletions of essential viral genes (8). HSV-1 *d*106S expresses GFP, which can be replaced by other genes of interest via homologous recombination. Using eleven different melanoma cell lines, we have shown that HSV-1 *d*106S is oncolytic, in particular if combined with plasmacytoid dendritic cells (PDC) (9). These cells are major producers of type I interferons (IFN) in the blood upon stimulation with herpes simplex or influenza viruses (10, 11). They surround and occasionally infiltrate primary melanoma lesions and sentinel lymph nodes (12–14).

Due to an immunosuppressive tumor microenvironment, infiltrating PDC are usually immature and tolerogenic, promoting regulatory immunity (15) and tumor progression (16, 17). Upon activation by Toll-like receptor (TLR) agonists, PDC induce a Th1-type immune response and contribute to T cell-mediated tumor regression. In this respect, we have shown that PDC develop strong killer-cell like activity against melanoma cells upon exposure to HSV-1 *d*106S (9). This was similarly observed by others using Toll-like receptor 7 and 9 agonists as well as viral vaccines for stimulation of PDC (18–26).

So far, evidence is accumulating that oncolytic herpes viruses are potent inducers of innate immune responses. Beyond that, robust anti-tumor immunity requires adaptive immune responses. Two recent proof-of-concept trials showed induction of strong (mostly CD4$^+$) T cell responses with subsequent delay in reappearance of new metastases in melanoma patients via injection of minigenes coding for different neoantigen-derived peptides (27) or via vaccination using respective peptides in the context of adjuvant (28).

With oncolytic viruses, induction of adaptive immunity is currently based on the uptake and cross-presentation of tumor-specific antigens released from dying tumor cells. To enhance antigen presentation, we envisaged to replace the transgene GFP in HSV-1 *d*106S by the melanoma-associated antigen MelanA/MART-1. We hypothesized that the expression of a tumor antigen in the context of the oncolytic HSV-1 *d*106S may provoke CD8$^+$ T cell responses against melanoma cells, combining oncolytic effects of the virus with enhanced expression of melanoma-associated antigens. Hence, such an oncolytic virus may target both innate and adaptive immune responses.

MATERIALS AND METHODS

Cloning of MelanA Into Transfer Plasmid pd27B

The transfer plasmid pd27B containing sequences homologous to HSV-1 *d*106S (8) and a MelanA expression plasmid (29) were propagated in *Escherichia coli* XL-1 Blue cells (Agilent, Böblingen, Germany) and isolated using the PureLink HiPure Plasmid Midiprep kit (Invitrogen/Life Technologies, Darmstadt, Germany). The coding sequence for MelanA was amplified using NheI-MelanA (5′-TAGATAGCTAGCATGCCAAGAGAA GATGCTC-3′) and MelanA-XbaI (5′-GTCCATTCTAGATTA AGGTGAATAAGGTGGTG-3′) (biomers.net, Ulm, Germany). The PCR product and pd27B were digested using NheI and XbaI (NEB, Frankfurt, Germany), followed by dephosphorylation of pd27B. Both products were purified using the QIAquick PCR purification kit (Qiagen, Hilden, Germany), ligated at room temperature overnight, and transformed into XL-1 Blue cells. Correct inserts were identified using T7-EEV-Prom (5′-AAGGCTAGAGTACTTAATACGA-3′; Promega, Mannheim, Germany) with primers 5′-CCGATGAGCAGTAAGACTC-3′; 5′-AGTTGTGGTTTGTCCAAACTC-3′; 5′-TGGATAAAAGTC TTCATGTTGG-3′.

Cultivation of HSV-1 *d*106S and HSV-1 *d*106S-MelanA

HSV-1 *d*106S is an infectious recombinant strain derived from the HSV-1 *d*106 virus (30). It expresses GFP under the control of a CMV promoter, has a restored susceptibility to aciclovir, and is replication-deficient due to deletions of essential viral genes and promoter regions (8). Complementing E11 cells providing ICP4 and ICP27/47 *in trans* were propagated in DMEM supplemented with 10% heat-inactivated FCS (Sigma-Aldrich, Munich, Germany), 90 U/ml streptomycin, 0.3 mg/ml glutamine, 200 U/ml penicillin, and periodic G418 selection (400 μg/ml). Infected at 90% confluency (MOI 0.1), cells were harvested at 50–60 h when they showed cytopathic effects but were still adherent. After three freeze-thaw cycles, cells were resuspended in DPBS. Supernatants were filtered through 0.45 μm pores and stored at

Abbreviations: HSV, Herpes simplex virus; IFN, interferon; ko, knockout; MOI, multiplicity of infection; PBMC, peripheral blood mononuclear cells; PCR, polymerase chain reaction; PDC, plasmacytoid dendritic cells; p.i., post infection; sg, single guide.

−80°C. The number of infectious HSV-1 particles was quantified using the 50% tissue culture infective dose ($TCID_{50}$) according to the method of Reed and Munch.

Isolation of HSV-1 *d*106S DNA

Viral DNA was prepared from nucleocapsids following a published protocol (31). Supernatants of infected cell cultures were loaded onto discontinuous OptiPrep gradients (Sigma-Aldrich) of 40% iodixanol overlayed with 20% iodixanol, and subjected to ultracentrifugation using SW41Ti Ultraclear tubes (Beckman Coulter, Krefeld, Germany) at 30,000 rpm for 2 h, without braking at 800 rpm. The visible whitish ring containing viral particles was harvested by side-puncture, transferred to a VTi65 ultraclear tube (Beckman Coulter), and filled with 30% iodixanol, forming a continuous gradient during ultracentrifugation at 55,000 rpm for 6 h. The visible ring was transferred to a SW41Ti ultraclear tube, filled with DPBS, and pelleted at 20,000 rpm for 90 min. Pellets were re-suspended in DPBS, filtered through 0.45 μm pores, and digested using 10× Taq DNA polymerase buffer containing proteinase K (Sigma-Aldrich) and 0.1% (v/v) Tween 20 at 56°C for 1 h. For all subsequent steps, shearing of viral DNA was minimized by cutting off pipet tips and gentle mixing of solutions. The digested pellet was transferred to a phase lock "light" gel tube (5 Prime, Hilden, Germany) and mixed with phenol-chloroform-isoamylalcohol. After centrifugation at 2,000 rpm for 5 min, the aqueous phase was transferred to another phase lock gel tube, recapitulating the step described above. Traces of phenol were eliminated by chloroform extraction. The aqueous solution was precipitated with 7.5 M ammonium acetate and ice-cold ethanol at −80°C overnight. DNA was pelleted at 15,000 rpm at 4°C for 45 min, washed with 70% ethanol, and resuspended in TE-buffer. Purified DNA was not frozen to avoid double-strand breaks. Purity and integrity was checked using NanoDrop UV-spectrophotometry and EcoRI-HF digestion (NEB).

Homologous Recombination

E11 cells were seeded into 6-well plates to obtain 90% confluency for transfection. pd27B-MelanA was linearized using SwaI (NEB), purified using the QiaQuick PCR purification kit, and mixed with HSV-1 *d*106S DNA at a ratio of 1:4 (w/w) in DMEM plus glutamine. The mixture was heated at 95°C for 3 min, chilled on ice, and mixed with FuGENE HD transfection reagent (Roche, Mannheim, Germany). After incubation at room temperature for 30 min, the mixture was added to E11 cells. Cytopathic effects were identified after 2 days. Non-fluorescent viral plaques were purified using limiting dilution and further analyzed for evidence of homologous recombination.

Isolation and Cultivation of Cells

PBMC were isolated from EDTA-anticoagulated blood of healthy donors using standard Biocoll density gradient centrifugation (Biochrom AG, Berlin, Germany), as approved by the Ethical Committee of the Medical Faculty, Friedrich-Alexander-Universität Erlangen-Nürnberg (Ref. no. 3299). PBMC were cultivated in RPMI 1640 with supplements described above. For generation of macrophages, PBMC were seeded into Nunc Lab-Tek chamber slides (Thermo Fisher Scientific) and cultivated in the presence of 15% heat-inactivated autologous serum, removing non-adherent cells by trypsin after 3 days. At 10–14 days, macrophages were infected with wild type HSV-1 (32), HSV-1 166v (33), HSV-1 *d*106S, and HSV-1 *d*106S-MelanA. MRC-5 fibroblasts (ATCC® CCL-171™) and melanoma cell lines (IGR-37, IGR-39, ARST-1, ICNI-5li, SK-MEL30, LIWE-7) were cultivated as described (9).

CRISPR-Cas9 Knockout

The MelanA gene was knocked out from SK-MEL30 cells using CRISPR-Cas9 technology (Addgene, Cambridge, MA). Sequences of single guide (sg) RNAs were taken from the GECKO library (sgMelanA1: 5′-GCACGGCCACTCTTACACCA-3′; sgMelanA2: 5′-TTGAACTTACTCTTCAGCCG-3′) (34) and inserted into LentiCRISPRv2 puro (#52961) (35). Lentiviral stocks were produced from 293T cells transfected with plasmids LentiCRISPRv2 puro, psPAX2 (#12259), and pMD2.G (#12260).

HLA Typing

High resolution HLA-A, -B, and -C genotyping was performed using the HLA SBT S4 HLA class I kit (Protrans GmbH, Hockenheim, Germany) according to the manufacturer's instructions in full compliance with the HLA typing standards of the European Federation for Immunogenetics (EFI).

MelanA-Specific T Cell Generation and Coculture

$CD8^+$ T cells were purified from PBMC of a HLA-A*02:01-positive donor using a CD8 cell isolation kit (Miltenyi Biotec, Bergisch-Gladbach, Germany) and stimulated using artificial antigen-presenting cells (36) loaded with MelanA/MART-$1^{27L26-34}$ peptide (ELAGIGILTV, GenScript, distributed by Biozol, Eching, Germany). The coculture was carried out in M' medium (37) supplemented with 5% autologous plasma and 3% T cell growth factor (38), kindly provided by Mathias Oelke. On day 7 and weekly thereafter until week 4, T cells were restimulated. Purity was assessed using HLA-A*02:01/MART-$1^{27L26-35}$ tetramers and found to be $> 95\%$. Coculture with HLA-matched fibroblast and melanoma cell lines was carried out in the presence of Alexa 488-labeled CD107a (eBiosciences/ThermoFisher, Frankfurt, Germany) and Golgi blockers brefeldin A and monensin (Sigma-Aldrich/Merck; 1:1,000) for 4 h. Prior to coculture, melanoma and MRC5 cells were plated at 90% confluency, infected with the respective viruses (MOI 1) for 20 h or loaded with peptide for 1 h, washed, and subsequently overlaid with a total of 1.5×10^5 $CD8^+$ T cells in 96-well plates. After FcR blocking, cells were stained with fixable viability dye eFluor 506 (eBiosciences) and anti-CD8 APC/Cy7 (BioLegend, Koblenz, Germany), and, after permeabilization using the BD Cytofix/Cytoperm™ Kit, with anti-IFN-gamma PE-Cy7 or the respective isotype (eBiosciences).

FACS Analysis

PBMC were exposed to HSV-1 *d*106S and HSV-1 *d*106S-MelanA for 24 h, washed, and incubated with FcR blocking reagent at 4°C for 10 min. Cell populations were stained at 4°C for 20 min, using a published protocol (39) with antibodies to CD3 (Alexa Fluor700; clone UCHT1; BioLegend, London, UK), CD4 (PE-Cy7; clone RPA-T4; BioLegend), CD11c (PE-Cy5; clone B-ly6, BD Biosciences, Heidelberg, Germany), CD14 (APC; clone HCD14; BioLegend), CD19 (APC-H7; clone SJ25C1; BD Biosciences), CD56 (BV-605; clone NCAM16.2; BD Biosciences), and CD304 (PE; clone AD5-17F6; Miltenyi Biotec). Dead cells were stained using PacificBlue (Invitrogen/Life Technologies). Cells were collected using multiparameter LSR-II flow cytometer with FACSDiva software (BD Biosciences) and FCS Express 3 Software (De Novo Software, Los Angeles, CA, USA). MelanA expression was studied in infected cells, using the BD Cytofix/Cytoperm kit with FITC-conjugated (clone A103, Santa Cruz, Heidelberg, Germany) or unconjugated murine anti-MelanA (clone A103, Dako, Hamburg, Germany) and the respective isotype controls followed by Alexa Fluor 555-conjugated goat anti-mouse $F(ab')_2$ (Invitrogen/Life Technologies).

Western Blot Analysis

Cells were lysed on ice for 30 min (50 mM TRIS, pH 8.0; 150 mM NaCl; 5 mM EDTA; 1% NP-40; 0.1 mM PMSF), heated in sample buffer containing SDS and ß-mercaptoethanol at 105°C for 10 min, separated on a 10% polyacrylamide gel, and transferred to a PVDF membrane (Merck Millipore, Darmstadt, Germany). After blocking with 5% milk powder plus 0.4% Tween 20, samples were incubated with unconjugated MelanA antibody (1:750) at room temperature for 1.5 h or at 4°C overnight, followed by HRP-conjugated rabbit polyclonal anti-mouse IgG (H+L) (DAKO Diagnostics GmbH, Hamburg; 1:1,000) at room temperature for 60 min. After adding ECL solution containing luminol (Sigma-Aldrich) for 1 min, luminescence was recorded using the Fujifilm LAS-1000 plus gel documentation system.

Immunofluorescence and Confocal Microscopy

E11/Vero cells and macrophages were infected in chamber slides using HSV-1 *d*106S and HSV-1 *d*106S-MelanA (MOI 10) for 16 h, and incubated in DPBS plus 0.3% Triton-X100 at 4°C for 20 min. After blocking in DPBS with 1% BSA (NEB) and 5% FCS, cells were stained with unconjugated anti-MelanA (diluted 1:75 in DPBS plus 1% BSA) at room temperature for 1 h and Alexa Fluor 555-conjugated goat anti-mouse $F(ab')_2$ (Invitrogen/Life Technologies, diluted 1:500 in DPBS plus 1% BSA) for 30 min. Slides were washed with DPBS containing DAPI and covered with VectaShield (Vector Laboratories, distributed by Biozol). In some experiments, cell membranes were stained using Alexa Fluor 555-labeled wheat germ agglutinin (5 μg/ml) (Life Technologies). Cells were analyzed using the DMI 6000B inverted microscope and the TCS SP5 laser scanning microscope equipped with the LAS-AF software (Leica Microsystems, Mannheim, Germany).

Cell Killing Assays

To investigate direct oncolytic effects of HSV-1 *d*106S and HSV-1 *d*106S-MelanA, 1×10^4 melanoma cells were infected with these viruses using different MOI (1 and 10). Cell viability was checked at day 1, 2, 3, and 4 p.i. using the MTT lysis assay according to the manufacturer's recommendations (Trevigen, R&D Systems, Nordenstadt, Germany). Oncolytic effects of MelanA-specific $CD8^+$ T-cells were studied in melanoma cells, which had been infected with HSV-1 *d*106S and HSV-1 *d*106S-MelanA (MOI 1) for 8 h, followed by $CD8^+$ T-cell coculture (ratio 1:8) for 16 h and subsequent MTT lysis assay. Peptide-loaded cells served as controls.

Statistics

In our statistical analysis, we used one-way ANOVA for multiple group comparisons with GraphPad Prism version 8. Two-sided $p < 0.05$ were considered significant.

RESULTS

Generation of HSV-1 *d*106S-MelanA

The infectious, but replication-deficient HSV-1 *d*106S expresses GFP under the control of a CMV promoter. To replace this transgene by MelanA, the coding sequence of MelanA was amplified from expression plasmid pcDNA3(+) MART-1 (29) (**Figure 1A**) and cloned into transfer plasmid pd27B (8). The clone used for homologous recombination was sequenced, revealing identity with the MelanA sequence in GenBank (accession no. NM_005511). After infection of E11 cells with HSV-1 *d*106S (**Figure 1B**), viral DNA was isolated from nucleocapsids. Purity and integrity of DNA were confirmed by spectrometry and digestion with EcoRI, which revealed distinct bands (**Figure 1C**). Cotransfection of SwaI-linearized pd27B-MelanA with HSV-1 *d*106S DNA into E11 cells resulted in mostly GFP-expressing (**Figure 1D**, upper part) and a few non-fluorescent viral plaques (**Figure 1D**, lower part), which indicated homologous recombination with replacement of GFP in a minority of transfected cells.

Characterization of HSV-1 *d*106S-MelanA

Two non-fluorescent viral plaques were purified via limiting dilution and used to infect E11 cells. The coding sequence of MelanA was detected in cells infected with both clones, but not in cells exposed to HSV-1 *d*106S, while all three infections were positive for the housekeeping ß-glucuronidase gene (**Figure 2A**). Western blotting detected MelanA protein in E11 cells infected with the two non-fluorescing clones, but not with HSV-1 *d*106S, while ß-actin was present in all three infections (**Figure 2B**). In flow cytometry, E11 cells infected with HSV-1 *d*106S expressed GFP, while cells infected with the two putative MelanA-expressing clones showed red fluorescence after intracellular staining of MelanA (**Figure 2C**). Vero cells, which do not support productive HSV-1 *d*106S replication, also expressed GFP or MelanA upon infection (**Figure 2D**) with mostly nuclear and cytoplasmic expression of GFP and MelanA, respectively, as evident from confocal microscopy. Altogether, we obtained a recombined HSV-1 *d*106S strain expressing MelanA, further termed HSV-1 *d*106S-MelanA.

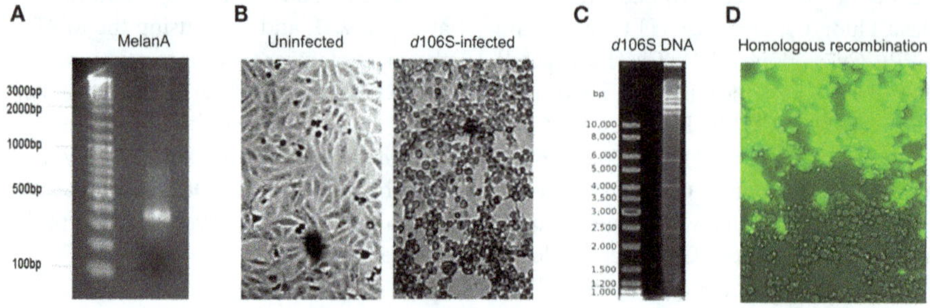

FIGURE 1 | Generation of HSV-1 *d*106S-MelanA. **(A)** Agarose gel image of full-length MelanA amplified from expression plasmid pcDNA3(+) MART-1 (29) using XbaI/NheI-containing primers. **(B)** Light microscopic images of uninfected E11 cells (left) and cytopathic effects induced in these cells 56 h post HSV-1 *d*106S infection (right). **(C)** EcoRI digestion of HSV-1 *d*106S DNA obtained from viral nucleocapsids showing distinct bands as evidence of DNA integrity. **(D)** Overlay of phase contrast and immunofluorescence microscopy of E11 cells harboring fluorescing (upper part) and non-fluorescing (lower part) viral plaques, representing HSV-1 *d*106S and HSV-1 *d*106S-MelanA, respectively, after cotransfection of the linearized transfer plasmid pd27B-MelanA and HSV-1 *d*106S DNA. Light and immunofluorescence microscopy were taken using the DMI 6000B inverted microscope (20 × magnification).

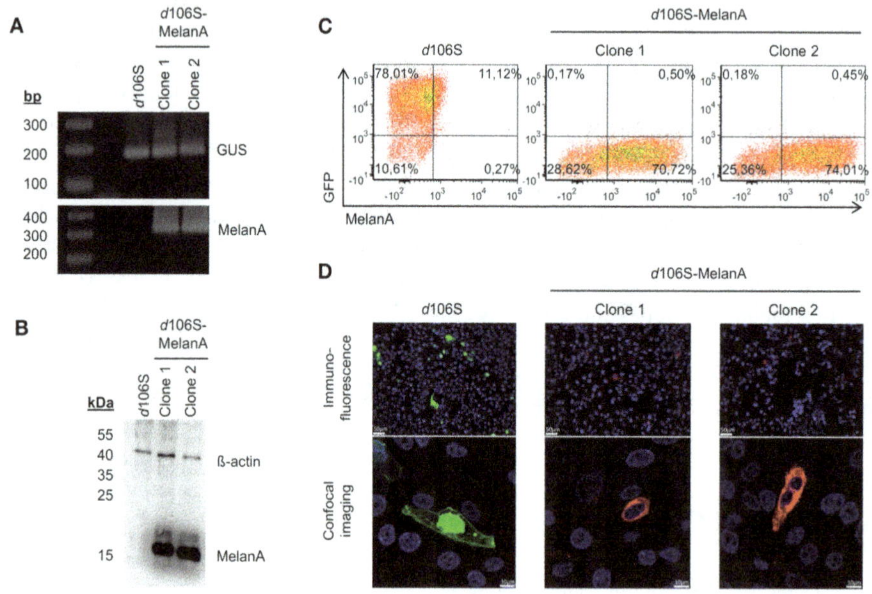

FIGURE 2 | Characterization of HSV-1 *d*106S-MelanA. MelanA expression in E11 cells infected with HSV-1 *d*106S and two non-fluorescent viral clones (MOI 10), which were obtained after cotransfection using HSV-1 *d*106S DNA and transfer plasmid pd27B-MelanA, as evident from **(A)** PCR, **(B)** Western blot, and **(C)** flow cytometry. Controls were **(A)** housekeeping gene ß-glucuronidase (GUS) and **(B)** ß-actin protein. **(D)** Expression of GFP and MelanA in Vero cells infected with HSV-1 *d*106S and two non-fluorescent HSV-1 *d*106S-MelanA clones, analyzed using immunofluorescence microscopy (upper panel) and confocal imaging (lower panel). The immunofluorescence and confocal images were taken using the DMI 6000B inverted microscope (20 × magnification) and the TCS SP5 laser scanning microscope (40 × magnification, 2.5 × zoom), respectively. Scale bars represent 50 and 10 μm in immunofluorescence and confocal images, respectively.

Expression of MelanA in Human Fibroblast and Melanoma Cell Lines

Melanoma cells frequently express MelanA, which may be lost upon immune escape (40). Three of our melanoma cells lines expressed MelanA (IGR-37, ARST-1, SK-MEL30), while three others were negative (LIWE-7, IGR-39, ICNI-5li). We analyzed whether MelanA expression may be restored in the latter upon infection with HSV-1 *d*106S-MelanA (MOI 1). At 20h p.i., IGR-37 and ARST-1 cells still expressed MelanA (**Figure 3A**), while transgene expression was induced in LIWE-7, IGR-39, and ICNI-5li cells (**Figure 3B**). Similarly, MelanA expression was induced in MRC-5 fibroblasts. MelanA protein expression was confirmed in IGR-37 and LIWE-7 cells using Western blotting (**Figure 3C**). These data indicated that melanoma cell lines which did not express MelanA *per se* could be induced to do so.

To exclude upregulation of endogenous MelanA in these cell lines, we used two CRISPR-Cas9 approaches targeting different regions of the MelanA gene (sgMelanA1, sgMelanA2) to knock out this gene in SK-MEL30 cells. Four weeks after lentiviral

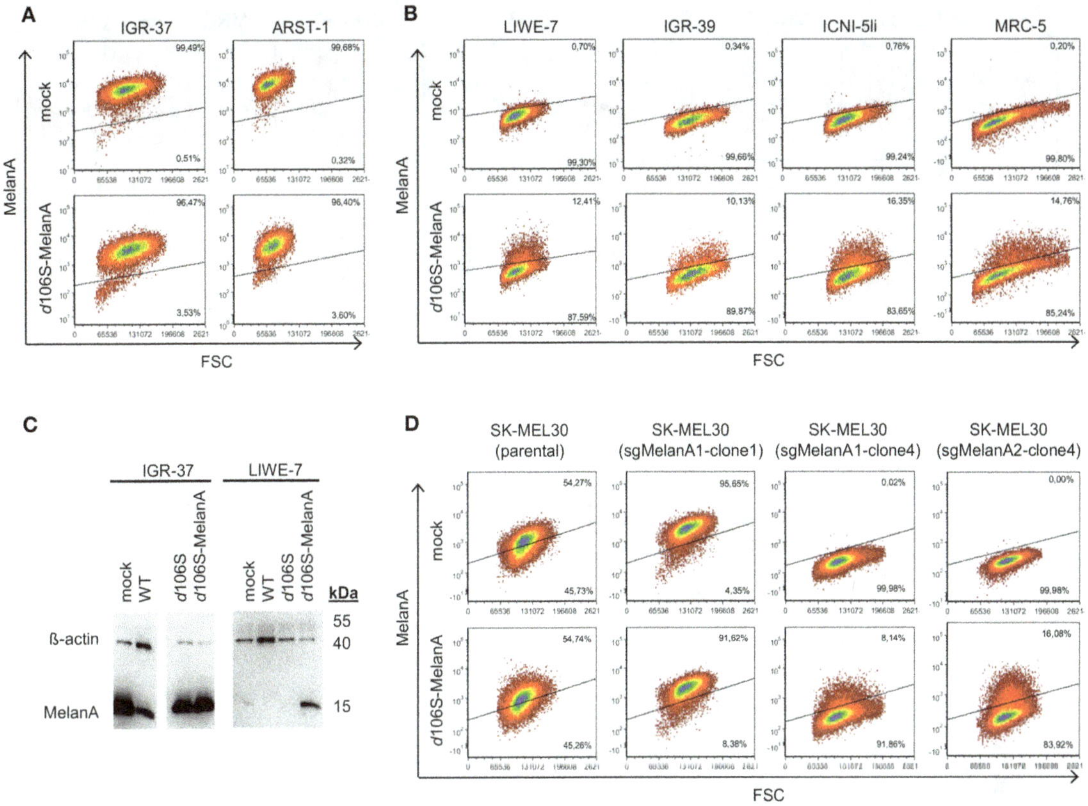

FIGURE 3 | Induction of MelanA expression in melanoma and fibroblast cell lines by HSV-1 *d*106S-MelanA. Expression of MelanA in **(A)** MelanA-positive (IGR-37, ARST-1) or **(B)** MelanA-negative melanoma cells (LIWE-7, IGR-39, ICNI-5li) and in MRC-5 fibroblast cells before (mock) and 20 h p.i. using HSV-1 *d*106S-MelanA. Data are representative of one (MRC-5, ICNI-5li), two (ARST-1, IGR-39), three (IGR-37), and four (LIWE-7) separate experiments. **(C)** Expression of MelanA and ß actin in melanoma cell lines IGR-37 and LIWE-7, analyzed by Western blotting after infection with HSV-1 wildtype (WT), HSV-1 *d*106S, and HSV-1 *d*106S-MelanA. **(D)** MelanA expression in parental SK-MEL30 cells and after CRISPR-Cas9 treatment resulting in loss of MelanA expression in two of the three analyzed cell clones (sgMelanA1-clone4, sgMelanA2-clone4), while in one cell clone the knockout was not successful (sgMelanA1-clone1). Upon HSV-1 *d*106S-MelanA infection, MelanA was re-expressed in the cell clones, which had lost MelanA expression.

transduction, MelanA was no longer detectable in 85% of cells. After single-cell sorting, two and five MelanA-negative cell clones were obtained for sgMelanA1 and sgMelanA2, respectively. Upon infection with HSV-1 *d*106S-MelanA, MelanA-negative cell clones (sgMelanA1-clone4, sgMelanA2-clone4) started to re-express MelanA, while MelanA expression was marginally downregulated in parental SK-MEL30 cells and a cell clone with ineffective MelanA knockout (sgMelanA1-clone1) (**Figure 3D**). These data indicated *de novo* expression of the transgene in the viral context.

Presentation of MelanA in Human Fibroblast and Melanoma Cell Lines

In further experiments, we investigated whether expression of MelanA in infected cell lines was followed by presentation of MelanA peptides within the HLA-A context. To this end, we cocultured HLA-A*02:01-positive fibroblast (MRC-5) and melanoma (SK-MEL30) cell lines with HLA-A*02:01/MART-$1^{27L26-34}$-specific CD8$^+$ T cells. As expected, MelanA-expressing SK-MEL30 cells induced CD8$^+$ T cell activation after 4 h of coculture, as evident from degranulation (CD107a) (**Figure 4A**) and IFN-gamma (**Figure 4B**) production, while MelanA-negative MRC-5 cells failed to do so. Similar results were obtained after infection of cell lines using HSV-1 *d*106S, confirming that virus infection *per se* did not induce CD8$^+$ T cell activation. Upon infection of MRC-5 cells with HSV-1 *d*106S-MelanA, however, CD8$^+$ T cells showed enhanced surface exposure of CD107a (**Figure 4A**) and, at least to some extent, IFN-gamma production (**Figure 4B**). These results indicated processing of virus-encoded MelanA with presentation of the respective peptide in the context of HLA-A in these cells. As a positive control for CD8$^+$ T cell activation, MRC-5 and SK-MEL30 cells were exogenously loaded with saturating concentrations of the optimized MelanA/MART-$1^{27L26-34}$ peptide.

To corroborate activation of CD8$^+$ T cells by virus-encoded MelanA in melanoma cells, we investigated SK-MEL30 knockout cells. A MelanA-negative cell clone obtained using sgMelanA1 (sgMelanA1-clone4) did not activate HLA-A*02:01/MART-$1^{27L26-34}$-specific CD8$^+$ T cells, while HSV-1

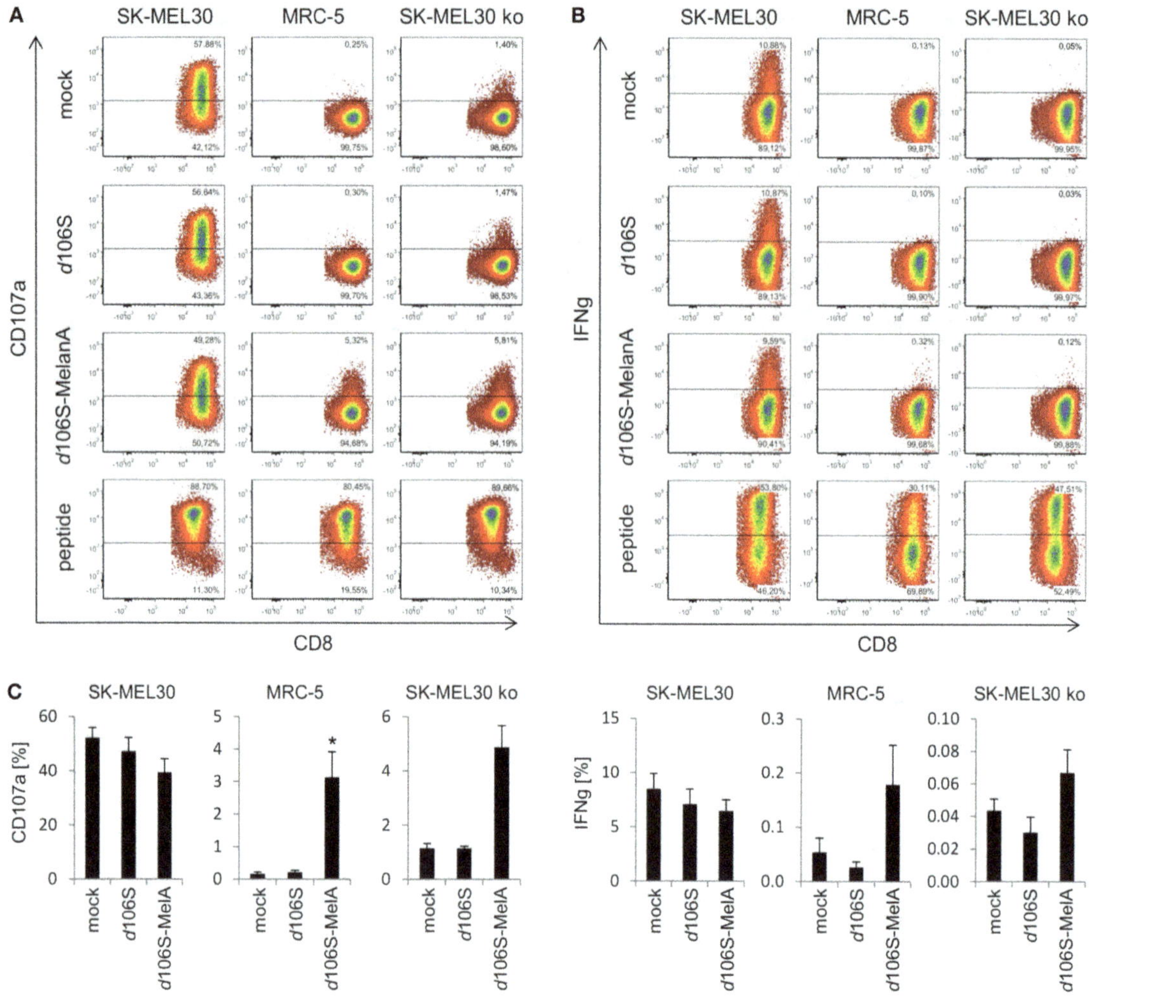

FIGURE 4 | Activation of $CD8^+$ T cells by HLA-matched melanoma and fibroblast cell lines infected with HSV-1 *d*106S-MelanA. Degranulation (CD107a) and IFN-gamma (IFNg) production in HLA-A*02:01/MART-$1^{27L26-34}$-specific $CD8^+$ T cells after coculture with HLA-matched SK-MEL30 melanoma and MRC-5 fibroblast cell lines for 4 h. In contrast to SK-MEL30 cells, MelanA was not expressed by MRC-5 and SK-MEL30 knockout (ko) cells (sgMelanA1-clone4). Cell lines were infected with HSV-1 *d*106S or HSV-1 *d*106S-MelanA for 20 h prior to coculture or loaded with MelanA peptide MART-$1^{27L26-34}$. T cells were identified as viable $CD8^+$ cells after exclusion of doublets. **(A)** One representative experiment and **(B)** mean and standard error of four, five, and **(C)** three separate experiments for SK-MEL30, MRC-5, and SK-MEL30 ko cells, respectively. Percentages of CD107a- and IFNg-expressing cells were compared to mock using one-way ANOVA for multiple group comparisons; $^*p < 0.05$.

*d*106S-MelanA infection of this cell clone induced degranulation as evident from the detection of CD107a at the surface of $CD8^+$ T cells (**Figure 4A**). A similar increase in $CD8^+$ T cell degranulation was observed after infection of another MelanA-negative SK-MEL30 clone obtained using sgMelanA2 (data not shown). In independent experiments, significant $CD8^+$ T cell degranulation was induced by HSV-1 *d*106S-MelanA-infected MRC-5 compared to uninfected cells (0.2% vs. 3.2%, $p = 0.03$) (**Figure 4C**). A similar trend was observed in SK-MEL30 knockout cells (1.1% vs. 4.9%, $p = 0.06$). Altogether, fibroblast and melanoma cells were induced to express tumor antigen and present respective peptides to tumor antigen-specific HLA-matched $CD8^+$ T cells.

Direct and $CD8^+$ T Cell-Mediated Oncolytic Effects of HSV-1 *d*106S-MelanA

To investigate direct effects of HSV-1 *d*106S and HSV-1 *d*106S-MelanA on tumor cell killing, SK-MEL30 wild type cells were infected using two different MOI. Oncolytic effects of both viruses on SK-MEL30 cells were comparable. Infection using a MOI of 10 resulted in a significantly stronger reduction of viability than infection using a MOI of 1 ($p < 0.001$ for *d*106S and $p < 0.01$ for *d*106S-MelanA at day 2 p.i.) (**Figure 5A**). MRC-5 cells were significantly less susceptible to this oncolytic effect (MOI 10) compared to SK-MEL30 cells at day 1 and 2 p.i. ($p < 0.05$).

In further experiments, we studied whether infection of MelanA-negative melanoma cells using HSV-1 *d*106S-MelanA

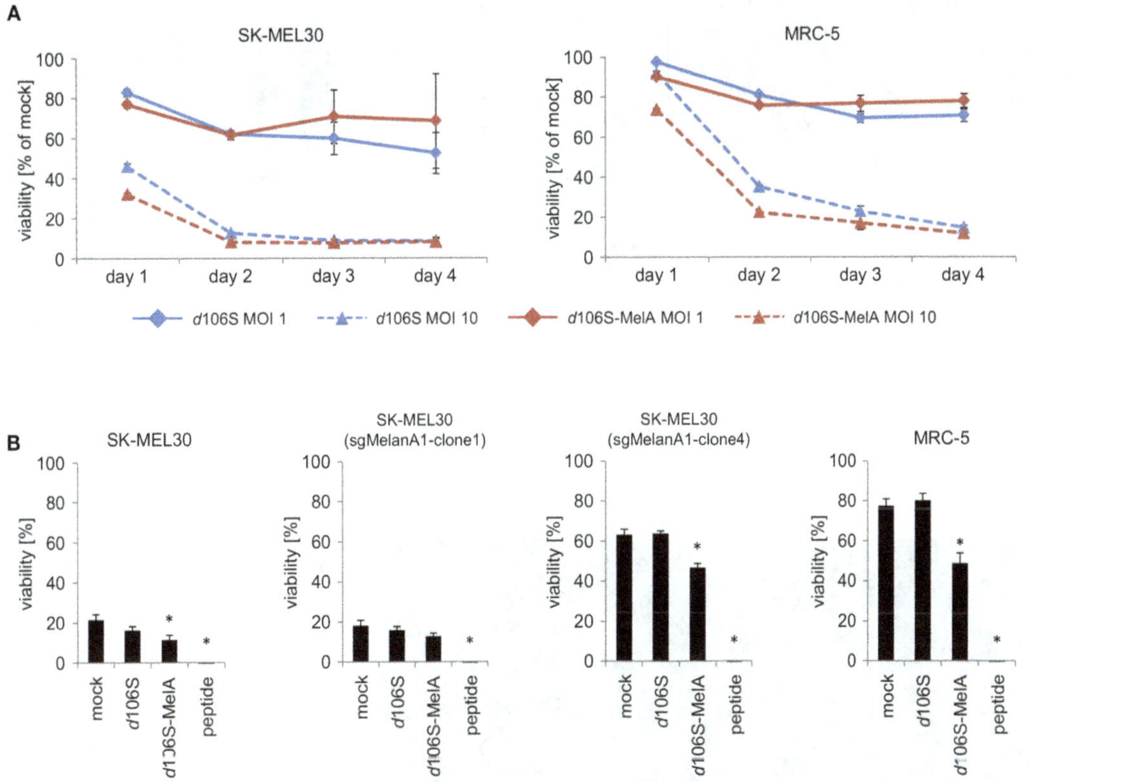

FIGURE 5 | Direct and indirect oncolytic effects of HSV-1 *d*106S-MelanA. **(A)** Viability of SK-MEL30 wild type cells and MRC-5 fibroblast cells was assessed after infection with HSV-1 *d*106S and HSV-1 *d*106S-MelanA (MOI 1 and 10) using MTT lysis assay at day 1, 2, 3, and 4 p.i. **(B)** Parental SK-MEL30 cells and sgMelanA1-clone1, which both expressed MelanA, as well as MelanA-negative sgMelanA1-clone4 and MRC-5 fibroblast cells were infected with HSV-1 *d*106S and HSV-1 *d*106S-MelanA (MOI 1) for 8 h or exposed to MelanA peptide for 1 h prior to coculture with $CD8^+$ T cells for another 16 h. MTT values were corrected for values of $CD8^+$ T cells only, and normalized to mock-infected cells incubated in the absence of $CD8^+$ T cells. Data show mean and standard error of three independent experiments. Viabilities were compared to mock using one-way ANOVA for multiple group comparisons; $^*p < 0.05$.

would contribute to the oncolytic effects of MelanA-specific $CD8^+$ T cells. SK-MEL30 wild type cells as well as sgMelanA1-clone1, which both expressed MelanA, were readily attacked, while MelanA-negative SK-MEL30 (sgMelanA1-clone 4) and MRC-5 cells remained mostly unaffected (**Figure 5B**). Exposure of all cell lines to MelanA peptide significantly increased cell death in comparison to untreated cells ($p < 0.05$). Notably, infection with HSV-1 *d*106S-MelanA significantly induced T cell-mediated killing of the MelanA-negative SK-MEL30 (sgMelanA1-clone4) and MRC-5 cells, and even enhanced lysis of the MelanA-expressing SK-MEL30 cell line ($p < 0.05$), whereas infection using HSV-1 *d*106S showed no effect. In sum, HSV-1 *d*106S-MelanA proved to be oncolytic via two effects: direct oncolysis of melanoma cells and induction of enhanced oncolytic activity by MelanA-specific $CD8^+$ T cells.

Expression of the Transgene GFP in Human PBMC and Antigen-Presenting Cells

We have shown that fibroblast and melanoma cell lines can be induced to express MelanA upon HSV-1 *d*106S-MelanA infection. To find out whether the transgene can also be expressed in antigen-presenting cells, we studied the infection of PBMC obtained from healthy volunteers. Because GFP is more readily detected compared to MelanA, we used HSV-1 *d*106S and focused on monocytes, which can differentiate into antigen-presenting cells. However, CD14 was downregulated at 24 h p.i., as reported previously (41), which precluded proper identification of monocytes. Therefore, antigen-presenting cells including monocytes were labeled using CD11c, which remained expressed at the cell surface. Upon infection with wild type HSV-1, PBMC did not display green fluorescence, while GFP was detected in a proportion of cells exposed to HSV-1 v166 (33) (**Figure 6A**). This virus codes for a VP22-GFP fusion protein, which is not only expressed but also secreted from infected cells. Therefore, cells with attached fluorescing viruses or VP22 cannot be discriminated from truly infected cells. In contrast, HSV-1 *d*106S expresses GFP under the control of a CMV promotor in infected cells only, and GFP is not incorporated into viral particles. This virus induced GFP expression in $CD11c^+$ PBMC, becoming more prominent with increasing MOI (**Figure 6A**). Individual cell populations were identified as T cells ($CD3^+$), B cells ($CD3^-$ $CD19^+$), NK cells ($CD3^-$ $CD19^-$ $CD56^+$), and $CD11c^+$ cells ($CD3^-$ $CD19^-$ $CD11c^+$) using a multicolor flow cytometry panel (**Supplementary Figure 1**). Again, green

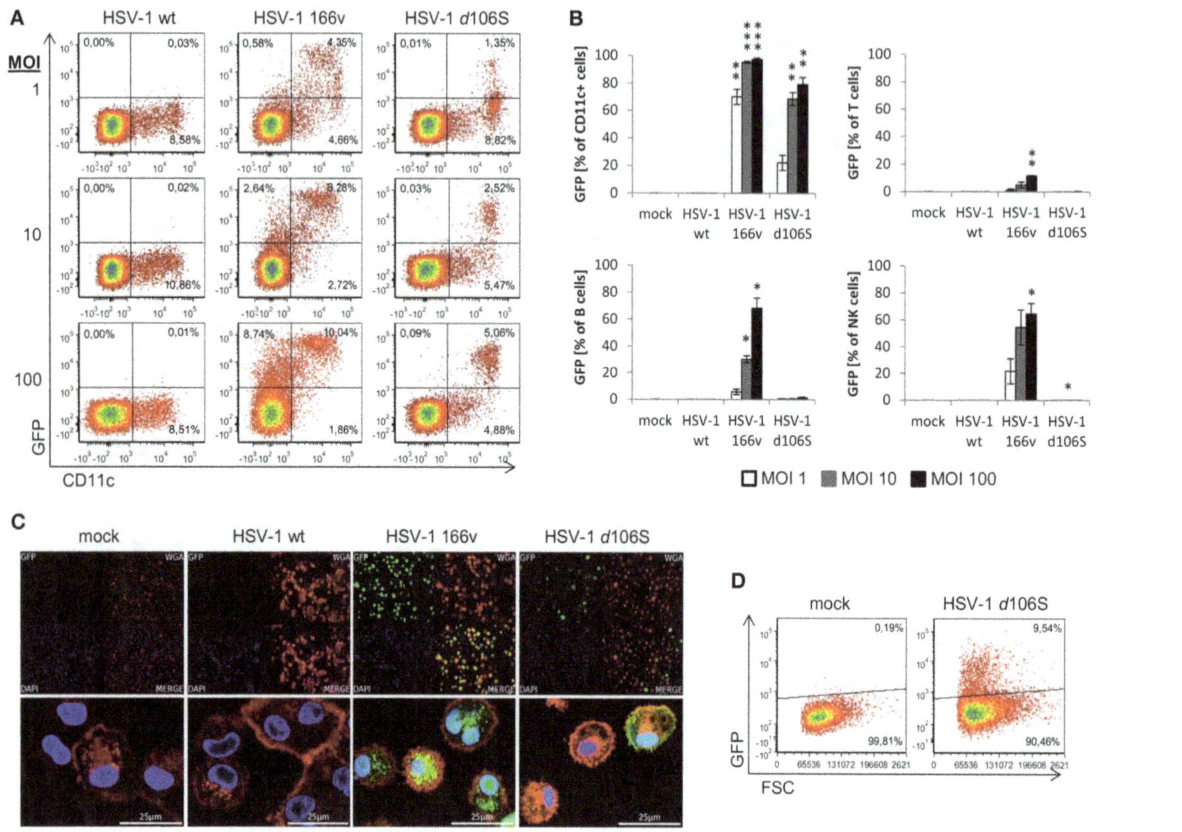

FIGURE 6 | Expression of GFP in human PBMC and macrophages after infection with HSV-1 *d*106S. **(A)** Expression of GFP in CD11c$^-$ and CD11c$^+$ viable PBMC after infection with HSV-1 wildtype (wt), HSV-1 166v, and HSV-1 *d*106S for 24h, using increasing multiplicities of infection (MOI). One representative experiment out of three is shown. **(B)** Percentage of GFP-expressing cells among CD11c$^+$ cells, T cells, B cells, and natural killer (NK) cells. T cells were identified as CD3$^+$ cells, B cells as CD3$^-$ CD19$^+$ cells, NK cells as CD3$^-$ CD19$^-$ CD56$^+$ cells, and CD11c$^+$ cells as CD3$^-$ CD19$^-$ CD11c$^+$ cells (for detailed gating strategy see **Supplementary Figure 1**). Data are shown as mean and standard deviation of three independent experiments using different donors. Expression of GFP in plasmacytoid dendritic cells was not evaluated due to low number of events. Percentages of GFP-expressing cells were compared to mock using one-way ANOVA for multiple group comparisons; $^*p < 0.05$, $^{**}p < 0.01$, $^{***}p < 0.001$. **(C)** Expression of GFP in macrophages obtained from a HSV-seronegative donor and exposed to HSV-1 wild type (WT), HSV-1 166v, and HSV-1 *d*106S for 24 h. Cellular membranes were stained using Alexa Fluor 555-labeled wheat germ agglutinin and visualized using confocal imaging. **(D)** Expression of GFP in macrophages exposed to HSV-1 *d*106S for 24 h. Flow cytometry data are representative for two HSV-seronegative donors studied in independent experiments.

fluorescence was not detected upon infection with wild type HSV-1, but upon infection with HSV-1 v166 (CD11c$^+$ cells > CD56$^+$ NK cells = CD19$^+$ B cells > CD3$^+$ T cells) **(Figure 6B)**. With HSV-1 *d*106S, GFP was detected in CD11c$^+$ cells only, resulting in 22.1, 68.3, and 79.2% of cells infected at MOI of 1, 10, and 100, respectively **(Figure 6B)**.

In addition to primary CD11c$^+$ cells, we studied macrophages generated from PBMC of HSV-seronegative donors in the presence of autologous serum. Adherent cells were differentiated into macrophages, which, upon exposure to HSV-1 *d*106S, expressed GFP in confocal imaging (**Figure 6C**) and flow cytometry (**Figure 6D**) comparable to the extent observed in fibroblast and melanoma cell lines. Overall, these data indicated expression of virus-encoded GFP in CD11c$^+$ cells and in macrophages. We further sought to confirm expression of the transgene upon HSV-1 *d*106S-MelanA infection. However, we were not able to verify MelanA expression in PBMC and macrophages in any of the experimental settings (data not shown).

DISCUSSION

Oncolytic viruses infect and replicate in tumor tissues. Subsequent lysis of infected cells releases tumor-specific antigens, which are taken up by antigen-presenting cells and induce anti-tumor immune responses via cross-presentation to T cells (42). We sought to optimize the induction of adaptive immune responses by incorporation of a tumor antigen into the viral genome. For this purpose, we used the infectious but replication-deficient HSV-1 *d*106S, which exerts oncolytic activity in particular in combination with PDC (9), and replaced the transgene GFP by MelanA via homologous recombination. Using flow cytometry, Western blotting, and immunofluorescence, protein expression was confirmed in complementing E11 and Vero cells. Upon HSV-1 *d*106S-MelanA infection, we detected transgene expression in MelanA-negative fibroblast and melanoma cells, and in SK-MEL30 cells with specific knockout of the MelanA gene using CRISPR-Cas9 technology. These data confirmed *de novo* expression of MelanA in the viral context.

Subsequent coculture of infected melanoma and fibroblast cell lines with HLA-matched MelanA-specific CD8$^+$ T cells verified MelanA-specific activation, as evident from CD8$^+$ T cell degranulation upon induced MelanA expression. The infection of parental MelanA-expressing SK-MEL30 cells induced a slightly reduced degranulation of CD8$^+$ T cells, most likely due to the oncolytic activity of the virus on target melanoma cells. Notably, we observed an increase after HSV-1 *d*106S-MelanA infection of MelanA-negative cells. It has to be admitted, though, that the degree of IFN-gamma secretion in CD8$^+$ T cells was very low. This was not due to a functional limitation of CD8$^+$ T cells, as evident from the control using an optimized MelanA peptide. It may rather be the result of the limited MelanA expression induced upon HSV-1 *d*106S-MelanA infection, which was not significantly enhanced using a higher MOI (*data not shown*). The reason may be the efficient oncolytic activity of this replication-deficient virus, resulting in depletion of MelanA-expressing target cells (**Figure 5A**). Importantly, we observed enhanced CD8$^+$ T cell mediated killing of MelanA-negative melanoma cells upon infection with HSV-1 *d*106S-MelanA, but not upon infection with HSV-1 *d*106S (**Figure 5B**). These data indicate that HSV-1 *d*106S-MelanA exerts direct and indirect oncolytic effects.

Altogether, our data confirmed that HSV-1 *d*106S-MelanA could re-express MelanA in melanoma cells which have escaped immune recognition via loss of tumor antigen expression. Loss of MelanA expression may be more frequent than previously thought, occurring in three of our 11 melanoma cell lines (**Figure 3** and data not shown). As a consequence, MelanA-specific CD8$^+$ T cells may be re-directed to infected tumor lesions, which will become re-accessible to this adaptive CD8$^+$ T cell response. In this case, an efficient oncolysis will be mediated by HSV-1 *d*106S-MelanA as well as by innate and adaptive immune cells. The apoptotic and necrotic tumor cells will serve as source for new tumor-associated antigens, which have evolved during tumor progression. In this respect, it has previously been shown that apoptotic cells, which were killed by infection with replication-deficient HSV, served as vaccines by pulsing DCs (43). Apoptotic debris will be phagocytosed by dendritic cells and cross-presented to T cells. In this respect, CD11c$^+$ cells and macrophages may also play an important role.

Our tumor vaccine may profit from incorporating other tumor antigens which are targets of cytotoxic CD8$^+$ T cells, like the MAGE-A family, tyrosinase, NY-ESO1, gp100 or neoantigens (44). With the incorporation of MelanA into HSV-1 *d*106S, however, viral stocks harbored slightly less infectious virions compared to the parental strain. The generation of infectious stocks may become increasingly challenging with the incorporation of additional tumor-associated antigens. The difficulty in inserting full-length sequences of tumor antigens may be overcome by introducing much smaller genomic information as minigenes coding for tumor antigen-derived peptides (27). It may also be worth cloning the coding sequences of tumor antigens or peptides into T-VEC, which is fully replicative and thus more virulent than HSV-1 *d*106S-MelanA.

The minor virulence of the non-replicative HSV-1 *d*106S-MelanA in comparison to the replication-competent T-VEC strain may be advantageous for the infection of antigen-presenting cells: a reduced cytotoxicity may facilitate the presentation of tumor peptides in the context of HLA-ABC. For these purposes, we infected PBMC with HSV-1 *d*106S, showing GFP expression in CD11c$^+$ antigen-presenting cells, but not in other immune cells. Subsequently, we noticed expression of GFP in macrophages comparable to the extent of MelanA expression in infected MRC-5 cells. However, we were not able to detect MelanA expression in any of the immune cells investigated, which was unexpected because both transgenes are expressed from the same CMV promoter. So far, it is unclear whether expression of MelanA in antigen-presenting cells is too low to be detected reliably, or whether MelanA is proteasomally degraded and presented on HLA-ABC immediately after mRNA translation.

More importantly, HSV-1 *d*106S has been shown to induce CD8$^+$ T cell responses *in vivo*. To this end, studies in mice and monkeys (45–47) revealed that HSV-1 *d*106S can not only activate, but also induce virus-specific CD8$^+$ T cells. This *de novo* induction may be more difficult with tumor-associated antigens (with the exception of neoantigens), which, as autoantigens, need to overcome self-tolerance. *De novo* induction can occur via direct presentation of the tumor antigen synthesized in the cytosol or via indirect cross-presentation after endocytosis of the tumor antigen, export into the cytosol and proteasomal degradation, transport to the endoplasmic reticulum and loading on HLA-ABC. Whether the vaccine HSV-1 *d*106S-MelanA can induce expansion of MelanA-specific CD8$^+$ T cells, and if so, which of the two mechanisms hold true, needs to be evaluated in further studies. It would be particularly valuable to study these effects *in vivo* using suitable animal models. The immune stimulation following intratumoral injection of the oncolytic virus *in vivo* may enhance the CMV promotor activity and thus contribute to a more efficient transgene expression.

A further prospect of our research is the combination of oncolytic viruses with other anti-cancer approaches like checkpoint inhibitors, chemotherapy, targeted therapy, and radiation therapy (42, 48, 49). It may even be interesting to test oncolytic viruses in combination with tumor-specific peptides. These conditions may reduce the immune-inhibitory activities of tumors and help tumor antigen-specific CD8$^+$ T cells to gain access to the malignant lesion. In addition, a new generation of oncolytic herpes viruses has been designed, which is less virulent due to deletion of ICP6 in addition to inactivation of neurovirulence factor γ34.5 and antagonist of the host cell's transporter associated with antigen presentation, ICP47. This oncolytic herpes virus allows a broader applicability and is currently being tested in glioblastoma and prostate cancer patients (7).

For these reasons, our approach to develop an oncolytic herpes virus which augments antitumor responses by coding for a tumor antigen appears to be promising for further combination immunotherapies against malignant melanoma. It may also be promising for other tumors. This may be true in particular for tumors which are known to be infiltrated by PDC, like head and neck squamous cell carcinoma (50), and ovarian (51, 52) and breast cancer (53, 54). A tumor antigen-expressing HSV-1 *d*106S may target both PDC and myeloid dendritic cells, which cooperate in inducing effective anti-tumor T cell responses (55).

AUTHOR CONTRIBUTIONS

JB, MW-K, DK, BS, and PS conceived the experiments. JB, ST, AR, MW-K, BS, and PS performed the experiments, analyzed and interpreted the data. DK and ND provided the parental HSV-1 *d*106S virus, transfer plasmid, and complementing cell line. BS-T and SG provided melanoma cell lines. JD and NS contributed the MelanA expression plasmid. MW-K contributed MelanA-specific $CD8^+$ T cells to the project. CB performed HLA-typing of cell lines and donors, and BS and PS wrote the manuscript. All authors were involved in critically reading of the manuscript and approved the final version of the manuscript.

ACKNOWLEDGMENTS

The present work was performed by JB in fulfillment of the requirements for obtaining the degree Dr. med. We thank Bernhard Fleckenstein and Thomas Stamminger, Erlangen, and André Gessner, Regensburg, for support, and Valerie Bezler and Konstanze Kühn for excellent assistance. Christiane Heilingloh, Department of Dermatology, Universitätsklinikum Erlangen, and Frank Neipel and Michael Mach, Institute of Clinical and Molecular Virology, Erlangen, are acknowledged for help in establishing protocols. We thank Gillian Elliot and Peter O'Hare, Section of Virology, Faculty of Medicine, Imperial College London, London, UK, for their generous contribution of HSV-1 166v. Plasmids lentiCRISPRv2 puro, pMD2.G, and psPAX2 were kind gifts from Feng Zhang and Didier Trono.

REFERENCES

1. Andtbacka RH, Kaufman HL, Collichio F, Amatruda T, Senzer N, Chesney J, et al. Talimogene laherparepvec improves durable response rate in patients with advanced melanoma. *J Clin Oncol.* (2015) 33:2780–8. doi: 10.1200/JCO.2014.58.3377
2. Andtbacka RH, Ross M, Puzanov I, Milhem M, Collichio F, Delman KA, et al. Patterns of Clinical response with talimogene laherparepvec (T-VEC) in patients with melanoma treated in the OPTiM phase III clinical trial. *Ann Surg Oncol.* (2016) 23:4169–77. doi: 10.1245/s10434-016-5286-0
3. Xia T, Konno H, Barber GN. Recurrent loss of STING signaling in melanoma correlates with susceptibility to viral oncolysis. *Cancer Res.* (2016) 76:6747–59. doi: 10.1158/0008-5472.CAN-16-1404
4. Ribas A, Dummer R, Puzanov I, VanderWalde AR, Andtbacka HI, et al. Oncolytic Virotherapy promotes intratumoral T cell infiltration and improves anti-PD-1 immunotherapy. *Cell* (2017) 170:1109–19 e10. doi: 10.1016/j.cell.2017.08.027
5. Sun L, Funchain P, Song JM, Rayman P, Tannenbaum C, Ko J, et al. Talimogene laherparepvec combined with anti-PD-1 based immunotherapy for unresectable stage III-IV melanoma: a case series. *J Immunother Cancer* (2018) 6:36. doi: 10.1186/s40425-018-0337-7
6. Watanabe D, Goshima F. Oncolytic virotherapy by HSV. *Adv Exp Med Biol.* (2018) 1045:63–84. doi: 10.1007/978-981-10-7230-7_4
7. Fukuhara H, Ino Y, Todo T. Oncolytic virus therapy: a new era of cancer treatment at dawn. *Cancer Sci.* (2016) 107:1373–9. doi: 10.1111/cas. 13027
8. Liu X, Broberg E, Watanabe D, Dudek T, Deluca N, Knipe DM. Genetic engineering of a modified herpes simplex virus 1 vaccine vector. *Vaccine* (2009) 27:2760–7. doi: 10.1016/j.vaccine.2009.03.003
9. Thomann S, Boscheinen JB, Vogel K, Knipe DM, DeLuca N, Gross S, et al. Combined cytotoxic activity of an infectious, but non-replicative herpes simplex virus type 1 and plasmacytoid dendritic cells against tumour cells. *Immunology* (2015) 146:327–38. doi: 10.1111/imm.12509
10. Cella M, Jarrossay D, Facchetti F, Alebardi O, Nakajima H, Lanzavecchia A, et al. Plasmacytoid monocytes migrate to inflamed lymph nodes and produce large amounts of type I interferon. *Nat Med.* (1999) 5:919–23. doi: 10.1038/11360
11. Siegal FP, Kadowaki N, Shodell M, Fitzgerald-Bocarsly PA, Shah K, Ho S, et al. The nature of the principal type 1 interferon-producing cells in human blood. *Science* (1999) 284:1835–7. doi: 10.1126/science.284.542 1.1835
12. Gerlini G, Urso C, Mariotti G, Di Gennaro P, Palli D, Brandani P, et al. Plasmacytoid dendritic cells represent a major dendritic cell subset in sentinel lymph nodes of melanoma patients and accumulate in metastatic nodes. *Clin Immunol.* (2007) 125:184–93. doi: 10.1016/j.clim.2007. 07.018
13. Salio M, Cella M, Vermi W, Facchetti F, Palmowski MJ, Smith CL, et al. Plasmacytoid dendritic cells prime IFN-gamma-secreting melanoma-specific CD8 lymphocytes and are found in primary melanoma lesions. *Eur J Immunol.* (2003) 33:1052–62. doi: 10.1002/eji.2003 23676
14. Vermi W, Bonecchi R, Facchetti F, Bianchi D, Sozzani S, Festa S, et al. Recruitment of immature plasmacytoid dendritic cells (plasmacytoid monocytes) and myeloid dendritic cells in primary cutaneous melanomas. *J Pathol.* (2003) 200:255–68. doi: 10.1002/path.1344
15. Aspord C, Leccia MT, Charles J, Plumas J. Plasmacytoid dendritic cells support melanoma progression by promoting Th2 and regulatory immunity through OX40L and ICOSL. *Cancer Immunol Res.* (2013) 1:402–15. doi: 10.1158/2326-6066.CIR-13-0114-T
16. Jensen TO, Schmidt H, Moller HJ, Donskov F, Hoyer M, Sjoegren P, et al. Intratumoral neutrophils and plasmacytoid dendritic cells indicate poor prognosis and are associated with pSTAT3 expression in AJCC

stage I/II melanoma. *Cancer* (2012) 118:2476–85. doi: 10.1002/cncr.26511

17. Labidi-Galy SI, Sisirak V, Meeus P, Gobert M, Treilleux I, Bajard A, et al. Quantitative and functional alterations of plasmacytoid dendritic cells contribute to immune tolerance in ovarian cancer. *Cancer Res.* (2011) 71:5423–34. doi: 10.1158/0008-5472.CAN-11-0367
18. Palamara F, Meindl S, Holcmann M, Luhrs P, Stingl G, Sibilia M. Identification and characterization of pDC-like cells in normal mouse skin and melanomas treated with imiquimod. *J Immunol.* (2004) 173:3051–61. doi: 10.4049/jimmunol.173.5.3051
19. Pashenkov M, Goess G, Wagner C, Hormann M, Jandl T, Moser A, et al. Phase II trial of a toll-like receptor 9-activating oligonucleotide in patients with metastatic melanoma. *J Clin Oncol.* (2006) 24:5716–24. doi: 10.1200/JCO.2006.07.9129
20. Drobits B, Holcmann M, Amberg N, Swiecki M, Grundtner R, Hammer M, et al. Imiquimod clears tumors in mice independent of adaptive immunity by converting pDCs into tumor-killing effector cells. *J Clin Invest.* (2012) 122:575–85. doi: 10.1172/JCI61034
21. Kalb ML, Glaser A, Stary G, Koszik F, Stingl G. TRAIL(+) human plasmacytoid dendritic cells kill tumor cells *in vitro*: mechanisms of imiquimod- and IFN-alpha-mediated antitumor reactivity. *J Immunol.* (2012) 188:1583–91. doi: 10.4049/jimmunol.1102437
22. Chaperot L, Blum A, Manches O, Lui G, Angel J, Molens JP, et al. Virus or TLR agonists induce TRAIL-mediated cytotoxic activity of plasmacytoid dendritic cells. *J Immunol.* (2006) 176:248–55. doi: 10.4049/jimmunol.176.1.248
23. Angel J, Chaperot L, Molens JP, Mezin P, Amacker M, Zurbriggen R, et al. Virosome-mediated delivery of tumor antigen to plasmacytoid dendritic cells. *Vaccine* (2007) 25:3913–21. doi: 10.1016/j.vaccine.2007.01.101
24. de Vries IJ, Tel J, Benitez-Ribas D, Torensma R, Figdor CG. Prophylactic vaccines mimic synthetic CpG oligonucleotides in their ability to modulate immune responses. *Mol Immunol.* (2011) 48:810–7. doi: 10.1016/j.molimm.2010.12.022
25. Tel J, Aarntzen EH, Baba T, Schreibelt G, Schulte BM, Benitez-Ribas D, et al. Natural human plasmacytoid dendritic cells induce antigen-specific T-cell responses in melanoma patients. *Cancer Res.* (2013) 73:1063–75. doi: 10.1158/0008-5472.CAN-12-2583
26. Schuster P, Donhauser N, Pritschet K, Ries M, Haupt S, Kittan NA, et al. Co-ordinated regulation of plasmacytoid dendritic cell surface receptors upon stimulation with herpes simplex virus type 1. *Immunology* (2010) 129:234–47. doi: 10.1111/j.1365-2567.2009.03176.x
27. Sahin U, Derhovanessian E, Miller M, Kloke BP, Simon P, Lower M, et al. Personalized RNA mutanome vaccines mobilize poly-specific therapeutic immunity against cancer. *Nature* (2017) 547:222–6. doi: 10.1038/nature23003
28. Ott PA, Hu Z, Keskin DB, Shukla SA, Sun J, Bozym DJ, et al. An immunogenic personal neoantigen vaccine for patients with melanoma. *Nature* (2017) 547:217–21. doi: 10.1038/nature22991
29. Shimizu K, Mizuno T, Shinga J, Asakura M, Kakimi K, Ishii Y, et al. Vaccination with antigen-transfected, NKT cell ligand-loaded, human cells elicits robust in situ immune responses by dendritic cells. *Cancer Res.* (2013) 73:62–73. doi: 10.1158/0008-5472.CAN-12-0759
30. Samaniego LA, Neiderhiser L, DeLuca NA. Persistence and expression of the herpes simplex virus genome in the absence of immediate-early proteins. *J Virol.* (1998) 72:3307–20.
31. Szpara ML, Tafuri YR, Enquist LW. Preparation of viral DNA from nucleocapsids. *J Vis Exp.* (2011) 54:3151. doi: 10.3791/3151
32. Kittan NA, Bergua A, Haupt S, Donhauser N, Schuster P, Korn K, et al. Impaired plasmacytoid dendritic cell innate immune responses in patients with herpes virus-associated acute retinal necrosis. *J Immunol.* (2007) 179:4219–30. doi: 10.4049/jimmunol.179.6.4219
33. Elliott G, O'Hare P. Live-cell analysis of a green fluorescent protein-tagged herpes simplex virus infection. *J Virol.* (1999) 73:4110–9.
34. Shalem O, Sanjana NE, Hartenian E, Shi X, Scott DA, Mikkelson T, et al. Genome-scale CRISPR-Cas9 knockout screening in human cells. *Science* (2014) 343:84–7. doi: 10.1126/science.1247005
35. Sanjana NE, Shalem O, Zhang F. Improved vectors and genome-wide libraries for CRISPR screening. *Nat Methods* (2014) 11:783–4. doi: 10.1038/nmeth.3047
36. Oelke M, Maus MV, Didiano D, June CH, Mackensen A, Schneck JP. *Ex vivo* induction and expansion of antigen-specific cytotoxic T cells by HLA-Ig-coated artificial antigen-presenting cells. *Nat Med.* (2003) 9:619–24. doi: 10.1038/nm869
37. Oelke M, Kurokawa T, Hentrich I, Behringer D, Cerundolo V, Lindemann A, et al. Functional characterization of CD8(+) antigen-specific cytotoxic T lymphocytes after enrichment based on cytokine secretion: comparison with the MHC-tetramer technology. *Scand J Immunol.* (2000) 52:544–9. doi: 10.1046/j.1365-3083.2000.00810.x
38. Oelke M, Moehrle U, Chen JL, Behringer D, Cerundolo V, Lindemann A, et al. Generation and purification of CD8+ melan-A-specific cytotoxic T lymphocytes for adoptive transfer in tumor immunotherapy. *Clin Cancer Res.* (2000) 6:1997–2005.
39. Maecker HT, McCoy JP, Nussenblatt R. Standardizing immunophenotyping for the human immunology project. *Nat Rev Immunol.* (2012) 12:191–200. doi: 10.1038/nri3158
40. Khong HT, Wang QJ, Rosenberg SA. Identification of multiple antigens recognized by tumor-infiltrating lymphocytes from a single patient: tumor escape by antigen loss and loss of MHC expression. *J Immunother.* (2004) 27:184–90. doi: 10.1097/00002371-200405000-00002
41. Vogel K, Thomann S, Vogel B, Schuster P, Schmidt B. Both plasmacytoid dendritic cells and monocytes stimulate natural killer cells early during human herpes simplex virus type 1 infections. *Immunology* (2014) 143:588–600. doi: 10.1111/imm.12337
42. Bommareddy PK, Shettigar M, Kaufman HL. Integrating oncolytic viruses in combination cancer immunotherapy. *Nat Rev Immunol.* (2018) 18:498–513. doi: 10.1038/s41577-018-0014-6
43. Benencia F, Courreges MC, Conejo-Garcia JR, Mohammed-Hadley A, Coukos G. Direct vaccination with tumor cells killed with ICP4-deficient HSVd120 elicits effective antitumor immunity. *Cancer Biol Ther.* (2006) 5:867–74. doi: 10.4161/cbt.5.7.2908
44. Loffler MW, Chandran PA, Laske K, Schroeder C, Bonzheim I, Walzer M, et al. Personalized peptide vaccine-induced immune response associated with long-term survival of a metastatic cholangiocarcinoma patient. *J Hepatol.* (2016) 65:849–55. doi: 10.1016/j.jhep.2016.06.027
45. Taylor TJ, Diaz F, Colgrove RC, Bernard KA, DeLuca NA, et al. Production of immunogenic West Nile virus like particles using a herpes simplex virus 1 recombinant vector. *Virology* (2016) 496:186–93. doi: 10.1016/j.virol.2016.06.006
46. Murphy CG, Lucas WT, Means RE, Czajak S, Hale CL, Lifson JD, et al. Vaccine protection against simian immunodeficiency virus by recombinant strains of herpes simplex virus. *J Virol.* (2000) 74:7745–54. doi: 10.1128/JVI.74.17.7745-7754.2000
47. Kaur A, Sanford HB, Garry D, Lang S, Klumpp SA, Watanabe D, et al. Ability of herpes simplex virus vectors to boost immune responses to DNA vectors and to protect against challenge by simian immunodeficiency virus. *Virology* (2007) 357:199–214. doi: 10.1016/j.virol.2006.08.007
48. Fend L, Yamazaki T, Remy C, Fahrner C, Gantzer M, Nourtier V, et al. Immune checkpoint blockade, immunogenic chemotherapy or IFN-alpha blockade boost the local and abscopal effects of oncolytic virotherapy. *Cancer Res.* (2017) 77:4146–57. doi: 10.1158/0008-5472.CAN-16-2165
49. Twumasi-Boateng K, Pettigrew JL, Kwok YE, Bell JC, Nelson BH. Oncolytic viruses as engineering platforms for combination immunotherapy. *Nat Rev Cancer* (2018) 18:419–32. doi: 10.1038/s41568-018-0009-4
50. Hartmann E, Wollenberg B, Rothenfusser S, Wagner M, Wellisch D, Mack B, et al. Identification and functional analysis of tumor-infiltrating plasmacytoid dendritic cells in head and neck cancer. *Cancer Res.* (2003) 63:6478–87.
51. Curiel TJ, Cheng P, Mottram P, Alvarez X, Moons L, Evdemon-Hogan M, et al. Dendritic cell subsets differentially regulate angiogenesis in human ovarian cancer. *Cancer Res.* (2004) 64:5535–8. doi: 10.1158/0008-5472.CAN-04-1272

52. Labidi-Galy SI, Treilleux I, Goddard-Leon S, Combes JD, Blay JY, Ray-Coquard I, et al. Plasmacytoid dendritic cells infiltrating ovarian cancer are associated with poor prognosis. *Oncoimmunology* (2012) 1:380–2. doi: 10.4161/onci.18801
53. Sisirak V, Faget J, Gobert M, Goutagny N, Vey N, Treilleux I, et al. Impaired IFN-alpha production by plasmacytoid dendritic cells favors regulatory T-cell expansion that may contribute to breast cancer progression. *Cancer Res.* (2012) 72:5188–97. doi: 10.1158/0008-5472.CAN-11-3468
54. Treilleux I, Blay JY, Bendriss-Vermare N, Ray-Coquard I, Bachelot T, Guastalla JP, et al. Dendritic cell infiltration and prognosis of early stage breast cancer. *Clin Cancer Res.* (2004) 10:7466–74. doi: 10.1158/1078-0432.CCR-04-0684
55. Lou Y, Liu C, Kim GJ, Liu YJ, Hwu P, Wang G. Plasmacytoid dendritic cells synergize with myeloid dendritic cells in the induction of antigen-specific antitumor immune responses. *J Immunol.* (2007) 178:1534–41. doi: 10.4049/jimmunol.178.3.1534

9

Dendritic Cell Targeting Using a DNA Vaccine Induces Specific Antibodies and $CD4^+$ T Cells to the Dengue Virus Envelope Protein Domain III

Arthur Baruel Zaneti[1], Marcio Massao Yamamoto[1], Fernando Bandeira Sulczewski[1], Bianca da Silva Almeida[1], Higo Fernando Santos Souza[1], Natália Soares Ferreira[1], Denicar Lina Nascimento Fabris Maeda[2], Natiely Silva Sales[2], Daniela Santoro Rosa[3,4], Luís Carlos de Souza Ferreira[2] and Silvia Beatriz Boscardin[1,4]*

[1] Department of Parasitology, Institute of Biomedical Sciences, University of São Paulo, São Paulo, Brazil, [2] Department of Microbiology, Institute of Biomedical Sciences, University of São Paulo, São Paulo, Brazil, [3] Department of Microbiology, Immunology and Parasitology, Federal University of São Paulo (UNIFESP/EPM), São Paulo, Brazil, [4] Institute for Investigation in Immunology (iii)-INCTiii, São Paulo, Brazil

***Correspondence:**
Silvia Beatriz Boscardin
sbboscardin@usp.br

Dengue fever has become a global threat, causing millions of infections every year. An effective vaccine against all four serotypes of dengue virus (DENV) has not been developed yet. Among the different vaccination strategies available today, DNA vaccines are safe and practical, but currently induce relatively weak immune responses in humans. In order to improve immunogenicity, antigens may be targeted to dendritic cells (DCs), the main antigen presenting cells and orchestrators of the adaptive immune response, inducing T and B cell activation. It was previously shown that a DNA vaccine encoding a fusion protein comprised of an antigen and a single-chain Fv antibody (scFv) specific for the DC endocytic receptor DEC205 induced strong immune responses to the targeted antigen. In this work, we evaluate this strategy to improve the immunogenicity of dengue virus (DENV) proteins. Plasmids encoding the scFv αDEC205, or an isotype control (scFv ISO), fused to the DENV2 envelope protein domain III (EDIII) were generated, and EDIII specific immune responses were evaluated in immunized mice. BALB/c mice were intramuscularly (i.m.) immunized three times with plasmid DNAs encoding either scDEC-EDIII or scISO-EDIII followed by electroporation. Analyses of the antibody responses indicated that EDIII fusion with scFv targeting the DEC205 receptor significantly enhanced serum anti-EDIII IgG titers that inhibited DENV2 infection. Similarly, mice immunized with the scDEC-EDIII plasmid developed a robust $CD4^+$ T cell response to the targeted antigen, allowing the identification of two linear epitopes recognized by the BALB/c haplotype. Taken together, these results indicate that targeting DENV2 EDIII protein to DCs using a DNA vaccine encoding the scFv αDEC205 improves both antibody and $CD4^+$ T cell responses. This strategy opens perspectives for the use of DNA vaccines that encode antigens targeted to DCs as a strategy to increase immunogenicity.

Keywords: dengue fever, dendritic cells, envelope protein domain III, single-chain Fv antibody, DNA vaccine

INTRODUCTION

Dengue virus (DENV) is the causative agent of dengue fever, an infection that has become a serious public health issue. In the last decades, the alarming increase in the number of cases [50–100 million per year, (1)] and also the increase in the incidence of more severe clinical forms of the disease (like dengue hemorrhagic fever, DHF or dengue shock syndrome, DSS) led the World Health Organization to prioritize the development of a vaccine against dengue (2). DENV is transmitted to humans by the bite of mosquitoes of the genus *Aedes* (such as *Aedes aegypti* and *Aedes albopictus*) infected with one of the four virus serotypes (DENV 1–4) (3).

The virus genome is translated into a polyprotein which is processed by virus and host proteases to produce three proteins that make up the viral particle: capsid (C), pre-membrane/membrane (prM/M) and envelope (E), and seven other non-structural proteins, NS1, NS2a, NS2b, NS3a, NS4a, NS4b, and NS5 (3). The E protein plays an important role in the protective immunity against DENV as it contains the majority of epitopes that elicit neutralizing antibodies (4–6). This protein can be divided into three domains: the central domain (EDI), the domain responsible for dimerization containing the fusion peptide (EDII), and the domain that binds to the surface cell receptor (EDIII) (2). EDIII has been extensively used in vaccine development for its ability to induce antibodies able to block DENV infection (7–9). In addition to neutralizing antibodies, T cell responses also play a relevant role in the development of protection. T cells limit the spread of viral infection because they kill infected cells and secrete pro-inflammatory cytokines (10, 11). IFNγ-secreting Th1 and CX3CR1$^+$ cytotoxic CD4$^+$ T cells are also associated with protection (12, 13).

Dendritic cells (DCs) are central for immunity induction, activating both T and B cells. These cells are excellent antigen presenting cells (APCs) because of their ability to acquire different antigens (either by pinocytosis, endocytosis, or phagocytosis), when compared to other cell types such as macrophages and B cells (14). To accomplish their role as APCs, DCs express a large number of extra and intercellular receptors that are responsible for their ability to "sense" the environment. When they encounter an antigen in the context of infection/inflammation, DCs undergo a maturation process that results in the up-regulation of co-stimulatory and MHCII molecules, and increases their ability to present antigens in the context of MHC I and II (15).

The last decades have proven to be extremely prolific for the study of DC biology and function, as different DC subsets were identified both in humans and in mice (16). Each subset is normally characterized by the expression of different surface markers. The DEC205 is an endocytic C-type lectin receptor expressed by murine and human DCs in different organs (17–20) that uptakes antigens and directs them to MHCII rich late endosomes, increasing antigen presentation to CD4$^+$ T cells (21). In mice, DEC205$^+$ DCs are resident in the T cell zone of lymphoid organs, and also express the CD8α marker (22). The DEC205$^+$CD8α^+ DCs were involved in the uptake of dying cells, and in the resistance to some viral infections (23–25). Antigens derived from different pathogens have been targeted to DEC205$^+$CD8α^+ DCs using chimeric anti-DEC205 monoclonal antibodies (mAbs) genetically fused to them, administered in the presence of a DC maturation stimulus (26–34).

The use of chimeric mAbs to target antigens to different endocytic receptors has become more spread, and this concept was employed in the development of more effective DNA vaccines. These vaccines are usually safe, cheap, easy to produce but may fail to induce strong immune responses, especially in humans (35). An improvement in the immune response was obtained after antigen targeting to the DEC205$^+$ DCs using DNA vaccines consisting of plasmids encoding a single chain variable fragment (scFv) fused to the antigen of interest (36–41). However, other groups have shown that antigen targeting to DEC205$^+$ DCs using DNA vaccines was also able to induce immune tolerance to the antigen of interest and consequently protect against experimental allergic encephalomyelitis (42).

In this work, we generated a DNA vaccine encoding the anti-DEC205 scFv fused to DENV2 EDIII (pscDEC-EDIII). Vaccine administration by intramuscular immunization followed by electroporation elicited high titers of anti-EDIII antibodies in mice immunized with pscDEC-EDIII capable of blocking DENV2 infection in VERO cells. In addition, EDIII targeting to DEC205$^+$ DCs within the context of a DNA vaccine elicited specific CD4$^+$ T cell proliferation and pro-inflammatory cytokine production.

MATERIALS AND METHODS

Plasmid Generation

Constructions of the pcDNA3 scDEC-OVA and scISO-OVA plasmids were described previously (37). We digested the DNA fragment encoding ovalbumin (OVA) with the restriction enzymes *Not*I and *Xba*I (New England Biolabs) and purified the open vectors with the "PureLink Quick Plasmid DNA" kit (Invitrogen). The sequence corresponding to the ectodomain of the DENV2 envelope protein (HQ026763, lineage DENV-2/BR0690/RJ/2008) was synthetized and cloned into the pUC57 plasmid (Genscript USA Inc.). We amplified the EDIII sequence (aa 297–394) with the primers sense 5′ GGCGGCCGCATGTCCTACTCTATGTGCAC 3′ and anti-sense 5′ TCTAGATCAGTGATGGTGATGGTGAT-GTTTCTTAAACCAATTCAGCTTC 3′ with the Phusion High Fidelity DNA Polymerase (New England Biolabs) according to the manufacturer's instructions. The anti-sense primer was also designed to insert a 6× His-tag at the end of the sequence. The PCR product was cloned into the pJET1.2/blunt vector (Thermo Scientific) and digested with the restriction enzymes *Not*I and *Xba*I (New England Biolabs). The digestion product was purified with the "PureLink Quick Plasmid DNA" kit (Invitrogen) and cloned in frame with the open reading frames of scDEC and scISO in the pcDNA3 vectors using the T4 DNA ligase enzyme (New England Biolabs). The final vectors, named pscDEC-EDIII and pscISO-EDIII were sequenced to confirm the presence of the EDIII sequence in frame with the antibody sequences. We transformed the plasmids into DH5α bacteria and purified the

DNA in large scale using the "EndoFree Plasmid Maxi Kit" (QIAGEN) for subsequently transfection of human embryonic kidney (HEK) 293T cells and mice immunization.

HEK 293T Transient Transfection

The transfection of HEK293T cells was performed as described previously (30). After 5 days in culture, the supernatants of cultures transfected with pscDEC-EDIII or pscISO-EDIII were collected, centrifuged at 1,000 × g for 30 min and filtered in 0.22 μM filters (Corning). The samples were concentrated in a dialysis membrane surrounded by sucrose and dialyzed twice in PBS for 4 h at 4°C.

Western Blotting

The scDEC-EDIII or scISO-EDIII containing samples were sorted in a 12% SDS-PAGE gel under reducing conditions. The proteins were transferred to a nitrocellulose membrane (GE Healthcare) and the membrane was blocked overnight at 4°C with PBS containing 0.05% Tween 20 (PBS-T 0.05%), 2.5% BSA and 5% non-fat milk. After three 5-min washes with PBS-T 0.05%, the membrane was incubated with 6x-HIS tag monoclonal antibody (1:5,000; Thermo Fisher Scientific) at room temperature (rt) for 2 h. Next, the membrane was incubated with goat anti-mouse total IgG-HRP antibody (1:2,000; Jackson ImmunoResearch Laboratories) for 2 h at rt and developed using quimioluminescence (ECL kit, GE Healthcare).

CHO-DEC Binding Assay

Transgenic CHO cells stably expressing the mouse DEC205 receptor (kindly provided by Dr. Michel Nussenzweig, The Rockefeller University, New York) were used for the binding assays. One hundred thousand cells were incubated with 4, 2, or 1 μg/mL of the scDEC-EDIII or scISO-EDIII scFvs for 40 min on ice. After two washes with FACS buffer (2% fetal bovine serum in PBS), cells were incubated with the 6x-HIS tag monoclonal antibody (1:5,000; Thermo Fisher Scientific) for 20 min on ice. The cells were washed two times again with FACS buffer and incubated with the anti-mouse IgG-Alexa488 antibody (1:2,000; Life technologies). After another round of washes, the cells were analyzed by flow cytometry and 20,000 events were acquired in the FACSCalibur™ flow cytometer (BD Biosciences).

Mice and Immunization

Six- to eight-weeks-old male BALB/c mice were bred at the Isogenic Mouse Facility of the Parasitology Department, University of São Paulo, Brazil. This study was carried out in accordance with the recommendations of the Federal Law 11.794 (2008), the Guide for the Care and Use of Laboratory Animals of the Brazilian National Council of Animal Experimentation (CONCEA) and the ARRIVE guidelines. The Institutional Animal Care and Use Committee (IACUC) of the University of São Paulo approved the protocol under the following number: 36/2016. Groups of eight animals were immunized with 100 μg of pscDEC-EDIII or pscISO-EDIII diluted in saline (0.9% NaCl). A control group consisting of 4 animals was injected with saline alone. Briefly, the animals were anesthetized by intraperitoneal (i.p) injection of a mixture of Ketamine and Xylazine (100 and 10 mg/kg, respectively). Next, the skin over the hind leg was sterilized with ethanol and the injections were carried out intramuscularly (i.m.) in the anterior tibial muscle of the mice followed immediately by electroporation. For the electroporation, two 130 V pulses with 1 ms duration and four 70 V pulses with 50 ms duration were applied with the CUY560-5-0.5 electrode using the NEPA21 Super Electroporator (Nepa Gene Co., Ltd.). The interval between each pulse was 450 ms. Three doses were administered in 2-week intervals. Animals were euthanized 2 weeks after the last dose, their sera were collected via cardiac puncture and the spleens were removed for subsequent analysis.

ELISA

We used sera collected from the different immunization groups for the detection of EDIII-specific antibodies by ELISA. High binding ELISA plates (Costar) were coated overnight at rt with 100 ng/well of the recombinant EDIII protein (43) diluted in PBS. In the following day, the plates were washed three times with PBS containing 0.02% Tween 20 (PBS-T 0.02%) and then blocked with PBS-T 0.02%, 1% BSA, and 5% non-fat milk for 1 h at rt. After three washes, serum samples were serially diluted in PBS-T 0.02%, 0.25% BSA, and 5% non-fat milk and incubated for 2 h at rt. Goat anti-mouse IgG antibody conjugated with horseradish peroxidase (HRP) (1:2,000; Jackson ImmunoResearch Laboratories) or HRP conjugated subclass-specific anti-mouse IgG (1:2,000; SouthernBiotech) were used as secondary antibodies, and plates were incubated for 2 h at rt. ELISA was developed with ortho-phenylenediaminedihydrochloride (Sigma) and H_2O_2 diluted in phosphate–citrate buffer, pH 4.7. The reaction was stopped with 4N H_2SO_4 and the OD_{490} was measured in a microplate reader (Biotek). Titers represent the highest serum dilution showing an $OD_{490} > 0.1$ normalized in a log10 scale. The IgG1/IgG2a ratio was calculated by dividing the mean values of the highest serum dilution obtained for IgG1 by the mean value of the highest serum dilution obtained for IgG2a without normalization. To determine the avidity of the antibodies, we performed an extra step before adding the secondary antibody. Fixed dilutions ($OD_{490} = 0.7$) of the samples were incubated with 7 M urea or PBS for 5 min. After three washes, the procedure continued exactly as described for the standard ELISA protocol. The avidity index was calculated by the sample's $OD_{490} \times 100$ in 7 M urea divided by the OD_{490} in PBS.

Virus Neutralization Assay and Competition Assays

Viral neutralization was assessed via a flow cytometry based assay adapted from (44). VERO cells (1×10^5 cells/well) were cultured in flat-bottomed 96-well plates (Costar) overnight at 37°C and 5% CO_2. Sera from immunized mice were heat inactivated at 56°C for 30 min. Two-fold serially diluted sera were incubated with virus particles of the DENV2 NGC strain (MOI of 0.1) for 30 min at 37°C and 5% CO_2. The sera/virus mixtures were then incubated with the cells for 1 h at 37°C and 5% CO_2. Next, the sera/virus mixtures were removed and DMEM containing 5% fetal bovine serum (FBS) was added to the cells that were then incubated for 24 h at 37°C and 5% CO_2. Trypsin was used to detach the cells that were resuspended in DMEM 5% FBS and transferred to V-bottomed 96-well plates. Cells were fixed and stained as described previously (45) using 4G2 (10 µg/mL; mouse anti-flavivirus envelope antibody) as a primary antibody and anti-mouse IgG-Alexa488 (1:2,000; Life technologies) as a secondary antibody. The cells were resuspended in FACS buffer and 20,000 events were acquired in the BD FACSCalibur™ flow cytometer (BD biosciences). The sera effect on virus neutralization was determined in comparison to a control infection with sera derived from mice injected with saline only.

For the competition assay, adapted from (43), a fixed dilution of the sera from the groups (1:20) was incubated with different molar concentrations of the recombinant EDIII protein for 30 min. The sera/protein mixture was then incubated with the DENV2 NGC strain for 30 min and the experiment continued as described above. Neutralization of infection was determined in comparison to a control infection with DENV2 incubated with recombinant EDIII plus sera from saline injected mice.

Imunofluorescence

VERO cells (25×10^3 cells/well) were cultured on glass coverslips inside 24-well plates (Costar) overnight at 37°C and 5% CO_2. Infections were performed with MOI of 0.1 with the DENV2 NGC strain for 1 h. After this period, supernatants containing the virus were discarded and the cells were incubated for 24 h in DMEM 5% FBS. Cells were fixed with ice-cold methanol for 5 min and the coverslips were blocked in PBS containing 1% BSA for 1 h at rt. Next, cells were incubated with pooled sera from the different mouse groups, or with the 4G2 mAb (as a positive control), during 1 h at rt, followed by another incubation with anti-mouse IgG-Alexa488 (1:2,000; Life technologies) in the same conditions. Nuclei were labeled with DAPI (1 µg/mL) and the images were acquired in a fluorescence microscope (Leica DMI6000B/AF6000, Buffalo Grove, IL, USA) coupled to a digital camera system (DFC 365 FX, Leica) and processed by the Leica Application Suite X (LAS X).

Splenocyte Isolation

Two weeks after the last vaccine dose, spleens were removed aseptically and processed exactly as previously described (30). Pools ($n = 4$; two pools per group) of bulk splenocytes were resuspended in R10 [RPMI supplemented with 10% of FBS (GIBCO), 2 mM L-glutamine (GIBCO), 10 mM Hepes (GIBCO), 1 mM sodium pyruvate (GIBCO), 1% vol/vol non-essential aminoacid solution (GIBCO), 1% vol/vol vitamin solution (GIBCO), 20 µg/mL of ciprobacter (Isofarma, Brazil) and 5×10^{-5} M 2-mercaptoetanol (GIBCO)]. Cell viability and concentration were estimated using the Countess™ Automated Cell Counter (Invitrogen).

Peptide Library

A peptide library comprising the DENV 2 E protein (HQ026763, lineage DENV-2/BR0690/RJ/2008) amino acids 161–404 was synthesized by GenScript USA Inc. This library contained 29 overlapping 20-mer peptides that were synthesized with more than 75% purity. Peptides were resuspended in water (10 mg/mL) and stored at −20°C. For *in vitro* stimulation experiments, peptides were divided into 3 pools as depicted in **Table 1**.

ELISpot

We used the mouse IFN gamma ELISPOT Ready-SET-Go!® (eBioscience) to detect IFN-γ producing splenocytes. The procedure was performed according to the manufacturer's instructions. Briefly, ELISpot plates (MAIPS4510; Millipore) were coated with the capture antibody and incubated overnight at 4°C. The plates were washed twice with PBS and blocked for 1 h with R10 at rt. Splenocytes were incubated in the presence of 2 µg/mL pooled EDIII or EDI/II (negative control) peptides for 20 h at 37°C with 5% CO_2. Unpulsed cells were used as controls for each group. After incubation, the plates were washed three times with PBS-T 0.05% and incubated for 2 h at rt with the biotinylated anti-IFN-γ antibody. Following

TABLE 1 | List of peptides derived from the E protein.

Peptide position	Peptide sequence*	Domain	Pool number
161–180	EIKITPQSSTTEAELTGYGT	EDI + EDII	1
169–188	STTEAELTGYGTVTMECSPR	EDI + EDII	1
177–196	GYGTVTMECSPRTGLDFNEM	EDI + EDII	1
185–204	CSPRTGLDFNEMVLLQMEDK	EDI + EDII	1
193–212	FNEMVLLQMEDKAWLVHRQW	EDI + EDII	1
201–220	MEDKAWLVHRQWFLDLPLPW	EDI + EDII	1
209–228	HRQWFLDLPLPWLPGADTQG	EDI + EDII	1
217–236	PLPWLPGADTQGSNWIQKET	EDI + EDII	1
225–244	DTQGSNWIQKETLVTFKNPH	EDI + EDII	1
233–252	QKETLVTFKNPHAKKQDVVV	EDI + EDII	1
241–260	KNPHAKKQDVVVLGSQEGAM	EDI + EDII	2
249–268	DVVVLGSQEGAMHTALTGAT	EDI + EDII	2
257–276	EGAMHTALTGATEIQMSSGN	EDI + EDII	2
265–284	TGATEIQMSSGNLLFTGHLK	EDI + EDII	2
273–292	SSGNLLFTGHLKCRLRMDKL	EDI + EDII	2
281–300	GHLKCRLRMDKLQLKG**MSYS**	EDI + EDII + EDIII	2
289–308	**MDKLQLKGMSYSMCTGKFKI**	EDIII	2
297–316	**MSYSMCTGKFKIVKEIAETQ**	EDIII	2
305–324	**KFKIVKEIAETQHGTIVIRV**	EDIII	2
313–332	**AETQHGTIVIRVQYEGDGSP**	EDIII	2
321–340	**VIRVQYEGDGSPCKIPFEIT**	EDIII	3
329–348	**DGSPCKIPFEITDLEKRHVL**	EDIII	3
337–356	**FEITDLEKRHVLGRLITVNP**	EDIII	3
345–364	**RHVLGRLITVNPIVTEKDSP**	EDIII	3
353–372	**TVNPIVTEKDSPVNIEAEPP**	EDIII	3
361–380	**KDSPVNIEAEPPFGDSYIIV**	EDIII	3
369–388	**AEPPFGDSYIIVGVEPGQLK**	EDIII	3
377–396	**YIIVGVEPGQLKLNWFKKGS**	EDIII	3
385–404	**GQLKLNWFKKGSSIGQMF**	EDIII	3

**Bold shows the EDIII amino acid sequence.*

another round of washes, the plates were incubated with avidin-HRP for 45 min at rt. Plates were washed three times with PBS-T 0.05% and the spots were developed with the "AEC substrate set" kit (BD biosciences). We used an automated stereomicroscope (KS ELISPOT, Zeiss, Oberkochem, Germany) to count the number of spots. The formula (# of spots in the pulsed well – # of spots in the unpulsed well) was used to calculate the number of IFN-γ producing cells/10^6 cells.

Proliferation and Intracellular Staining (ICS)

To analyze T cell proliferation, splenocytes from mice were labeled with carboxyfluoresceinsuccinimidyl ester (CFSE). Briefly, 50 × 10^6 splenocytes were resuspended in pre-heated PBS and labeled with 1.25 μM of CFSE for 10 min at 37°C. Cells were then washed, resuspended in R10 and 3 × 10^5 cells/well were incubated at 37°C and 5% CO_2 in 96-well round-bottomed plates with 2 μg/mL of pooled EDIII or EDI/II (negative control) peptides. Unpulsed cells were used as controls for each group. After 3 days in culture, cells were restimulated with the same peptide pools plus 2 μg/mL of αCD28. After 1 h incubation at 37°C and 5% CO_2, 0.5 μg of Golgi Plug (Brefeldin A, BD Pharmingen) was added per well, and the plate was incubated for 12 h at 37°C and 5% CO_2. After the incubation period, the cells were washed with FACS buffer and transferred to V-bottomed 96 well plates. Cells were stained with LIVE/DEAD® dye (Life Technologies) and αCD4-PerCP (clone RM4-5) for 40 min on ice and in the dark. After 4 washes with FACS Buffer, the cells were fixed and permeabilized using the Cytofix/Cytoperm kit (BD Pharmingen) according to the manufacturer's instructions. The cells were then washed three times with PermWash buffer (BD Pharmingen). The intracellular staining was performed using αCD3-APC/Cy7 (clone 145-2C11), αIFNγ-APC (clone XMG1.2), αIL2-PE (clone JES6-5H4), and αTNFα-PE/Cy7 (clone MP6-XT22) for 40 min on ice and in the dark. The cells were washed twice and resuspended in FACS Buffer. All antibodies were purchased from BD Pharmingen. Flow cytometer readings were carried out with 200,000 events acquired in the BD LSRFortessa flow cytometer (BD Biosciences) and analyzed using FlowJo software (version 9.3, Tree Star, San Carlo, CA). The analysis of proliferating ($CFSE^{low}$) cells producing different combinations of cytokines (IFNγ, IL-2, and TNFα) was performed with the Boolean gating platform (FlowJo Software). The percentages of proliferating or/and cytokine-producing cells were calculated by subtracting the values obtained with unpulsed cells.

Data Analysis

We used the Prism 7 software (GraphPad Software Inc, LA Jolla, CA) for all tests. Statistical differences were considered significant when $p \leq 0.05$. One-way ANOVA followed by Tukey's honestly significantly different (HSD) were used for the ELISA data and Two-way ANOVA followed by Bonferroni correction was used for the ELISpot, CFSE and ICS data. The NT_{50} values for the neutralization assays were determined with the non-linear regression (curve fit) analysis.

RESULTS

Production of the Recombinant scFvs

The DENV2 EDIII nucleotide sequence (encoding amino acids 297–394) was cloned in frame into plasmids encoding the variable regions of the heavy and light chains of the anti-DEC205 (clone NLDC145) and the isotype control (clone III/10) as previously described (37). **Figure 1A** shows a schematic representation of pscDEC-EDIII and pscISO-EDIII that were then used to transfect HEK293T cells. Western blot analyses of concentrated cell culture supernatants confirmed secretion of scDEC-EDIII and scISO-EDIII by transfected cells (~46 kDa, **Figure 1B**). To demonstrate that scDEC-EDIII retained the capacity to bind to the DEC205 receptor, CHO cells stably expressing the murine DEC205 receptor were incubated with different concentrations of either scDEC-EDIII or scISO-EDIII. **Figure 1C** shows that only the scDEC-EDIII bound to DEC205 receptor in a concentration dependent manner. Taken together, these results indicate that both scFvs were successfully secreted from transiently transfected cells, and that the scDEC-EDIII preserved its binding capacity to the DEC205 receptor.

In vivo EDIII Targeting to DCs Improves Antibody Responses

Next, we assessed if immunization with pscDEC-EDIII could improve the anti-EDIII antibody response. For that purpose, mice received three doses of each plasmid administered i.m. followed by electroporation (**Figure 2A**). Twelve days after the administration of the first and second doses, and 14 days after the third dose, mice were bled and the sera were tested individually for reactivity against the recombinant EDIII produced in bacteria. **Supplementary Figure 1** shows an increase in anti-EDIII antibody titers in mice immunized with both plasmids, especially after the administration of the third dose. Moreover, the anti-EDIII antibody titers observed in the animals immunized the pscDEC-EDIII were higher than those observed in mice immunized with pscISO-EDIII (**Figure 2B**). When IgG subclasses present in the sera of immunized mice were analyzed, IgG1, IgG2a, and IgG2b but not IgG3 were detected (**Figure 2C**). Notably, the IgG1/IgG2a ratio detected in mice immunized with pscDEC-EDIII was approximately 10× higher (6.62) than the one obtained in mice immunized with pscISO-EDIII (0.60). When antibody avidity was measured, we noticed that it was higher in sera from mice immunized with pscDEC-EDIII than in mice immunized with pscISO-EDIII (**Figure 2D**). Anti-EDIII antibodies were also tested for binding to the viral E protein by immunofluorescence and, as expected, sera collected from mice immunized with pscDEC-EDIII or pscISO-EDIII reacted with VERO cells previously infected with DENV2 (**Figure 2E**). The labeling patterns were similar to those observed in infected cells stained with 4G2 mAb that recognizes the E protein of Flaviviruses. These results indicate that there are differences in the magnitude, and in the quality of anti-EDIII antibodies raised after immunization with pscDEC-EDIII or pscISO-EDIII.

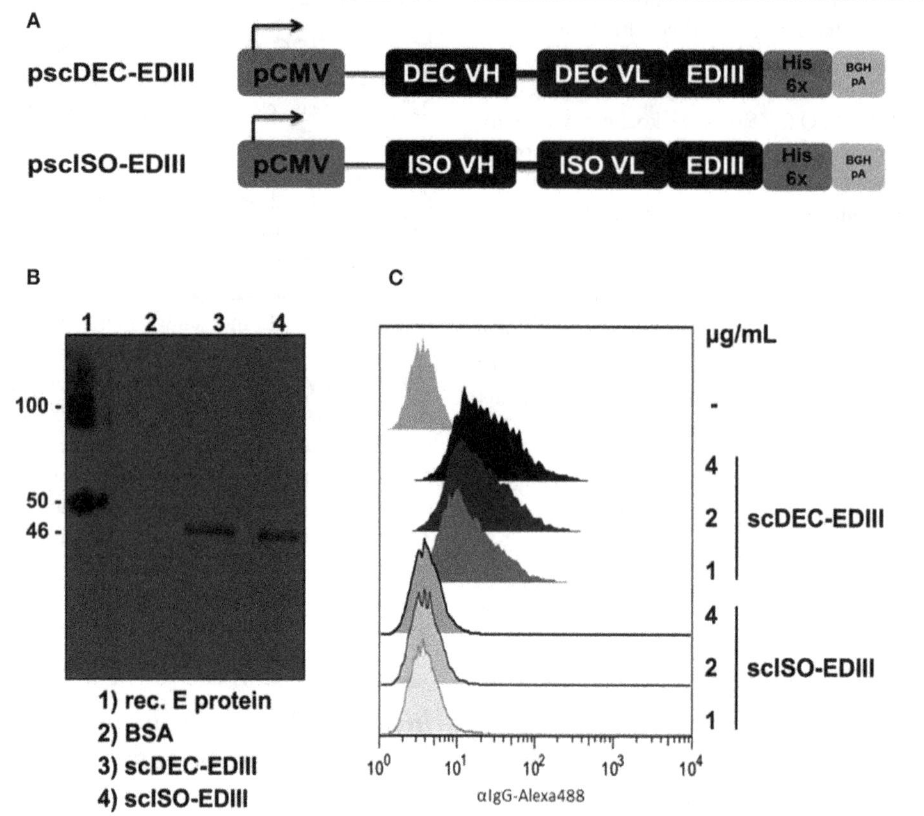

FIGURE 1 | Construction and characterization of the plasmids encoding the EDIII antigen genetically fused with scFvs. **(A)** Map of the plasmid vectors encoding the scFvs fused to the EDIII antigen. The EDIII DNA sequence was cloned in frame with the C-terminal portion of the variable light-chain (VL) after the linker sequence GGSSGGSGGGGSGGGGR. The variable heavy-chain (VH) is connected to the VL via a linker $(GGGGS)_3$. pCMV: Cytomegalovirus promoter; His 6x: polyhistidine tag; BGH pA: bovine growth hormone polyadenylation signal. **(B)** Western blotting with the supernatant of HEK293T cells transfected with pscDEC-EDIII and psclSO-EDIII. The membrane was incubated with a 6x-HIS tag mAb followed by incubation with goat anti-mouse total IgG-HRP. E protein: DENV2 envelope protein; BSA: bovine serum albumin. Numbers on the side indicate the molecular weight (kDa). **(C)** Binding of scDEC-EDIII or sclSO-EDIII to the DEC205 receptor constitutively expressed by CHO cells. One hundred thousand CHO cells were incubated with 4, 2 or 1 µg/mL of either scFv. Cells were labeled with a 6x-HIS tag mAb followed by incubation with goat anti-mouse IgG-Alexa488. Analysis was performed using the FlowJo software (version 9.3, Tree Star).

Anti-EDIII Antibodies Raised in Immunized Mice Inhibit DENV2 Infection

Anti-EDIII antibodies were shown to be effective to block virus entry into eukaryotic cells (7–9, 46, 47). We then analyzed if anti-EDIII antibodies present in the sera of immunized mice were able to block DENV2 infection. **Figure 3A** shows that antibodies raised in mice immunized with both scFvs plasmids inhibited virus entry with the same efficiency and in a dilution dependent manner. The 50% neutralization titers (NT_{50}) were also similar for sera derived from pscDEC-EDIII (1.66) or from pscISO-EDIII (1.69) immunized mice. To verify if the anti-EDIII antibodies were able to block DENV2 infectivity by binding to EDIII, we performed a competition assay using different concentrations of recombinant EDIII and a fixed serum dilution. Sera derived from mice immunized with pscDEC-EDIII, or pscISO-EDIII were then incubated with increasing amounts of EDIII. We observed a reduction in the sera capacity to inhibit DENV infection as the amount of EDIII was increased (**Figure 3B**). Of note, although we noticed a difference in the slope of the curves between the two groups, no statistical significance was observed, indicating that the anti-EDIII antibodies induced in both groups bound equally well to recombinant EDIII.

These results indicate that immunization with a DC targeted DNA vaccine was able to elicit higher anti-EDIII antibody titers with higher avidity. However, their blocking capacity did not differ from the blocking capacity of anti-EDIII antibodies induced by the vaccine that did not target DCs.

DC-Targeted DNA Vaccine Elicits Specific IFNγ Production and CD4$^+$ T Cell Proliferation

We also investigated if EDIII targeting to DCs would impact cellular immune responses, particularly CD4$^+$ T cells. Splenocytes harvested 14 days after the administration of the last immunization dose were incubated with three peptide pools containing peptides derived from a library comprising EDI/II and EDIII 20-mer overlapping peptides (**Table 1**). Pool 1 contained 10 peptides restricted to EDI/II domains (not present

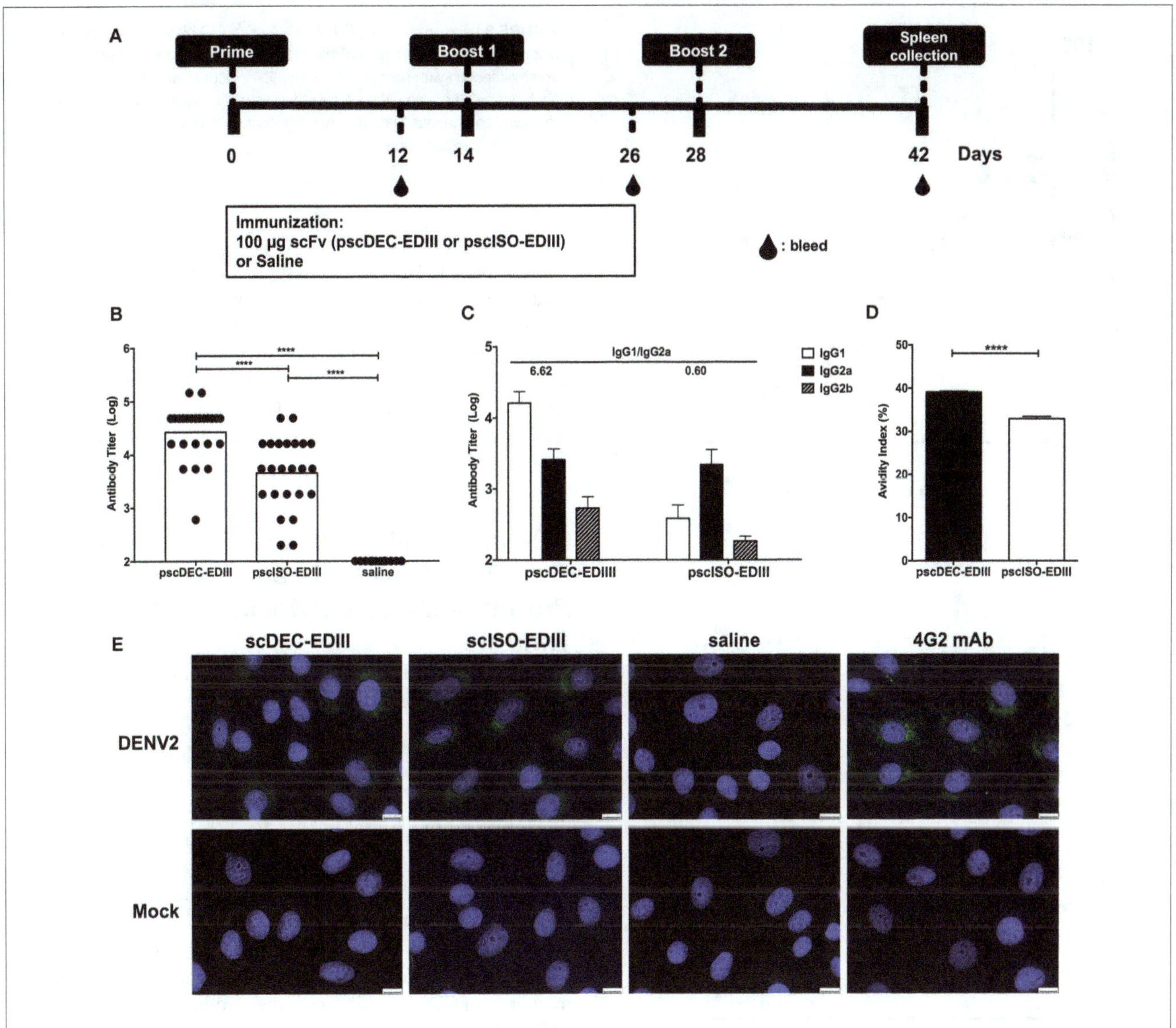

FIGURE 2 | Anti-EDIII antibody responses in mice immunized with pscDEC-EDIII and pscISO-EDIII. **(A)** Immunization regimen. Groups of BALB/c mice were immunized i.m. with the plasmids followed by electroporation. Three doses were given in 2-weeks intervals. **(B)** Total anti-EDIII IgG antibody titers and **(C)** IgG subclasses, 14 days after the administration of the third vaccine dose ($n = 24$; pscDEC-EDIII and pscISO-EDIII and $n = 12$; Saline, from three independent experiments). ELISAs were performed using recombinant EDIII as antigen and developed using a goat anti-mouse total or subclass specific IgG-HRP antibodies. Graphs show the antibody titers in normalized log10 scale. **(D)** Avidity of the anti-EDIII antibodies. Fixed dilutions of the pooled group samples were incubated with 7 M urea or PBS. The avidity index was calculated by the sample's $OD_{490} \times 100$ in 7M urea divided by the OD_{490} in PBS. Symbols represent individual mice, columns, and bars represent the mean and SD for each group. Data were analyzed by a one-way ANOVA followed by the post-test HSD Tukey **(B)** or by unpaired *t*-test **(D)**. *P*-value indicators **** refer to $p < 0.0001$. **(E)** Recognition of the DENV2 virus by the sera from mice immunized with pscDEC-EDIII and pscISO-EDIII. VERO cells were infected with DENV2 NGC strain or mock (medium). Cells were fixed with methanol and incubated with the sera from mice immunized with either scFv. The virus/sera and nuclei were labeled with the anti-mouse IgG-Alexa488 (green) and DAPI (blue), respectively. The 4G2 mAb was used as a control. Results shown are representative of two independent experiments. Scale bar, 10 µm.

in the EDIII sequence encoded by the DNA vaccine plasmids), pool 2 contained five peptides derived from EDI/II and five peptides derived from EDIII sequence, and pool 3 contained nine peptides derived from EDIII amino acid sequence. All three pools were used to stimulate splenocytes from mice immunized with pscDEC-EDIII, pscISO-EDIII or saline. ELISpot assays showed that the number of IFNγ-producing splenocytes derived from mice immunized with pscDEC-EDIII was higher than that observed in mice immunized with the isotype control DNA vaccine or saline (**Figure 4A**). In addition, the response was mainly directed to a peptide(s) contained in pool 3 (**Figure 4A**). There was also a statistically significant difference in the number of IFNγ-expressing cells derived from mice immunized with pscDEC-EDIII after stimulation with peptide pool 2. This result suggests that pools 2 and 3 contain peptides able to bind to the BALB/c H-$2K^d$ haplotype. When $CD4^+$ T cell proliferation (representative gating strategy shown in **Supplementary Figure 2**, $CFSE^{low}$

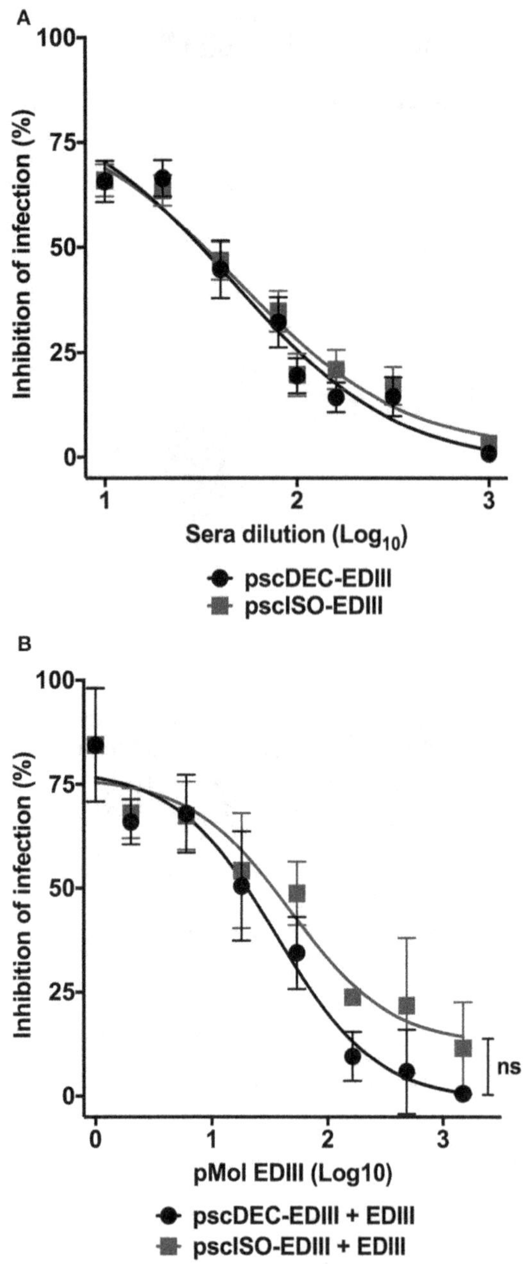

FIGURE 3 | Antibodies from mice immunized with pscDEC-EDIII and pscISO-EDIII partially inhibit DENV infection by binding to EDIII. **(A)** Neutralization in VERO cells. Pooled sera from mice immunized as described in **Figure 2** were heat inactivated at 56°C for 30 min. Two-fold serially diluted sera were incubated with the DENV2 particles for 30 min at 37°C and 5% CO_2. The sera/virus mixture was then incubated with the cells for 1 h at 37°C and 5% CO_2. The cultures supernatant was replaced by DMEM 5% FBS followed by another incubation at the same conditions for 24 h. Cells were stained with the 4G2 (mouse anti-flavivirus envelope antibody) and anti-mouse IgG-Alexa488. The neutralization of infection was determined in comparison to a control infection. Results are represented by means and SEM from pooled data of four independent experiments. **(B)** Competition assay with the recombinant EDIII protein. A fixed dilution (1:20) of sera was incubated with increasing molar concentrations of EDIII protein prior to incubation with the virus. The cells were resuspended in FACS buffer and 20,000 events were *(Continued)*

FIGURE 3 | acquired in the BD FACSCalibur™ (BD biosciences) flow cytometer. The neutralization of infection was determined in comparison to a control infection with sera derived from mice injected with saline. Data were analyzed by a two-way ANOVA for repetitive measures followed by Sidak's multiple comparisons test. ns = not-significant. Representative of three independent experiments.

panel) was analyzed, we also detected a higher frequency of $CD3^+CD4^+CFSE^{low}$ cells in the DC-targeted DNA vaccine group when compared to the groups immunized with the isotype control plasmid or saline (**Figure 4B**). Similarly to the previous experiment, the highest frequency of proliferation was directed against pool 3. As expected, pool 1 (comprising unrelated peptides derived from EDI/II domain) elicited a lower response in mice immunized with scFv plasmids that was not different from the response induced in animals that received saline.

DC-Targeted DNA Vaccine Induces $CD4^+$ T Cells That Proliferate and Produce Pro-Inflammatory Cytokines at the Same Time

We next assessed if $CD4^+$ T cells that proliferated in response to pools 2 and 3 were also able to produce the pro-inflammatory cytokines IFNγ, IL-2, and TNFα (representative gating strategy shown in **Supplementary Figure 3**). As shown in **Figure 5A**, the frequency of $CD4^+$ T cells that proliferated and produced IFNγ was higher in animals immunized with pscDEC-EDIII pulsed with pools 2 and 3 when compared to animals that received saline. For pool 3, as observed in the ELISpot assay, the frequency of $CD4^+CFSE^{low}$ that produced IFNγ was also higher in mice immunized with pscDEC-EDIII than in the group immunized with pscISO-EDIII. We did not observe significant differences among the groups when we compared the frequency of $CD4^+CFSE^{low}$ cells that produced IL-2 (**Figure 5B**). TNFα production by proliferating $CD4^+$ T cells was also higher in cells derived from pscDEC-EDIII immunized mice, especially when they were incubated with pool 3. A higher response against pool 2 was also observed, but it did not reach statistical significance when compared to the other two groups (**Figure 5C**).

The results in **Figure 5** showed that immunization with pscDEC-EDIII induced $CD4^+$ T cells that proliferated and produced three pro-inflammatory cytokines mainly to peptides contained in pools 2 and 3. To explore this response in more detail, we performed a Boolean analysis of the data (representative gating strategy shown in **Supplementary Figure 2**, $CFSE^{low}$ and $cytokine^+$ panels), and showed that the $CD4^+CFSE^{low}$ cells were polyfunctional and able to produce combinations of the tested cytokines. For example, proliferating $CD4^+$ T cells from mice immunized with pscDEC-EDIII produced all three cytokines simultaneously when pulsed with pool 2 (**Figure 6A**). Despite not statistically significant, we also observed an increase in the frequencies of $CD4^+$ T cells that proliferated and produced IL-2/TNFα,

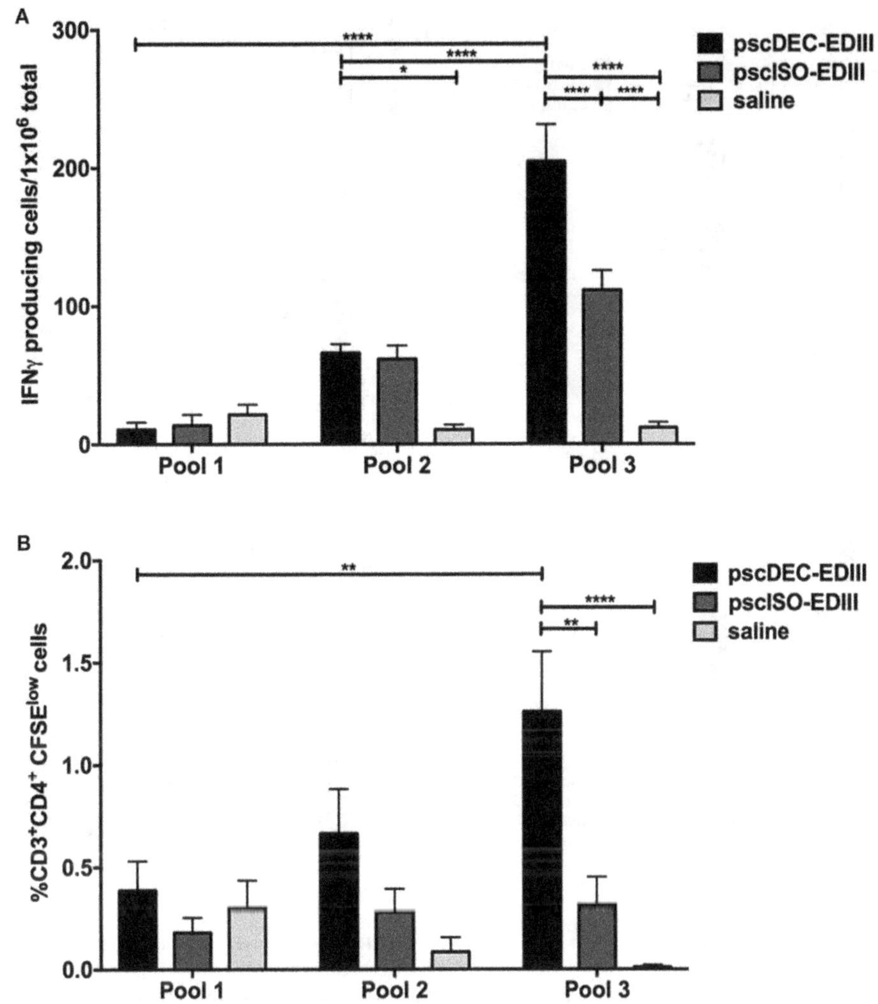

FIGURE 4 | Vaccination with pscDEC-EDIII induces IFNγ production and CD4$^+$ T cell proliferation. Groups of mice were immunized as described in **Figure 2**. **(A)** IFNγ ELISpot. Splenocytes were stimulated with 2 μg/mL of the peptides pools (**Table 1**). **(B)** Proliferation of CD3$^+$CD4$^+$ cells measured after CFSE staining. Splenocytes were stained with CFSE and stimulated with the same peptide pools (**Table 1**). After 3 days in culture, cells were pulsed again with the pools and with the αCD28 mAb. The frequency of cells that lost CFSE was determined by flow cytometry on the 4th day. The gating strategy is shown in **Supplementary Figure 2**. Columns and bars in both graphs represent the mean and SEM of pooled data from three independent experiments. The amount of spots/proliferation was determined after subtraction of values obtained in non-stimulated samples. Data were analyzed by a two-way ANOVA followed by the post-test HSD Tukey. *P*-value indicators *, ** and **** refer to $p < 0.05$, $p < 0.01$, and $p < 0.0001$, respectively.

or only IL-2 or TNFα in pscDEC-EDIII immunized animals. The only exception was due to the IFNγ/TNFα double positive cells whose frequency was higher in pscISO-EDIII immunized animals. Similar results were observed in assays using pool 3 (**Figure 6B**). Mice immunized with pscDEC-EDIII showed a statistically significant increase in the frequency of triple positive CD4$^+$ T cells when compared to the group that received saline. Moreover, the percentage of CD3$^+$CD4$^+$ cells that proliferated and produced only TNFα was statistically higher in mice immunized with pscDEC-EDIII than in those that received pscISO-EDIII or saline. Despite not significant, we observed that animals immunized with pscDEC-EDIII presented a higher frequency of cells positive for IFNγ/TNFα, only IFNγ, or only IL-2 when compared with the other two groups. Taken together, these results indicate that EDIII targeting to DCs using a DNA vaccine was able to elicit a polyfunctional CD4$^+$ T cell response.

Identification of EDIII-Specific Epitopes Recognized by CD4$^+$ T Cells Elicited in Mice Immunized With pscDEC-EDIII

In order to identify the peptide(s) present in the pools able to specifically activate CD4$^+$ T cell responses in mice immunized with pscDEC-EDIII, we performed an ELISpot assay using individual peptides comprising the complete EDIII sequence plus two control peptides derived from EDI/EDII (EIKITPQSSTTEAELTGYGT and STTEAELTGYGTVTMECSPR). Splenocytes from mice

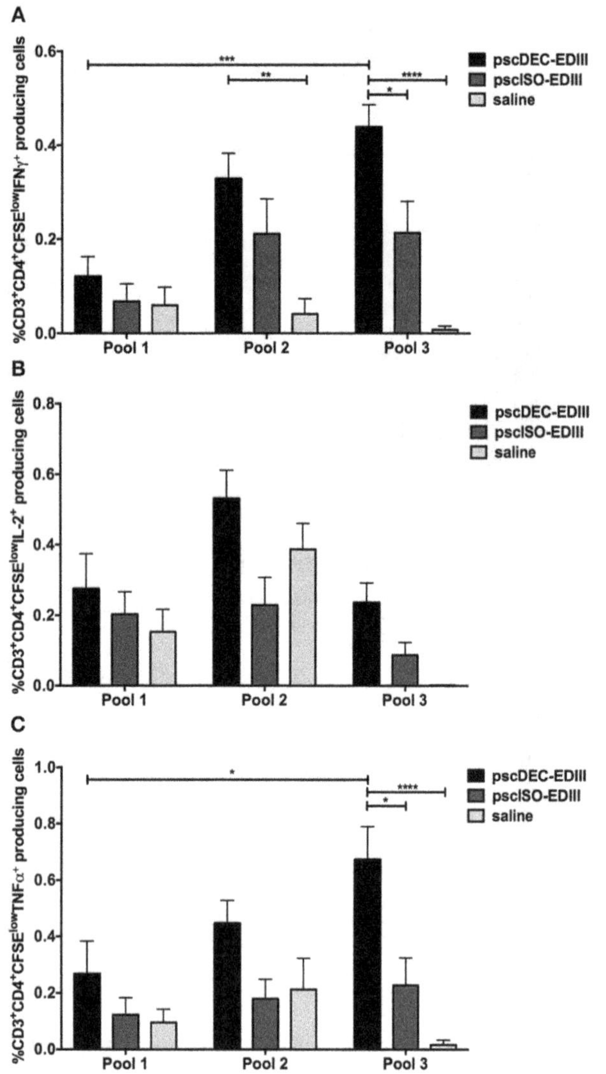

FIGURE 5 | The pscDEC-EDIII vaccine induces pro-inflammatory cytokines in proliferating CD4$^+$ T cells. Groups of mice were immunized as described in **Figure 2** and cytokine production was evaluated by intracellular cytokine staining. **(A–C)** Splenocytes were stimulated with 2 μg/mL of peptide pools (**Table 1**). After 3 days in culture, the cells were pulsed again with the pools and with the αCD28 mAb. The frequency of CD3$^+$CD4$^+$ cells that produced **(A)** IFNγ, **(B)** IL-2 or **(C)** TNFα within the CFSE^{low} population was determined by flow cytometry on the 4th day. The gating strategy is shown in **Supplementary Figure 3**. Columns and bars in both graphs represent the mean and SEM of pooled data from three independent experiments. The percentage of CFSE^{low} cells producing cytokines was determined after subtraction of values obtained in non-stimulated samples. Data were analyzed by a two-way ANOVA followed by the post-test HSD Tukey. *P*-value indicators *, **, *** and **** refer to $p < 0.05$, $p < 0.01$, $p < 0.001$ and $p < 0.0001$, respectively.

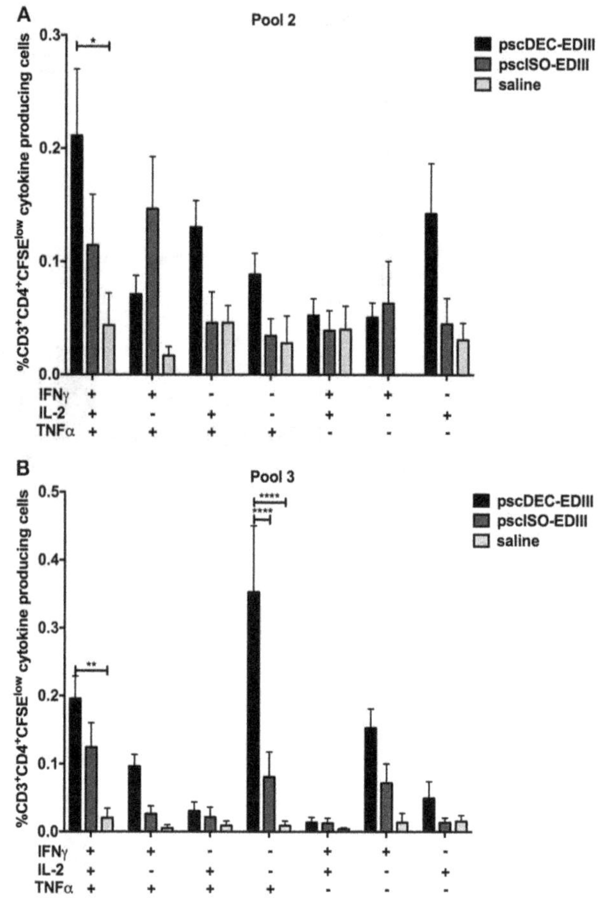

FIGURE 6 | Boolean analysis of the CD3$^+$CD4$^+$CFSE^{low} cells producing different combinations of IFNγ, IL-2, and TNFα. Groups of mice were immunized as described in **Figure 2**. Splenocytes were stimulated with 2 μg/mL of peptide pool 2 **(A)** or 3 **(B)**. After 3 days in culture, cells were pulsed again with the peptide pools and αCD28 mAb. Proliferation and IFNγ, IL-2, and TNFα production were evaluated by CFSE staining and ICS, respectively. The Boolean gating platform was used to analyze all the different possible combinations of CD3$^+$CD4$^+$CFSE^{low} cells expressing each or combinations of the cytokines. The gating strategy is shown in **Supplementary Figure 2**. Columns and bars in both graphs represent the mean and SEM of pooled data from two independent experiments. The frequencies of CFSE^{low} cells producing cytokines were determined after subtraction of values obtained in non-stimulated samples. Data were analyzed by a two-way ANOVA followed by the post-test HSD Tukey. *P*-value indicators *, **, and **** refer to $p < 0.05$, $p < 0.01$ and $p < 0.0001$, respectively.

immunized with pscDEC-EDIII were pulsed with each individual peptide and the number of IFNγ producing splenocytes/10^6 total cells was recorded. **Figure 7** indicates that the response was mainly directed to two peptides: MDKLQLKGMSYSMCTGKFKI present in pool 2, and RHVLGRLITVNPIVTEKDSP in pool 3. In addition, we observed that peptide RHVLGRLITVNPIVTEKDSP represented the immunodominant epitope since the response directed to it was almost three times higher than that detected after stimulation with peptide MDKLQLKGMSYSMCTGKFKI.

DISCUSSION

Dengue infection has become a major public health concern as the disease outbreaks and complications have increased substantially in the last five decades (48). Since then, the development of a vaccine has become a global health priority.

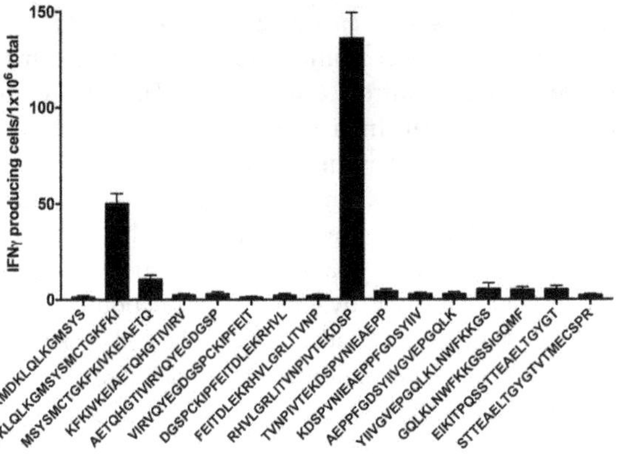

FIGURE 7 | Two peptides from the EDIII sequence induce IFNγ production. Groups of mice were immunized as described in **Figure 2** and an IFNγ ELISpot was performed. Splenocytes from mice immunized with pscDEC-EDIII were stimulated with 2 μg/mL of peptides spanning the entire EDIII sequence. Peptides EIKITPQSSTTEAELTGYGT and STTEAELTGYGTVTMECSPR from EDI/II sequence were used as negative controls. Columns and bars represent the mean and SEM of pooled data from two independent experiments. The number of spots was determined after subtraction of values obtained in non-stimulated samples.

The challenge is enormous as dengue is caused by four different serotypes and a previous immune response against one particular serotype can exacerbate the disease caused by another (8). Different approaches are being evaluated and two vaccines based on live attenuated viruses have reached phase III trials: the CYD-TDV by Sanofi Pasteur and the TV003/TV005 by US National Institutes of Health (49). However, results of the CYD-TDV vaccine indicating that the risk of severe disease could increase in seronegative individuals led WHO to recommend that the vaccine would only be administered in populations with dengue serological prevalence rates above 80% (50). In this way, other approaches are currently being developed.

Antigen targeting to DCs through the use of chimeric mAbs has been a promising strategy to induce either humoral or cellular immune responses against different antigens such as: ovalbumin (26–28), *Plasmodium yoelii* circumsporozoite protein (27), *Yersinia pestis* LcrV (29), DENV2 non-structural protein 1 (30), *Trypanosoma cruzi* amastigote surface protein 2 (31), *Plasmodium vivax* merozoite surface protein 1 (32, 33), and HIV gag (51, 52), among others.

However, the production of such mAbs is time consuming and expensive. DNA vaccines, on the other hand, are cheap, safe and easier to produce and purify, but in general are less immunogenic (35). Different approaches have been developed to increase the immunogenicity of DNA vaccines. Among them are the use of electroporation (53, 54) and the use of plasmids encoding scFv specific for the DEC205 receptor coupled to the antigen of interest.

Although EDIII has been recently used in a DNA immunization strategy (9), in this work we sought to produce a DNA vaccine able to target EDIII from DENV2 to the DEC205$^+$ DCs *in vivo*. This was accomplished when we fused the sequence of anti-DEC205 scFv to the EDIII, generating the DNA plasmid named pscDEC-EDIII. As a negative control, we also fused the scFv of a control mAb that was not able to bind to DCs (pscISO-EDIII). Interestingly, a similar construct was engineered by Coconi-Linares et al. that expressed a scFvDEC-EDIII in the plant *Nicotiana benthamiana* (55). In this case, the authors purified the recombinant scFvDEC205-EDIII protein and immunized BALB/c mice in the presence of anti-CD40 and poly (I:C). Their results showed that the scFvDEC205-EDIII was immunogenic, inducing antibodies with neutralization capacity and proliferating T cells. Nonetheless, a more detailed evaluation of the antibody and T cell responses was not performed.

We decided to use the pscDEC-EDIII as a DNA vaccine for its simplicity and potential to induce strong immune responses when administered together with electroporation. Initially we showed that both plasmids (pscDEC-EDIII or its isotype control) were able to drive the production of chimeric scFvs when transfected in HEK293T cells. More importantly, the scFvs were successfully secreted from the cells, indicating availability in the extracellular medium and possible targeting to the DEC205$^+$ DCs. Indeed, scDEC-EDIII showed a concentration dependent binding to the DEC205 receptor. Similar results were obtained with other antigens coupled to the same scFvs (37, 56).

Once production and DEC205 receptor specific binding were confirmed for scDEC-EDIII, we used scFv plasmids to immunize mice. We showed that the anti-E antibody titers after the administration of three doses were higher in the group immunized with pscDEC-EDIII when compared to the non-targeted control. Others obtained similar results using different antigens like ovalbumin, HIV gag p41 (37), HER2/neu (38), hepatitis B virus (57), human respiratory syncytial virus (40), and botulinum neurotoxin (39). Although the number of doses varied as well as the amount of plasmid DNA, all these studies used electroporation following intramuscular injection. Interestingly, when we analyzed the IgG isotypes elicited by immunization with the scFvs, we noticed that there was a difference in the IgG1/IgG2a ratio in the sera of mice immunized with pscDEC-EDIII or pscISO-EDIII. Although some groups, using different antigens, also obtained similar results (37, 58), others showed differences when both groups were compared (38). Despite the differences from one study to another, it has become clear that antigen targeting to the DEC205$^+$ DCs modulates the humoral immune response differently than the non-targeted antigen. We also noticed a significant increase in the avidity of the anti-E antibodies raised in mice immunized with pscDEC-EDIII, while antibodies derived from both immunized groups recognized infected cells. A similar recognition pattern was also obtained after intradermal immunization with a DNA plasmid encoding EDIII (9). This result indicated that the EDIII recognized by the mice sera presented a similar conformation when compared to the EDIII present in the viral particle.

EDIII has been previously described as a target for neutralizing antibodies (46, 47, 59, 60). We then decided to analyze if sera from scFv immunized animals were able to block virus invasion *in vitro*. The results showed that sera from mice immunized with pscDEC-EDIII or with pscISO-EDIII blocked DENV2 infection in a dilution dependent manner.

This result contrasted with our previous results showing higher titers and avidity in the sera of mice immunized with pscDEC-EDIII. A positive correlation between neutralization capacity and higher avidity to the viral particle was observed previously on dengue-infected patients (61). In contrast, other results using HIV envelope proteins showed that higher avidity not always correlates with neutralization capacity (62). More importantly, when sera from these mice were previously incubated with different amounts of recombinant EDIII, we observed a reversion in the sera capacity to block infection. This result more clearly demonstrated that the antibodies directed to EDIII mediate DENV infection inhibition in this model. Similar results were also obtained when an EDIII recombinant protein was administered in the presence of the heat-labile toxin (LT) or its non-toxic B subunit (43), or when a chimeric protein containing EDIII was administered to monkeys (63).

Our group and others described that antigen targeting to the DEC205$^+$ DCs is a very efficient way of elicit CD4$^+$ T cell responses (27, 30–34, 51, 64, 65). We then sought to analyze the CD4$^+$ T cell response induced after immunization with plasmids encoding scFvs genetically fused to EDIII. We took advantage of a peptide library comprising overlapping peptides derived from the E protein amino acids 161 to 404. Our data showed that the pscDEC-EDIII immunization induced CD4$^+$ T cells that proliferated when pulsed with peptide pools comprising the EDIII portion of the molecule. An analysis of pro-inflammatory cytokines produced by the animals immunized with pscDEC-EDIII showed a higher frequency of IFNγ and TNFα producing CD4$^+$ T cells when compared to the animals immunized with the isotype control, although IL-2 levels were comparable. Interestingly, there was a difference in the magnitude of the response when splenocytes were pulsed with pools 2 or 3. The frequency of CD4$^+$ T cells that proliferated and produced IFNγ or TNFα was higher after pulse with pool 3, indicating the presence of an immunodominant epitope(s) capable of binding the BALB/c haplotype (H-2K^d). A more detailed analysis showed that pscDEC-EDIII immunization elicited polyfunctional CD4$^+$ T cells producing one, two, or three pro-inflammatory cytokines, even though statistical significance in comparison to the isotype control group was only reached when single TNFα producers were compared. CD4$^+$ T cells producing the same combination of pro-inflammatory cytokines were also observed in animals immunized with scDEC-HIV p41 (37) or with scDEC-HER2 (38). The presence of polyfunctional CD4$^+$ T cells with protective capacity was first described in a mouse model testing a vaccine against *Leishmania major* (66). After that, many groups set out to investigate if polyfunctional CD4$^+$ T cells could be related with protection in other models. Studies with HIV-1 infected individuals showed that those displaying polyfunctional CD4$^+$ T cells were able to better control disease (67, 68). In dengue infection, one study showed that CD4$^+$ T cells that produced either IFNγ or IL-2 correlated with protection from secondary virus infection in children (69). Polyfunctional CD4$^+$ T cells were also identified in individuals submitted to a DENV-1 vaccine candidate, although protection against infection was not investigated in this particular study (70).

Worth mentioning is the fact that, in some cases, DNA vaccination with a scFv encoding the scDEC205 fused with an antigen elicited weaker immune responses when compared to the non-targeted controls (56, 58, 71). The reason for these results is still unclear. In fact, DEC205 targeting using chimeric anti-DEC205 mAbs has been known to induce tolerance if the antigen is delivered in the absence of a DC maturation stimulus (72). However, electroporation facilitates DNA uptake and makes more DNA available for detection by intracellular DNA sensors, thereby activating the production of cytokines as an innate reaction (73). In addition, the plasmid backbone should also be considered. As a mechanistic explanation is still elusive, additional studies are necessary.

Finally, we attempted to map the epitopes responsible for the CD4$^+$ T cell proliferation and cytokine production. When splenocytes from mice immunized with pscDEC-EDIII were pulsed with each individual peptide, we identified two peptides that were probably responsible for the response observed against pools 2 and 3: MDKLQLKGMSYSMCTGKFKI and RHVLGRLITVNPIVTEKDSP, respectively. Peptide RHVLGRLITVNPIVTEKDSP comprises the sequence of peptide RHVLGRLITVNPIVT that was shown to induce IFNγ production when this peptide was used to immunize C57BL/6J mice (74). In addition, the same peptide was also shown to bind to HLA-DRB1*08:02 in patients from Nicaragua (75) and Sri Lanka (76). This result indicates that our immunization strategy may have the potential to induce CD4$^+$ T cells in humans. Peptide MDKLQLKGMSYSMCTGKFKI is contained in the sequence of peptide SGNLLFTGHLKCRLRMDKLQLKGMSYSMCTG, which was previously used to immunize BALB/c mice. Proliferation and release of IL-2 were detected in this case (77). As DEC205 targeting greatly improves CD4$^+$ T cell responses, it is relatively easy to map antigenic peptides. CD4$^+$ T cell epitopes derived from different proteins have been more easily mapped in samples derived from animals submitted to antigen targeting to DCs. CD4$^+$ T cells epitopes were detected in the *Plasmodium yoelii* circunsporozoite protein (27), in the HIV p24 gag (51), in the *Leishmania major* LACK antigen (64), in the *Yersinia pestis* LcrV antigen (65) and in the *Trypanosoma cruzi* ASP-2 protein (31).

The role of CD4$^+$ T cells in dengue infection is still not very well defined. CD4$^+$ T cells from infected patients were found to have *ex vivo* specific cytolytic activity against DENV (13). Individuals vaccinated with an experimental live attenuated DENV1 vaccine exhibited CD4$^+$ T cells with cytotoxic and proliferative capacities *in vitro* (78, 79). In mouse models, a DNA vaccine encoding the NS1 protein induced protection via CD4$^+$ T cells and antibodies (80). Immunization with a chimeric αDEC205 mAb fused to NS1 was also able to induce CD4$^+$ T cells that contributed for protection (30). Yauch et al. showed that vaccination with CD4$^+$ peptides in an IFN-α/βR$^{-/-}$ mouse model reduced viral loads. Interestingly, CD4$^+$ T cells did not seem to have an impact on antibody neutralization of the virus measured by infection of C6/36 cells (81). Further studies will be needed to address the role of CD4$^+$ T cells in our model.

Although in the literature CD8α^+ DCs are described as playing an important role in the uptake of apoptotic cells and in antigen cross-presentation in the context of MHC Class I (82, 83), we did not detect a robust $CD8^+$ T cell response induced by our scFv DNA vaccines (data not shown). One reason for that might be related to the choice of the EDIII as an antigen, as most $CD8^+$ T cell epitopes are localized on the non-structural proteins, especially NS3 and NS5 (84). Our group has previously demonstrated that NS1 targeting to DCs via DEC205 induced protection partially mediated by $CD8^+$ T cells (30). In addition, studies mapping $CD8^+$ T cell epitopes usually use peptides of no more than 12-15 amino acids. Our peptide library consisted of 20-mers, which might have restricted the identification of $CD8^+$ T cell responses.

Taken together, our results show that antigen targeting to $CD8\alpha^+$ DCs using DNA vaccines is a promising strategy to induce cellular and humoral responses and may be used in the development of more efficient dengue vaccines.

AUTHOR CONTRIBUTIONS

AZ and SB designed the experiments. AZ, FS, BA, HS, NF, NS, and MY conducted most of the experiments. AZ and SB analyzed the data. AZ and SB prepared the figures and wrote the manuscript. LF, DM, and DR contributed reagents. DR, LF, FS, NS, and MY revised the manuscript. All authors read and approved the final version of the manuscript.

ACKNOWLEDGMENTS

The authors would like to thank Danielle Chagas, Anderson Domingos Silva and Doroty Nunes da Silva for assistance in the animal facility, and Dr. Mauro Javier Cortéz Veliz for the use of the immunofluorescence microscope.

REFERENCES

1. Bhatt S, Gething PW, Brady OJ, Messina JP, Farlow AW, Moyes CL, et al. The global distribution and burden of dengue. *Nature* (2013) 496:504–7. doi: 10.1038/nature12060nature12060
2. Whitehead SS, Blaney JE, Durbin AP, Murphy BR. Prospects for a dengue virus vaccine. *Nat Rev Microbiol.* (2007) 5:518–28. doi: 10.1038/nrmicro1690
3. Lindenbach BD, Rice CM. Flaviviridae: the viruses and their replication, In: Knipe DM, Howley PM, editors. *Fields Virology.* 4th ed. Philadelphia, PA: Lippincott Williams & Wilkins (2001). p. 991–1042.
4. Kurane I. Dengue hemorrhagic fever with special emphasis on immunopathogenesis. *Comp Immunol Microbiol Infect Dis.* (2007) 30:329–40. doi: 10.1016/j.cimid.2007.05.010
5. Zhang ZS, Yan YS, Weng YW, Huang HL, Li SQ, He S, et al. High-level expression of recombinant dengue virus type 2 envelope domain III protein and induction of neutralizing antibodies in BALB/C mice. *J Virol Methods* (2007) 143:125–31. doi: 10.1016/j.jviromet.2007.02.012
6. Block OK, Rodrigo WW, Quinn M, Jin X, Rose RC, Schlesinger JJ. A tetravalent recombinant dengue domain III protein vaccine stimulates neutralizing and enhancing antibodies in mice. *Vaccine* (2010) 28:8085–94. doi: 10.1016/j.vaccine.2010.10.004
7. Crill WD, Roehrig JT. Monoclonal antibodies that bind to domain III of dengue virus E glycoprotein are the most efficient blockers of virus adsorption to Vero cells. *J Virol.* (2001) 75:7769–73. doi: 10.1128/JVI.75.16.7769-7773.2001
8. Wahala WM, Silva AM. The human antibody response to dengue virus infection. *Viruses* (2011) 3:2374–95. doi: 10.3390/v3122374
9. Poggianella M, Slon Campos JL, Chan KR, Tan HC, Bestagno M, Ooi EE, et al. Dengue E protein domain III-based DNA immunisation induces strong antibody responses to all four viral serotypes. *PLoS Negl Trop Dis.* (2015) 9:e0003947. doi: 10.1371/journal.pntd.0003947
10. Bukowski JF, Kurane I, Lai CJ, Bray M, Falgout B, Ennis FA. Dengue virus-specific cross-reactive $CD8^+$ human cytotoxic T lymphocytes. *J Virol.* (1989) 63:5086–91.
11. Kurane I, Meager A, Ennis FA. Dengue virus-specific human T cell clones. Serotype crossreactive proliferation, interferon gamma production, and cytotoxic activity. *J Exp Med.* (1989) 170:763–75.
12. Rothman AL. Dengue: defining protective versus pathologic immunity. *J Clin Invest.* (2004) 113:946–51. doi: 10.1172/JCI21512
13. Weiskopf D, Bangs DJ, Sidney J, Kolla RV, De Silva AD, de Silva AM, et al. Dengue virus infection elicits highly polarized $CX3CR1^+$ cytotoxic $CD4^+$ T cells associated with protective immunity. *Proc Natl Acad Sci USA.* (2015) 112:E4256–63. doi: 10.1073/pnas.1505956112
14. Banchereau J, Steinman RM. Dendritic cells and the control of immunity. *Nature* (1998) 392 245–52. doi: 10.1038/32588
15. Delamarre L, Holcombe H, Mellman I. Presentation of exogenous antigens on major histocompatibility complex (MHC) class I and MHC class II molecules is differentially regulated during dendritic cell maturation. *J Exp Med.* (2003) 198:111–22. doi: 10.1084/jem.20021542
16. Merad M, Sathe P, Helft J, Miller J, Mortha A. The dendritic cell lineage: ontogeny and function of dendritic cells and their subsets in the steady state and the inflamed setting. *Annu Rev Immunol.* (2013) 31:563–604. doi: 10.1146/annurev-immunol-020711-074950
17. Inaba K, Swiggard WJ, Inaba M, Meltzer J, Mirza A, Sasagawa T, et al. Tissue distribution of the DEC-205 protein that is detected by the monoclonal antibody NLDC-145. I Expression on dendritic cells and other subsets of mouse leukocytes. *Cell Immunol.* (1995) 163:148–56.
18. Witmer-Pack MD, Swiggard WJ, Mirza A, Inaba K, Steinman RM. Tissue distribution of the DEC-205 protein that is detected by the monoclonal antibody NLDC-145. II Expression in situ in lymphoid and nonlymphoid tissues *Cell Immunol.* (1995) 163:157–62.
19. Guo M, Gong S, Maric S, Misulovin Z, Pack M, Mahnke K, et al. A monoclonal antibody to the DEC-205 endocytosis receptor on human dendritic cells. *Hum Immunol.* (2000) 61:729–38. doi: 10.1016/S0198-8859(00)00144-0
20. Ebner S, Ehammer Z, Holzmann S, Schwingshackl P, Forstner M, Stoitzner P, et al. Expression of C-type lectin receptors by subsets of dendritic cells in human skin. *Int Immunol* (2004) 16:877–87. doi: 10.1093/intimm/dxh088
21. Mahnke K, Guo M, Lee S, Sepulveda H, Swain SL, Nussenzweig M, et al. The dendritic cell receptor for endocytosis, DEC-205, can recycle and enhance antigen presentation via major histocompatibility complex class II-positive lysosomal compartments. *J Cell Biol* (2000) 151:673–84. doi: 10.1083/jcb.151.3.673
22. Vremec D, Pooley J, Hochrein H, Wu L, Shortman K. CD4 and CD8 expression by dendritic cell subtypes in mouse thymus and spleen. *J Immunol.* (2000) 164:2978–86. doi: 10.4049/jimmunol.164.6.2978
23. den Haan JM, Lehar SM, Bevan MJ. $CD8^+$ but not $CD8^-$ dendritic cells cross-prime cytotoxic T cells *in vivo*. *J Exp Med.* (2000) 192:1685–96. doi: 10.1084/jem.192.12.1685
24. Iyoda T, Shimoyama S, Liu K, Omatsu Y, Akiyama Y, Maeda Y, et al. The $CD8^+$ dendritic cell subset selectively endocytoses dying cells in culture and *in vivo*. *J Exp Med.* (2002) 195:1289–302. doi: 10.1084/jem.20020161
25. Allan RS, Smith CM, Belz GT, van Lint AL, Wakim LM, Heath WR, et al. Epidermal viral immunity induced by $CD8alpha^+$ dendritic cells but not by Langerhans cells. *Science* (2003) 301:1925–8. doi: 10.1126/science.1087576
26. Bonifaz LC, Bonnyay DP, Charalambous A, Darguste DI, Fujii S, Soares H, et al. *In vivo* targeting of antigens to maturing dendritic cells via the DEC-205 receptor improves T cell vaccination. *J Exp Med.* (2004) 199:815–24. doi: 10.1084/jem.20032220

27. Boscardin SB, Hafalla JC, Masilamani RF, Kamphorst AO, Zebroski HA, Rai U, et al. Antigen targeting to dendritic cells elicits long-lived T cell help for antibody responses. *J Exp Med.* (2006) 203:599–606. doi: 10.1084/jem.20051639
28. Dudziak D, Kamphorst AO, Heidkamp GF, Buchholz VR, Trumpfheller C, Yamazaki S, et al. Differential antigen processing by dendritic cell subsets *in vivo*. *Science* (2007) 315:107–11. doi: 10.1126/science.1136080
29. Do Y, Koh H, Park CG, Dudziak D, Seo P, Mehandru S, et al. Targeting of LcrV virulence protein from Yersinia pestis to dendritic cells protects mice against pneumonic plague. *Eur J Immunol.* (2010) 40:2791–6. doi: 10.1002/eji.201040511
30. Henriques HR, Rampazo EV, Goncalves AJ, Vicentin EC, Amorim JH, Panatieri RH, et al. Targeting the non-structural protein 1 from dengue virus to a dendritic cell population confers protective immunity to lethal virus challenge. *PLoS Negl Trop Dis.* (2013) 7:e2330. doi: 10.1371/journal.pntd.0002330
31. Rampazo EV, Amorim KN, Yamamoto MM, Panatieri RH, Rodrigues MM, Boscardin SB. Antigen targeting to dendritic cells allows the identification of a CD4 T-cell epitope within an immunodominant trypanosoma cruzi antigen. *PLoS ONE* (2015) 10:e0117778. doi: 10.1371/journal.pone.0117778
32. Amorim KN, Rampazo EV, Antonialli R, Yamamoto MM, Rodrigues MM, Soares IS, et al. The presence of T cell epitopes is important for induction of antibody responses against antigens directed to DEC205^{+} dendritic cells. *Sci Rep.* (2016) 6:39250. doi: 10.1038/srep39250
33. Antonialli R, Sulczewski FB, Amorim K, Almeida BDS, Ferreira NS, Yamamoto MM, et al. CpG Oligodeoxinucleotides and flagellin modulate the immune response to antigens targeted to CD8alpha(+) and CD8alpha(−) conventional dendritic cell subsets. *Front Immunol.* (2017) 8:1727. doi: 10.3389/fimmu.2017.01727
34. Apostolico JS, Lunardelli VA, Yamamoto MM, Souza HF, Cunha-Neto E, Boscardin SB, et al. Dendritic cell targeting effectively boosts T cell responses elicited by an HIV multiepitope DNA vaccine. *Front Immunol.* (2017) 8:101. doi: 10.3389/fimmu.2017.00101
35. Rosa DS, Apostólico JS, Boscardin SB. DNA vaccines: how much have we accomplished in the last 25 years? *J Vaccines Vaccin.* (2015) 6:283. doi: 10.4172/2157-7560.1000283
36. Demangel C, Zhou J, Choo AB, Shoebridge G, Halliday GM, Britton WJ. Single chain antibody fragments for the selective targeting of antigens to dendritic cells. *Mol Immunol.* (2005) 42:979–85. doi: 10.1016/j.molimm.2004.09.034
37. Nchinda G, Kuroiwa J, Oks M, Trumpfheller C, Park CG, Huang Y, et al. The efficacy of DNA vaccination is enhanced in mice by targeting the encoded protein to dendritic cells. *J Clin Invest.* (2008) 118:1427–36. doi: 10.1172/JCI34224
38. Cao J, Jin Y, Li W, Zhang B, He Y, Liu H, et al. DNA vaccines targeting the encoded antigens to dendritic cells induce potent antitumor immunity in mice. *BMC Immunol.* (2013) 14:39. doi: 10.1186/1471-2172-14-39
39. Chen BY, Zhou G, Li QL, Lu JS, Shi DY, Pang XB, et al. Enhanced effects of DNA vaccine against botulinum neurotoxin serotype A by targeting antigen to dendritic cells. *Immunol Lett.* (2017) 190:118–24. doi: 10.1016/j.imlet.2017.08.004
40. Hua Y, Jiao YY, Ma Y, Peng XL, Fu YH, Zhang XJ, et al. Enhanced humoral and CD8^{+} T cell immunity in mice vaccinated by DNA vaccine against human respiratory syncytial virus through targeting the encoded F protein to dendritic cells. *Int Immunopharmacol.* (2017) 46:62–9. doi: 10.1016/j.intimp.2017.02.023
41. Ngu LN, Nji NN, Ambada G, Ngoh AA, Njambe Priso GD, Tchadji JC, et al. Dendritic cell targeted HIV-1 gag protein vaccine provides help to a recombinant Newcastle disease virus vectored vaccine including mobilization of protective CD8^{+} T cells. *Immun Inflamm Dis.* (2018) 6:163–75. doi: 10.1002/iid3.209
42. Ring S, Maas M, Nettelbeck DM, Enk AH, Mahnke K. Targeting of autoantigens to DEC205(+) dendritic cells *in vivo* suppresses experimental allergic encephalomyelitis in mice. *J Immunol.* (2013) 191:2938–47. doi: 10.4049/jimmunol.1202592
43. Maeda D, Batista MT, Pereira LR, de Jesus Cintra M, Amorim JH, Mathias-Santos C, et al. Adjuvant-mediated epitope specificity and enhanced neutralizing activity of antibodies targeting dengue virus envelope protein. *Front Immunol.* (2017) 8:1175. doi: 10.3389/fimmu.2017.01175
44. Lambeth CR, White LJ, Johnston RE, de Silva AM. Flow cytometry-based assay for titrating dengue virus. *J Clin Microbiol.* (2005) 43:3267–72. doi: 10.1128/JCM.43.7.3267-3272.2005
45. Medina F, Medina JF, Colon C, Vergne E, Santiago GA, Munoz-Jordan JL. Dengue virus: isolation, propagation, quantification, and storage. *Curr Protoc Microbiol* (2012). Chapter 15, Unit 15D.12. doi: 10.1002/9780471729259.mc15d02s27
46. Beltramello M, Williams KL, Simmons CP, Macagno A, Simonelli L, Quyen NT, et al. The human immune response to dengue virus is dominated by highly cross-reactive antibodies endowed with neutralizing and enhancing activity. *Cell Host Microbe.* (2010) 8:271–83. doi: 10.1016/j.chom.2010.08.007
47. Shrestha B, Brien JD, Sukupolvi-Petty S, Austin SK, Edeling MA, Kim T, et al. The development of therapeutic antibodies that neutralize homologous and heterologous genotypes of dengue virus type 1. *PLoS Pathog.* (2010) 6:e1000823. doi: 10.1371/journal.ppat.1000823
48. WHO (Ed.). *Global Strategy for Dengue Prevention and Control 2012-2020.* France: WHO Library Cataloguing-in-Publication Data (2012).
49. Vannice KS, Durbin A, Hombach J. Status of vaccine research and development of vaccines for dengue. *Vaccine* (2016) 34:2934–8. doi: 10.1016/j.vaccine.2015.12.073
50. Wilder-Smith A, Hombach J, Ferguson N, Selgelid M, O'Brien K, Vannice K, et al. Deliberations of the strategic advisory group of experts on immunization on the use of CYD-TDV dengue vaccine. *Lancet Infect Dis.* (2018) 19:e31–8. doi: 10.1016/S1473-3099(18)30494-8
51. Trumpfheller C, Finke JS, Lopez CB, Moran TM, Moltedo B, Soares H, et al. Intensified and protective CD4^{+} T cell immunity in mice with anti-dendritic cell HIV gag fusion antibody vaccine. *J Exp Med.* (2006) 203:607–17. doi: 10.1084/jem.20052005
52. Trumpfheller C, Caskey M, Nchinda G, Longhi MP, Mizenina O, Huang Y, et al. The microbial mimic poly IC induces durable and protective CD4^{+} T cell immunity together with a dendritic cell targeted vaccine. *Proc Natl Acad Sci USA* (2008) 105:2574–9. doi: 10.1073/pnas.0711976105
53. Sardesai NY, Weiner DB. Electroporation delivery of DNA vaccines: prospects for success. *Curr Opin Immunol.* (2011) 23:421–9. doi: 10.1016/j.coi.2011.03.008
54. Sales NS, Silva JR, Aps L, Silva MO, Porchia B, Ferreira LCS, et al. *In vivo* electroporation enhances vaccine-mediated therapeutic control of human papilloma virus-associated tumors by the activation of multifunctional and effector memory CD8(+) T cells. *Vaccine* (2017) 35:7240–9. doi: 10.1016/j.vaccine.2017.11.011
55. Coconi-Linares N, Ortega-Davila E, Lopez-Gonzalez M, Garcia-Machorro J, Garcia-Cordero J, Steinman RM, et al. Targeting of envelope domain III protein of DENV type 2 to DEC-205 receptor elicits neutralizing antibodies in mice. *Vaccine* (2013) 31:2366–71. doi: 10.1016/j.vaccine.2013.03.009
56. Tenbusch M, Ignatius R, Nchinda G, Trumpfheller C, Salazar AM, Topfer K, et al. Immunogenicity of DNA vaccines encoding simian immunodeficiency virus antigen targeted to dendritic cells in rhesus macaques. *PLoS ONE* (2012) 7:e39038. doi: 10.1371/journal.pone.0039038
57. Yu D, Liu H, Shi S, Dong L, Wang H, Wu N, et al. A novel dendritic-cell-targeting DNA vaccine for hepatitis B induces T cell and humoral immune responses and potentiates the antivirus activity in HBV transgenic mice. *Immunol Lett.* (2015) 168:293–9. doi: 10.1016/j.imlet.2015.10.007
58. Niezold T, Storcksdieck Genannt Bonsmann M, Maaske A, Temchura V, Heinecke V, Hannaman D, et al. DNA vaccines encoding DEC205-targeted antigens: immunity or tolerance? *Immunology* (2015) 145:519–33. doi: 10.1111/imm.12467
59. Sukupolvi-Petty S, Austin SK, Purtha WE, Oliphant T, Nybakken GE, Schlesinger JJ, et al. Type- and subcomplex-specific neutralizing antibodies against domain III of dengue virus type 2 envelope protein recognize adjacent epitopes. *J Virol* (2007) 81:12816–26. doi: 10.1128/JVI.00432-07
60. Sukupolvi-Petty S, Austin SK, Engle M, Brien JD, Dowd KA, Williams KL, et al. Structure and function analysis of therapeutic monoclonal antibodies against dengue virus type 2. *J Virol.* (2010) 84:9227–39. doi: 10.1128/JVI.01087-10

61. Puschnik A, Lau L, Cromwell EA, Balmaseda A, Zompi S, Harris E. Correlation between dengue-specific neutralizing antibodies and serum avidity in primary and secondary dengue virus 3 natural infections in humans. *PLoS Negl Trop Dis.* (2013) 7:e2274. doi: 10.1371/journal.pntd.0002274
62. Alexander MR, Ringe R, Sanders RW, Voss JE, Moore JP, Klasse PJ. What do chaotrope-based avidity assays for antibodies to HIV-1 envelope glycoproteins measure? *J Virol.* (2015) 89:5981–95. doi: 10.1128/JVI.00320-15
63. Valdes I, Gil L, Romero Y, Castro J, Puente P, Lazo L, et al. The chimeric protein domain III-capsid of dengue virus serotype 2 (DEN-2) successfully boosts neutralizing antibodies generated in monkeys upon infection with DEN-2. *Clin Vaccine Immunol.* (2011) 18:455–9. doi: 10.1128/CVI.00382-10
64. Soares H, Waechter H, Glaichenhaus N, Mougneau E, Yagita H, Mizenina O, et al. A subset of dendritic cells induces $CD4^+$ T cells to produce IFN-gamma by an IL-12-independent but $CD70^-$ dependent mechanism *in vivo. J Exp Med.* (2007) 204:1095–106. doi: 10.1084/jem.20070176
65. Do Y, Park CG, Kang YS, Park SH, Lynch RM, Lee H, et al. Broad T cell immunity to the LcrV virulence protein is induced by targeted delivery to DEC-205/CD205-positive mouse dendritic cells. *Eur J Immunol.* (2008) 38:20–9. doi: 10.1002/eji.200737799
66. Darrah PA, Patel DT, De Luca PM, Lindsay RW, Davey DF, Flynn BJ, et al. Multifunctional TH1 cells define a correlate of vaccine-mediated protection against Leishmania major. *Nat Med.* (2007) 13:843–50. doi: 10.1038/nm1592
67. Emu B, Sinclair E, Favre D, Moretto WJ, Hsue P, Hoh R, et al. Phenotypic, functional, and kinetic parameters associated with apparent T-cell control of human immunodeficiency virus replication in individuals with and without antiretroviral treatment. *J Virol.* (2005) 79:14169–78. doi: 10.1128/JVI.79.22.14169-14178.2005
68. Owen RE, Heitman JW, Hirschkorn DF, Lanteri MC, Biswas HH, Martin JN, et al. HIV+ elite controllers have low HIV-specific T-cell activation yet maintain strong, polyfunctional T-cell responses. *AIDS* (2010) 24:1095–105. doi: 10.1097/QAD.0b013e3283377a1e
69. Hatch S, Endy TP, Thomas S, Mathew A, Potts J, Pazoles P, et al. Intracellular cytokine production by dengue virus-specific T cells correlates with subclinical secondary infection. *J Infect Dis.* (2011) 203:1282–91. doi: 10.1093/infdis/jir012jir012
70. Lindow JC, Borochoff-Porte N, Durbin AP, Whitehead SS, Fimlaid KA, Bunn JY, et al. Primary vaccination with low dose live dengue 1 virus generates a proinflammatory, multifunctional T cell response in humans. *PLoS Negl Trop Dis.* (2012) 6:e1742. doi: 10.1371/journal.pntd.0001742
71. Tenbusch M, Nchinda G, Storcksdieck genannt Bonsmann M, Temchura V, Uberla K. Targeting the antigen encoded by adenoviral vectors to the DEC205 receptor modulates the cellular and humoral immune response. *Int Immunol.* (2013) 25:247–58. doi: 10.1093/intimm/dxs112dxs112
72. Hawiger D, Inaba K, Dorsett Y, Guo M, Mahnke K, Rivera M, et al. Dendritic cells induce peripheral T cell unresponsiveness under steady state conditions *in vivo. J Exp Med.* (2001) 194:769–79. doi: 10.1084/jem.194.6.769
73. Takaoka A, Wang Z, Choi MK, Yanai H, Negishi H, Ban T, et al. DAI (DLM-1/ZBP1) is a cytosolic DNA sensor and an activator of innate immune response. *Nature* (2007) 448:501–5. doi: 10.1038/nature06013
74. Li S, Peng L, Zhao W, Zhong H, Zhang F, Yan Z, et al. Synthetic peptides containing B- and T-cell epitope of dengue virus-2 E domain III provoked B- and T-cell responses. *Vaccine* (2011) 29:3695–702. doi: 10.1016/j.vaccine.2011.03.002
75. Grifoni A, Angelo MA, Lopez B, O'Rourke PH, Sidney J, Cerpas C, et al. Global Assessment of Dengue Virus Specific CD4(+) T cell responses in dengue-endemic areas. *Front Immunol.* (2017) 8:1309. doi: 10.3389/fimmu.2017.01309
76. Weiskopf D, Angelo MA, Grifoni A, O'Rourke PH, Sidney J, Paul S, et al. HLA-DRB1 alleles are associated with different magnitudes of dengue virus-specific $CD4^+$ T-Cell responses. *J Infect Dis.* (2016) 214:1117–24. doi: 10.1093/infdis/jiw309
77. Roehrig JT, Risi PA, Brubaker JR, Hunt AR, Beaty BJ, Trent DW, et al. T-helper cell epitopes on the E-glycoprotein of dengue 2 Jamaica virus. *Virology* (1994) 198:31–8. doi: 10.1006/viro.1994.1005
78. Kurane I, Innis BL, Nisalak A, Hoke C, Nimmannitya S, Meager A, et al. Human T cell responses to dengue virus antigens. Proliferative responses and interferon gamma production. *J Clin Invest.* (1989) 83:506–13. doi: 10.1172/JCI113911
79. Green S, Kurane I, Edelman R, Tacket CO, Eckels KH, Vaughn DW, et al. Dengue virus-specific human $CD4^+$ T-lymphocyte responses in a recipient of an experimental live-attenuated dengue virus type 1 vaccine: bulk culture proliferation, clonal analysis, and precursor frequency determination. *J Virol.* (1993) 67:5962–7.
80. Goncalves AJ, Oliveira ER, Costa SM, Paes MV, Silva JF, Azevedo AS, et al. Cooperation between $CD4^+$ T Cells and humoral immunity is critical for protection against dengue using a DNA vaccine based on the NS1 antigen. *PLoS Negl Trop Dis.* (2015) 9:e0004277. doi: 10.1371/journal.pntd.0004277
81. Yauch LE, Prestwood TR, May MM, Morar MM, Zellweger RM, Peters B, et al. $CD4^+$ T cells are not required for the induction of dengue virus-specific $CD8^+$ T cell or antibody responses but contribute to protection after vaccination. *J Immunol.* (2010) 185:5405–16. doi: 10.4049/jimmunol.1001709
82. Pooley JL, Heath WR, Shortman K. Cutting edge: intravenous soluble antigen is presented to CD4 T cells by $CD8^-$ dendritic cells, but cross-presented to CD8 T cells by $CD8^+$ dendritic cells. *J Immunol.* (2001) 166:5327–30. doi: 10.4049/jimmunol.166.9.5327
83. den Haan JM, Bevan MJ. Constitutive versus activation-dependent cross-presentation of immune complexes by $CD8^+$ and $CD8^-$ dendritic cells *in vivo. J Exp Med.* (2002) 196:817–27. doi: 10.1084/jem.20020295
84. Rivino L, Kumaran EA, Jovanovic V, Nadua K, Teo EW, Pang SW, et al. Differential targeting of viral components by $CD4^+$ versus $CD8^+$ T lymphocytes in dengue virus infection. *J Virol.* (2013) 87:2693–706. doi: 10.1128/JVI.02675-12

10

Sources of Type I Interferons in Infectious Immunity: Plasmacytoid Dendritic Cells Not Always in the Driver's Seat

Shafaqat Ali[1,2], *Ritu Mann-Nüttel*[1], *Anja Schulze*[1], *Lisa Richter*[1], *Judith Alferink*[2,3] and *Stefanie Scheu*[1*]

[1] *Institute of Medical Microbiology and Hospital Hygiene, University of Düsseldorf, Düsseldorf, Germany,* [2] *Cluster of Excellence EXC 1003, Cells in Motion, Münster, Germany,* [3] *Department of Psychiatry, University of Münster, Münster, Germany*

***Correspondence:**
Stefanie Scheu
stefanie.scheu@uni-duesseldorf.de

Type I Interferons (IFNs) are hallmark cytokines produced in immune responses to all classes of pathogens. Type I IFNs can influence dendritic cell (DC) activation, maturation, migration, and survival, but also directly enhance natural killer (NK) and T/B cell activity, thus orchestrating various innate and adaptive immune effector functions. Therefore, type I IFNs have long been considered essential in the host defense against virus infections. More recently, it has become clear that depending on the type of virus and the course of infection, production of type I IFN can also lead to immunopathology or immunosuppression. Similarly, in bacterial infections type I IFN production is often associated with detrimental effects for the host. Although most cells in the body are thought to be able to produce type I IFN, plasmacytoid DCs (pDCs) have been termed the natural "IFN producing cells" due to their unique molecular adaptations to nucleic acid sensing and ability to produce high amounts of type I IFN. Findings from mouse reporter strains and depletion experiments in *in vivo* infection models have brought new insights and established that the role of pDCs in type I IFN production *in vivo* is less important than assumed. Production of type I IFN, especially the early synthesized IFNβ, is rather realized by a variety of cell types and cannot be mainly attributed to pDCs. Indeed, the cell populations responsible for type I IFN production vary with the type of pathogen, its tissue tropism, and the route of infection. In this review, we summarize recent findings from *in vivo* models on the cellular source of type I IFN in different infectious settings, ranging from virus, bacteria, and fungi to eukaryotic parasites. The implications from these findings for the development of new vaccination and therapeutic designs targeting the respectively defined cell types are discussed.

Keywords: type I interferon, plasmacytoid dendritic cells, interferon producing cells, infection, pathogen, virus, immunopathology, immune activation

INTRODUCTION

The cytokine family of type I IFNs fulfills key functions in anti-viral immunity but is also produced in the immune responses to other classes of pathogens covering viruses, bacteria, parasites, and fungi (1). Additionally, these cytokines are functionally involved in the pathogenesis of inflammatory autoimmune diseases (2).

Together with IFNβ, type I IFNs comprise multiple IFNα subtypes (11 in mice and 13 in humans), IFNε, IFNκ, and IFNω in most mammals. In addition, IFNδ, IFNζ (limitin), and IFNτ have been detected exclusively in pigs, mice, and ruminants, respectively (3–6). Type I IFNs are encoded by intronless genes clustered in mice on chromosome 4 and in humans on chromosome 9 (3–6). Induction of type I IFN expression is facilitated after activation of a diverse set of pathogen sensing pattern recognition receptor (PRR) pathways by binding of IFN regulatory factors (IRFs) and NF-κB to acute response elements in the promoters of type I IFN gene loci (7). All type I IFNs bind to a common heterodimeric IFNα receptor (IFNAR), which is composed of the IFNAR1 and IFNAR2 subunits and is expressed by virtually all nucleated cells of the body. Following IFNAR engagement by its ligands, canonical type I IFN signaling activates the Janus kinase (JAK)-signal transducer and activator of transcription (STAT) pathway, leading to transcription of IFN-stimulated genes (ISGs) (5, 8). ISG-encoded proteins mediate induction of cell-intrinsic antimicrobial states in infected and neighboring cells that limit the spread of infectious agents, particularly viral pathogens. Additionally, ISGs influence innate and adaptive immune responses by promoting antigen presentation and NK cell functions, modulating inflammatory cytokine production, and activating high-affinity antigen-specific T and B cell responses and immunological memory (9). Type I IFN production, however, can also have deleterious roles in chronic viral and bacterial infections, and can lead to immunopathologies such as inflammatory disorders and autoimmunity (1, 2, 10, 11).

IFNβ was originally defined as the antiviral factor produced by fibroblasts after viral infections (12) and has been thought to be produced by virtually all cells of the body. Later pDCs specialized in the rapid secretion of high amounts of type I IFN have been termed the natural "IFN producing cells" (IPCs). Recent findings, however, indicate that production of type I IFN, especially the early synthesized IFNβ, in anti-infectious immune responses can occur independently of pDCs and that the cell type responsible for type I IFN production rather depends on the specific infectious setting. In this review we summarize the recent findings on the identity and function of type I IFN producing cells in infection by focusing on insights gained from *in vivo* mouse models covering type I IFN reporter mice and models of cell type specific ablation.

Pathways of Type I IFN Activation in Different Cell Types

To devise novel anti-infectious treatment regimens targeting a specific cellular subtype, it is crucial to know the identity of the cells responsible for the production of type I IFN in the course of an infection. Early on, pDCs were considered primary producers of IFNα during virus infections (13, 14). For human pDCs it has been reported that IFNα/β transcripts account for an astounding 50% of all mRNAs in the cell after viral activation (15). More than 40 years ago, pDCs were first described in humans as natural IPCs that activate NK cells upon exposure to viruses (16, 17). The murine equivalent was described in 2001 as type I IFN producing cells with plasmacytoid morphology (18–20). These cells detect RNA and DNA viruses through two endosomal sensors, TLR7 and TLR9, respectively, which induce secretion of type I IFN through the MyD88-IRF7 signaling pathway (21–24). Specifically, TLR7/9-ligand interactions in early endosomes result in type I IFN production while ligand recognition in late endosomes or lysosomes rather leads to inflammatory cytokine production and pDC maturation (25, 26). At least in the mouse, TLR7 and 9 are also expressed by monocytes, conventional DCs (cDCs), and B cells (27, 28). Therefore, the contribution of those cell types to type I IFN production triggered via the TLR7/9-MyD88-IRF7 pathway has to be considered. B cells, for instance, have recently been shown to produce type I IFN *in vivo* after optimized stimulation conditions using the TLR9 ligand CpG-A (29). A specific feature of pDCs is that they can produce type I IFN independently of IFNAR mediated feedback signaling (30). However, they do respond to type I IFN by generating an autocrine circuit through IFNAR, which augments type I IFN secretion and induces their activation and migration (31, 32).

In humans, pDCs, monocytes, and other myeloid cells also produce type I IFN after stimulation of the TLR8-MyD88-IRF7 pathway by viral single-stranded RNA (ssRNA) (33, 34). The mouse TLR8 was initially considered non-functional (33, 34). More recently it has been shown that mouse TLR8 can be stimulated by a combination of oligodeoxynucleotides (ODNs) and human TLR8 ligands. Further, mouse pDCs produce type I IFN after stimulation with vaccinia virus (VV) in a TLR8 dependent way (35, 36). Two additional TLRs, TLR3 and 4, are able to induce type I IFN expression independently of the MyD88 pathway via recruiting the TIR domain-containing adaptor protein inducing interferon beta (TRIF; also known as TIR domain-containing adapter molecule 1, TICAM-1). This activates the transcription factor IRF3 thus initiating type I IFN, in particular IFNβ expression (37, 38). TLR3 is absent in mouse pDCs but highly expressed in endosomes of murine CD8α$^+$ and CD103$^+$ and human CD141$^+$ cDCs of the DC1 subtype that are efficient in cross-presenting (39, 40). It recognizes double-stranded RNA (dsRNA) as viral replication intermediates as well as ssRNA containing stem loops (41). In addition to DCs, TLR3 activation can lead to type I IFN expression in macrophages, fibroblasts, and epithelial cells (42). While TLR3 exclusively signals via the TRIF pathway, TLR4 utilizes MyD88 as well as TRIF signaling routes after recognizing its cognate ligand bacterial lipopolysaccharide (LPS). Analogous to TLR3 activation, LPS binding to TLR4 induces type I IFN expression via TRIF-IRF3 (43). The majority of hematopoietic cells of the myeloid and lymphoid lineage, with the exception of human pDCs, and few other cell types such as pancreatic β-cells express TLR4 (44).

In contrast to pDCs, cDCs, and macrophages mainly produce type I IFN in response to virus challenge by utilizing retinoic acid-inducible gene I (RIG-I)-like helicases (RLHs) (43, 45–47). RLHs, including RIG-I and melanoma differentiation-associated gene 5 (MDA5), are cytoplasmic dsRNA receptors that transmit their signal through the mitochondrial antiviral-signaling protein, virus-induced signaling adapter (MAVS, aka *IFNb* promoter stimulator (IPS)-1 or Cardif). This activates IRF3 and IRF7 to induce the transcription of type I IFN and other antiviral genes (48–50).

Finally, soluble sensors in the cytoplasm detect dsDNA in a sequence-independent manner, exhibit a broad expression spectrum including pDCs, cDCs, macrophages, and mouse embryonic fibroblasts (MEFs), and activate signaling pathways leading to type I IFN expression (47, 51). These sensors include the cyclic GMP-AMP synthase (cGAS)/STING pathway, the RNA polymerase III/RIG-I/MAVS pathway, DNA-dependent activator of IRFs (DAI), IFNγ-inducible protein 16 (IFI16), and the DDX family (47, 51–58).

Mouse Models and *in vivo* Experimental Strategies for the Definition of the Cellular Source of Type I IFNs in Infection

Several models of cytokine reporter mice have been developed for the detection of type I IFN production *in vivo*, as intracellular staining is not sensitive in most cases (**Table 1** and **Figure 1**). Earlier published IFNβ knock-out mouse lines already contained reporter elements to detect *Ifnb* promoter-driven gene transcription. For example, coding sequences for the mouse immunoglobulin λ2 chain, a green fluorescent protein (GFP), or the human CD2 had been inserted immediately downstream of the *Ifnb* promoter to visualize IFNβ expression on a cellular level (73–75). However, the reporter features in these mouse strains have not been used *in vivo* so far.

More recently, a mouse line expressing GFP under the control of the *Ifna6* promoter (Ifna6$^{gfp/+}$) recapitulates the expression of various IFNα genes and has been employed to define the cellular source of IFNα in virus infection models (32, 46, 76). Also, for IFNβ a fluorescence reporter-knock-in mouse model (IFNβ$^{mob/mob}$) has been generated. Here, yellow fluorescent protein (YFP) is expressed from a bicistronic mRNA linked by an internal ribosomal entry site (IRES) to the endogenous IFNβ mRNA (59). Ifna6$^{gfp/+}$ as well as IFNβ$^{mob/mob}$ reporter mice have each been shown to report for the majority of type I IFNs. However, *in vitro* analyses on BM-derived DCs from the double reporter mouse line generated by intercrossing the Ifna6$^{gfp/+}$ and IFNβ$^{mob/mob}$ reporter strains revealed that specific type I IFN subtypes can be produced by distinct cell subpopulations (77).

In an alternative reporter mouse system, a firefly luciferase reporter gene has been placed under the control of the *Ifnb* promoter (IFN-β$^{+/\Delta\beta-luc}$). Rather than IFNβ expression on a single cell level, this model detects *in vivo* kinetics of IFNβ expression in the mouse paralleling the spread of pathogens through the organism under infectious conditions (60). Additionally, in this mouse line the IFNβ coding sequence is flanked by *loxP* sites (IFN-β$^{flox\beta-luc/flox\beta-luc}$) providing the possibility to characterize the impact of IFNβ production by a given cell type on the pathophysiology of various infections via tissue- or cell-specific Cre-mediated deletion of IFNβ (60).

Methods and Models for Assessing the Impact of Type I IFN Producing Cell Populations *in vivo*

Several experimental strategies have been developed to determine the *in vivo* contribution of a specific cell type to the type I IFN response during infections (78). Initially, antibody mediated depletion has been utilized frequently to ablate pDCs and monocytes (79). Antibodies against Ly6G/C (also known as Gr1) and CD317 (also known as BST-2) have been used to deplete pDCs *in vivo* and *in vitro* (18, 79–87). However, these antibodies generally target multiple cell types in addition to pDCs: The antibody RB6-8C5 directed against Ly6G/C reacts strongly with neutrophil-specific Ly6G antigen, but cross-reacts also with the Ly6C Ag (88) expressed on pDCs as well as on monocytes/macrophages, activated T cells, NK cells, plasma cells, and endothelial cells (89–92). Likewise, CD317 is recognized by the three different antibody clones 120G8.04, JF05-1C2.4.1 (also known as PDCA-1), and eBio927, and is expressed in naïve mice by pDCs, but also plasma cells. Following stimulation with type I IFNs and IFNγ CD317 is upregulated, additionally, on several other myeloid and lymphoid cells (79, 93). Finally, *in vivo* treatment with clodronate-containing liposomes depletes phagocytes in mice, but also disturbs the microarchitecture of secondary lymphoid organs (94, 95).

In the past years, several genetically modified mouse lines with a constitutive or inducible lack of specific cell types attributed to produce type I IFN have become available (**Table 1** and **Figure 1**) (78). For pDCs, already several mouse models exist for constitutive or inducible ablation. Mice carrying a hypomorphic mutation at the *Ikaros* locus express low levels of the transcription factor Ikaros (Ik$^{L/L}$) and therefore lack peripheral pDCs, but no other DC subsets (61). When using this line as a "pDC-less" model, one has to take into account that other hematopoietic lineages including T and B cells and neutrophils are also affected by the Ik$^{L/L}$ mutation, and that Ik$^{L/L}$ mice start to develop thymic lymphomas by 10 weeks of age (62, 96, 97). Constitutive deletion of E2-2, the basic helix-loop-helix transcription factor, also known as TCF4, that controls development and maintenance of pDCs, results in perinatal lethality in mice (98). To overcome this lethality and to specifically ablate the pDC lineage, mice harboring a constitutively deleted and a floxed *Tfc4* allele (Tcf4$^{flox/-}$) have been crossed to Itgax-Cre (CD11c-Cre) or Rosa26-CreER mice in which Cre is expressed in DCs or can be induced ubiquitously after tamoxifen administration, respectively (63, 64, 99, 100). Another strategy uses Diphtheria toxin receptor (DTR)-mediated conditional and targeted cell depletion. CLEC4A-DTR-tg mice express DTR under the human pDC specific promotor of the C-type lectin domain family 4 member A (CLEC4A; also known as blood dendritic cell antigen 2, BDCA2). Administration of diphtheria toxin (DT) in these CLEC4A-DTR-tg mice results in transient but specific depletion of pDCs (65). In an alternative approach, a cDNA encoding the human DTR fused to the enhanced green fluorescent protein (EGFP) and preceded by an IRES was inserted into the 3′ untranslated region of the *Siglech* gene. This Siglech$^{dtr/dtr}$ mouse model allows specific elimination of pDCs *in vivo* via injection of DT (66). An analogous mouse line termed SiglecH-DTR-tg was generated using bacterial artificial chromosome (BAC) transgenic technology (67). SiglecH represents a sialic acid-binding Ig-like lectin that exerts immunomodulatory roles in antiviral immune responses. In SiglecH$^{eGFP/+}$mice, heterozygous for the reporter gene, it was shown that in addition to pDCs, SiglecH was

TABLE 1 | Genetically modified mouse models to visualize or define the function of type I IFN producing cells.

Function	Name(s)	Genetic modification	References
IFNα6-GFP reporter mouse	$Ifna6^{gfp/+}$	Knock-in of a GFP reporter gene into the *Ifna6* locus behind the *Ifna6* promoter; endogenous IFNα6 expression retained in homozygous reporter mouse	(46)
IFNβ-YFP reporter mouse	$IFN\beta^{mob/mob}$ (B6.129-Ifnb1tm1Lky/J)	Knock-in of an IRES-driven YFP reporter cassette behind the Stop codon of the *Ifnb1* gene; endogenous IFNβ expression retained in homozygous reporter mouse	(59)
IFNβ-luciferase reporter and conditional IFNβ knock-out	$IFN\text{-}\beta^{+/\Delta\beta-luc}$ and $IFN\text{-}\beta^{flox\beta-luc/flox\beta-luc}$	Knock-in of firefly luciferase reporter gene into the *Ifnb1* locus behind the *Ifnb1* promoter; endogenous IFNβ expression retained in homozygous reporter mouse; IFNβ coding sequence has been flanked by *loxP* sites.	(60)
Constitutive pDC ablation (*caveat*: T and B cells, and neutrophils affected)	$Ik^{L/L}$	Knock-in of the βgal coding sequence in-frame into exon-2 of the *Ikaros* gene resulting in a hypomorphic mutation	(61, 62)
Constitutive pDC ablation	$Tcf4^{flox/-}$ $Itgax\text{-}Cre^{+}$	Floxed *Tcf4* gene crossed to DC specific Itgax-CRE mice	(63, 64)
Inducible pDC ablation	$Tcf4^{flox/-}$ *R26*-$CreER^{+}$	Floxed *Tcf4* gene crossed to tamoxifen-inducible *R26*-CreER mice	(64)
Inducible transient pDC depletion after diphtheria toxin (DT) administration	CLEC4A-DTR-tg (BDCA2-DTR tg)	Transgene containing a 5 kb fragment upstream of the ATG of the human *CLEC4A* (BDCA-2) gene followed by the diphtheria toxin receptor (DTR) cDNA	(65)
Inducible transient pDC depletion after DT administration	$Siglech^{dtr/dtr}$	Knock-in of an IRES-driven cDNA encoding the human DTR fused to the enhanced green fluorescent protein (EGFP) into the 3' untranslated region of the *Siglech* gene	(66)
Inducible transient pDC depletion after DT administration (*caveat*: MZM and pre-pDC affected)	SiglecH-DTR-tg	BAC transgene, modified BAC encoding the complete *Siglech* gene locus (RPA24-163A12), bicistronic cassette containing cDNAs for human DTR and EGFP inserted into *Siglech* exon I, after the second triplet of the open reading frame	(67)
pDC-specific Cre expression (*caveat*: Cre mediated recombination detected in a minor fraction of $SiglecH^{-}$ B-, T-, NK-, and NK-T cells and splenic cDC and $CD11c^{int}$ BM cells)	pDCre	BAC transgene, modified BAC encoding the complete *Siglech* gene locus (RP24-396N13), bicistronic cassette containing cDNAs for Cre and mCherry inserted into *Siglech* exon I, after the ATG	(68)
Constitutive restriction of type I IFN production to pDCs and tamoxifen inducible pDC specific Cre expression	$pDC{:}IRF7^{+}$ ($Siglech^{Irf7/+}$; $Irf3^{-/-}$; $Irf7^{-/-}$)	Knock-in of bicistronic cassette containing the *irf7* gene locus stretching (protein coding exons) and the cDNA for Cre fused to the mutated ligand binding domain of the human estrogen receptor (ERT2), backcrossed $Irf3^{-/-}$; $Irf7^{-/-}$ double knockout mice	(69)
Inducible transient cDC depletion after DT administration	CD11c-DTR-tg	Transgene containing the murine CD11c promoter followed by a cDNA coding for a DTR-EGFP fusion protein	(70)
Inducible transient monocyte depletion after DT administration	CD11b-DTR-tg	Transgene containing the human CD11b promoter followed by a cDNA coding for a DTR-EGFP fusion protein	(71)
Inducible transient monocyte depletion of marginal metallophilic macrophages in the spleen and subcapsular sinus macrophages in the lymph nodes after DT administration	CD169-DTR-tg	Knock-in of the cDNA for the human DTR into the endogenous gene locus, behind the promoter for CD169.	(72)

expressed in specialized macrophage subsets, such as marginal zone macrophages (MZM), lymph node medullary macrophages, and microglia. SiglecH was also found in immediate precursors of pDCs (pre-pDCs) in the BM, which have the plasticity to differentiate into pDCs and cDCs (67, 101). Despite of SiglecH expression on above described other cell types Loschko et al. showed pDC specific antigen delivery in mice by using SiglecH as a target structure (102) suggesting the usability of SiglecH as a lead molecule for the generation of pDC specific transgenic animals. A side by side comparison showed a higher susceptibility to *Listeria monocytogenes* infection in DT-treated SiglecH-DTR-tg vs. CLEC4A-DTR-tg mice. This finding was attributed to the additional lack of MZM in SiglecH-DTR-tg mice after DT treatment which was not observed in CLEC4A-DTR-tg mice (67).

With the aim to specifically express the Cre recombinase in pDCs a BAC-tg "pDCre" mouse line was generated which expresses Cre under the control of the *Siglech* promoter (68). By crossing these mice with a reporter mouse line that indicates Cre activity via red fluorescent protein (RFP) expression the authors found ~30% of $SiglecH^{+}$ pDCs terminally labeled with RFP. Additionally, RFP expression was observed in a minor fraction of $SiglecH^{-}$ B-, T-, NK-, and NK-T cells and splenic cDCs and $CD11c^{int}$ BM cells suggesting that a small fraction of early lymphoid progenitors actively transcribes the SiglecH locus. Thus, the broader expression pattern of SiglecH should be considered when using SiglecH-DTR-tg mice to evaluate pDC functions *in vivo*.

Recently, a novel mouse model has been described in which type I IFN production is restricted to pDCs. In this knock-in model Irf7 expression is driven by the *Siglech* promoter ($Siglech^{Irf7/+}$). The $Siglech^{Irf7/+}$ mice were then backcrossed onto $Irf3^{-/-}$/$Irf7^{-/-}$ double knock-out mice which are deficient

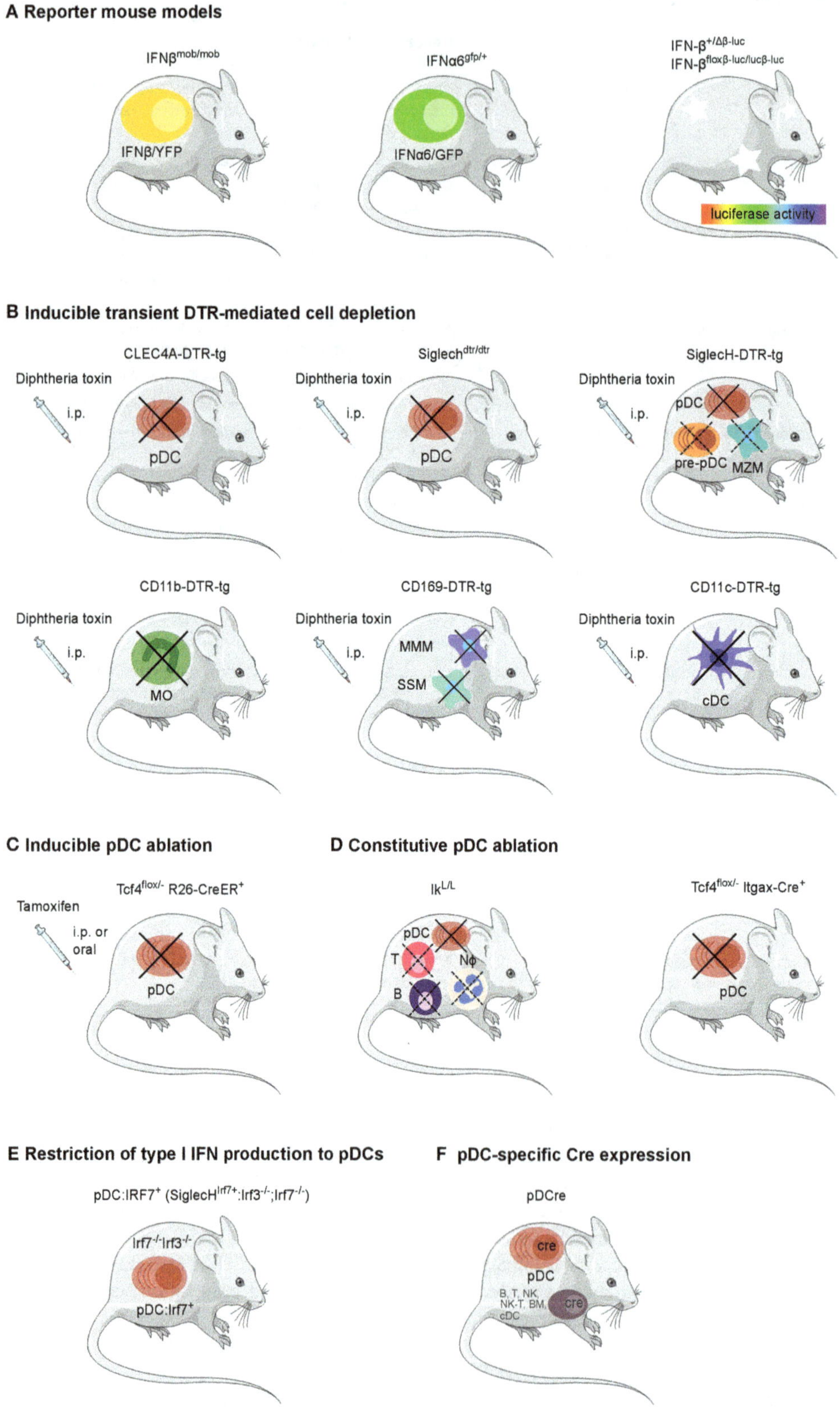

FIGURE 1 | Overview of genetically modified mouse models available to define the cellular source and impact of type I IFNs. **(A)** Reporter mouse models for the detection of type I IFN producing cells, **(B)** mouse strains for the transient DTR-mediated cell depletion and **(C)** inducible and **(D)** constitutive ablation of pDCs, **(E)** pDC-specific Cre expression, and **(F)** a mouse line with a restriction of the type I IFN production to pDCs have been employed in various infection settings *in vivo*.

(Continued)

FIGURE 1 | Each model system harbors specific advantages and caveats as further described in **Table 1**. B, B cell; BM, bone marrow cell; cDC, conventional dendritic cell; MMM, marginal metallophilic macrophage; MZM, marginal zone macrophage; MO, monocyte; NK, natural killer cell; Nφ, neutrophil; SSM, subcapsular sinus macrophage; T, T cell; pDC, plasmacytoid dendritic cell. The figure was created using Servier Medical Art according to Creative Commons Attribution 3.0 Unported License (https://creativecommons.org/licenses/by/3.0/). Changes were made to the original cartoons.

in type I IFN production. This yielded animals (referred to as "pDC:Irf7^{+}" mice) in which IRF7 signaling required for type I IFN expression is functional exclusively in pDCs (69). Additionally, in these mice an IRES site followed by coding sequences for Cre fused to the mutated ligand binding domain of the human estrogen receptor (ERT2) (103) was inserted behind the *Irf7* gene into the *Siglech* gene locus (69). Therefore, this mouse line can potentially be used in the future for tamoxifen inducible pDC specific Cre expression and thus pDC specific gene deletion when crossed to the respective floxed mouse lines.

Also, for other cell types than pDCs, the DTR-mediated depletion approach has been employed. In recent years, mice expressing the DTR under the control of the CD11b-, CD11c-, and CD169-promoters have been generated and successfully used for depletion of monocytes, cDCs, and CD169^{+} macrophage subpopulations such as MZMs and subcapsular sinus macrophages in the spleen and lymph nodes (70–72, 104–109).

In the following sections we will discuss approaches designed to define the type I IFN producing cell types in infection using the *in vivo* mouse models described above.

VIRAL INFECTIONS

In this chapter we will focus on more recent findings from *in vivo* models aimed at visualizing IFNα/β producing cell types and defining their contribution to the overall type I IFN production and their impact on the course of viral infections (**Table 2**). For a more generalized overview of the cellular sources of type I IFN in viral infections we kindly refer to an expert review by Swiecki et al. (127).

DNA Viruses

Findings on the cellular sources of type I IFN during relevant infection models for DNA viruses and the respective *in vivo* experimental strategies are highlighted in the following sections.

Human and Mouse Cytomegalovirus

Infection with the human cytomegalovirus (HCMV) causes mostly asymptomatic, latent infections in the immunocompetent host. In immunosuppressed individuals or newborns infected *in utero*, an infection with this virus can lead to severe illness and permanent organ damage. The murine cytomegalovirus (MCMV) exhibits high structural and biological similarity to HCMV and is thus widely used as a model system for antiviral immune responses (128). MCMV induces a biphasic type I IFN response, with peak expressions occurring at 8 h and 36–72 h p.i. which are triggered by the initial virus contact and viral particles entering the system after completion of the first viral replication cycle, respectively (110). Early type I IFN expression is independent of TLR signaling and predominantly generated by stromal cells infected by the virus (110). Using IFNβ$^{mob/mob}$ reporter mice, IFNβ production was detected in splenic pDCs as early as 6–12 h p.i. (59, 111). After *in vivo* depletion of pDCs by anti-CD317 or anti-Ly6G/C treatment IFNα serum levels were severely reduced 36 h after MCMV infection (18, 80, 81, 113). Under these conditions, however, other cell types secrete IL-12 and ensure sufficient IFNγ and NK cell responses leading to control of MCMV infection (18, 80). Of note, 44 h after MCMV infection IFNα serum levels in pDC depleted mice were no longer reduced as compared to untreated mice (113). Similar observations were made in Ik$^{L/L}$ mice that lack pDCs (61) or CLEC4A-DTR-tg mice that have been transiently depleted of pDCs (65, 113). Thus, transient type I IFN production at the first day of MCMV infection was pDC-dependent, while cells other than pDCs are responsible for the type I IFN levels measured at later timepoints, at least when relatively high inocula of MCMV are used. In contrast, at lower doses of MCMV which are presumably closer to a natural infection setting, pDCs can limit viral burden in the spleen and liver. Here, pDCs have been shown to promote NK cell activation and cytotoxicity in the early phase of MCMV infection (65). While it is well-established that pDCs sense the MCMV via the TLR9 and TLR7 mediated pathways (18, 80, 113, 129, 130), also the TLR3 and TLR2 pathways which are functionally used by other cells than pDCs have been shown to be involved in the induction of type I IFN production (104, 131, 132). These findings are in accordance with multiple observations that defects in MyD88 signaling have a more severe impact on anti-MCMV immune responses than TLR9 deficiency or pDC depletion (113, 129). So far, the identity of the non-pDC cell types involved in anti-MCMV type I IFN response remain incompletely defined.

Vaccinia Virus

One report indicated that vaccinia virus (VV) and to a lesser extend MCMV induce type I IFN in CD11c^{-} CD11b^{+} Ly6C^{+} inflammatory monocytes, but not macrophages or other types of DCs, in a TLR2 dependent way using IFNβ$^{mob/mob}$ reporter mice. Further, CD11b-DTR-tg mice depleted of monocytes exhibited increased viral titers in the liver and decreased serum levels of type I IFN after VV infection (104). This is similar to other studies using footpad infection of modified vaccinia virus Ankara (MVA) and pDC depletion in the CLEC4A-DTR-tg mouse model, where type I IFN levels in the draining lymph nodes were comparable to control mice indicating that pDCs are not required for mounting an intact type I IFN response after local infection with this dsDNA virus (118).

Adenovirus

The dsDNA adenovirus is used as a vector for the development of gene therapy applications but can also cause severe disease in immunocompromised individuals. By using CD11c-DTR-tg

TABLE 2 | Cellular sources of type I IFN production in viral infections *in vivo*.

Virus	Type I IFN producing cells	Model systems and assay methods	Observations in the absence of cell type
Murine cytomegalovirus (MCMV)	Splenic stroma cells	RT-PCR from *ex vivo* purified splenic stroma cells 8 h p.i. (110)	n.d.
	pDCs	FACS and immunohistochemistry of the spleen of IFNβ$^{mob/mob}$ reporter mice 12h p.i. (59, 111), ELISA from SN of *ex vivo* sorted Ly6G/C^{+} DCs 36h p.i. (112)	n.d.
		pDC depletion by anti-CD317 or anti-Ly6G/C (18, 80, 81, 113) or in CLEC4A-DTR-tg mice (65), pDC-deficient Ikaros$^{L/L}$ mice (113)	↓↓ IFNα serum levels until 36 h p.i.; ↑ Viral burden in the absence of pDCs only at low viral inoculation
	non-pDCs	pDC depletion by anti-Ly6G/C (113) or in CLEC4A-DTR-tg mice (65), pDC-deficient Ikaros$^{L/L}$ mice (113)	= IFNα serum levels starting 42 h p.i.
Herpes simplex virus-1 (HSV-1)	pDCs	Subcutaneous infection, pDC depletion by anti-CD317 or anti-Ly6G/C (82)	↑ viral titers in the draining LNs day 7 p.i.; type I IFN levels not measured
		i.v. infection, pDC depletion in Siglech$^{dtr/dtr}$ (66) or CLEC4A-DTR-tg mice (65, 114)	↑ Viral titers day 6 p.i. ↓ IFNα serum levels 6 h p.i.
	non-pDCs	Subcutaneous infection, pDC depletion in CLEC4A-DTR-tg mice (65, 114)	No viral titers measurable in the draining LNs day 7 p.i. in depleted or control mice, comparable CTL activation; type I IFN levels not measured
		i.v. infection, TLR3$^{-/-}$ mice (114)	↓ IFNα serum levels 12 h p.i.
Herpes simplex virus-2 (HSV-2)	pDCs	i.v. infection, pDC depletion by anti-CD317 (115, 116) or in CLEC4A-DTR-tg mice (65, 114)	↓ Serum IFNα levels 6/8 h p.i. ↑ viral titers in the liver ↓ survival
		Intravaginal infection, pDC depletion by anti-CD317 (117)	↓ Survival ↓ Local IFNα levels
	non-pDCs	Intravaginal infection, pDC depletion in CLEC4A-DTR-tg mice (65, 114)	= Survival = Local IFNα levels
Vaccinia virus (VV)	Inflammatory monocytes	Monocyte depletion in CD11b-DTR-tg mice (71, 104)	↓ Type I IFN serum levels ↑ Viral titers
Modified vaccinia virus Ankara (MVA)	Cells other than pDCs	Footpad infection, pDC depletion in CLEC4A-DTR-tg mice (118)	= Type I IFN levels in draining lymph nodes
Ectromelia virus	Inflammatory monocytes	i.p. infection, monocyte depletion by clodronate liposomes or pDC depletion by anti-BST2 mAb 927; *ex vivo* sorting of inflammatory monocytes and RT-PCR for type I IFN (119)	↓ Type I IFN levels in draining LN after clodronate treatment = Type IFN I serum levels after pDC depletion
Adenovirus and adenoviral vectors	cDCs	pDC depletion by anti PDCA-1 and cDC depletion in CD11c-DTR-tg mice (70, 105)	↓ Type I IFN serum levels after cDC depletion = Type IFN I serum levels after pDC depletion
influenza virus	pDCs	Intranasal infection, pDC-deficient Ikaros$^{L/L}$ mice (120)	= Virus titers = Weight loss as compared to WT; type I IFN levels not assessed
Thogoto virus	CD11b^{+} F4/80^{+} myeloid cells	i.p. infection, FACS analysis and luciferase of peritoneal exudate cells from IFNβ$^{mob/mob}$ and IFN-β$^{+/\Delta\beta-luc}$ reporter mice 6 and 18 h p.i. (59, 60, 121)	n.d.
Encephalomyocarditis virus (EMCV-D)	cDCs	cDC depletion in CD11c-DTR-tg mice (70, 106)	↓ Type I IFN serum levels ↑ Viral titers ↑ Diabetes
La Crosse virus, Rabies virus, Theiler's murine encephalomyelitis, vesicular stomatitis virus (VSV)	Astrocytes (to a lesser extent microglia/macrophages and neurons)	histology in IFN-β$^{+/\Delta\beta-luc}$ and IFN-β$^{flox\beta-luc/flox\beta-luc}$ immunostaining and RNA *in situ* hybridization (122, 123)	n.d.
Vesicular stomatitis virus (VSV)	pDCs	i.v. injection, pDCs depletion in CLEC4A-DTR-tg mice (65)	↓ IFNα serum levels ↑ viral titers 6 h p.i. but not at 12 or 24 h p.i.
	Macrophages, pDCs	s.c. infection, pDC depletion by anti-PDCA1 or LN macrophage depletion by clodronate liposomes or in CD11c-DTR-tg mice (70, 108)	↓↓ IFNα (90%) in macrophage depleted LNs ↓ IFNα (50%) in pDC depleted LNs

(Continued)

TABLE 2 | Continued

Virus	Type I IFN producing cells	Model systems and assay methods	Observations in the absence of cell type
La Crosse virus	Astrocytes, microglia, neurons	i.p. infection, histology in IFN-$\beta^{+/\Delta\beta-luc}$ and IFN-$\beta^{flox\beta-luc/flox\beta-luc}$ immunostaining and RNA *in situ* hybridization (122, 123)	n.d.
Newcastle disease virus (NDV)	pDCs, cDCs, macrophages, monocytes	systemic NDV infection, FACS analyses in Ifna6$^{gfp/+}$ reporter mice (46)	n.d.
	Alveolar macrophages	intranasal NDV infection, FACS analyses in Ifna6$^{gfp/+}$ reporter mice (46)	n.d.
Mouse hepatitis virus (MHV)	pDCs	i.p. infection, pDC depletion anti-CD317 or absence of pDCs in Itgax-Cre^{+} Tcf4$^{flox/-}$ mice (100, 124)	↓ IFNα serum levels ↑ Viral titers increased 48 h p.i.
Lymphocytic choriomeningitis virus (LCMV)	pDCs (and macrophages and cDCs)	WE, i.v. infection, 24–48 h p.i., Ifna6$^{gfp/+}$ reporter mice (76)	n.d.
	Non-pDCs	Armstrong and Clone13, i.v. infection, pDC depletion in CLEC4A-DTR-tg mice (65, 125)	↓ IFNα serum levels 16 h p.i. = At later timepoints
	Non-pDCs	Armstrong and WE, i.v. infection, pDC depletion by anti-Ly6G/C or absence of pDCs in Itgax-Cre^{+} Tcf4$^{flox/-}$ mice (81, 100)	= IFNα serum levels 48h p.i., virus cleared from organs day 8 p.i.
	Non-pDCs	Docile, i.v. infection, high dose, absence of pDCs in Itgax-Cre^{+} Tcf4$^{flox/-}$ mice (100)	Persistent serum virus titers
	Cells other than macrophages	WE, i.v., 48 h p.i., phagocyte depletion by clodronate liposomes, FACS analysis IFNβ$^{mob/mob}$ mice (94)	= IFNα serum levels
	Phagocytic cells	Armstrong, i.v., 48 h p.i., phagocyte depletion by clodronate liposomes (95)	↓↓ IFNα serum levels
	CD169^{+} macrophages	marginal metallophilic macrophage and subcapsular sinus macrophage depletion in CD169-DTR-tg mice (72, 107)	↓ Type I IFN from day 4 p.i. on, persistent virus titers
Chikungunya virus	pDCs	s.c. infection, restriction of type I IFN expression to pDCs in pDC:Irf7^{+} mice (69)	pDC:Irf7^{+} mice protected against infection, 100% lethal in IRF3/7 double deficient mice
Dengue virus	pDCs and cells other than pDCs	i.v. infection, restriction of type I IFN expression to pDCs in pDC:Irf7^{+} mice (69)	↓ Viral titers in pDC:Irf7^{+} as compared to IRF3/7 double deficient mice transiently 42–72 p p.i.
Respiratory syncytial virus (RSV)	pDCs	Intratracheal infection, pDC depletion by anti-CD317 (126)	↑ Viral titers ↑ Immunopathology in the lung day 9 p.i., ⌀ IFNα production in the lung

mice and anti-CD317 treatment to ablate cDCs vs. pDCs *in vivo* it has been shown that wildtype (WT) adenovirus as well as adenoviral vectors induce rapid IFNα/β production almost exclusively in splenic cDCs rather than in pDCs (105).

Herpes Simplex Virus

For Herpes Simplex Virus (HSV) local (subcutaneous or genital) as well as systemic (i.v.) infection models have been analyzed. After subcutaneous HSV-1 infection, pDCs were shown to provide type I IFN necessary for licensing of cDCs which in turn induce effective cytotoxic T cell responses. Here, mice depleted for pDCs by anti-Ly6G/C treatment displayed increased viral titers in the draining lymph nodes at day 7 p.i. as compared to controls (82). Similarly, in a genital HSV-2 herpes model, mice depleted for pDCs using anti-CD317 antibodies succumbed earlier to the infection and exhibited reduced local IFNα levels, while the Th1 response in draining lymph nodes developed normally (117). In contrast to findings from antibody-mediated depletion, in pDC depleted CLEC4A-DTR-tg mice neither differences in viral burden nor survival after vaginal HSV-2 infection was found nor were pDCs found to contribute significantly to antiviral CD8 T cell responses after subcutaneous HSV-1 inoculation (114). These contradicting findings have been explained by the antibody-mediated depletion of additional cell types other than pDCs in contrast to the more restricted depletion in the CLEC4A-DTR-tg genetic mouse model. On the other hand, it cannot be excluded that DTR mediated depletion is less effective and therefore a residual pDC activity retained after DT administration. Slight differences in the respective experimental settings might contribute as well as e.g. after antibody-mediated pDC depletion IFNα levels were measured in vaginal washes while in the genetic depletion model total protein amount was assessed in the vaginal and cervical tissue itself. As for MCMV, TLR3-expressing cells, such as CD8^{+} DCs or other hematopoietic and non-hematopoietic cells, are essential for type I IFN production in local HSV infection at later timepoints rather than pDCs (114).

After systemic challenge with UV-irradiated HSV in an early study immunohistological stainings for IFNα/β indicated that the majority of type I IFN producing cells in the spleen represent marginal metallophilic macrophages and to a lesser extend MZMs (133). However, IFNα levels were markedly reduced in pDC depleted Siglech$^{dtr/dtr}$ mice 6 h after i.v. infection with HSV-1 and viral titers were found increased in the spleen as compared to control animals pointing toward pDCs as the major type I IFN producers in this situation (66). Similar results were obtained in pDC depleted CLEC4A-DTR-tg mice, with the exception that no viral replication was detectable in the spleens of either DT-treated CLEC4A-DTR-tg or control mice (114). This discrepancy may reflect differences in the strains of HSV-1 used or differences in the promoters used to drive DTR expression (CLEC4A vs. SiglecH) with a slightly divergent expression pattern as discussed above. For systemic HSV-2 infections, results from antibody depletion and pDC ablation in CLEC4A-DTR-tg mice corresponded well since in both cases a reduction of IFNα serum levels were observed together with increased viral titers and reduced survival (114–116). Thus, similar to vaccinia virus the cell type responsible for the production of type I IFN in HSV infection may depend on the route of pathogen entry with pDCs controlling the infection once the virus has spread systemically.

Ectromelia Virus

Ectromelia virus (ECTV), a large DNA orthopoxvirus, is the causative agent of mousepox, the mouse homolog of human smallpox. ECTV causes systemic disease after s.c. infection of the footpad. *In vivo* it was shown by clodronate and anti-CD317 mediated depletion of monocytes vs. pDCs and *ex vivo* sorting and RT-PCR analyses that infected inflammatory monocytes are the major producers of type I IFN in the draining lymph nodes (119).

In summary, the cellular source for type I IFN production during DNA virus infection depends on the virus type itself, the dosage, timepoint as well as route of infection. Early after infection with MCMV pDCs are the primary source of type I IFN production capable of reducing virus titers at low concentrations of the virus. However, at later timepoints of infection CD8$^+$ DCs rather than pDCs become the key source of type I IFN production. In addition to pDCs, other cell types such as cDCs in adenovirus infection, metallophilic macrophages and MZMs during HSV exposure, stromal cells in MCMV infection and inflammatory monocytes in response to ECTV are an essential source of type I IFN.

RNA Viruses

A recent meta-transcriptomics survey defined 196 vertebrate-specific RNA virus species the majority of which is able to infect humans and cause diseases of varying severity (134, 135). At the moment only few mouse models are available to elucidate the host immune response to these viruses. In this chapter we summarize the *in vivo* model studies aimed at visualizing type I IFN producing cell types and defining their contribution to the type I IFN production and RNA virus control.

Newcastle Disease Virus

For systemic infections with RNA viruses, such as after i.v. inoculation with the paramyxovirus Newcastle disease virus (NDV), it has been shown that pDCs and also cDCs, macrophages, and monocytes, produced IFNα (46). Here, pDCs mount an antiviral type I IFN response in a viral replication-independent manner through virus recognition by TLR7 and the activation of the type I IFN positive feedback loop. Only in the absence of this type I IFN positive feedback, the virus infects and also replicates in pDCs. In this case, type I IFN induction occurs in pDCs via cytoplasmic RLHs (32). However, other ssRNA viruses have been reported to induce type I IFN expression in pDCs in a replication dependent manner (136, 137). Especially for vesicular stomatitis virus (VSV), the capture of the replicating virus in the autophagosome is required for its transfer to the TLR7 containing endosomal compartment (137). After local infection with NDV, here after intranasal infection, the IFNα-producing cells shifted from pDCs to alveolar macrophages and cDCs that utilize the RLH system for type I IFN induction (46).

Vesicular Stomatitis Virus

Upon s.c. VSV infection, draining LNs contained ~90% less IFNα when depleted of macrophages by clodronate liposomes. However, when pDCs were depleted by anti-CD317 treatment, IFNα levels induced by VSV were reduced only by half as compared to controls. It was concluded that infected CD169$^+$ subcapsular sinus macrophages produce IFNα, yet half of the type I IFN is produced by pDCs stimulated directly or indirectly by the infected macrophages (108). Later it was shown that CD169$^+$ macrophages in the spleen represent a compartment of enhanced viral replication (138). Thus, it is conceivable that CD169$^+$ macrophages potentiate the type I IFN response indeed indirectly via activating pDCs. When VSV was inoculated i.v. in CLEC4A-DTR-tg mice transiently depleted for pDCs, IFNα was found reduced and viral titers increased only at very early timepoints, again pointing to a rather transient role of pDCs in anti-viral immunity (65).

Dengue and Chikungunya Virus

For the distantly related arboviruses Dengue (DENV) and Chikungunya (CHIKV) virus it was recently shown that pDCs are sufficient to control these viruses via IRF7-regulated type I IFN responses in both systemic as well as local infection settings. In this report novel pDC:Irf7$^+$ mice were introduced in which IRF7-driven type I IFN production is restricted to pDCs and were compared to IRF3/7 double deficient mice that are completely devoid of type I IFN expression (69). After i.v. infection with DENV pDC:Irf7$^+$ mice exhibited a lower viral load than Irf3/7 double deficient mice. However, as compared to WT mice higher viral tiers were detected in pDC:Irf7$^+$ mice (69). After s.c. infection with CHIKV Irf3/7 double deficient mice succumb to the virus while 100% of pDC:Irf7$^+$ mice survive the infection exhibiting no overt clinical symptoms similar to WT mice. Early control of viremia in pDC:Irf7$^+$ mice was reduced as compared to WT but still improved as compared to Irf3/7 double deficient mice. Thus, analogous to findings from other virus infection models also for these RNA viruses, antiviral response mounted by pDCs controls infection once the virus spreads systemically.

La Crosse Virus, Rabies Virus, and Theiler's Murine Encephalomyelitis Virus

In infection models with RNA viruses exhibiting a specific tropism, pDCs play only a minor role. In the brain of mice infected with the ssRNA La Crosse virus, IFNβ production was assessed by the IFN-$\beta^{+/\Delta\beta-luc}$ luciferase reporter mouse model (60) and detected in astrocytes, microglia, and to a lesser extend also in infected neurons (122). This confirmed earlier findings where IFNα/β expression in these cell types after La Crosse virus infection was visualized by immunostaining and RNA *in situ* hybridization (123). Utilizing the conditional reporter activity of the IFN-$\beta^{flox\beta-luc/flox\beta-luc}$ mice it was shown for several neurotropic viruses such as rabies virus (RABV), Theiler's murine encephalomyelitis virus (TMEV), and VSV that astrocytes are the main producers of IFNβ after infection of the brain (139).

Encephalomyocarditis Virus

Another example for type I IFN expression by non-myeloid cells represent β-islet cells. The encephalomyocarditis virus (EMCV) strain D, an ssRNA picornavirus with tropism for the insulin-producing β cells of the pancreas, can induce diabetes and myocarditis in certain mouse strains. CD11c$^+$ cells in this model have been shown to be protective as DT treated CD11c-DTR-tg mice developed diabetes and exhibited increased viral titers in the pancreas, spleen, and heart associated with reduced type I IFN levels as compared to non-depleted controls (106).

Pneumonia Virus of Mice

Pneumonia virus of mice (PVM) infection led to a marked infiltration of pDCs and increased expression of type I IFN in WT but not TLR7- or MyD88-deficient mice. Transfer of TLR7-competent, but not TLR7-deficient pDCs led to a significantly diminished virus recovery in TLR7$^{-/-}$ animals on day 7 after infection with PVM indicating that TLR7-mediated signaling by pDC is required for appropriate innate responses to acute PVM infection (140).

Respiratory Syncytial Virus

For intratracheal infection with respiratory syncytial virus (RSV) it has been shown that anti-CD317 mediated depletion of pDCs completely abolished IFNα expression and protein levels in the lungs. This correlated with increased viral titers and exacerbated immunopathology of the lungs of pDC depleted mice (126). Thus, pDCs fulfill a substantial protective role during local RSV infection.

Influenza Virus and Influenza Virus-Like Orthomyxovirus Thogoto Virus

Initial *in vitro* studies showed that spleen cells from mice that were depleted for pDCs by anti-Ly6G/C injection did not produce IFNα in response to stimulation with inactivated influenza virus in contrast to splenocytes from untreated animals (18). IFNα production *in vitro* could be attributed to the CD317$^+$ CD11c$^+$ pDC population of sorted mouse spleen cells (86). However, *in vivo* intranasal infection with sublethal doses of influenza virus in pDC-deficient Ikaros$^{L/L}$ and WT mice revealed a similar course of disease, as determined e.g. by weight loss and viral titers (120). Thus, pDCs are able to produce type I IFN after stimulation by influenza but are dispensable for a successful antiviral immune response. Albeit, type I IFN levels *in vivo* were not assessed for this infection model.

For the influenza virus-like orthomyxovirus Thogoto virus (THOV) type I IFN production in the peritoneal cavity was mainly attributed to CD11b$^+$ F4/80$^+$ myeloid cells that was independent of the type I IFN receptor mediated feedback loop and coincided with the tropism of this virus (121).

Mouse Hepatitis Virus

After i.p. infection with Mouse hepatitis virus (MHV), pDC depletion by anti-CD317 was accompanied by severely diminished IFNα serum levels (124). The transient pDC depletion did not lead to lethality following the low-dose MHV infection used in this study. Nevertheless, initial viral titers in spleens were found increased more than 1,000-fold in pDC-depleted compared to control mice (124). Very similar observations were made in Itgax-Cre$^+$ Tcf4$^{flox/-}$ mice lacking pDCs. These mice show reduced serum IFNα levels and elevated viral loads in the liver and spleen (100). Thus, pDCs appear to be essential for type IFN I mediated protection against systemic infection with the prototypical acute cytopathic coronavirus MHV.

Lymphocytic Choriomeningitis Virus

Lymphocytic choriomeningitis virus (LCMV) infection is widely used to study acute as well as chronic infections. In an acute infection setting in Ifna6$^{gfp/+}$ reporter mice pDCs were found to be the major type I IFN producers after infection with the WE strain of LCMV. Additionally, few cDCs and macrophages specifically in the spleen exhibited GFP-reporter activity (76). Also, in IFN$\beta^{mob/mob}$ reporter mice macrophages could be excluded as major type I IFN producers and depletion of phagocytic cells by clodronate liposomes did not affect type I IFN serum levels (94). In contrast, another study using the Armstrong strain of LCMV reported severely reduced IFNα/β serum levels after clodronate treatment (95). Specifically, a small population of CD169$^+$ macrophages in the spleen and lymph nodes has recently been shown to release high amounts of type I IFN after LCMV infection. Selective depletion of these cells in CD169-DTR-tg mice resulted in reduced type I IFN levels from day 4 p.i. onward and persistent viral titers. As a consequence, CD169 depleted mice exhibited severe immunopathology and died quickly after infection (107). In line with this, production of serum type I IFN was not reduced in LCMV infected mice treated with the pDC depleting anti-Ly6G/C antibody as compared to those injected with control antibody (81). Also, in congenitally pDC-deficient Itgax-Cre$^+$ Tcf4$^{flox/-}$ mice, virus titers early after infection were comparable to WT controls confirming that pDCs are dispensable for the control of acute LCMV infection (100). Still, pDCs have been shown to be a transient source of type I IFN as pDC depletion in CLEC4A-DTR-tg mice led to reduced serum IFNα levels at 16 h p.i. with LCMV Armstrong or clone 13, but not at later timepoints (125). Contrasting the observations in acute LCMV infection, in a chronic infection setup using LCMV

Docile the virus persisted until day 53 in the blood of Itgax-Cre^{+} Tcf4$^{flox/-}$ mice while the virus was cleared between day 21 and 28 in WT mice. This was attributed to a failure of sufficient CD4^{+} and CD8^{+} T cell activation in the absence of pDCs and indicated that pDCs are essential for generating a functional adaptive immunity to chronic viral infections (100).

Taken together, pDCs are a major source of type I IFN and are required for type I IFN mediated protection against systemic infection in most of the RNA virus infections such as NDV, VSV, DENV, CHIKV, PVM, RSV, MHV, and LCMV. However, contribution of pDCs in type I IFN release and type I IFN mediated protection depends on the titer of the virus, time after infection, and the route of the infection. In addition to pDCs, other cell types such as cDCs, macrophages, and monocytes in NDV, macrophages in VSV, astrocytes, microglia, and neurons in La Crosse virus, astrocytes in RABV, TMEV, and VSV, β-islet cells and cDCs in EMCV, and cDCs and macrophages in LCMV infection significantly contribute to type I IFN production. Thus, similar to infection with DNA viruses, also after infection with RNA viruses pDCs are functionally involved in type I IFN production mostly early during infection but are dispensable for virus control during later stages of infection. In chronic infection, however, pDCs provide type I IFN to support and preserve T cell functions.

Retroviruses

HIV activates pDCs to produce high levels of IFNα most likely via activation of TLR7 (141). Also, it is assumed that type I IFNs are produced during HIV infection predominantly by pDCs as decreased IFNα production in HIV-infected patients correlates with numerical and functional deficiencies in circulating pDCs (142). A direct assessment of the contribution of pDCs to type I IFN levels in HIV-infection, however, has not been performed. Although type I IFNs are known to mediate antiviral immunity, there has always been caution toward a detrimental role of type I IFNs during HIV/AIDS because of their proinflammatory nature (11, 143, 144). Thus, many studies have shown that pDCs are a source of type I IFN in retroviral and other virus infections *in vivo*. However, additional cellular sources of type I IFN are required to fully control viral infections. In summary, pDCs are a known source of type I IFN in retroviral infection. However, the relative contribution of pDCs vs. other type I IFN producers to the overall type I IFN response and immune control or pathology after retrovirus infection, is not fully understood.

BACTERIAL INFECTIONS

While a considerable number of studies have been undertaken to define the cellular source of type I IFN and the functions of these cell types in viral infections, fewer data exist for non-viral infections. In bacterial infections, type I IFNs can act as activators of protective immune responses or mediate immunosuppressive functions leading to exacerbation of the infection. This ambivalent role of type I IFN has been reviewed recently (1, 11, 145). In this chapter we will focus on the efforts to clarify the identity and impact of type I IFN producing cells as knowledge on these has increased significantly paralleling the availability of newly developed mouse models.

Mycobacteria

It has been well established that CD4 T cells as well as secreted effector cytokines TNF, IL-12, and IFNγ exert protective functions in host resistance to the intracellular bacterial pathogen *Mycobacterium tuberculosis* (*Mtb*) (146). In contrast, the role of type I IFN during *Mtb* infection appears to promote infection instead of controlling infection. Type I IFNs downregulate IFNGR1 expression and thereby suppress IFNγ signaling (147, 148) and IFNAR-deficient mice displayed increased bacterial clearance to infection with *Mtb*, although bacterial growth in the lung was unaffected (149). In *in vitro* studies, BM-derived macrophages and DCs have been identified as a possible source of type I IFN in response to *Mtb* (149, 150). Also, human peripheral blood mononuclear cell (PBMC)-derived macrophages and especially DCs were shown to produce type I IFN after *in vitro* infection with *Mtb* (151, 152).

Similar to *Mtb*, IFNγ promotes antimicrobial activity against *Mycobacterium leprae* whereas type I IFNs contribute to pathogenesis (153). Here, PBMC-derived monocytes expressed IFNβ and IFN-stimulated genes including the immunosuppressive cytokine IL-10 during *M. leprae* infection *in vitro* (153). So far the cell type expressing type I IFN in the context of mycobacterial infections *in vivo* as well as definition of the functional impact of these cells await clarification.

Listeria monocytogenes

Type I IFN not only inhibits antibacterial signaling pathways and promotes infection in the case of mycobacteria. Also, *L. monocytogenes* has evolved mechanisms to activate the type I IFN pathway for the benefit of this intracellular pathogen. Mice deficient in IFNAR signaling are more resistant to systemic *L. monocytogenes* infection as compared to WT controls. Mechanistically, type I IFNs enhance susceptibility to systemic *Listeria* infection by reducing responsiveness to IFNγ, decreasing the number of pro-inflammatory myeloid cells, promoting the expression of proapoptotic genes, and enhancing T cell sensitivity to apoptosis (148, 154–156). Of note, in intragastric or foodborne infection with *L. monocytogenes* type I IFN receptor mediated signaling contributed positively to survival of infected mice or did not have an impact at all, respectively (157, 158). This emphasizes again, that the route of infection contributes significantly to differences in the impact of type I IFN in infection.

Four distinct cell types have been reported as sources for type I IFN production during systemic *L. monocytogenes* infection *in vivo* (**Table 3**). For one, a FACS-purified splenic cell population from infected mice that displays surface antigens typical of macrophages and not pDCs was identified as the main producer of type I IFN (159). Also, the apathogenic *Listeria* mutant lacking listeriolysin O which is unable to escape from the phagolysosome into the cytoplasm of the infected cell, does not stimulate IFNβ synthesis (164, 165). Later, Tip-DCs, an effector subtype of Mac-3^{hi} inflammatory monocytes, which produce TNF and iNOS were identified as the major IFNβ-producing cells *in vivo* in systemic *L. monocytogenes* infections using IFN$\beta^{mob/mob}$ and IFN-$\beta^{+/\Delta\beta-luc}$ reporter mice (160, 161). IFNβ-producing TiP-DCs harbored high bacterial loads and were located within the foci of infection in the splenic white pulp ideally positioned to activate T cells as well as NK cells via type I IFN (160). Bacterial loads in the spleen were severely increased in mice deficient in CCR2 and thus lacking TiP-DCs (162). Thus, this subtype of inflammatory monocytes has been attributed an important role in early containment of *L. monocytogenes* infection (162, 166). The overall role of TiP-DCs in this infection may therefore be ambiguous, having a regulatory function in controlling the balance between containment of infection and at the same time mediating detrimental effects of type I IFN on the host. Interestingly, in the spleens of *Listeria*-infected CCR2$^{-/-}$ mice increased levels of type I IFN were observed indicating that alternative cell types produce type I IFN in the absence of TiP-DCs which are triggered additionally by increased bacterial load. Along this line, a detrimental role for pDCs in controlling *L. monocytogenes* infection was demonstrated in *Siglech*$^{dtr/dtr}$ mice where ablation of pDCs caused significantly increased survival and decreased bacterial burden at day 3 p.i., while type I IFN levels themselves were not analyzed under these conditions (66). At earlier timepoints, however, anti-PDCA-1 mediated depletion of pDCs did not lead to a difference in bacterial load or levels of type I IFN in the spleen as compared to control animals (161). In one report, CD317^{+} SiglecH^{-} CD19^{+} B cells have been found to be able to induce IFNα after stimulation with heat-killed *L. monocytogenes* (163). *Ex vivo* isolated CD317^{+} SiglecH^{-} CD19^{+} B cells activated cytotoxic function of NK cells in an IFNα-dependent manner. *In vivo*, this B cell subset contributed positively to resistance to *L. monocytogenes* infection as Btk$^{-/-}$ mice deficient for B-cells and unable to generate CD317^{+} CD19^{+} B cells displayed increased susceptibility to *L. monocytogenes* infection, while adoptive transfer of CD317^{+} CD19^{+} B cells to Btk$^{-/-}$ mice normalized their resistance to *L. monocytogenes* infection (163).

TABLE 3 | Cellular sources of type I IFN production in *Listeria monocytogenes* infection *in vivo*.

Type I IFN producing cells	Model systems and assay methods	Observations in the absence of cell type
Macrophages	i.p. infection, RT-PCR for type I IFN from *ex vivo* FACS sorted cell populations (159)	n.d.
Tip-DCs	i.v. and i.p. infection, FACS analysis and histology in IFN$\beta^{mob/mob}$ and luciferase activity in IFN-$\beta^{+/\Delta\beta-luc}$ reporter mice (59, 60, 160, 161)	n.d.
Non-TiP-DCs	i.v. infection, TiP-DC deficient CCR2$^{-/-}$ mice (162)	↑ Bacterial load ↑ Type I IFN in the spleen
pDCs	i.p. infection, pDC depletion in *Siglech*$^{dtr/dtr}$ mice (66)	↑ Survival ↓ Proinflammatory cytokines
PDCA-1^{+} SiglecH^{-} CD19^{+} B cells	i.p. infection, B cell deficient Btk$^{-/-}$ mice (163)	↓ Survival

RT-PCR analyses from sorted cells, while no IFNα subtypes were detected (169).

In summary, type I IFN production has a detrimental effect for the host after infection with intracellular bacteria such as mycobacteria and *L. monocytogenes*. BMDCs and PBMC-derived DCs and macrophages are the responsible cell types for type I IFN production during mycobacteria infection. For *L. monocytogenes*, four cell types have been identified as type I IFN producers, namely macrophages, Tip-DCs, inflammatory monocytes, and B cells. In the case of extracellular bacteria, the cell types identified as type I IFN producers include macrophages and BMDCs. However, with the exception of the intracellular model organism *L. monocytogenes*, the knowledge on the cellular source of type I IFN in bacterial infection is rather scarce.

Extracellular Bacteria

As for intracellular bacteria also for extracellularly replicating bacterial pathogens type I IFN can either be detrimental or essential for host defense (145). Group B streptococci (GBS) are important neonatal pathogens and type I IFN receptor signaling is reported to contribute to host resistance against this pathogen (167). Mice i.p. infected with GBS express elevated levels of IFNβ and IFNα4 mRNA in the spleen. *In vitro*, GBS activated type I IFN expression in peritoneal macrophages, BM-derived cDCs and to a lesser extent also in macrophages, while pDCs were completely unable to produce type I IFN after GBS stimulation (167, 168).

In contrast to GBS, type I IFN induction in the mixed bacterial sepsis model of colon ascendens stent peritonitis (CASP) has been shown to have a detrimental effect on the host. Septic peritonitis induced in IFNAR$^{-/-}$ mice showed improved survival and bacterial clearance as compared to WT controls. Splenic CD11b^{+} CD11c^{-} macrophage-like cells could be identified as major producers of IFNβ *ex vivo* by

FUNGAL INFECTIONS

As for bacterial infections, the effect of type I IFN in mouse models for infections with pathogenic fungi has been reported as beneficial or detrimental for the host depending on the fungal species and the route of infection. Additionally, controversial results obtained from very similar infection settings have been explained by the possible impact of differences in the microbiome in the respective mouse colonies (1, 11). The cell type responsible for type I IFN production in fungal infections *in vivo*, however, awaits clarification. To our knowledge only for the important opportunistic fungal pathogen *Aspergillus fumigatus in vivo* studies in this direction have been undertaken. The type I IFN response triggered by *A. fumigatus* was analyzed initially in human pDCs isolated from PBMCs. When these cells were stimulated *in vitro* with *A. fumigatus* hyphae IFNα was detected in the supernatant (170). IFNAR$^{-/-}$ mice or mice depleted of pDCs by anti-CD317 treatment exhibited an increased susceptibility to pulmonary or i.v. infection with *A. fumigatus* conidia. A direct impact of pDC depletion on type I IFN levels *in vivo* after infection, however, has not been analyzed in this study (170). Therefore, the hypothesis that pDCs mediate their protective function in this fungal infection directly via type I IFN remains to be tested.

INFECTIONS WITH PROTOZOAN PARASITES

Infection with a wide variety of protozoan parasites can trigger type I IFN expression in mammalian hosts as reviewed recently (171, 172). For *Plasmodium*, *Leishmania*, and *Trypanosoma in vivo* infection models several studies have been carried out in the last few years which allowed the identification of cellular sources of type I IFN in response to intracellular parasite infections. This will be the focus of the following chapter and summarized in **Table 4**.

Plasmodium

Malaria is an important parasitic disease predominantly in tropical and subtropical African regions. It is caused by the protozoan parasite *Plasmodium* with *P. falciparum* being responsible for its most severe forms. In humans, malarial parasites are transmitted at sporozoite-stage by infected mosquitoes (182). The transmitted sporozoites rapidly travel to the liver, where they infect hepatocytes and initiate clinically silent but immunologically active liver-stage infection (171). Well-established *in vivo* mouse models include the lethal *Plasmodium yoelii* YM and *P. berghei* ANKA leading to high parasitemia and cerebral malaria (CM), respectively, after inoculation with *Plasmodium*-infected erythrocytes. Further, *P. chabaudi* is used as a chronic infection model. Various cellular sources for type I IFNs have been proposed after *Plasmodium* infection *in vitro* (182–184).

After inoculation with *P. berghei* ANKA infected erythrocytes *in vivo*, isolated splenic pDCs as well as CD8$^-$ cDCs expressed type I IFN (173, 174). Using anti-CD317 mediated pDC depletion and cDC depletion in CD11c-DTR-tg mice it was shown that cDCs but not pDCs are required for the induction of CM (173). Additionally, cDCs require IFNAR dependent signaling for systemic IFNα production in this model as indicated by substantially lower levels of serum IFNα in CD11c-Cre Ifnar1$^{fl/fl}$ mice, compared to those in infected *Ifnar1$^{fl/fl}$* littermate controls (174).

In contrast to the *P. berghei* ANKA model, *P. chabaudi* infection did not induce IFNα in splenic cDCs but rather in pDCs via the TLR9 sensing pathway (175). However, pDCs were not essential for parasite clearance in *P. chabaudi* infection (175). Direct *in vivo* analysis performed in IFNβ$^{mob/mob}$ reporter mice (59) revealed that in *P. chabaudi* infection about 75% of IFN producing cells are pDCs (176). In addition to pDCs, splenic red pulp macrophages (RPMs) can generate significant quantities of IFNβ in response to *P. chabaudi* infection. Contribution of both cell types to the type I IFN response in this system was defined by pDC depletion via anti-CD317 treatment and in RPM deficient SpiC$^{-/-}$ mice (176).

In the lethal malaria mouse model of *P. yoelii YM* infection, type I IFN enhances inflammatory blood leukocyte activation and lethal outcome (177). IFNβ$^{mob/mob}$ reporter mice indicated here that type I IFN is produced in high amounts by BM and blood pDCs and to lesser extent by tissue resident pDCs (177). Depletion of pDCs by anti-CD317 or using pDC specific CLEC4A-DTR-tg mice confirmed pDCs as the major cellular source of type I IFN in this severe malaria model (177, 178). However, depletion of pDCs also resulted in a slight but significant increase of parasitemia (178). Further, priming of pDCs by plasmodium activated CD169$^+$ macrophages was essential (177). It was proposed that in *in vivo* settings the low levels of secreted type I IFN produced by monocytes and macrophages prime pDCs for systemic production of type I IFN in malaria.

From data available so far, pDCs as well as cDCs and macrophage subtypes are the cell types responsible for the generation of the type I IFN response, depending on the *Plasmodium* species. Similar to LCMV, *Mycobacteria*, or *Listeria* infections (153, 156, 185), it is thought that early robust production of type I IFN in the first 24 h is essential to induce protective innate and adaptive immunity against *Plasmodium*, while late production of type I IFN impairs host anti-malaria immune responses by induction of negative immune regulators such as PD-L1 and IL-10 (178).

Leishmania

Leishmania spp. are transmitted to mammalian organisms by the bite of infected sand flies (186). The parasites preferentially infect macrophages, but can also be found in other cell types, such as fibroblasts, neutrophils, and DCs (172). Depending on the parasite species and strain *Leishmania* causes a mild to severe cutaneous, mucocutaneous or visceral leishmaniasis (171, 187). Increased production of type I IFN has been observed in local tissues and in the draining lymph nodes of *L. major* infected mice (187, 188). There are diverging reports about the role of type I IFN production in the control of parasite burden and development of disease pathology. Depending on the time course of infection and type I IFN induction it can exert detrimental or protective effects for the host in Leishmaniasis (189). Most of the studies addressing the cellular source of type I IFN in *Leishmania* infection were performed *in vitro*. For example, infection of murine macrophages with *L. major* or *L. amazonensis* lead to type I IFN production (188, 190). *In vitro* exposure of BM-derived as well as splenic pDCs to *L. major*, *L. infantum*, or *L. braziliensis* promastigotes induces release of IFNα and IFNβ in a TLR9-dependent manner (191). Intriguingly, the amounts of type I IFN produced in response to *Leishmania* spp. are comparable to the type I IFN levels produced in response to stimulation with CpG ODNs in these experiments (191). Recently *in vitro* exposure to the parasite *L. donovani* was reported to trigger IFNβ production in splenic B cells. Here, also high levels of type I IFN mRNA were detected in splenic B cells purified from *in vivo L. donovani* infected mice (179). Taken together, depending on the *Leishmania* subtypes, pDCs and B cells are the source of type I IFN when the cells are directly exposed to the pathogen *in vitro*. Information on the type I IFN producers *in vivo* remain

TABLE 4 | Cellular sources of type I IFN production in intracellular parasite infections *in vivo*.

Parasite	Type I IFN producing cells	Model systems and assay methods	Observations in the absence of cell type
Plasmodium berghei ANKA	pDCs and ($CD8^-$) cDCs	RT-PCR from *ex vivo* purified splenic pDCs and cDCs (173, 174)	n.d.
	cDCs	Phagocyte depletion by clodronate liposomes, cDC specific IFNAR deficiency in CD11c-Cre Ifnar1$^{fl/fl}$ mice	↓ IFNα serum levels
Plasmodium chabaudi	pDCs	RT-PCR for type I IFN from *ex vivo* purified splenic pDCs; pDC depletion by anti-CD317 (175)	= Parasite clearance
	pDCs and red pulp macrophages (RPMs)	FACS analysis in IFNβ$^{mob/mob}$ reporter mice, RT-PCR from *ex vivo* purified splenic cell populations, pDCs; pDC depletion by anti-CD317, RPM deficient SpiC$^{-/-}$ mice (176)	↓ IFNα levels in the spleen = Parasite clearance
Plasmodium yoelii YM	pDCs	FACS analysis in IFNβ$^{mob/mob}$ reporter mice (59, 177), pDC depletion by anti-CD317 (178) or CLEC4A-DTR-tg mice (65, 177)	↓ IFNα serum levels, ↑ Parasitemia
Leishmania donovani	B cells	RT-PCR for type I IFN from *ex vivo* purified B cells (179)	n.d.
Toxoplasma gondii	Intestinal epithelial or lamina propria cells	RT-PCR for type I IFN from *ex vivo* purified intestinal epithelial or lamina propria cells (180)	n.d.
	Inflammatory monocytes	RT-PCR for type I IFN from *ex vivo* depleted cell populations (181)	n.d.

scarce so far for this important protozoan parasite model but could be increased significantly making use of the now available mouse models.

Toxoplasma

Toxoplasma gondii is an intracellular protozoan parasite that has infected at least 50% of the human population. It causes severe toxoplasmosis in immune-suppressed patients. *T. gondii* can infect a wide range of warm-blooded animals, is able to invade any nucleated cell but survives outside of the mammalian host as well (171, 172). The gut epithelium is a strategic barrier to prevent or limit parasite dissemination upon oral infection with *T. gondii*. In the initial phase of oral *T. gondii* infection elevated IFNβ mRNA levels were observed in the small intestine. Intestinal epithelial cells (IECs) and cells from the lamina propria are the source of local IFNβ production in early infection as assessed by real-time PCR performed on cells isolated from infected mice (180). In *in vitro* infection, *T. gondii* has been reported to induce or suppress type I IFN induction depending on the host species, the cell type, and the parasite strain analyzed. One publication showed that BM-derived murine pDCs produce IFNα after infection with *T. gondii* (192). Murine pDCs recognized *T. gondii* profilin via TLR11 and TLR12 and produce type I IFN in a MyD88 dependent fashion (192, 193). In contrast to murine pDCs, human pDCs lack TLR11 and TLR12 and are unable to produce type I IFN despite of direct infection with *T. gondii*. Active infection with *T. gondii in vitro* rather functionally inactivates human pDCs (194). In particular macrophages and DCs serve as reservoirs of *T. gondii* infection and facilitate early dissemination (195). Most of the *Toxoplasma* strains tested are unable to induce type I IFN production in murine BM-derived macrophages after *in vitro* infection (196, 197). *T. gondii* mediated suppression of type I IFN expression has been reported also for monocytes, macrophages, and several DC subsets *in vitro* (181, 195, 196). On the other hand, few atypical *Toxoplasma* strains such as COUGAR and RUB can induce IFNβ production in murine BM-derived macrophages as well as in human skin fibroblasts in *in vitro* infection systems (196). In a physiological oral infection mouse model *ex vivo* isolated inflammatory monocytes in the gut-draining mesenteric lymph nodes were identified the major producers of IFNβ. The expression of IFNβ by inflammatory monocytes required phagocytic uptake of *T. gondii,* while active invasion did not trigger IFNβ induction (181). Thus, depending on the host species, the cell type, and the parasite strain, *T. gondii* may induce or suppress type I IFN production. Epithelial, skin fibroblasts, pDCs, macrophages and inflammatory monocytes here are known cellular sources of type I IFN. In *T. gondii* infection most of the knowledge about the cellular sources of type I IFN is deduced from *in vitro* experiments. Analysis of type I IFN reporter mouse models with and without ablation of different cell types is missing, so far.

Taken together, the major type I IFN producing cell types and their contribution to immunity against many protozoan parasites remain to be defined. To our knowledge, no direct study to elucidate the cellular sources of type I IFN in multicellular parasite such as helminth infections *in vivo* has been published. In order to understand the cellular sources of type I IFN and their relevance with regard to disease elimination in multicellular parasites such as helminths, type I IFN reporter mouse models and cell specific depletion models remain to be analyzed. As for the other pathogen types reviewed above, parasite numbers and the site of infection might influence the sensing pathway and cell type activated to produce type I IFN.

CONCLUDING REMARKS AND FUTURE PERSPECTIVES

In recent years the generation of novel animal models has remarkably advanced our understanding of the mode of action of IFNs and the cell type responsible for its production in the context of an infection. The existing knowledge does not allow to depict any cell type as a single cell type responsible for the entire type I IFN production in the course of any infection. Rather, depending on the type of infection a wide variety of cells have exhibited the capacity to produce type I IFN. Decisive factors for the type of cell initiating type I IFN production are the type and amount of pathogen and the site and stage of the infection. Additionally, the genetic background of the mouse model and its microbiome status contribute as well and need to be further analyzed.

Even though pDCs are more specialized than other cell types in type I IFN production, it is getting increasingly clear that *in vivo* their contribution to antiviral immunity and also to immune responses to bacterial, fungal, and parasitic infection exhibits restricted patterns in time of induction and duration. The importance of pDCs as the source of type I IFN early in virus infections does not hold true at later timepoints when other host cells take over as dominant producers of type I IFNs. The impact of pDCs also depends on the route of infection. While pDCs provide an important source of type I IFN in systemic infections, their requirement for I IFN-mediated antiviral immune responses in local tissues seems to be necessary only if other lines of defense are broken. However, there are exceptions to the rule as shown for local infections with MHV and HSV-2 where pDC-derived type I IFN in mice is critical for viral control and survival. Indeed, the limitation of pDC responses is caused by an upregulation of pro-apoptotic molecules and apoptosis induction in pDCs in a type I IFN-dependent manner during systemic viral infections (198). This has been suggested as a mechanism to prevent immunopathology due to sustained pDC-mediated type I IFN production. Besides pDCs, mainly macrophages, inflammatory monocytes and cDCs are able to mount significant anti-infectious type I IFN responses *in vivo*. Instead of a single specialized cell type, it is rather the orchestrated type I IFN expression by multiple cellular sources that ensures protective anti-infectious immune responses mediated by type I IFN. To elucidate synergisms and redundancies between the different type I IFN producing cells will be a topic of future studies.

Advanced single cell functional profiling and systems biology approaches will contribute significantly in the near future to identify the exact functions of specific cell types, even cell subtypes, in the different stages of an infection. The spatio-temporal interaction of the type I IFN producing cell with the pathogen and the immune cells that are activated by type I IFN could help to better dissect the diverse functions of type I IFN in the immune response at different stages of infection. Importantly, due to the severe side effects of type I IFN treatment, there is a dire need to better control its activity and thereby increase its beneficial net effect. Strategies such as modifying the affinity of type I IFNs or modulating its time of availability have been reviewed recently (199). These new approaches to develop and improve vaccination strategies and to define novel therapeutic leads for infectious diseases are urgently called for in a time where antibiotic resistances are projected to increase rapidly.

AUTHOR CONTRIBUTIONS

SA, RM-N, AS, LR, JA, and SS wrote the manuscript. SA, RM-N, and SS designed and generated tables. RM-N designed and generated the figure. All authors read and approved the final manuscript.

FUNDING

This work was supported by the Deutsche Forschungsgemeinschaft (RTG 2158 Natural products and natural product analogs against therapy-resistant tumors and microorganisms: new lead structures and modes of action), the Manchot Graduate School Molecules of Infection II and III, the Research Commission of the Medical Faculty of the University of Düsseldorf, Germany (30/2016) (to SS) and by the Deutsche Forschungsgemeinschaft (FOR 2107, AL 1145/5-2), the IZKF (Alf3/018/16), the DFG EXC 1003, Grant FF-2014-01 Cells in Motion–Cluster of Excellence, Münster, Germany, and the Alzheimer Forschung Initiative e.V. (14835) (to JA).

REFERENCES

1. McNab F, Mayer-Barber K, Sher A, Wack A, O'Garra A. Type I interferons in infectious disease. *Nat Rev Immunol.* (2015) 15:87–103. doi: 10.1038/nri3787
2. Kretschmer S, Lee-Kirsch MA. Type I interferon-mediated autoinflammation and autoimmunity. *Curr Opin Immunol.* (2017) 49:96–102. doi: 10.1016/j.coi.2017.09.003
3. Decker T, Muller M, Stockinger S. The yin and yang of type I interferon activity in bacterial infection. *Nat Rev Immunol.* (2005) 5:675–87. doi: 10.1038/nri1684
4. Hardy MP, Owczarek CM, Jermiin LS, Ejdeback M, Hertzog PJ. Characterization of the type I interferon locus and identification of novel genes. *Genomics.* (2004) 84:331–45. doi: 10.1016/j.ygeno.2004.03.003
5. Platanias LC. Mechanisms of type-I- and type-II-interferon-mediated signalling. *Nat Rev Immunol.* (2005) 5:375–86. doi: 10.1038/nri1604
6. van Pesch V, Lanaya H, Renauld JC, Michiels T. Characterization of the murine alpha interferon gene family. *J Virol.* (2004) 78:8219–28. doi: 10.1128/JVI.78.15.8219-8228.2004
7. Honda K, Takaoka A, Taniguchi T. Type I interferon [corrected] gene induction by the interferon regulatory factor family of transcription factors. *Immunity.* (2006) 25:349–60. doi: 10.1016/j.immuni.2006.08.009
8. Ivashkiv LB, Donlin LT. Regulation of type I interferon responses. *Nat Rev Immunol.* (2014) 14:36–49. doi: 10.1038/nri3581
9. Schneider WM, Chevillotte MD, Rice CM. Interferon-stimulated genes: a complex web of host defenses. *Annu Rev Immunol.* (2014) 32:513–45. doi: 10.1146/annurev-immunol-032713-120231
10. Trinchieri G. Type I interferon: friend or foe? *J Exp Med.* (2010) 207:2053–63. doi: 10.1084/jem.20101664
11. Stifter SA, Feng CG. Interfering with immunity: detrimental role of type I IFNs during infection. *J Immunol.* (2015) 194:2455–65. doi: 10.4049/jimmunol.1402794
12. Isaacs A, Lindenmann J. Virus interference. I. The interferon. *Proc R Soc Lond B Biol Sci.* (1957) 147:258–67. doi: 10.1098/rspb.1957.0048
13. Theofilopoulos AN, Baccala R, Beutler B, Kono DH. Type I interferons (alpha/beta) in immunity and autoimmunity. *Annu Rev Immunol.* (2005) 23:307–36. doi: 10.1146/annurev.immunol.23.021704.115843
14. Cella M, Jarrossay D, Facchetti F, Alebardi O, Nakajima H, Lanzavecchia A, et al. Plasmacytoid monocytes migrate to inflamed lymph nodes and

produce large amounts of type I interferon. *Nat Med.* (1999) 5:919–23. doi: 10.1038/11360

15. Ito T, Kanzler H, Duramad O, Cao W, Liu YJ. Specialization, kinetics, and repertoire of type 1 interferon responses by human plasmacytoid predendritic cells. *Blood.* (2006) 107:2423–31. doi: 10.1182/blood-2005-07-2709
16. Trinchieri G, Santoli D. Anti-viral activity induced by culturing lymphocytes with tumor-derived or virus-transformed cells. Enhancement of human natural killer cell activity by interferon and antagonistic inhibition of susceptibility of target cells to lysis. *J Exp Med.* (1978) 147:1314–33. doi: 10.1084/jem.147.5.1314
17. Trinchieri G, Santoli D, Dee RR, Knowles BB. Anti-viral activity induced by culturing lymphocytes with tumor-derived or virus-transformed cells. Identification of the anti-viral activity as interferon and characterization of the human effector lymphocyte subpopulation. *J Exp Med.* (1978) 147:1299–313. doi: 10.1084/jem.147.5.1299
18. Asselin-Paturel C, Boonstra A, Dalod M, Durand I, Yessaad N, Dezutter-Dambuyant C, et al. Mouse type I IFN-producing cells are immature APCs with plasmacytoid morphology. *Nat Immunol.* (2001) 2:1144–50. doi: 10.1038/ni736
19. Bjorck P. Isolation and characterization of plasmacytoid dendritic cells from Flt3 ligand and granulocyte-macrophage colony-stimulating factor-treated mice. *Blood.* (2001) 98:3520–6. doi: 10.1182/blood.V98.13.3520
20. Nakano H, Yanagita M, Gunn MD. CD11c(+)B220(+)Gr-1(+) cells in mouse lymph nodes and spleen display characteristics of plasmacytoid dendritic cells. *J Exp Med.* (2001) 194:1171–8. doi: 10.1084/jem.194.8.1171
21. Blasius AL, Beutler B. Intracellular toll-like receptors. *Immunity.* (2010) 32:305–15. doi: 10.1016/j.immuni.2010.03.012
22. Kawai T, Akira S. The role of pattern-recognition receptors in innate immunity: update on Toll-like receptors. *Nat Immunol.* (2010) 11:373–84. doi: 10.1038/ni.1863
23. Reizis B, Bunin A, Ghosh HS, Lewis KL, Sisirak V. Plasmacytoid dendritic cells: recent progress and open questions. *Annu Rev Immunol.* (2011) 29:163–83. doi: 10.1146/annurev-immunol-031210-101345
24. Kawai T, Sato S, Ishii KJ, Coban C, Hemmi H, Yamamoto M, et al. Interferon-alpha induction through Toll-like receptors involves a direct interaction of IRF7 with MyD88 and TRAF6. *Nat Immunol.* (2004) 5:1061–8. doi: 10.1038/ni1118
25. Guiducci C, Ott G, Chan JH, Damon E, Calacsan C, Matray T, et al. Properties regulating the nature of the plasmacytoid dendritic cell response to Toll-like receptor 9 activation. *J Exp Med.* (2006) 203:1999–2008. doi: 10.1084/jem.20060401
26. Honda K, Ohba Y, Yanai H, Negishi H, Mizutani T, Takaoka A, et al. Spatiotemporal regulation of MyD88-IRF-7 signalling for robust type-I interferon induction. *Nature.* (2005) 434:1035–40. doi: 10.1038/nature03547
27. Gururajan M, Jacob J, Pulendran B. Toll-like receptor expression and responsiveness of distinct murine splenic and mucosal B-cell subsets. *PLoS ONE.* (2007) 2:e863. doi: 10.1371/journal.pone.0000863
28. Iwasaki A, Medzhitov R. Toll-like receptor control of the adaptive immune responses. *Nat Immunol.* (2004) 5:987–95. doi: 10.1038/ni1112
29. Akkaya M, Akkaya B, Miozzo P, Rawat M, Pena M, Sheehan PW, et al. B cells produce Type 1 IFNs in response to the TLR9 agonist CpG-A conjugated to cationic lipids. *J Immunol.* (2017) 199:931–40. doi: 10.4049/jimmunol.1700348
30. Barchet W, Cella M, Odermatt B, Asselin-Paturel C, Colonna M, Kalinke U. Virus induced interferon alpha production by a dendritic cell subset in the absence of feedback signaling *in vivo*. *J Exp Med.* (2002) 195:507–16. doi: 10.1084/jem.20011666
31. Asselin-Paturel C, Brizard G, Chemin K, Boonstra A, O'Garra A, Vicari A, et al. Type I interferon dependence of plasmacytoid dendritic cell activation and migration. *J Exp Med.* (2005) 201:1157–67. doi: 10.1084/jem.20041930
32. Kumagai Y, Kumar H, Koyama S, Kawai T, Takeuchi O, Akira S. Cutting Edge: TLR-dependent viral recognition along with type I IFN positive feedback signaling masks the requirement of viral replication for IFN-{alpha} production in plasmacytoid dendritic cells. *J Immunol.* (2009) 182:3960–4. doi: 10.4049/jimmunol.0804315
33. Heil F, Hemmi H, Hochrein H, Ampenberger F, Kirschning C, Akira S, et al. Species-specific recognition of single-stranded RNA via toll-like receptor 7 and 8. *Science.* (2004) 303:1526–9. doi: 10.1126/science.1093620
34. Jurk M, Heil F, Vollmer J, Schetter C, Krieg AM, Wagner H, et al. Human TLR7 or TLR8 independently confer responsiveness to the antiviral compound R-848. *Nat Immunol.* (2002) 3:499. doi: 10.1038/ni0602-499
35. Gorden KK, Qiu XX, Binsfeld CC, Vasilakos JP, Alkan SS. Cutting edge: activation of murine TLR8 by a combination of imidazoquinoline immune response modifiers and polyT oligodeoxynucleotides. *J Immunol.* (2006) 177:6584–7. doi: 10.4049/jimmunol.177.10.6584
36. Martinez J, Huang X, Yang Y. Toll-like receptor 8-mediated activation of murine plasmacytoid dendritic cells by vaccinia viral DNA. *Proc Natl Acad Sci USA.* (2010) 107:6442–7. doi: 10.1073/pnas.0913291107
37. Oshiumi H, Matsumoto M, Funami K, Akazawa T, Seya T. TICAM-1, an adaptor molecule that participates in Toll-like receptor 3-mediated interferon-beta induction. *Nat Immunol.* (2003) 4:161–7. doi: 10.1038/ni886
38. Yamamoto M, Sato S, Hemmi H, Hoshino K, Kaisho T, Sanjo H, et al. Role of adaptor TRIF in the MyD88-independent toll-like receptor signaling pathway. *Science.* (2003) 301:640–3. doi: 10.1126/science.1087262
39. Jelinek I, Leonard JN, Price GE, Brown KN, Meyer-Manlapat A, Goldsmith PK, et al. TLR3-specific double-stranded RNA oligonucleotide adjuvants induce dendritic cell cross-presentation, CTL responses, and antiviral protection. *J Immunol.* (2011) 186:2422–9. doi: 10.4049/jimmunol.1002845
40. Azuma M, Ebihara T, Oshiumi H, Matsumoto M, Seya T. Cross-priming for antitumor CTL induced by soluble Ag + polyI:C depends on the TICAM-1 pathway in mouse CD11c(+)/CD8alpha(+) dendritic cells. *Oncoimmunology.* (2012) 1:581–92. doi: 10.4161/onci.19893
41. Tatematsu M, Nishikawa F, Seya T, Matsumoto M. Toll-like receptor 3 recognizes incomplete stem structures in single-stranded viral RNA. *Nat Commun.* (2013) 4:1833. doi: 10.1038/ncomms2857
42. Matsumoto M, Funami K, Tanabe M, Oshiumi H, Shingai M, Seto Y, et al. Subcellular localization of Toll-like receptor 3 in human dendritic cells. *J Immunol.* (2003) 171:3154–62. doi: 10.4049/jimmunol.171.6.3154
43. Akira S, Uematsu S, Takeuchi O. Pathogen recognition and innate immunity. *Cell.* (2006) 124:783–801. doi: 10.1016/j.cell.2006.02.015
44. Vaure C, Liu Y. A comparative review of toll-like receptor 4 expression and functionality in different animal species. *Front Immunol.* (2014) 5:316. doi: 10.3389/fimmu.2014.00316
45. Barchet W, Krug A, Cella M, Newby C, Fischer JA, Dzionek A, et al. Dendritic cells respond to influenza virus through TLR7- and PKR-independent pathways. *Eur J Immunol.* (2005) 35:236–42. doi: 10.1002/eji.200425583
46. Kumagai Y, Takeuchi O, Kato H, Kumar H, Matsui K, Morii E, et al. Alveolar macrophages are the primary interferon-alpha producer in pulmonary infection with RNA viruses. *Immunity.* (2007) 27:240–52. doi: 10.1016/j.immuni.2007.07.013
47. Wu J, Chen ZJ. Innate immune sensing and signaling of cytosolic nucleic acids. *Annu Rev Immunol.* (2014) 32:461–88. doi: 10.1146/annurev-immunol-032713-120156
48. Kumar H, Kawai T, Kato H, Sato S, Takahashi K, Coban C, et al. Essential role of IPS-1 in innate immune responses against RNA viruses. *J Exp Med.* (2006) 203:1795–803. doi: 10.1084/jem.20060792
49. Takeuchi O, Akira S. MDA5/RIG-I and virus recognition. *Curr Opin Immunol.* (2008) 20:17–22. doi: 10.1016/j.coi.2008.01.002
50. Reikine S, Nguyen JB, Modis Y. Pattern recognition and signaling mechanisms of RIG-I and MDA5. *Front Immunol.* (2014) 5:342. doi: 10.3389/fimmu.2014.00342
51. Stetson DB, Medzhitov R. Recognition of cytosolic DNA activates an IRF3-dependent innate immune response. *Immunity.* (2006) 24:93–103. doi: 10.1016/j.immuni.2005.12.003
52. Holm CK, Paludan SR, Fitzgerald KA. DNA recognition in immunity and disease. *Curr Opin Immunol.* (2013) 25:13–8. doi: 10.1016/j.coi.2012.12.006
53. Sun L, Wu J, Du F, Chen X, Chen ZJ. Cyclic GMP-AMP synthase is a cytosolic DNA sensor that activates the type I interferon pathway. *Science.* (2013) 339:786–91. doi: 10.1126/science.1232458
54. Paludan SR, Bowie AG. Immune sensing of DNA. *Immunity.* (2013) 38:870–80. doi: 10.1016/j.immuni.2013.05.004

55. Takaoka A, Wang Z, Choi MK, Yanai H, Negishi H, Ban T, et al. DAI (DLM-1/ZBP1) is a cytosolic DNA sensor and an activator of innate immune response. *Nature.* (2007) 448:501–5. doi: 10.1038/nature06013
56. Unterholzner L, Keating SE, Baran M, Horan KA, Jensen SB, Sharma S, et al. IFI16 is an innate immune sensor for intracellular DNA. *Nat Immunol.* (2010) 11:997–1004. doi: 10.1038/ni.1932
57. Ablasser A, Goldeck M, Cavlar T, Deimling T, Witte G, Rohl I, et al. cGAS produces a 2'-5'-linked cyclic dinucleotide second messenger that activates STING. *Nature.* (2013) 498:380–4. doi: 10.1038/nature12306
58. Crowl JT, Gray EE, Pestal K, Volkman HE, Stetson DB. Intracellular nucleic acid detection in autoimmunity. *Annu Rev Immunol.* (2017) 35:313–36. doi: 10.1146/annurev-immunol-051116-052331
59. Scheu S, Dresing P, Locksley RM. Visualization of IFNbeta production by plasmacytoid versus conventional dendritic cells under specific stimulation conditions *in vivo*. *Proc Natl Acad Sci USA.* (2008) 105:20416–21. doi: 10.1073/pnas.0808537105
60. Lienenklaus S, Cornitescu M, Zietara N, Lyszkiewicz M, Gekara N, Jablonska J, et al. Novel reporter mouse reveals constitutive and inflammatory expression of IFN-beta *in vivo*. *J Immunol.* (2009) 183:3229–36. doi: 10.4049/jimmunol.0804277
61. Allman D, Dalod M, Asselin-Paturel C, Delale T, Robbins SH, Trinchieri G, et al. Ikaros is required for plasmacytoid dendritic cell differentiation. *Blood.* (2006) 108:4025–34. doi: 10.1182/blood-2006-03-007757
62. Kirstetter P, Thomas M, Dierich A, Kastner P, Chan S. Ikaros is critical for B cell differentiation and function. *Eur J Immunol.* (2002) 32:720–30. doi: 10.1002/1521-4141(200203)32:3<720::AID-IMMU720>3.0.CO;2-P
63. Caton ML, Smith-Raska MR, Reizis B. Notch-RBP-J signaling controls the homeostasis of CD8- dendritic cells in the spleen. *J Exp Med.* (2007) 204:1653–64. doi: 10.1084/jem.20062648
64. Cisse B, Caton ML, Lehner M, Maeda T, Scheu S, Locksley R, et al. Transcription factor E2-2 is an essential and specific regulator of plasmacytoid dendritic cell development. *Cell.* (2008) 135:37–48. doi: 10.1016/j.cell.2008.09.016
65. Swiecki M, Gilfillan S, Vermi W, Wang Y, Colonna M. Plasmacytoid dendritic cell ablation impacts early interferon responses and antiviral NK and CD8(+) T cell accrual. *Immunity.* (2010) 33:955–66. doi: 10.1016/j.immuni.2010.11.020
66. Takagi H, Fukaya T, Eizumi K, Sato Y, Sato K, Shibazaki A, et al. Plasmacytoid dendritic cells are crucial for the initiation of inflammation and T cell immunity *in vivo*. *Immunity.* (2011) 35:958–71. doi: 10.1016/j.immuni.2011.10.014
67. Swiecki M, Wang Y, Riboldi E, Kim AH, Dzutsev A, Gilfillan S, et al. Cell depletion in mice that express diphtheria toxin receptor under the control of SiglecH encompasses more than plasmacytoid dendritic cells. *J Immunol.* (2014) 192:4409–16. doi: 10.4049/jimmunol.1303135
68. Puttur F, Arnold-Schrauf C, Lahl K, Solmaz G, Lindenberg M, Mayer CT, et al. Absence of Siglec-H in MCMV infection elevates interferon alpha production but does not enhance viral clearance. *PLoS Pathog.* (2013) 9:e1003648. doi: 10.1371/journal.ppat.1003648
69. Webster B, Werneke SW, Zafirova B, This S, Coleon S, Decembre E, et al. Plasmacytoid dendritic cells control dengue and Chikungunya virus infections via IRF7-regulated interferon responses. *Elife.* (2018) 7:e34273. doi: 10.7554/eLife.34273
70. Jung S, Unutmaz D, Wong P, Sano G, De los Santos K, Sparwasser T, et al. *In vivo* depletion of CD11c+ dendritic cells abrogates priming of CD8+ T cells by exogenous cell-associated antigens. *Immunity.* (2002) 17:211–20. doi: 10.1016/S1074-7613(02)00365-5
71. Cailhier JF, Partolina M, Vuthoori S, Wu S, Ko K, Watson S, et al. Conditional macrophage ablation demonstrates that resident macrophages initiate acute peritoneal inflammation. *J Immunol.* (2005) 174:2336–42. doi: 10.4049/jimmunol.174.4.2336
72. Miyake Y, Asano K, Kaise H, Uemura M, Nakayama M, Tanaka M. Critical role of macrophages in the marginal zone in the suppression of immune responses to apoptotic cell-associated antigens. *J Clin Invest.* (2007) 117:2268–78. doi: 10.1172/JCI31990
73. Erlandsson L, Blumenthal R, Eloranta ML, Engel H, Alm G, Weiss S, et al. Interferon-beta is required for interferon-alpha production in mouse fibroblasts. *Curr Biol.* (1998) 8:223–6. doi: 10.1016/S0960-9822(98)70086-7
74. Deonarain R, Alcami A, Alexiou M, Dallman MJ, Gewert DR, Porter AC. Impaired antiviral response and alpha/beta interferon induction in mice lacking beta interferon. *J Virol.* (2000) 74:3404–9. doi: 10.1128/JVI.74.7.3404-3409.2000
75. Takaoka A, Mitani Y, Suemori H, Sato M, Yokochi T, Noguchi S, et al. Cross talk between interferon-gamma and -alpha/beta signaling components in caveolar membrane domains. *Science.* (2000) 288:2357–60. doi: 10.1126/science.288.5475.2357
76. Jung A, Kato H, Kumagai Y, Kumar H, Kawai T, Takeuchi O, et al. Lymphocytoid choriomeningitis virus activates plasmacytoid dendritic cells and induces a cytotoxic T-cell response via MyD88. *J Virol.* (2008) 82:196–206. doi: 10.1128/JVI.01640-07
77. Frenz T, Graalmann L, Detje CN, Doring M, Grabski E, Scheu S, et al. Independent of plasmacytoid dendritic cell (pDC) infection, pDC triggered by virus-infected cells mount enhanced type I IFN responses of different composition as opposed to pDC stimulated with free virus. *J Immunol.* (2014) 193:2496–503. doi: 10.4049/jimmunol.1400215
78. Reizis B. Plasmacytoid dendritic cells: development, regulation, and function. *Immunity.* (2019) 50:37–50. doi: 10.1016/j.immuni.2018.12.027
79. Swiecki M, Colonna M. Unraveling the functions of plasmacytoid dendritic cells during viral infections, autoimmunity, and tolerance. *Immunol Rev.* (2010) 234:142–62. doi: 10.1111/j.0105-2896.2009.00881.x
80. Krug A, French AR, Barchet W, Fischer JA, Dzionek A, Pingel JT, et al. TLR9-dependent recognition of MCMV by IPC and DC generates coordinated cytokine responses that activate antiviral NK cell function. *Immunity.* (2004) 21:107–19. doi: 10.1016/j.immuni.2004.06.007
81. Dalod M, Salazar-Mather TP, Malmgaard L, Lewis C, Asselin-Paturel C, Briere F, et al. Interferon alpha/beta and interleukin 12 responses to viral infections: pathways regulating dendritic cell cytokine expression *in vivo*. *J Exp Med.* (2002) 195:517–28. doi: 10.1084/jem.20011672
82. Yoneyama H, Matsuno K, Toda E, Nishiwaki T, Matsuo N, Nakano A, et al. Plasmacytoid DCs help lymph node DCs to induce anti-HSV CTLs. *J Exp Med.* (2005) 202:425–35. doi: 10.1084/jem.20041961
83. Kuwajima S, Sato T, Ishida K, Tada H, Tezuka H, Ohteki T. Interleukin 15-dependent crosstalk between conventional and plasmacytoid dendritic cells is essential for CpG-induced immune activation. *Nat Immunol.* (2006) 7:740–6. doi: 10.1038/ni1348
84. Goubier A, Dubois B, Gheit H, Joubert G, Villard-Truc F, Asselin-Paturel C, et al. Plasmacytoid dendritic cells mediate oral tolerance. *Immunity.* (2008) 29:464–75. doi: 10.1016/j.immuni.2008.06.017
85. Shen H, Iwasaki A. A crucial role for plasmacytoid dendritic cells in antiviral protection by CpG ODN-based vaginal microbicide. *J Clin Invest.* (2006) 116:2237–43. doi: 10.1172/JCI28681
86. Asselin-Paturel C, Brizard G, Pin JJ, Briere F, Trinchieri G. Mouse strain differences in plasmacytoid dendritic cell frequency and function revealed by a novel monoclonal antibody. *J Immunol.* (2003) 171:6466–77. doi: 10.4049/jimmunol.171.12.6466
87. Loschko J, Schlitzer A, Dudziak D, Drexler I, Sandholzer N, Bourquin C, et al. Antigen delivery to plasmacytoid dendritic cells via BST2 induces protective T cell-mediated immunity. *J Immunol.* (2011) 186:6718–25. doi: 10.4049/jimmunol.1004029
88. Fleming TJ, Fleming ML, Malek TR. Selective expression of Ly-6G on myeloid lineage cells in mouse bone marrow. RB6-8C5 mAb to granulocyte-differentiation antigen (Gr-1) detects members of the Ly-6 family. *J Immunol.* (1993) 151:2399–408.
89. Jutila MA, Kroese FG, Jutila KL, Stall AM, Fiering S, Herzenberg LA, et al. Ly-6C is a monocyte/macrophage and endothelial cell differentiation antigen regulated by interferon-gamma. *Eur J Immunol.* (1988) 18:1819–26. doi: 10.1002/eji.1830181125
90. Sato N, Yahata T, Santa K, Ohta A, Ohmi Y, Habu S, et al. Functional characterization of NK1.1 + Ly-6C+ cells. *Immunol Lett.* (1996) 54:5–9. doi: 10.1016/S0165-2478(96)02632-6
91. Takahama Y, Sharrow SO, Singer A. Expression of an unusual T cell receptor (TCR)-V beta repertoire by Ly-6C+ subpopulations of CD4+ and/or CD8+ thymocytes. Evidence for a developmental relationship between Ly-6C+ thymocytes and CD4-CD8-TCR-alpha beta+ thymocytes. *J Immunol.* (1991) 147:2883–91.

92. Wrammert J, Kallberg E, Agace WW, Leanderson T. Ly6C expression differentiates plasma cells from other B cell subsets in mice. *Eur J Immunol.* (2002) 32:97–103. doi: 10.1002/1521-4141(200201)32:1<97::AID-IMMU97>3.0.CO;2-Y
93. Blasius AL, Giurisato E, Cella M, Schreiber RD, Shaw AS, Colonna M. Bone marrow stromal cell antigen 2 is a specific marker of type I IFN-producing cells in the naive mouse, but a promiscuous cell surface antigen following IFN stimulation. *J Immunol.* (2006) 177:3260–5. doi: 10.4049/jimmunol.177.5.3260
94. Lang PA, Recher M, Honke N, Scheu S, Borkens S, Gailus N, et al. Tissue macrophages suppress viral replication and prevent severe immunopathology in an interferon-I-dependent manner in mice. *Hepatology.* (2010) 52:25–32. doi: 10.1002/hep.23640
95. Louten J, van Rooijen N, Biron CA. Type 1 IFN deficiency in the absence of normal splenic architecture during lymphocytic choriomeningitis virus infection. *J Immunol.* (2006) 177:3266–72. doi: 10.4049/jimmunol.177.5.3266
96. Dumortier A, Jeannet R, Kirstetter P, Kleinmann E, Sellars M, dos Santos NR, et al. Notch activation is an early and critical event during T-Cell leukemogenesis in Ikaros-deficient mice. *Mol Cell Biol.* (2006) 26:209–20. doi: 10.1128/MCB.26.1.209-220.2006
97. Dumortier A, Kirstetter P, Kastner P, Chan S. Ikaros regulates neutrophil differentiation. *Blood.* (2003) 101:2219–26. doi: 10.1182/blood-2002-05-1336
98. Zhuang Y, Cheng P, Weintraub H. B-lymphocyte development is regulated by the combined dosage of three basic helix-loop-helix genes, E2A, E2-2, and HEB. *Mol Cell Biol.* (1996) 16:2898–905. doi: 10.1128/MCB.16.6.2898
99. Bergqvist I, Eriksson M, Saarikettu J, Eriksson B, Corneliussen B, Grundstrom T, et al. The basic helix-loop-helix transcription factor E2-2 is involved in T lymphocyte development. *Eur J Immunol.* (2000) 30:2857–63. doi: 10.1002/1521-4141(200010)30:10<2857::AID-IMMU2857>3.0.CO;2-G
100. Cervantes-Barragan L, Lewis KL, Firner S, Thiel V, Hugues S, Reith W, et al. Plasmacytoid dendritic cells control T-cell response to chronic viral infection. *Proc Natl Acad Sci USA.* (2012) 109:3012–7. doi: 10.1073/pnas.1117359109
101. Schlitzer A, Heiseke AF, Einwachter H, Reindl W, Schiemann M, Manta CP, et al. Tissue-specific differentiation of a circulating CCR9-pDC-like common dendritic cell precursor. *Blood.* (2012) 119:6063–71. doi: 10.1182/blood-2012-03-418400
102. Loschko J, Heink S, Hackl D, Dudziak D, Reindl W, Korn T, et al. Antigen targeting to plasmacytoid dendritic cells via Siglec-H inhibits Th cell dependent autoimmunity. *J Immunol.* (2011) 187:6346–56. doi: 10.4049/jimmunol.1102307
103. Feil R, Wagner J, Metzger D, Chambon P. Regulation of Cre recombinase activity by mutated estrogen receptor ligand-binding domains. *Biochem Biophys Res Commun.* (1997) 237:752–7. doi: 10.1006/bbrc.1997.7124
104. Barbalat R, Lau L, Locksley RM, Barton GM. Toll-like receptor 2 on inflammatory monocytes induces type I interferon in response to viral but not bacterial ligands. *Nat Immunol.* (2009) 10:1200–7. doi: 10.1038/ni.1792
105. Fejer G, Drechsel L, Liese J, Schleicher U, Ruzsics Z, Imelli N, et al. Key role of splenic myeloid DCs in the IFN-alphabeta response to adenoviruses *in vivo*. *PLoS Pathog.* (2008) 4:e1000208. doi: 10.1371/journal.ppat.1000208
106. McCartney SA, Vermi W, Lonardi S, Rossini C, Otero K, Calderon B, et al. RNA sensor-induced type I IFN prevents diabetes caused by a beta cell-tropic virus in mice. *J Clin Invest.* (2011) 121:1497–507. doi: 10.1172/JCI44005
107. Shaabani N, Duhan V, Khairnar V, Gassa A, Ferrer-Tur R, Haussinger D, et al. CD169(+) macrophages regulate PD-L1 expression via type I interferon and thereby prevent severe immunopathology after LCMV infection. *Cell Death Dis.* (2016) 7:e2446. doi: 10.1038/cddis.2016.350
108. Iannacone M, Moseman EA, Tonti E, Bosurgi L, Junt T, Henrickson SE, et al. Subcapsular sinus macrophages prevent CNS invasion on peripheral infection with a neurotropic virus. *Nature.* (2010) 465:1079–83. doi: 10.1038/nature09118
109. Sapoznikov A, Fischer JA, Zaft T, Krauthgamer R, Dzionek A, Jung S. Organ-dependent in vivo priming of naive CD4+, but not CD8+, T cells by plasmacytoid dendritic cells. *J Exp Med.* (2007) 204:1923–33. doi: 10.1084/jem.20062373
110. Schneider K, Loewendorf A, De Trez C, Fulton J, Rhode A, Shumway H, et al. Lymphotoxin-mediated crosstalk between B cells and splenic stroma promotes the initial type I interferon response to cytomegalovirus. *Cell Host Microbe.* (2008) 3:67–76. doi: 10.1016/j.chom.2007.12.008
111. Bauer J, Dress RJ, Schulze A, Dresing P, Ali S, Deenen R, et al. Cutting edge: IFN-beta expression in the spleen is restricted to a subpopulation of plasmacytoid dendritic cells exhibiting a specific immune modulatory transcriptome signature. *J Immunol.* (2016) 196:4447–51. doi: 10.4049/jimmunol.1500383
112. Dalod M, Hamilton T, Salomon R, Salazar-Mather TP, Henry SC, Hamilton JD, et al. Dendritic cell responses to early murine cytomegalovirus infection: subset functional specialization and differential regulation by interferon alpha/beta. *J Exp Med.* (2003) 197:885–98. doi: 10.1084/jem.20021522
113. Delale T, Paquin A, Asselin-Paturel C, Dalod M, Brizard G, Bates EE, et al. MyD88-dependent and -independent murine cytomegalovirus sensing for IFN-alpha release and initiation of immune responses *in vivo*. *J Immunol.* (2005) 175:6723–32. doi: 10.4049/jimmunol.175.10.6723
114. Swiecki M, Wang Y, Gilfillan S, Colonna M. Plasmacytoid dendritic cells contribute to systemic but not local antiviral responses to HSV infections. *PLoS Pathog.* (2013) 9:e1003728. doi: 10.1371/journal.ppat.1003728
115. Stout-Delgado HW, Du W, Shirali AC, Booth CJ, Goldstein DR. Aging promotes neutrophil-induced mortality by augmenting IL-17 production during viral infection. *Cell Host Microbe.* (2009) 6:446–56. doi: 10.1016/j.chom.2009.09.011
116. Stout-Delgado HW, Yang X, Walker WE, Tesar BM, Goldstein DR. Aging impairs IFN regulatory factor 7 up-regulation in plasmacytoid dendritic cells during TLR9 activation. *J Immunol.* (2008) 181:6747–56. doi: 10.4049/jimmunol.181.10.6747
117. Lund JM, Linehan MM, Iijima N, Iwasaki A. Cutting Edge: Plasmacytoid dendritic cells provide innate immune protection against mucosal viral infection *in situ*. *J Immunol.* (2006) 177:7510–4. doi: 10.4049/jimmunol.177.11.7510
118. Brewitz A, Eickhoff S, Dahling S, Quast T, Bedoui S, Kroczek RA, et al. CD8(+) T cells orchestrate pDC-XCR1(+) dendritic cell spatial and functional cooperativity to optimize priming. *Immunity.* (2017) 46:205–19. doi: 10.1016/j.immuni.2017.01.003
119. Xu RH, Wong EB, Rubio D, Roscoe F, Ma X, Nair S, et al. Sequential activation of two pathogen-sensing pathways required for type I interferon expression and resistance to an acute DNA virus infection. *Immunity.* (2015) 43:1148–59. doi: 10.1016/j.immuni.2015.11.015
120. Wolf AI, Buehler D, Hensley SE, Cavanagh LL, Wherry EJ, Kastner P, et al. Plasmacytoid dendritic cells are dispensable during primary influenza virus infection. *J Immunol.* (2009) 182:871–9. doi: 10.4049/jimmunol.182.2.871
121. Kochs G, Anzaghe M, Kronhart S, Wagner V, Gogesch P, Scheu S, et al. *In vivo* conditions enable IFNAR-independent type I interferon production by peritoneal CD11b+ cells upon thogoto virus infection. *J Virol.* (2016) 90:9330–7. doi: 10.1128/JVI.00744-16
122. Kallfass C, Ackerman A, Lienenklaus S, Weiss S, Heimrich B, Staeheli P. Visualizing production of beta interferon by astrocytes and microglia in brain of La Crosse virus-infected mice. *J Virol.* (2012) 86:11223–30. doi: 10.1128/JVI.01093-12
123. Delhaye S, Paul S, Blakqori G, Minet M, Weber F, Staeheli P, et al. Neurons produce type I interferon during viral encephalitis. *Proc Natl Acad Sci USA.* (2006) 103:7835–40. doi: 10.1073/pnas.0602460103
124. Cervantes-Barragan L, Zust R, Weber F, Spiegel M, Lang KS, Akira S, et al. Control of coronavirus infection through plasmacytoid dendritic-cell-derived type I interferon. *Blood.* (2007) 109:1131–7. doi: 10.1182/blood-2006-05-023770
125. Wang Y, Swiecki M, Cella M, Alber G, Schreiber RD, Gilfillan S, et al. Timing and magnitude of type I interferon responses by distinct sensors impact CD8 T cell exhaustion and chronic viral infection. *Cell Host Microbe.* (2012) 11:631–42. doi: 10.1016/j.chom.2012.05.003
126. Smit JJ, Rudd BD, Lukacs NW. Plasmacytoid dendritic cells inhibit pulmonary immunopathology and promote clearance of respiratory syncytial virus. *J Exp Med.* (2006) 203:1153–9. doi: 10.1084/jem.20052359
127. Swiecki M, Colonna M. Type I interferons: diversity of sources, production pathways and effects on immune responses. *Curr Opin Virol.* (2011) 1:463–75. doi: 10.1016/j.coviro.2011.10.026
128. Alcami A, Koszinowski UH. Viral mechanisms of immune evasion. *Mol Med Today.* (2000) 6:365–72. doi: 10.1016/S1357-4310(00)01775-5

129. Zucchini N, Bessou G, Traub S, Robbins SH, Uematsu S, Akira S, et al. Cutting edge: Overlapping functions of TLR7 and TLR9 for innate defense against a herpesvirus infection. *J Immunol.* (2008) 180:5799–803. doi: 10.4049/jimmunol.180.9.5799
130. Doring M, Lessin I, Frenz T, Spanier J, Kessler A, Tegtmeyer P, et al. M27 expressed by cytomegalovirus counteracts effective type I interferon induction of myeloid cells but not of plasmacytoid dendritic cells. *J Virol.* (2014) 88:13638–50. doi: 10.1128/JVI.00216-14
131. Szomolanyi-Tsuda E, Liang X, Welsh RM, Kurt-Jones EA, Finberg RW. Role for TLR2 in NK cell-mediated control of murine cytomegalovirus *in vivo*. *J Virol.* (2006) 80:4286–91. doi: 10.1128/JVI.80.9.4286-4291.2006
132. Tabeta K, Georgel P, Janssen E, Du X, Hoebe K, Crozat K, et al. Toll-like receptors 9 and 3 as essential components of innate immune defense against mouse cytomegalovirus infection. *Proc Natl Acad Sci USA.* (2004) 101:3516–21. doi: 10.1073/pnas.0400525101
133. Eloranta ML, Alm GV. Splenic marginal metallophilic macrophages and marginal zone macrophages are the major interferon-alpha/beta producers in mice upon intravenous challenge with herpes simplex virus. *Scand J Immunol.* (1999) 49:391–4. doi: 10.1046/j.1365-3083.1999.00514.x
134. ME JW, Adair K, Brierley L. RNA viruses: a case study of the biology of emerging infectious diseases. *Microbiol Spectr.* (2013) 1:1–11. doi: 10.1128/microbiolspec.OH-0001-2012
135. Shi M, Lin XD, Chen X, Tian JH, Chen LJ, Li K, et al. The evolutionary history of vertebrate RNA viruses. *Nature.* (2018) 556:197–202. doi: 10.1038/s41586-018-0012-7
136. Hornung V, Schlender J, Guenthner-Biller M, Rothenfusser S, Endres S, Conzelmann KK, et al. Replication-dependent potent IFN-alpha induction in human plasmacytoid dendritic cells by a single-stranded RNA virus. *J Immunol.* (2004) 173:5935–43. doi: 10.4049/jimmunol.173.10.5935
137. Lee HK, Lund JM, Ramanathan B, Mizushima N, Iwasaki A. Autophagy-dependent viral recognition by plasmacytoid dendritic cells. *Science.* (2007) 315:1398–401. doi: 10.1126/science.1136880
138. Honke N, Shaabani N, Cadeddu G, Sorg UR, Zhang DE, Trilling M, et al. Enforced viral replication activates adaptive immunity and is essential for the control of a cytopathic virus. *Nat Immunol.* (2011) 13:51–7. doi: 10.1038/ni.2169
139. Pfefferkorn C, Kallfass C, Lienenklaus S, Spanier J, Kalinke U, Rieder M, et al. Abortively infected astrocytes appear to represent the main source of interferon beta in the virus-infected brain. *J Virol.* (2016) 90:2031–8. doi: 10.1128/JVI.02979-15
140. Davidson S, Kaiko G, Loh Z, Lalwani A, Zhang V, Spann K, et al. Plasmacytoid dendritic cells promote host defense against acute pneumovirus infection via the TLR7-MyD88-dependent signaling pathway. *J Immunol.* (2011) 186:5938–48. doi: 10.4049/jimmunol.1002635
141. O'Brien M, Manches O, Bhardwaj N. Plasmacytoid dendritic cells in HIV infection. *Adv Exp Med Biol.* (2013) 762:71–107. doi: 10.1007/978-1-4614-4433-6_3
142. Feldman S, Stein D, Amrute S, Denny T, Garcia Z, Kloser P, et al. Decreased interferon-alpha production in HIV-infected patients correlates with numerical and functional deficiencies in circulating type 2 dendritic cell precursors. *Clin Immunol.* (2001) 101:201–10. doi: 10.1006/clim.2001.5111
143. Herbeuval JP, Shearer GM. HIV-1 immunopathogenesis: how good interferon turns bad. *Clin Immunol.* (2007) 123:121–8. doi: 10.1016/j.clim.2006.09.016
144. Hosmalin A, Lebon P. Type I interferon production in HIV-infected patients. *J Leukoc Biol.* (2006) 80:984–93. doi: 10.1189/jlb.0306154
145. Kovarik P, Castiglia V, Ivin M, Ebner F. Type I interferons in bacterial infections: a Balancing Act. *Front Immunol.* (2016) 7:652. doi: 10.3389/fimmu.2016.00652
146. O'Garra A, Redford PS, McNab FW, Bloom CI, Wilkinson RJ, Berry MP. The immune response in tuberculosis. *Annu Rev Immunol.* (2013) 31:475–527. doi: 10.1146/annurev-immunol-032712-095939
147. Kearney SJ, Delgado C, Eshleman EM, Hill KK, O'Connor BP, Lenz LL. Type I IFNs downregulate myeloid cell IFN-gamma receptor by inducing recruitment of an early growth response 3/NGFI-A binding protein 1 complex that silences ifngr1 transcription. *J Immunol.* (2013) 191:3384–92. doi: 10.4049/jimmunol.1203510
148. Rayamajhi M, Humann J, Penheiter K, Andreasen K, Lenz LL. Induction of IFN-alphabeta enables Listeria monocytogenes to suppress macrophage activation by IFN-gamma. *J Exp Med.* (2010) 207:327–37. doi: 10.1084/jem.20091746
149. Stanley SA, Johndrow JE, Manzanillo P, Cox JS. The Type I IFN response to infection with Mycobacterium tuberculosis requires ESX-1-mediated secretion and contributes to pathogenesis. *J Immunol.* (2007) 178:3143–52. doi: 10.4049/jimmunol.178.5.3143
150. Mayer-Barber KD, Andrade BB, Barber DL, Hieny S, Feng CG, Caspar P, et al. Innate and adaptive interferons suppress IL-1alpha and IL-1beta production by distinct pulmonary myeloid subsets during *Mycobacterium tuberculosis* infection. *Immunity.* (2011) 35:1023–34. doi: 10.1016/j.immuni.2011.12.002
151. Giacomini E, Iona E, Ferroni L, Miettinen M, Fattorini L, Orefici G, et al. Infection of human macrophages and dendritic cells with Mycobacterium tuberculosis induces a differential cytokine gene expression that modulates T cell response. *J Immunol.* (2001) 166:7033–41. doi: 10.4049/jimmunol.166.12.7033
152. Remoli ME, Giacomini E, Lutfalla G, Dondi E, Orefici G, Battistini A, et al. Selective expression of type I IFN genes in human dendritic cells infected with *Mycobacterium tuberculosis*. *J Immunol.* (2002) 169:366–74. doi: 10.4049/jimmunol.169.1.366
153. Teles RM, Graeber TG, Krutzik SR, Montoya D, Schenk M, Lee DJ, et al. Type I interferon suppresses type II interferon-triggered human anti-mycobacterial responses. *Science.* (2013) 339:1448–53. doi: 10.1126/science.1233665
154. Auerbuch V, Brockstedt DG, Meyer-Morse N, O'Riordan M, Portnoy DA. Mice lacking the type I interferon receptor are resistant to Listeria monocytogenes. *J Exp Med.* (2004) 200:527–33. doi: 10.1084/jem.20040976
155. Carrero JA, Calderon B, Unanue ER. Listeriolysin O from Listeria monocytogenes is a lymphocyte apoptogenic molecule. *J Immunol.* (2004) 172:4866–74. doi: 10.4049/jimmunol.172.8.4866
156. O'Connell RM, Saha SK, Vaidya SA, Bruhn KW, Miranda GA, Zarnegar B, et al. Type I interferon production enhances susceptibility to Listeria monocytogenes infection. *J Exp Med.* (2004) 200:437–45. doi: 10.1084/jem.20040712
157. Kernbauer E, Maier V, Rauch I, Muller M, Decker T. Route of infection determines the impact of type I interferons on innate immunity to listeria monocytogenes. *PLoS ONE.* (2013) 8:e65007. doi: 10.1371/journal.pone.0065007
158. Pitts MG, Myers-Morales T, D'Orazio SE. Type I IFN does not promote susceptibility to foodborne listeria monocytogenes. *J Immunol.* (2016) 196:3109–16. doi: 10.4049/jimmunol.1502192
159. Stockinger S, Kastner R, Kernbauer E, Pilz A, Westermayer S, Reutterer B, et al. Characterization of the interferon-producing cell in mice infected with Listeria monocytogenes. *PLoS Pathog.* (2009) 5:e1000355. doi: 10.1371/journal.ppat.1000355
160. Dresing P, Borkens S, Kocur M, Kropp S, Scheu S. A fluorescence reporter model defines "Tip-DCs" as the cellular source of interferon beta in murine listeriosis. *PLoS ONE.* (2010) 5:e15567. doi: 10.1371/journal.pone.0015567
161. Solodova E, Jablonska J, Weiss S, Lienenklaus S. Production of IFN-beta during Listeria monocytogenes infection is restricted to monocyte/macrophage lineage. *PLoS ONE.* (2011) 6:e18543. doi: 10.1371/journal.pone.0018543
162. Serbina NV, Salazar-Mather TP, Biron CA, Kuziel WA, Pamer EG. TNF/iNOS-producing dendritic cells mediate innate immune defense against bacterial infection. *Immunity.* (2003) 19:59–70. doi: 10.1016/S1074-7613(03)00171-7
163. Bao Y, Han Y, Chen Z, Xu S, Cao X. IFN-alpha-producing PDCA-1+ Siglec-H- B cells mediate innate immune defense by activating NK cells. *Eur J Immunol.* (2011) 41:657–68. doi: 10.1002/eji.201040840
164. O'Riordan M, Yi CH, Gonzales R, Lee KD, Portnoy DA. Innate recognition of bacteria by a macrophage cytosolic surveillance pathway. *Proc Natl Acad Sci USA.* (2002) 99:13861–6. doi: 10.1073/pnas.202476699
165. Stockinger S, Materna T, Stoiber D, Bayr L, Steinborn R, Kolbe T, et al. Production of type I IFN sensitizes macrophages to cell death induced by Listeria monocytogenes. *J Immunol.* (2002) 169:6522–9. doi: 10.4049/jimmunol.169.11.6522

166. Serbina NV, Shi C, Pamer EG. Monocyte-mediated immune defense against murine Listeria monocytogenes infection. *Adv Immunol.* (2012) 113:119–34. doi: 10.1016/B978-0-12-394590-7.00003-8
167. Mancuso G, Midiri A, Biondo C, Beninati C, Zummo S, Galbo R, et al. Type I IFN signaling is crucial for host resistance against different species of pathogenic bacteria. *J Immunol.* (2007) 178:3126–33. doi: 10.4049/jimmunol.178.5.3126
168. Mancuso G, Gambuzza M, Midiri A, Biondo C, Papasergi S, Akira S, et al. Bacterial recognition by TLR7 in the lysosomes of conventional dendritic cells. *Nat Immunol.* (2009) 10:587–94. doi: 10.1038/ni.1733
169. Weighardt H, Kaiser-Moore S, Schlautkotter S, Rossmann-Bloeck T, Schleicher U, Bogdan C, et al. Type I IFN modulates host defense and late hyperinflammation in septic peritonitis. *J Immunol.* (2006) 177:5623–30. doi: 10.4049/jimmunol.177.8.5623
170. Ramirez-Ortiz ZG, Lee CK, Wang JP, Boon L, Specht CA, Levitz SM. A nonredundant role for plasmacytoid dendritic cells in host defense against the human fungal pathogen *Aspergillus fumigatus*. *Cell Host Microbe.* (2011) 9:415–24. doi: 10.1016/j.chom.2011.04.007
171. Beiting DP. Protozoan parasites and type I interferons: a cold case reopened. *Trends Parasitol.* (2014) 30:491–8. doi: 10.1016/j.pt.2014.07.007
172. Silva-Barrios S, Stager S. Protozoan parasites and type I IFNs. *Front Immunol.* (2017) 8:14. doi: 10.3389/fimmu.2017.00014
173. deWalick S, Amante FH, McSweeney KA, Randall LM, Stanley AC, Haque A, et al. Cutting edge: conventional dendritic cells are the critical APC required for the induction of experimental cerebral malaria. *J Immunol.* (2007) 178:6033–7. doi: 10.4049/jimmunol.178.10.6033
174. Haque A, Best SE, Montes de Oca M, James KR, Ammerdorffer A, Edwards CL, et al. Type I IFN signaling in CD8- DCs impairs Th1-dependent malaria immunity. *J Clin Invest.* (2014) 124:2483–96. doi: 10.1172/JCI70698
175. Voisine C, Mastelic B, Sponaas AM, Langhorne J. Classical CD11c+ dendritic cells, not plasmacytoid dendritic cells, induce T cell responses to *Plasmodium chabaudi* malaria. *Int J Parasitol.* (2010) 40:711–9. doi: 10.1016/j.ijpara.2009.11.005
176. Kim CC, Nelson CS, Wilson EB, Hou B, DeFranco AL, DeRisi JL. Splenic red pulp macrophages produce type I interferons as early sentinels of malaria infection but are dispensable for control. *PLoS ONE.* (2012) 7:e48126. doi: 10.1371/journal.pone.0048126
177. Spaulding E, Fooksman D, Moore JM, Saidi A, Feintuch CM, Reizis B, et al. STING-licensed macrophages prime type I IFN production by plasmacytoid dendritic cells in the bone marrow during severe *Plasmodium yoelii* malaria. *PLoS Pathog.* (2016) 12:e1005975. doi: 10.1371/journal.ppat.1005975
178. Yu X, Cai B, Wang M, Tan P, Ding X, Wu J, et al. Cross-regulation of two type I interferon signaling pathways in plasmacytoid dendritic cells controls anti-malaria immunity and host mortality. *Immunity.* (2016) 45:1093–107. doi: 10.1016/j.immuni.2016.10.001
179. Silva-Barrios S, Smans M, Duerr CU, Qureshi ST, Fritz JH, Descoteaux A, et al. Innate immune B cell activation by *Leishmania donovani* exacerbates disease and mediates hypergammaglobulinemia. *Cell Rep.* (2016) 15:2427–37. doi: 10.1016/j.celrep.2016.05.028
180. Minns LA, Menard LC, Foureau DM, Darche S, Ronet C, Mielcarz DW, et al. TLR9 is required for the gut-associated lymphoid tissue response following oral infection of *Toxoplasma gondii*. *J Immunol.* (2006) 176:7589–97. doi: 10.4049/jimmunol.176.12.7589
181. Han SJ, Melichar HJ, Coombes JL, Chan SW, Koshy AA, Boothroyd JC, et al. Internalization and TLR-dependent type I interferon production by monocytes in response to *Toxoplasma gondii*. *Immunol Cell Biol.* (2014) 92:872–81. doi: 10.1038/icb.2014.70
182. Sebina I, Haque A. Effects of type I interferons in malaria. *Immunology.* (2018) 155:176–85. doi: 10.1111/imm.12971
183. Pichyangkul S, Yongvanitchit K, Kum-arb U, Hemmi H, Akira S, Krieg AM, et al. Malaria blood stage parasites activate human plasmacytoid dendritic cells and murine dendritic cells through a Toll-like receptor 9-dependent pathway. *J Immunol.* (2004) 172:4926–33. doi: 10.4049/jimmunol.172.8.4926
184. Liehl P, Zuzarte-Luis V, Chan J, Zillinger T, Baptista F, Carapau D, et al. Host-cell sensors for Plasmodium activate innate immunity against liver-stage infection. *Nat Med.* (2014) 20:47–53. doi: 10.1038/nm.3424
185. Wilson EB, Yamada DH, Elsaesser H, Herskovitz J, Deng J, Cheng G, et al. Blockade of chronic type I interferon signaling to control persistent LCMV infection. *Science.* (2013) 340:202–7. doi: 10.1126/science.1235208
186. Beignon AS, McKenna K, Skoberne M, Manches O, DaSilva I, Kavanagh DG, et al. Endocytosis of HIV-1 activates plasmacytoid dendritic cells via Toll-like receptor-viral RNA interactions. *J Clin Invest.* (2005) 115:3265–75. doi: 10.1172/JCI26032
187. Schleicher U, Liese J, Justies N, Mischke T, Haeberlein S, Sebald H, et al. Type I interferon signaling is required for CpG-Oligodesoxynucleotide-induced control of *Leishmania major*, but not for spontaneous cure of subcutaneous primary or secondary *L. major* infection. *Front Immunol.* (2018) 9:79. doi: 10.3389/fimmu.2018.00079
188. Diefenbach A, Schindler H, Donhauser N, Lorenz E, Laskay T, MacMicking J, et al. Type 1 interferon (IFNalpha/beta) and type 2 nitric oxide synthase regulate the innate immune response to a protozoan parasite. *Immunity.* (1998) 8:77–87. doi: 10.1016/S1074-7613(00)80460-4
189. Bogdan C, Mattner J, Schleicher U. The role of type I interferons in non-viral infections. *Immunol Rev.* (2004) 202:33–48. doi: 10.1111/j.0105-2896.2004.00207.x
190. Vivarini Ade C, Pereira Rde M, Teixeira KL, Calegari-Silva TC, Bellio M, Laurenti MD, et al. Human cutaneous leishmaniasis: interferon-dependent expression of double-stranded RNA-dependent protein kinase (PKR) via TLR2. *FASEB J.* (2011) 25:4162–73. doi: 10.1096/fj.11-185165
191. Schleicher U, Liese J, Knippertz I, Kurzmann C, Hesse A, Heit A, et al. NK cell activation in visceral leishmaniasis requires TLR9, myeloid DCs, and IL-12, but is independent of plasmacytoid DCs. *J Exp Med.* (2007) 204:893–906. doi: 10.1084/jem.20061293
192. Pepper M, Dzierszinski F, Wilson E, Tait E, Fang Q, Yarovinsky F, et al. Plasmacytoid dendritic cells are activated by Toxoplasma gondii to present antigen and produce cytokines. *J Immunol.* (2008) 180:6229–36. doi: 10.4049/jimmunol.180.9.6229
193. Koblansky AA, Jankovic D, Oh H, Hieny S, Sungnak W, Mathur R, et al. Recognition of profilin by Toll-like receptor 12 is critical for host resistance to *Toxoplasma gondii*. *Immunity.* (2013) 38:119–30. doi: 10.1016/j.immuni.2012.09.016
194. Pierog PL, Zhao Y, Singh S, Dai J, Yap GS, Fitzgerald-Bocarsly P. *Toxoplasma gondii* inactivates human plasmacytoid dendritic cells by functional Mimicry of IL-10. *J Immunol.* (2018) 200:186–95. doi: 10.4049/jimmunol.1701045
195. Leng J, Butcher BA, Denkers EY. Dysregulation of macrophage signal transduction by Toxoplasma gondii: past progress and recent advances. *Parasite Immunol.* (2009) 31:717–28. doi: 10.1111/j.1365-3024.2009.01122.x
196. Melo MB, Nguyen QP, Cordeiro C, Hassan MA, Yang N, McKell R, et al. Transcriptional analysis of murine macrophages infected with different Toxoplasma strains identifies novel regulation of host signaling pathways. *PLoS Pathog.* (2013) 9:e1003779.
197. Beiting DP, Peixoto L, Akopyants NS, Beverley SM, Wherry EJ, Christian DA, et al. Differential induction of TLR3-dependent innate immune signaling by closely related parasite species. *PLoS ONE.* (2014) 9:e88398. doi: 10.1371/journal.pone.0088398
198. Swiecki M, Wang Y, Vermi W, Gilfillan S, Schreiber RD, Colonna M. Type I interferon negatively controls plasmacytoid dendritic cell numbers *in vivo*. *J Exp Med.* (2011) 208:2367–74. doi: 10.1084/jem.20110654
199. Tomasello E, Pollet E, Vu Manh TP, Uze G, Dalod M. Harnessing mechanistic knowledge on beneficial versus deleterious IFN-I effects to design innovative immunotherapies targeting cytokine activity to specific cell types. *Front Immunol.* (2014) 5:526. doi: 10.3389/fimmu.2014.00526

11

What Makes a pDC: Recent Advances in Understanding Plasmacytoid DC Development and Heterogeneity

*Andrea Musumeci, Konstantin Lutz, Elena Winheim and Anne Barbara Krug**

Institute for Immunology, Biomedical Center, Ludwig-Maximilian-University, Munich, Germany

***Correspondence:**
Anne Barbara Krug
anne.krug@med.uni-muenchen.de

Dendritic cells (DCs) are professional antigen presenting cells (APCs) that originate in the bone marrow and are continuously replenished from hematopoietic progenitor cells. Conventional DCs (cDCs) and plasmacytoid DCs (pDCs) are distinguished by morphology and function, and can be easily discriminated by surface marker expression, both in mouse and man. Classification of DCs based on their ontology takes into account their origin as well as their requirements for transcription factor (TF) expression. cDCs and pDCs of myeloid origin differentiate from a common DC progenitor (CDP) through committed pre-DC stages. pDCs have also been shown to originate from a lymphoid progenitor derived IL-7R^{+} FLT3^{+} precursor population containing cells with pDC or B cell potential. Technological advancements in recent years have allowed unprecedented resolution in the analysis of cell states, down to the single cell level, providing valuable information on the commitment, and dynamics of differentiation of all DC subsets. However, the heterogeneity and functional diversification of pDCs still raises the question whether different ontogenies generate restricted pDC subsets, or fully differentiated pDCs retain plasticity in response to challenges. The emergence of novel techniques for the integration of high-resolution data in individual cells promises interesting discoveries regarding DC development and plasticity in the near future.

Keywords: plasmacytoid dendritic cells, hematopoiesis, dendritic cell development, DC progenitor, plasticity, heterogeneity

INTRODUCTION

Plasmacytoid dendritic cells (pDCs) and two major subsets of conventional dendritic cells (cDC1 and cDC2) have been identified in mice and humans as well as other mammalian species including non-human primates and pigs, with high similarities between species (1–3). cDC subsets recognize both extracellular and intracellular pathogens, efficiently process and present exogenous antigens to naive CD4^{+} and CD8^{+} T cells and elicit effective adaptive immunity. pDCs are highly effective in sensing intracellular viral or self DNA and RNA mainly via Toll-like receptors (TLRs) and rapidly producing large amounts of type I and III interferons (IFNs) (4). Thus, they play an important role in antiviral immunity and systemic autoimmunity (5–8). pDCs are distinguished from cDC subsets by expression of surface markers CD45R (B220), CD45RA, Ly-6C, Siglec-H, and BST2 (CD317) in the mouse and CD303 (BDCA2), CD304 (BDCA4), CD123 (IL-3R), and CD45RA in humans.

DC subpopulations originate from proliferating progenitor cells in the bone marrow (BM) and require fms-like tyrosine kinase 3 ligand (FLT3L)–FLT3 interaction for their development. Lin^- $FLT3^+$ c-$Kit^{low/int}$ M-$CSFR^+$ murine BM cells, so called common DC progenitors (CDP), which are derived from the myeloid macrophage DC progenitors (MDP) or lymphoid primed multipotent progenitors (LMPP), were shown to be DC-committed and to generate pDCs, cDC1 and cDC2 [**Figure 1**, (9, 10)]. Clonal assays and subsequent single cell transcriptome and imaging analyses demonstrated that the majority of CDPs are already pre-committed to pDC or cDC subsets (9–13). This is also the case for the pre-cDCs, which already contain pre-cDC1, and pre-cDC2 (13, 14). In contrast, pDCs are also produced from a lymphoid progenitor (LP) (15) in the steady state whereas this happens for cDCs only in situation of cDC ablation (16).

DC subpopulations can be defined by their ontogeny and by the requirement of specific transcription factors (TF) for their development. pDCs require high-level expression of IRF-8, TCF-4 (also known as E2-2) and BCL-11A for their development, functional specification and maintenance (17–21). Expression of DNA-binding protein inhibitor ID-2, which prevents the activity of the major pDC TF E2-2, needs to be suppressed to allow the generation of pDCs from CDPs (22, 23). On the other hand, the major cDC branches can be distinguished by distinct requirements for IRF-8 (for cDC1) and IRF-4 (for cDC2) (14, 24–27).

DC subpopulations are also distinguished by a high degree of functional specialization (28). While cDC1 efficiently cross-present antigens to $CD8^+$ T cells (27, 29, 30) and produce high levels of IL-12p70, thus promoting cytotoxic T cells and Th1 cells (31, 32), cDC2 are superior in presenting antigens on MHC class II, supporting Th1, Th2, and Th17 polarization (26, 27, 33). pDCs participate in the first line of defense against viral infections by acting as innate effector cells, which initiate IFN-induced antiviral responses in adjacent cells and recruit cytotoxic NK cells (5). Resting pDCs are weak antigen presenting cells and in contrast to cDCs do not prime naïve T cells. After activation, pDCs can acquire the capacity to present antigens and activate T cells directly. Their ability to prime T cells, thus performing truly like DCs, is debated and complicated by the finding that pDC-like cells, which were shown to be related to cDCs (13, 15, 34, 35) have been included in the pDC population in many functional studies, as discussed below. By producing cytokines and chemokines activated pDCs modulate T cell responses elicited by cDCs (5). During viral infection pDCs were shown to cooperate with cDC1 in lymph nodes, promoting their maturation and cross-presentation activity to induce antiviral $CD8^+$ T cells (36). But there is also evidence for a role of pDCs in the induction of immune tolerance by generation of hyporesponsive and regulatory T cells (37–39).

Recent technological developments have allowed unprecedented resolution, down to the single cell level, in the analysis of cell transcriptomes as well as in *in vivo* lineage tracing, overcoming the limitations of discrimination based solely on surface markers (40–44). The characterization of transcriptional profiles of individual cells (13, 42, 45) and more recently the integrated analysis of single cell transcriptome and chromatin accessibility (46) has revealed unexpected heterogeneity and signs of very early lineage priming of individual hematopoietic BM progenitor cells, which were previously considered multi- or oligopotent. For example, single cell barcoding and tracing showed that DC and even pDC commitment can already be imprinted in early LMPP and at the HSPC stage (12, 41, 47). cDC subtype specification was detected already at the CDP and pre-cDC stage of development (12–14). In some instances, these analyses led to the definition of more stringent surface marker combinations that allow the discrimination of largely committed progenitor cells within the "oligopotent" population (13, 15).

Combining CRISPR/Cas9-based genomic perturbation with transcriptome profiling in the same cells revealed differentiation trajectories and regulatory networks during hematopoiesis (40, 48). Integration of clonal labeling and lineage tracing experiments and single cell time-lapse imaging experiments may lead to a better understanding of immune cell differentiation dynamics and regulation in the future (11, 40, 43, 49).

PLASMACYTOID DENDRITIC CELL DEVELOPMENT FROM MYELOID AND LYMPHOID PROGENITORS

Early works indicated that DCs can be derived from both $FLT3^+$ CMP and CLP (50, 51). Competitive *in vivo* transfer experiments with CMPs and CLPs showed that pDCs can also be generated from both, but are mainly of "myeloid" origin (52). Subsequent studies indicated that CMP and CLP-derived pDCs differ in their ability to produce type I IFN and to stimulate T cells (53, 54). Interestingly, a significant proportion of pDCs expresses recombination activation genes (*Rag1*/*Rag2*) and undergoes immunoglobulin D_H-J_H rearrangement indicating a "lymphoid" past. But the expression of Rag genes and detection of Ig rearrangements in pDCs derived from both CMP and CLP suggested that these are by-products of a "lymphoid" transcriptional program expressed only transiently in the pDC lineage (55, 56). However, the issue was revisited by Sathe et al. who found that RAG1 expression and Ig rearrangement are mainly found in CLP-derived pDCs (54). pDC generation from CLPs but not CDPs required constitutive type I IFN signals for upregulation of FLT3, suggesting differential requirements for instructive cytokines for the two developmental pathways (57). After the discovery that myeloid progenitor derived CDPs generate both cDCs and pDCs, research mostly focused on the branching of pDC and cDC development.

We found that $CCR9^{low}$ pDC-like precursor cells (CD11c+ Siglec H+ BST2+ B220lo/hi), which express lower levels of E2-2 and higher levels of Id2 than pDCs, can be generated from murine CDPs and these can give rise to $CCR9^{high}$ pDCs as well as cDCs [**Figure 1**, (11, 58, 59)]. The $CCR9^{low}$ pDC-like precursor population in the BM contains only a small fraction of proliferating cells indicating heterogeneity within this population regarding differentiation stage (58). It remains to be determined if this population, which can also be detected in lymphoid organs at low frequency contains differentiated cells

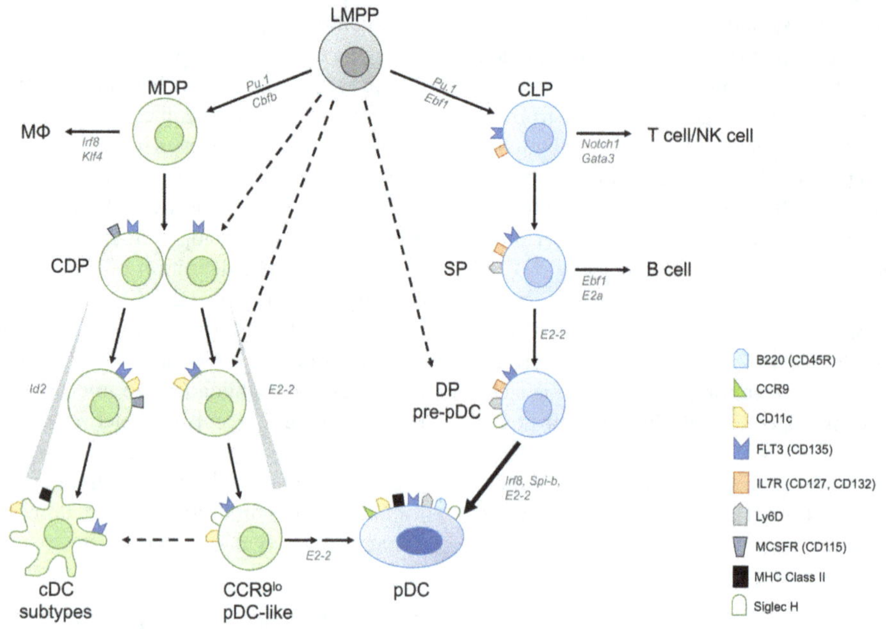

FIGURE 1 | Converging plasmacytoid dendritic cell differentiation pathways. Plasmacytoid dendritic cells (pDCs) can be derived from both myeloid and lymphoid progenitors. Common DC progenitors (CDPs) arise from lymphoid primed multipotent progenitors (LMPPs) either directly or via macrophage-DC progenitors (MDPs). CDPs contain precursor cells committed to conventional DC (cDC) and plasmacytoid DC fates, and M-CSFR$^-$ CDPs have higher pDC potential than M-CSFR$^+$ CDPs. A fraction of CDPs can give rise to CCR9^{low} pDC-like precursor cells and then CCR9^{high} pDCs in an E2-2 dependent manner. pDC-like cells retain the potential to differentiate into cDCs as well as CCR9^{high} mature pDCs. Inhibitor of DNA binding 2 (Id2), which inhibits E2-2 activity, needs to be suppressed to allow pDC differentiation. pDCs are also generated via the lymphoid pathway, from IL-7R$^+$ lymphoid progenitors (LPs) which give rise to Ly-6D single positive (SP) LP and subsequently to Ly-6D Siglec-H double positive (DP) pre-pDC, terminally committed to the pDC fate.

with plasticity to develop into pDCs and cDCs or precursors with dual potential or both. Interestingly, pDC-like cells with a similar phenotype accumulated in the BM of Mtg16-deficient mice, which failed to downregulate Id2 expression, thereby blocking the activity of E2-2 and further pDC differentiation (60). In addition, Zeb2 has been identified as an important regulator of Id2 expression, which allows pDC development from CDPs by suppressing the alternative cDC1 fate at a common precursor stage (22, 23). More recently Etv6 was shown to cooperate with IRF8 to refine cDC1-specific gene expression and repress the pDC gene expression signature indicating the close relationship between cDC1 and pDCs (61). Siglec-H, a canonical marker distinguishing mature pDCs from cDCs, is expressed at very early stages of differentiation, but does not denote a plasmacytoid commitment. Within the CDP and the pre-DC fraction in the BM, Siglec-H$^+$ cells expressing TF Zbtb46 are exclusively committed to cDCs (62) and were shown to contain precursors committed to cDC1 and cDC2 (13, 14). Similarly, Siglec-H$^+$ Ly-6C$^+$ cells in the pre-DC compartment (defined as Lin$^-$ CD135$^+$ CD11c$^+$ MHCII$^-$ CD172α^-) were shown to give rise to both subsets of cDCs, whereas Siglec-H$^+$ Ly-6C$^-$ pre-DCs gave rise to cDC subsets and pDCs (13). Using the single cell imaging and tracking method we could show that CDP progeny transit through a CD11c$^+$ CCR9^{low} Siglec-H$^+$ pDC-like stage during their development into CCR9^{high} pDCs (11). The CDP-derived pDC-committed precursor, which must be present within this population, is still a missing link. M-CSFR$^+$ CDPs give rise to pDCs, however their output is rather low. Interestingly, Onai et al. found that the pDC potential was higher in the M-CSFR$^-$ E2-2$^+$ fraction of CDPs in murine BM (12, 63). They also demonstrated that E2-2^{high} cells within M-CSFR$^-$ IL-7R$^-$ CDPs gave rise exclusively to pDCs in spleen and lymph nodes, but also to cDCs in the small intestine, showing the plasticity of this pDC-primed CDP subset or its progeny in the local tissue environment (63).

More recently Rodrigues et al. found that FLT3$^+$ IL-7R (CD127)$^+$ CD117$^{lo/int}$ lymphoid progenitor (LP) cells in murine BM, which differ from CDPs only by expression of IL-7R and lack of M-CSFR expression, have a 5-fold higher output of pDCs compared to CDPs (15). Within this LP pool, three subpopulations were distinguished by diverse expression of Siglec-H and Ly-6D. Of these, only the Siglec-H Ly-6D double positive (DP) population had exclusive pDC potential, while the Ly-6D single positive (SP) population generated both B cells and pDCs, congruent with the results of a recently published computational fate mapping analysis of single cell RNAseq data (64). Further analysis showed the SP population to contain cells committed either to B cell or to pDC differentiation. The model proposed by Rodrigues et al. suggests that IL-7R$^+$ Siglec-H and Ly-6D DN LPs proceed to upregulate Ly-6D (SP) and, under the influence of lineage defining TFs IRF8 and EBF1 induced by FLT3L and IL-7 respectively, proceed either to the pDC lineage or towards B cells (**Figure 1**). Interestingly, mice lacking Zeb2 in CD11c^{+} cells were shown to have a severe defect in pDC numbers, which was attributed to failed repression of Id2 leading to diversion of precursors to cDC1 (22, 23). Since a substantial proportion of pDCs was shown to be derived from the LP which lacks cDC potential in the steady state (65), it remains to be investigated if the transcriptional repressor Zeb2 is also involved in suppressing alternative cell fates in the LP.

Functionally, the IL-7R^{+} DP cells described by Rodriguez et al. as pDC precursors can be considered immature progenitors, as they do not yet express genes important for pDC function (such as *Irf7* and *Spib*) and require further cell divisions to generate mature pDCs (15). In contrast to the CDP-derived CD11c^{+} Siglec-H^{+} CCR9^{low} pDC-like precursors, the IL-7R^{+} DP cells lack CD11c and B220 expression and fail to produce type I IFNs in response to TLR9 stimulation by CpG-A, a hallmark of the pDC-lineage, but acquire this capacity after culture with FLT3L (15).

IL-7R^{+} Siglec-H^{+} Ly-6D^{+} pDC-committed precursors make a substantial contribution to the pool of differentiated pDCs. Thus, pDC generation seems to be regulated by the cell fate decision between pDC and cDC1, but also by the pDC versus B cell dichotomy. The contribution of the two pathways to pDC generation under conditions of inflammation or infection and the functional consequences of the distinct ontogeny of pDCs remain to be investigated.

HETEROGENEITY OF pDCs AND pDC-LIKE CELLS IN MURINE LYMPHOID ORGANS

Different subsets of pDCs have been identified in the BM, mostly differing in their degree of differentiation and their capacity to produce type I IFNs or pro-inflammatory cytokines (4, 66). Markers such as CCR9, SCA-1, CD9, and Ly-49Q, which are expressed by the majority of peripheral mouse pDCs, can be used to discriminate these subsets (59, 67, 68). More recently, single cell RNAseq analysis confirmed the presence of two subsets within Lin^{-} CD11c^{+} BST2^{+} Siglec-H^{+} cells in spleen and BM (15). The "pDC-like cells" described in this paper express several genes characteristic of cDCs and other myeloid cells (including *Zbtb46*) but lack or express low levels of *Ccr9*, *Ly6d*, and *Dntt*. By gene expression profile and surface phenotype (lower levels of Siglec-H, BST2, MHCII, higher levels of CD11c, Ly-6C, and CX3CR1 compared to pDCs) they greatly resemble the CCR9^{low} MHCII^{low} CX3CR1^{+} pDC-like precursors described previously in BM (58, 59) and are a subset of those. Interestingly, Rodrigues et al. also found that the minor subset of pDC-like cells (defined as Zbtb46-eGFP^{+} Siglec-H^{int} BST2^{+}), responded with IFN-α production to CpG-A and showed better antigen processing and presenting ability than "regular" pDCs. It was also previously shown that IFN-β production in the spleen is limited to a small subset of CD9^{-} cells within the CCR9^{+} mature pDC population in murine spleen (69).

These works suggest the existence of minor subsets of pDCs in peripheral organs, differing in the extent of IFN-I production and the capacity of antigen processing and presentation. Considering that these subsets identified by differential expression of surface markers are largely overlapping and often very rare, it remains unclear whether the functional differences observed are due to functional specialization or are the result of lineage imprinting, or whether they are simply sequential stages of pDC differentiation leading to the mature pDC.

REVISITING THE DEFINITION OF HUMAN pDCs

The pDC-like cells described in the mouse which express pDC markers and TFs, but rapidly give rise to cDCs and behave like cDCs in antigen presentation assays greatly resemble the subset of CD123^{+} CD45RA^{+} CD33^{+} CX3CR1^{+} pre-DCs recently identified in human blood (35) and the AXL^{+} SIGLEC6^{+} human blood DC subset (AS-DC) described by Villani et al. (34). These "pDC-like cells," which are hidden in the pDC population as defined by surface marker expression (Lin^{-} HLA-DR^{+} CD123^{+} CD45RA^{+} CD303^{+}), are functionally distinct from pDC in that they do not produce type I IFN in response to TLR7 and 9 stimulation. In that respect they are different from the Zbtb46^{+} Siglec-H^{+} pDC-like cells found in murine spleen. As to their classification as precursors of cDCs, it is based mainly on the observation that the pre-DCs acquire cDC phenotype and function in culture (35). The human pre-DC population contains pre-cDC1 and pre-cDC2 (35, 70). However, these cells are not proliferating in the steady state and appear to be functionally mature and could therefore actively participate in immune responses (34, 35). Cells in human blood, BM and tonsil defined as a CD2^{+} CD5^{+} (and CD81^{+}) subpopulation of human pDCs were studied previously and were found to produce IL-12 but not IFN-α and to stimulate naïve CD4^{+} T cells (71–74). This population is largely overlapping with the recently described pre-DC and AS-DC (34, 35). It is currently not resolved to which extent cytokine responses and T cell activation capacity attributed to human pDCs in earlier studies were influenced by contamination by cDC precursors, especially because most studies were performed with pDCs that had been stimulated e.g., with IL-3, CD40L or viruses (75–77). It was shown recently that human blood pDCs diversify into functionally distinct and stable subsets after activation by influenza virus or CpG even after prior exclusion of contaminating pre-DCs demonstrating great functional plasticity of this cell type (78). In the light of these recent findings the functional properties of *bona fide* pDCs in innate and adaptive immune responses need to be reexamined.

FUTURE PERSPECTIVES

Technological advances including single cell transcriptome, epigenome, and mass cytometry analyses as well as single cell tracking methods have revealed that development and functional specification of DC subpopulations is much more complex than anticipated. Several questions regarding pDC development and functional plasticity remain unanswered. It would be important to address the contribution of the CDP and LP to pDCs during infections or inflammation and to clarify if the developmental history of pDCs is really relevant for their function. Furthermore, it is unclear at this point, which functions ascribed to human pDCs are mediated by *bona fide* pDCs and which are mediated by the contaminating pre-DCs. This is especially important for developing pDC-targeted or adoptive transfer therapies for induction of immunity or tolerance. Similarly, the functional diversification of pDCs after activation and also the phenomenon of pDC exhaustion during chronic infection (79) are important topics for further study. An exciting area of research is the correlation of gene expression with chromatin accessibility and epigenetic modifications on the single cell level and the integration of all this data (80), which will allow to unravel the transcriptional regulation of cell fate decisions leading to pDC development and functional diversification. Combined with CRISPR/Cas9-based genetic screening and functional assays these new single cell analysis methods will lead to a thorough understanding of development, plasticity and function of DC subpopulations with implications for DC targeted therapy.

AUTHOR CONTRIBUTIONS

All authors listed have made a substantial, direct and intellectual contribution to the work, and approved it for publication.

REFERENCES

1. Auray G, Keller I, Python S, Gerber M, Bruggmann R, Ruggli N, et al. Characterization and transcriptomic analysis of porcine blood conventional and plasmacytoid dendritic cells reveals striking species-specific differences. *J Immunol.* (2016) 197:4791–806. doi: 10.4049/jimmunol.1600672
2. Guilliams M, Dutertre CA, Scott CL, McGovern N, Sichien D, Chakarov S, et al. Unsupervised high-dimensional analysis aligns dendritic cells across tissues and species. *Immunity.* (2016) 45:669–84. doi: 10.1016/j.immuni.2016.08.015
3. Heidkamp GF, Sander J, Lehmann CHK, Heger L, Eissing N, Baranska A, et al. Human lymphoid organ dendritic cell identity is predominantly dictated by ontogeny, not tissue microenvironment. *Sci Immunol.* (2016) 1:eaai7677.doi: 10.1126/sciimmunol.aai7677
4. Swiecki M, Colonna M. The multifaceted biology of plasmacytoid dendritic cells. *Nat Rev Immunol.* (2015) 15:471–85. doi: 10.1038/nri3865
5. Swiecki M, Gilfillan S, Vermi W, Wang Y, Colonna M. Plasmacytoid dendritic cell ablation impacts early interferon responses and antiviral NK and CD8(+) T cell accrual. *Immunity.* (2010) 33:955–66. doi: 10.1016/j.immuni.2010.11.020
6. Rowland SL, Riggs JM, Gilfillan S, Bugatti M, Vermi W, Kolbeck R, et al. Early, transient depletion of plasmacytoid dendritic cells ameliorates autoimmunity in a lupus model. *J Exp Med.* (2014) 211:1977–91. doi: 10.1084/jem.20132620
7. Sisirak V, Ganguly D, Lewis KL, Couillault C, Tanaka L, Bolland S, et al. Genetic evidence for the role of plasmacytoid dendritic cells in systemic lupus erythematosus. *J Exp Med.* (2014) 211:1969–76. doi: 10.1084/jem.20132522
8. Ah Kioon MD, Tripodo C, Fernandez D, Kirou KA, Spiera RF, Crow MK, et al. Plasmacytoid dendritic cells promote systemic sclerosis with a key role for TLR8. *Sci Transl Med.* (2018) 10:eaam8458. doi: 10.1126/scitranslmed.aam8458
9. Naik SH, Sathe P, Park H-Y, Metcalf D, Proietto AI, Dakic A, et al. Development of plasmacytoid and conventional dendritic cell subtypes from single precursor cells derived *in vitro* and *in vivo. Nat Immunol.* (2007) 8:1217–26. doi: 10.1038/ni1522
10. Onai N, Obata-Onai A, Schmid MA, Ohteki T, Jarrossay D, Manz MG. Identification of clonogenic common Flt3+M-CSFR+ plasmacytoid and conventional dendritic cell progenitors in mouse bone marrow. *Nat Immunol.* (2007) 8:1207–16. doi: 10.1038/ni1518
11. Dursun E, Endele M, Musumeci A, Failmezger H, Wang S-H, Tresch A, et al. Continuous single cell imaging reveals sequential steps of plasmacytoid dendritic cell development from common dendritic cell progenitors. *Scient Rep.* (2016) 6:37462. doi: 10.1038/srep37462
12. Onai N, Kurabayashi K, Hosoi-Amaike M, Toyama-Sorimachi N, Matsushima K, Inaba K, et al. A clonogenic progenitor with prominent plasmacytoid dendritic cell developmental potential. *Immunity.* (2013) 38:943–57. doi: 10.1016/j.immuni.2013.04.006
13. Schlitzer A, Sivakamasundari V, Chen J, Sumatoh HRB, Schreuder J, Lum J, et al. Identification of cDC1- and cDC2-committed DC progenitors reveals early lineage priming at the common DC progenitor stage in the bone marrow. *Nat Immunol.* (2015) 16:718–28. doi: 10.1038/ni.3200
14. Grajales-Reyes GE, Iwata A, Albring J, Wu X, Tussiwand R, KC W, et al. Batf3 maintains autoactivation of Irf8 for commitment of a CD8α(+) conventional DC clonogenic progenitor. *Nat Immunol.* (2015) 16:708–17. doi: 10.1038/ni.3197
15. Rodrigues PF, Alberti-Servera L, Eremin A, Grajales-Reyes GE, Ivanek R, Tussiwand R. Distinct progenitor lineages contribute to the heterogeneity of plasmacytoid dendritic cells. *Nat Immunol.* (2018) 392:245. doi: 10.1038/s41590-018-0136-9
16. Salvermoser J, van Blijswijk J, Papaioannou NE, Rambichler S, Pasztoi M, Pakalniskyte D, et al. Clec9a-mediated ablation of conventional dendritic cells suggests a lymphoid path to generating dendritic cells *in vivo. Front Immunol.* (2018) 9:699. doi: 10.3389/fimmu.2018.00699
17. Ippolito GC, Dekker JD, Wang YH, Lee BK, Shaffer AL III, Lin J, et al. Dendritic cell fate is determined by BCL11A. *Proc Natl Acad Sci USA.* (2014) 111:E998–1006. doi: 10.1073/pnas.1319228111
18. Cisse B, Caton ML, Lehner M, Maeda T, Scheu S, Locksley R, et al. Transcription factor E2-2 is an essential and specific regulator of plasmacytoid dendritic cell development. *Cell.* (2008) 135:37–48. doi: 10.1016/j.cell.2008.09.016
19. Ghosh HS, Cisse B, Bunin A, Lewis KL, Reizis B. Continuous expression of the transcription factor E2-2 maintains the cell fate of mature plasmacytoid dendritic cells. *Immunity.* (2010) 33:905–16. doi: 10.1016/j.immuni.2010.11.023
20. Grajkowska LT, Ceribelli M, Lau CM, Warren ME, Tiniakou I, Nakandakari Higa S, et al. Isoform-specific expression and feedback regulation of E protein TCF4 control dendritic cell lineage specification. *Immunity.* (2017) 46:65–77. doi: 10.1016/j.immuni.2016.11.006
21. Sichien D, Scott CL, Martens L, Vanderkerken M, Van Gassen S, Plantinga M, et al. IRF8 transcription factor controls survival and function of terminally differentiated conventional and plasmacytoid dendritic cells, respectively. *Immunity.* (2016) 45:626–40. doi: 10.1016/j.immuni.2016.08.013
22. Scott CL, Soen B, Martens L, Skrypek N, Saelens W, Taminau J, et al. The transcription factor Zeb2 regulates development of conventional and plasmacytoid DCs by repressing Id2. *J Exp Med.* (2016) 213:897–911. doi: 10.1084/jem.20151715
23. Wu X, Briseño CG, Grajales-Reyes GE, Haldar M, Iwata A, Kretzer NM, et al. Transcription factor Zeb2 regulates commitment to plasmacytoid dendritic cell and monocyte fate. *Proc Natl Acad Sci USA.* (2016) 113:14775–80. doi: 10.1073/pnas.1611408114
24. Murphy TL, Grajales-Reyes GE, Wu X, Tussiwand R, Briseño CG, Iwata A, et al. Transcriptional control of dendritic cell development. *Annu Rev Immunol.* (2016) 34:93–119. doi: 10.1146/annurev-immunol-032713-120204

25. Miller JC, Brown BD, Gautier EL, Jojic V, Cohain A, Pandey G, et al. Deciphering the transcriptional network of the dendritic cell lineage. *Nat Immunol.* (2012) 13:888–99. doi: 10.1038/ni.2370
26. Schlitzer A, McGovern N, Teo P, Zelante T, Atarashi K, Low D, et al. IRF4 transcription factor-dependent CD11b+ dendritic cells in human and mouse control mucosal IL-17 cytokine responses. *Immunity.* (2013) 38:970–83. doi: 10.1016/j.immuni.2013.04.011
27. Williams JW, Tjota MY, Clay BS, Vander Lugt B, Bandukwala HS, Hrusch CL, et al. Transcription factor IRF4 drives dendritic cells to promote Th2 differentiation. *Nat Commun.* (2013) 4:2990. doi: 10.1038/ncomms3990
28. Dress RJ, Wong AY, Ginhoux F. Homeostatic control of dendritic cell numbers and differentiation. *Immunol Cell Biol.* (2018) 96:463–76. doi: 10.1111/imcb.12028
29. den Haan JMM, Lehar SM, Bevan MJ. Cd8+but not Cd8–dendritic cells cross-prime cytotoxic T cells *in vivo. J Exp Med.* (2000) 192:1685–96. doi: 10.1084/jem.192.12.1685
30. Segura E, Amigorena S. Cross-presentation by human dendritic cell subsets. *Immunol Lett.* (2014) 158:73–8. doi: 10.1016/j.imlet.2013.12.001
31. Nizzoli G, Krietsch J, Weick A, Steinfelder S, Facciotti F, Gruarin P, et al. Human CD1c+ dendritic cells secrete high levels of IL-12 and potently prime cytotoxic T-cell responses. *Blood.* (2013) 122:932–42. doi: 10.1182/blood-2013-04-495424
32. Shortman K, Heath WR. The CD8+ dendritic cell subset. *Immunol Rev.* (2010) 234:18–31. doi: 10.1111/j.0105-2896.2009.00870.x
33. Dudziak D, Kamphorst AO, Heidkamp GF, Buchholz VR, Trumpfheller C, Yamazaki S, et al. Differential antigen processing by dendritic cell subsets *in vivo. Science.* (2007) 315:107–11. doi: 10.1126/science.1136080
34. Villani AC, Satija R, Reynolds G, Sarkizova S, Shekhar K, Fletcher J, et al. Single-cell RNA-seq reveals new types of human blood dendritic cells, monocytes, and progenitors. *Science.* (2017) 356:eaah4573. doi: 10.1126/science.aah4573
35. See P, Dutertre C-A, Chen J, Günther P, McGovern N, Irac SE, et al. Mapping the human DC lineage through the integration of high-dimensional techniques. *Science.* (2017) 356:eaag3009. doi: 10.1126/science.aag3009
36. Brewitz A, Eickhoff S, Dahling S, Quast T, Bedoui S, Kroczek RA, et al. CD8(+) T cells orchestrate pDC-XCR1(+) dendritic cell spatial and functional cooperativity to optimize priming. *Immunity.* (2017) 46:205–19. doi: 10.1016/j.immuni.2017.01.003
37. Loschko J, Heink S, Hackl D, Dudziak D, Reindl W, Korn T, et al. Antigen targeting to plasmacytoid dendritic cells via Siglec-H inhibits Th cell-dependent autoimmunity. *J Immunol.* (2011) 187:6346–56. doi: 10.4049/jimmunol.1102307
38. Irla M, Kupfer N, Suter T, Lissilaa R, Benkhoucha M, Skupsky J, et al. MHC class II-restricted antigen presentation by plasmacytoid dendritic cells inhibits T cell-mediated autoimmunity. *J Exp Med.* (2010) 207:1891–905. doi: 10.1084/jem.20092627
39. Hadeiba H, Lahl K, Edalati A, Oderup C, Habtezion A, Pachynski R, et al. Plasmacytoid dendritic cells transport peripheral antigens to the thymus to promote central tolerance. *Immunity.* (2012) 36:438–50. doi: 10.1016/j.immuni.2012.01.017
40. Giladi A, Paul F, Herzog Y, Lubling Y, Weiner A, Yofe I, et al. Single-cell characterization of haematopoietic progenitors and their trajectories in homeostasis and perturbed haematopoiesis. *Nat Cell Biol.* (2018) 20:836–46. doi: 10.1038/s41556-018-0121-4
41. Naik SH, Perie L, Swart E, Gerlach C, van Rooij N, de Boer RJ, et al. Diverse and heritable lineage imprinting of early haematopoietic progenitors. *Nature.* (2013) 496:229–32. doi: 10.1038/nature12013
42. Paul F, Arkin Ya, Giladi A, Jaitin DA, Kenigsberg E, Keren-Shaul H, et al. Transcriptional heterogeneity and lineage commitment in myeloid progenitors. *Cell.* (2015) 163:1663–77. doi: 10.1016/j.cell.2015.11.013
43. Pei W, Feyerabend TB, Rossler J, Wang X, Postrach D, Busch K, et al. Polylox barcoding reveals haematopoietic stem cell fates realized *in vivo. Nature.* (2017) 548:456–60. doi: 10.1038/nature23653
44. Schraml BU, van Blijswijk J, Zelenay S, Whitney PG, Filby A, Acton SE, et al. Genetic tracing via DNGR-1 expression history defines dendritic cells as a hematopoietic lineage. *Cell.* (2013) 154:843–58. doi: 10.1016/j.cell.2013.07.014
45. Perie L, Duffy KR, Kok L, de Boer RJ, Schumacher TN. The branching point in erythro-myeloid differentiation. *Cell.* (2015) 163:1655–62. doi: 10.1016/j.cell.2015.11.059
46. Buenrostro JD, Corces MR, Lareau CA, Wu B, Schep AN, Aryee MJ, et al. Integrated single-cell analysis maps the continuous regulatory landscape of human hematopoietic differentiation. *Cell.* (2018) 173:1535–48 e16. doi: 10.1016/j.cell.2018.03.074
47. Lin DS, Kan A, Gao J, Crampin EJ, Hodgkin PD, Naik SH. DiSNE movie visualization and assessment of clonal kinetics reveal multiple trajectories of dendritic cell development. *Cell Rep.* (2018) 22:2557–66. doi: 10.1016/j.celrep.2018.02.046
48. Jaitin DA, Weiner A, Yofe I, Lara-Astiaso D, Keren-Shaul H, David E, et al. Dissecting immune circuits by linking CRISPR-pooled screens with single-cell RNA-Seq. *Cell.* (2016) 167:1883–96 e15. doi: 10.1016/j.cell.2016.11.039
49. Hoppe PS, Coutu DL, Schroeder T. Single-cell technologies sharpen up mammalian stem cell research. *Nat Cell Biol.* (2014) 16:919–27. doi: 10.1038/ncb3042
50. Karsunky H, Merad M, Cozzio A, Weissman IL, Manz MG. Flt3 ligand regulates dendritic cell development from Flt3+ lymphoid and myeloid-committed progenitors to Flt3+ dendritic cells *in vivo. J Exp Med.* (2003) 198:305–13. doi: 10.1084/jem.20030323
51. Manz MG, Traver D, Miyamoto T, Weissman IL, Akashi K. Dendritic cell potentials of early lymphoid and myeloid progenitors. *Blood.* (2001) 97:3333–41. doi: 10.1182/blood.V97.11.3333
52. Karsunky H, Merad M, Mende I, Manz MG, Engleman EG, Weissman IL. Developmental origin of interferon-alpha-producing dendritic cells from hematopoietic precursors. *Exp Hematol.* (2005) 33:173–81. doi: 10.1016/j.exphem.2004.10.010
53. Yang G-X, Lian Z-X, Kikuchi K, Moritoki Y, Ansari AA, Liu Y-J, et al. Plasmacytoid dendritic cells of different origins have distinct characteristics and function: studies of lymphoid progenitors versus myeloid progenitors. *J Immunol.* (2005) 175:7281–7. doi: 10.4049/jimmunol.175.11.7281
54. Sathe P, Vremec D, Wu L, Corcoran L, Shortman K. Convergent differentiation: myeloid and lymphoid pathways to murine plasmacytoid dendritic cells. *Blood.* (2013) 121:11–9. doi: 10.1182/blood-2012-02-413336
55. Pelayo R, Hirose J, Huang J, Garrett KP, Delogu A, Busslinger M, et al. Derivation of 2 categories of plasmacytoid dendritic cells in murine bone marrow. *Blood.* (2005) 105:4407–15. doi: 10.1182/blood-2004-07-2529
56. Shigematsu H, Reizis B, Iwasaki H, Mizuno S-i, Hu D, Traver D, et al. Plasmacytoid dendritic cells activate lymphoid-specific genetic programs irrespective of their cellular origin. *Immunity.* (2004) 21:43–53. doi: 10.1016/j.immuni.2004.06.011
57. Chen Y-L, Chen T-T, Pai L-M, Wesoly J, Bluyssen HAR, Lee C-K. A type I IFN-Flt3 ligand axis augments plasmacytoid dendritic cell development from common lymphoid progenitors. *J Exp Med.* (2013) 210:2515–22. doi: 10.1084/jem.20130536
58. Schlitzer A, Heiseke AF, Einwächter H, Reindl W, Schiemann M, Manta C-P, et al. Tissue-specific differentiation of a circulating CCR9-pDC-like common dendritic cell precursor. *Blood.* (2012) 119:6063–71. doi: 10.1182/blood-2012-03-418400
59. Schlitzer A, Loschko J, Mair K, Vogelmann R, Henkel L, Einwächter H, et al. Identification of CCR9- murine plasmacytoid DC precursors with plasticity to differentiate into conventional DCs. *Blood.* (2011) 117:6562–70. doi: 10.1182/blood-2010-12-326678
60. Ghosh HS, Ceribelli M, Matos I, Lazarovici A, Bussemaker HJ, Lasorella A, et al. ETO family protein Mtg16 regulates the balance of dendritic cell subsets by repressing Id2. *J Exp Med.* (2014) 211:1623–35. doi: 10.1084/jem.20132121
61. Lau CM, Tiniakou I, Perez OA, Kirkling ME, Yap GS, Hock H, et al. Transcription factor Etv6 regulates functional differentiation of cross-presenting classical dendritic cells. *J Exp Med.* (2018) 215:2265–78. doi: 10.1084/jem.20172323
62. Satpathy AT, KC W, Albring JC, Edelson BT, Kretzer NM, Bhattacharya D, et al. Zbtb46 expression distinguishes classical dendritic cells and their committed progenitors from other immune lineages. *J Exp Med.* (2012) 209:1135–52. doi: 10.1084/jem.20120030
63. Onai N, Asano J, Kurosaki R, Kuroda S, Ohteki T. Flexible fate commitment of E2–2high common DC progenitors implies

tuning in tissue microenvironments. *Int Immunol.* (2017) 29:443–56. doi: 10.1093/intimm/dxx058

64. Herman JS, Sagar, Grun D. FateID infers cell fate bias in multipotent progenitors from single-cell RNA-seq data. *Nat Methods.* (2018) 15:379–86. doi: 10.1038/nmeth.4662
65. Rodriguez-Fraticelli AE, Wolock SL, Weinreb CS, Panero R, Patel SH, Jankovic M, et al. Clonal analysis of lineage fate in native haematopoiesis. *Nature.* (2018) 553:212–6. doi: 10.1038/nature25168
66. Macri C, Pang ES, Patton T, O'Keeffe M. Dendritic cell subsets. *Semin Cell Dev Biol.* (2017) 84:11–21. doi: 10.1016/j.semcdb.2017.12.009
67. Niederquell M, Kurig S, Fischer JAA, Tomiuk S, Swiecki M, Colonna M, et al. Sca-1 expression defines developmental stages of mouse pDCs that show functional heterogeneity in the endosomal but not lysosomal TLR9 response. *Eur J Immunol.* (2013) 43:2993–3005. doi: 10.1002/eji.201343498
68. Kamogawa-Schifter Y, Ohkawa J, Namiki S, Arai N, Arai K-I, Liu Y. Ly49Q defines 2 pDC subsets in mice. *Blood.* (2005) 105:2787–92. doi: 10.1182/blood-2004-09-3388
69. Bauer J, Dress RJ, Schulze A, Dresing P, Ali S, Deenen R, et al. Cutting Edge: IFN-beta expression in the spleen is restricted to a subpopulation of plasmacytoid dendritic cells exhibiting a specific immune modulatory transcriptome signature. *J Immunol.* (2016) 196:4447–51. doi: 10.4049/jimmunol.1500383
70. Breton G, Zheng S, Valieris R, Tojal da Silva I, Satija R, Nussenzweig MC. Human dendritic cells. (DCs) are derived from distinct circulating precursors that are precommitted to become CD1c+ or CD141+ DCs. *J Exp Med.* (2016) 213:2861–70. doi: 10.1084/jem.20161135
71. Bryant C, Fromm PD, Kupresanin F, Clark G, Lee K, Clarke C, et al. A CD2 high-expressing stress-resistant human plasmacytoid dendritic-cell subset. *Immunol Cell Biol.* (2016) 94:447–57. doi: 10.1038/icb.2015.116
72. Matsui T, Connolly JE, Michnevitz M, Chaussabel D, Yu CI, Glaser C, et al. CD2 distinguishes two subsets of human plasmacytoid dendritic cells with distinct phenotype and functions. *J Immunol.* (2009) 182:6815–23. doi: 10.4049/jimmunol.0802008
73. Zhang H, Gregorio JD, Iwahori T, Zhang X, Choi O, Tolentino LL, et al. A distinct subset of plasmacytoid dendritic cells induces activation and differentiation of B and T lymphocytes. *Proc Natl Acad Sci USA.* (2017) 114:1988–93. doi: 10.1073/pnas.1610630114
74. Zhang X, Lepelley A, Azria E, Lebon P, Roguet G, Schwartz O, et al. Neonatal plasmacytoid dendritic cells. (pDCs) display subset variation but can elicit potent anti-viral innate responses. *PLoS ONE.* (2013) 8:e52003. doi: 10.1371/journal.pone.0052003
75. Cella M, Facchetti F, Lanzavecchia A, Colonna M. Plasmacytoid dendritic cells activated by influenza virus and CD40L drive a potent TH1 polarization. *Nat Immunol.* (2000) 1:305–10. doi: 10.1038/79747
76. Grouard G, Rissoan MC, Filgueira L, Durand I, Banchereau J, Liu YJ. The enigmatic plasmacytoid T cells develop into dendritic cells with interleukin. (IL)-3 and CD40-ligand. *J Exp Med.* (1997) 185:1101–11. doi: 10.1084/jem.185.6.1101
77. Hoeffel G, Ripoche AC, Matheoud D, Nascimbeni M, Escriou N, Lebon P, et al. Antigen crosspresentation by human plasmacytoid dendritic cells. *Immunity.* (2007) 27:481–92. doi: 10.1016/j.immuni.2007.07.021
78. Alculumbre SG, Saint-André V, Di Domizio J, Vargas P, Sirven P, Bost P, et al. Diversification of human plasmacytoid predendritic cells in response to a single stimulus. *Nat Immunol.* (2017) 19:63–75. doi: 10.1038/s41590-017-0012-z
79. Macal M, Jo Y, Dallari S, Chang AY, Dai J, Swaminathan S, et al. Self-renewal and toll-like receptor signaling sustain exhausted plasmacytoid dendritic cells during chronic viral infection. *Immunity.* (2018) 48:730–44 e5. doi: 10.1016/j.immuni.2018.03.020
80. Stuart T, Satija R. Integrative single-cell analysis. *Nat Rev Genet.* (2019) 20:257–72. doi: 10.1038/s41576-019-0093-7

12

Harnessing Dendritic Cells for Poly (D,L-lactide-*co*-glycolide) Microspheres (PLGA MS)—Mediated Anti-Tumor Therapy

*Julia Koerner[1], Dennis Horvath[1] and Marcus Groettrup[1,2]**

[1] *Division of Immunology, Department of Biology, University of Konstanz, Konstanz, Germany,* [2] *Biotechnology Institute Thurgau at the University of Konstanz, Kreuzlingen, Switzerland*

Correspondence:
Marcus Groettrup
marcus.groettrup@uni-konstanz.de

With emerging success in fighting off cancer, chronic infections, and autoimmune diseases, immunotherapy has become a promising therapeutic approach compared to conventional therapies such as surgery, chemotherapy, radiation therapy, or immunosuppressive medication. Despite the advancement of monoclonal antibody therapy against immune checkpoints, the development of safe and efficient cancer vaccine formulations still remains a pressing medical need. Anti-tumor immunotherapy requires the induction of antigen-specific CD8+ cytotoxic T lymphocyte (CTL) responses which recognize and specifically destroy tumor cells. Due to the crucial role of dendritic cells (DCs) in initiating anti-tumor immunity, targeting tumor antigens to DCs has become auspicious in modern vaccine research. Over the last two decades, micron- or nanometer-sized particulate delivery systems encapsulating tumor antigens and immunostimulatory molecules into biodegradable polymers have shown great promise for the induction of potent, specific and long-lasting anti-tumor responses *in vivo*. Enhanced vaccine efficiency of the polymeric micro/nanoparticles has been attributed to controlled and continuous release of encapsulated antigens, efficient targeting of antigen presenting cells (APCs) such as DCs and subsequent induction of CTL immunity. Poly (D, L-lactide-*co*-glycolide) (PLGA), as one of these polymers, has been extensively studied for the design and development of particulate antigen delivery systems in cancer therapy. This review provides an overview of the current state of research on the application of PLGA microspheres (PLGA MS) as anti-tumor cancer vaccines in activating and potentiating immune responses attempting to highlight their potential in the development of cancer therapeutics.

Keywords: PLGA, microspheres, cancer vaccine, dendritic cell, anti-tumor response, spray drying, immunotherapy, CTL

INTRODUCTION

With an annual incidence of several million new cases worldwide, cancer represents one of the most prevalent malignancies and leading causes of pain and mortality. Conventional treatment options usually include a combination of primary resection, radiotherapy and/or chemotherapy. However, cancer patients suffer from devastating adverse side-effects and poor quality of life after chemo- or radiation therapy. Moreover, therapeutic failure of standard therapeutics results in increased risk of tumor relapse and metastasis formation (1). Hence, there is an urgent need for safe and effective vaccine development against this life-threating group of diseases. With the identification of multiple unique cancer antigens (tumor-associated antigens, TAA) and the investigation of manifold immune evasion pathways of tumors, immunotherapy has become a growing focus in clinical research.

Cancer immunotherapy encompasses therapeutic modulation of the host's immune system to defend against foreign or self-antigens that have gone awry in tumor development. Cancer vaccines aim at triggering immune activation to specifically target and eliminate tumor cells. Ideally, a memory response is generated to impede metastasis formation and further spread of the disease. In contrast to passive immunotherapy which aims at delivering neutralizing antibodies, active forms of immunotherapy are supposed to induce multi-faceted cell mediated immunity by simultaneous activation of APCs, CD4+ and CD8+ T cells, as well as B cells and innate immune cells, as for instance NK cells, granulocytes and macrophages. Compared to standard tumor therapies, immunotherapeutic anti-tumor vaccines offer distinct advantages, namely: increased specificity and reduced toxicity by activation of antigen-specific CTL responses. Effector CTLs are able to decrease large tumor masses and induce long-term protection against tumor recurrence through induction of immunological memory (2). Recent advances in cancer immunotherapy have paved the way for the discovery of versatile methods for prevention or treatment of various types of cancer. As a result, several cancer vaccines are currently investigated in clinical trials. However, most of them have not progressed beyond phase III studies. Although antigen-specific responses were generated and increases in overall survival rates were obtained, there is no consistency in clinical benefit. Most of the approaches were presented with major drawbacks in vaccine delivery and efficacy. Administration of soluble antigenic formulations, e.g. synthetic peptides or purified tumor-associated antigens was not promising due to poor immunogenicity, limited bioavailability, short half-life and rapid degradation or elimination of the antigens *in vivo*, demanding the need for repeated injections (3).

Due to the unique ability of DCs to prime and activate naïve T cells (4, 5), DC-based vaccination strategies have shown to be a promising approach in the development of polyvalent cancer vaccines. The first promising results have been achieved using *ex vivo* derived autologous tumor cells or DCs that have been pulsed with various tumor-associated proteins or peptides (6). However, major drawbacks were seen in suboptimal antigen presenting capacity of isolated DCs or simple lack of autologous tumor samples (7, 8). Several promising immunotherapeutic advances came across with the use of allogeneic tumor-lysate pulsed DCs, loading of DCs with MHC class I restricted tumor antigens (9–11), or via transfection of cDNA encoding TAAs (8, 12). Whole tumor lysate contains a large repertoire of tumor antigens capable of inducing immune responses against a broad spectrum of multiple epitopes including those that are unique to the patient's tumor. The development of DC-based vaccination has led to the first therapeutic cancer vaccine. In April 2010, Provenge® (Sipuleucel-T) was approved by the FDA for treatment of castration-resistant, metastatic prostate cancer (13). This immunotherapy involves *ex vivo* stimulation of autologous, blood-derived antigen presenting cells from prostate cancer patients that are pulsed with a prostate cancer-associated antigen [PAP (prostate acid phosphatase)–GM-CSF fusion protein]. DCs were subsequently re-introduced into patients to stimulate an immune response against PAP-expressing prostate cancer cells. These well-tolerated approaches using *ex vivo* loaded DCs were tested in a variety of experimental models and clinical trials [reviewed in Tacken et al. (14)], and seemed to be encouraging due to good safety records, the generation of enhanced T cell responses and partial reduction of tumor load. However, clinical application is still limited as these *ex vivo* procedures are laborious and time-consuming, extremely expensive and lack universal applicability (15). More importantly, the overall clinical response rates in cancer patients were only 7% (16).

To circumvent the limitations associated with *in vitro* manipulation of cells, direct *in vivo* targeting of DCs along with appropriate adjuvants for simultaneous activation of dendritic cells has gained major focus. Particulate delivery systems have shown to overcome the main obstacles related to traditional cancer therapeutics. Instead of causing the risk to induce systemic, adverse immunity, vaccine antigens are delivered to DCs in a targeted manner. We and others have established the use of PLGA MS as an efficient vaccine delivery system for dendritic cell targeting. Subsequent induction of potent immune responses has led to remarkable protective and therapeutic anti-tumor activity *in vivo*. In this article we review how DCs can be antigen charged and matured with PLGA MS *in vitro* and *in vivo* and how microspheres can be produced and formulated to optimally be taken up by DCs. Moreover, we discuss the parameters how antigen presentation and T cell stimulation by PLGA MS-loaded DCs can be improved to elicit a vigorous and effective anti-tumor immune response.

COMPARISON OF PARTICULATE ANTIGEN DELIVERY SYSTEMS

At present, several particulate drug delivery systems for cancer immunotherapy–other than PLGA based particles–have passed pre-clinical investigations and are currently tested for human application, such as liposomes, virosomes, immune-stimulatory complexes (ISCOMs) or gold particles. These systems are reviewed elsewhere (17) and are beyond the scope of this article. Furthermore, detailed analysis of nano-sized particulate vaccine delivery systems has been already extensively reviewed (18–20) and is only of specialized focus in this review.

Multiple different natural or synthetic polyesters have been reported for the development of (sub)micron sized colloidal drug delivery systems, such as poly(lactic acid) (PLA), poly(glycolic acid) (PGA), poly(ε-caprolactone) (PCL), poly(methyl methacrylate) (PMMA), poly(β-amino esters) as well as other ester derivates [poly(anhydrides), poly(orthoesters), poly(phosphoesters), poly(phosphazenes) or poly(cyanoacrylate)]. Due to their excellent bioavailability,

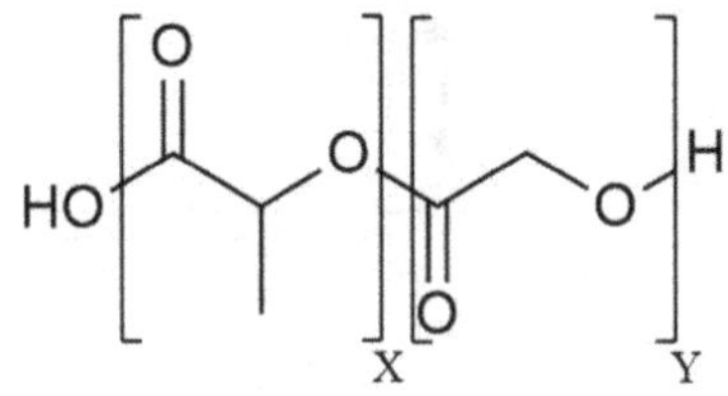

FIGURE 1 | Chemical structure of the poly (D,L – lactide-*co*-glycolide) (PLGA) co-polymer.

biodegradable and biocompatible properties, controlled release and low toxicity, these polymers have been extensively studied as delivery systems of various therapeutic vaccines as well as for cancer immunotherapy in preclinical settings (21–23). Based on the method of preparation, different types of polymeric particles can be designed: spheres, capsules, cubes and other shapes. While the active compound of micro/nanocapsules is contained inside a cavity underneath the polymeric layer, micro/nanospheres homogenously entrap the encapsulated materials into the inner polymer matrix core (24).

The aliphatic co-polymer PLGA is one of the most frequently used and explored polymers for controlled delivery of bioactive molecules in microspheres and nanoparticles (NP) (25). The amorphous PLGA is composed of varying proportions of lactic and glycolic acids (**Figure 1**). Due to its ideal *in vivo* properties of biodegradability, biocompatibility and its clear safety records, PLGA has been licensed by the U.S. Food and Drug Administration (FDA) and European Medicines Agency (EMA) for use in pharmaceutical application via parenteral (subcutaneous, intradermal, intramuscular) and mucosal routes as well as for suspension formulations of biomedical devices including surgical sutures and bone implants (26). At present, there are 12 PLGA-based microparticle cancer vaccine formulations approved by the FDA for clinical use. Most of these PLGA MS systems are targeting prostate cancer, for example Pamorelin LA® which encapsulates the gonadotropin releasing hormone (GnRH) agonist triptorelin pamoate for palliative treatment of advanced prostate cancer (27). Of note, not a single nanoparticulate vehicle has reached clinical approval due to associated toxicity issues (28) as discussed later in this review.

PROPERTIES OF PLGA PARTICLES

A wide range of biologically active compounds including hormones, antibiotics, and drugs can be encapsulated into PLGA particles (29, 30). Thus, PLGA micro- and nanoparticles have been well-established as delivery systems of innumerable antigens such as proteins, peptides, lipopeptides, viral or bacterial DNA as well as immunomodulatory molecules (31–37). PLGA particles exhibit a vast array of advantages over soluble vaccine formulations. At first, GMP (good manufacturing practice) grade polymer is commercially available (for example, PLGA Resomer® from Evonik Industries) meeting the GMP requirements of regulatory authorities. Encapsulation within PLGA particles protects the encapsulated bioactive molecules from premature degradation by proteolytic enzymes or metabolic turnover and minimizes loss of therapeutic activity prior to delivery. The enhanced bioavailability is due to sustained and controlled release of encapsulated substances over extended time periods of several weeks to months thus creating a depot effect at the site of injection. Prolonged antigen presentation and continuous T cell stimulation would circumvent the need for conventional multiple dose immunization schedules, e.g. prime-boost vaccination (38, 39). Hence, PLGA MS would provide a valuable approach for single administration vaccine design so that clinical intervention is only limited to one therapeutic injection. Encapsulation of peptides into PLGA MS was shown to enhance and extend antigen presentation on MHC class I and II by DCs and macrophages (29, 38) which is possibly due to higher total load of antigens and prolonged degradation time of larger microparticles compared to nanoparticles (40). Furthermore, entrapment of proteins or peptides into biodegradable PLGA microspheres increases the immunogenicity of poorly immunogenic antigens, e.g. weak self-antigens in tumor tissue. While soluble peptide immunizations elicited only very poor CD8+ T cell responses, microencapsulation of the HLA-A*0201 restricted immunodominant epitope STEAP 1 (six transmembrane epithelial antigen of the prostate) was shown to induce potent prostate cancer peptide-specific CTL activation and cytotoxic effector function (36, 41).

Release and Encapsulation Qualities of PLGA Microspheres

Upon encountering aqueous medium, PLGA is slowly hydrolyzed into its original monomeric components. The resulting products lactic and glycolic acid are physiological metabolites of the citric acid cycle and thus completely eliminated from the human body as carbon dioxide and water (42). The degradation rate and subsequent drug release is primarily dependent on the PLGA polymer composition and the molecular weight of the polymer. These two factors also impact hydrophilicity, the hydration rate as well as the glass transition temperature (Tg) of the respective polymer type, which in turn also affect the release profile (43). A high content of glycolic acid in the co-polymer leads to higher hydrolysis rates and a more rapid release, as glycolic acid is slightly more hydrophilic than the crystalline lactic acid, which fosters water permeability into the polymer matrix. Several other factors contribute to release rates of PLGA MS including concentration of the polymer in the organic solvent during PLGA MS fabrication, PLGA particle size and morphology, as well as storage conditions such as temperature and humidity and of course, the encapsulated material itself. The PLGA 50:50 polymer is preferred over other PLGA polymers with different lactic:glycolic ratios (65:35; 75:25; 80:20) in controlled release vaccine formulation since encapsulated molecules are homogenously dispersed inside the polymer matrix. Additionally, it is slightly more hydrophilic and thus possesses the fastest degradation rate resulting in complete degradation within 30 to 60 days in aqueous medium (44). It also occupies the least crystallinity hence being more prone to (enzyme-independent) hydrolysis and bulk erosion. Only when the PLGA polymer becomes porous and hydrated, encapsulated material of high molecular weight can be released. This will prevent early release of antigens or adjuvants before internalization of the particles by DCs and thus reduces systemic distribution of the encapsulated molecules. The release profile of PLGA degradation encompasses two phases with an initial burst that is followed by progressive release of the encapsulated material. The burst release is likely attributed to weakly bound or adsorbed proteins on the PLGA particle surface that are rapidly dispersed upon submersion into aqueous media (45). Noticeably, about 30% of the entrapped material can be released within a few days, though the percentage markedly depends on the physical properties of the microparticles (46).

Physico-Chemical Characteristics of PLGA Particles

A major advantage of using PLGA polymers is attributed to its great flexibility and ease to manipulate and modify its physicochemical properties such as: molecular mass of the polymer, hydrophilicity and crystallinity (monomer ratio), end-group chemistry, particle size and surface charge. All these factors can be modified to obtain desired and suitable degradation rates and subsequent release patterns for individual treatment regimen. Furthermore, these properties also dictate intracellular trafficking and can thus be individually adjusted to the needs of the encapsulated material (47). The main improvement of using PLGA particles as vaccine delivery system relies on the ability to simultaneously stimulate innate and adaptive immunity through directing intracellular antigen processing toward the cross-presentation pathway. Furthermore, maintenance of integrity and thus activity of the encapsulated material ensures their bioavailability and their ability to mount effective immune responses (48).

PRODUCTION METHODS FOR PLGA MS

There are several methods employed to produce micro- and nanoparticles such as emulsification-solvent-evaporation, organic phase separation (coacervation), nano-precipitation (diafiltration), and newer strategies such as supercritical microfluidics, coaxial electrospray or the PRINT (particle replication in non-wetting templates) technology (49). However, major drawbacks of the most widely used single or double emulsification solvent evaporation techniques is poor encapsulation efficiency, which either requires increased drug loading or the use of surfactants (e.g. PVA, poly-vinyl alcohol) to stabilize the oil-in-water emulsion until particles have been formed. Moreover, high shear or cavitation forces, excessive use of energy or freezing and drying cycles cause significant risk of aggregation or degradation of encapsulated material of these particles, thereby rendering emulsion techniques difficult for mass production (50). Furthermore, the initial burst is very high due to poor drug loading into the particles while adsorption onto the particle surface is very common (22). Nevertheless, we have used and optimized the spray-drying technology in our laboratory.

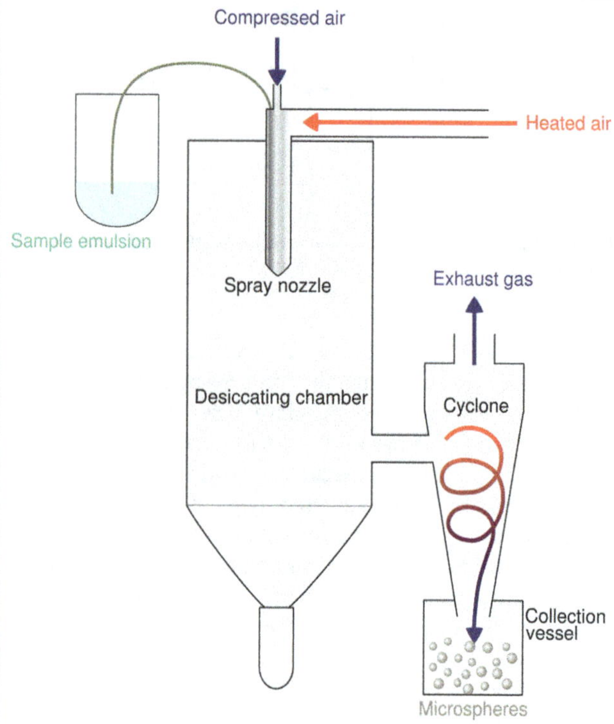

FIGURE 2 | Schematic illustration of the spray drying process for preparation of PLGA microspheres. The sample emulsion is spray-atomized into small droplets at the nozzle. These droplets in the heated dry air flow are transformed into dry particles by evaporation of the organic solvent. The particles are then separated from the drying medium and collected under constant low pressure as dry powder in the lower collection vessel.

Microencapsulation by Spray Drying

Spray-drying is a very suitable and rapid one-step process for encapsulation of both hydrophobic as well as hydrophilic proteins and peptides into PLGA particles. The principle is based on nebulization of a solid-in-oil dispersion or water-in-oil-emulsion composed of antigen and adjuvants in an aqueous phase that is mixed with the volatile, water-immiscible organic solvent [e.g. dichloromethane (DCM)] used to dissolve the PLGA polymer. The fluid is spray-atomized into a gas stream of compressed air or compressed nitrogen into a desiccating chamber, where liquid droplets pass a current of warm air-stream subsequently creating microparticles at the spray nozzle by evaporation of the organic solvent (51, 52). Evaporation keeps the product temperature at low levels, thus only little temperature deterioration occurs (53). As the fluid is converted into a dry powder in the drying chamber, the particle-loaded air stream enters tangentially into the cyclone, which results in a centrifugal force that creates a downward spiral movement in the cyclone causing particle deposition at the bottom of the cyclone separator and the collecting vessel (54) (see **Figure 2**).

This microencapsulation process warrants stability and the biological activity of the encapsulated epitopes and guarantees high yield and encapsulation efficiencies of more than 85% (55). The low preparation temperature of the spray drying method avoids thermal denaturation of encapsulated compounds. The produced microspheres do not exhibit aggregation and show good suspensibility in injection solution. Spray drying usually produces particles with a particle size distribution of about 500 nm–5 μm. Besides process parameters such as the liquid feed rate, the drying air flow rate or the inlet air temperature, molecular weight and concentration of the polymer in the organic solvent critically determines particle size and affects microsphere morphology and subsequently degradation and drug release of PLGA MS (56). The spray-drying method has been successfully used with several biodegradable polymers such as PLA, PCL, gelatin, and polysaccharides or related biopolymers (57–59). It has several advantages over other particle production methods such as lower residual organic solvent, higher yield, and higher encapsulation efficiency or prolonged sustained release. Mentionable, particle sizes can now be easily controlled by using the nano-spray drying method based on the vibrating mesh technology (60, 61). Sticky adhesion of PLGA microparticles to the interior surface of the spray-drier's glass ware, as always referred to a salient drawback of spray drying (62), has been overcome by the use of the non-ionic surfactant Poloxamer® 188 to wash out spray-dried particles.

The optimized drying procedure after spray drying by vacuum drying over several days reduces the residual amount of organic solvent to a minimum (63). The authorized pharmaceutical limit for residual organic volatile impurities of DCM by the U.S. (USP) and European Pharmacopeia (PhEur) is 0.06%. This is pertinent, as incomplete solvent removal or solvent impurities may cause chemical degradation of the encapsulated compounds within the polymer matrix. By efficient removal of the solvent, spray-dried PLGA MS are highly stable as dry powder for long-term storage without degradation of the encapsulated compounds thus preserving therapeutic activity. Furthermore, spray drying can be easily scaled up to produce large batches. Polymer-drug solutions of high volumes are rapidly spray-dried within minutes, which would facilitate industrial production processes for potential clinical application.

In vivo Uptake of PLGA Particles by APCs

Without specific recognition, PLGA MS provide non-specific and untargeted antigen delivery toward APCs (mainly DCs, but also macrophages) because particle sizes of 0.5–5 μm exhibit similar dimensions to pathogens (44, 64). Conceptionally, the particulate matter facilitates cellular uptake and internalization by APCs and allows for faster degradation and rapid intracellular release of the antigenic cargo (25). Thus, encapsulated antigens are better processed and presented by APCs compared to antigens in soluble form. Consequently, PLGA MS-mediated antigen delivery induces a more efficient recognition of presented epitopes by the immune systems (65, 66). DCs, but also macrophages, are highly phagocytic cells being equally able to internalize large, micron-sized particles and small nanoparticles. Several studies indicate that the majority of DCs are able to take up PLGA MS (as well as PLGA nanoparticles) within 24 h. Although, the ideal particle size for uptake by APCs still remains a matter of debate, the particle size critically influences cellular uptake mechanisms but also dictates fate of intracellular endocytic pathways and DC activation and thus affects the generated immune response (20).

Particle Size Influences the Immunogenicity of PLGA Particles

It has been demonstrated that DCs preferably engulf smaller, submicron- or virus-sized particles of 20–200 nm, whereas large particulate vaccines of bacterial size (>500 nm; e.g. microspheres) are mainly taken up by macrophages (67, 68). PLGA particle uptake by human DCs *in vitro* was less efficient at sizes exceeding 500 nm (69). A comparative study by Joshi et al. analyzed OVA (ovalbumin) -specific CTLs in blood after *in vivo* administration of PLGA particles containing OVA/CpG of 300 nm, 1, 7, and 17 μm size. The smallest particles induced the highest antigen specific T cell response suggesting that the smaller the particle the stronger the response (70). Noteworthy, PLGA particles were injected intraperitoneally and tetramer-positive signals were analyzed after two booster vaccinations–incomparable to our vaccination regimen and analysis of peak T cell response on day 6 after PLGA MS vaccination *in vivo* (71). In fact, it was reported, that immature DCs (iDCs) are also able to internalize larger particles by either phagocytosis or micropinocytosis (72, 73). As well, Gutierro et al. have demonstrated increased access of large sized PLGA particles (1 μm) to APCs which in turn elicited a higher total IgG response and increased IFN-γ production of T cells (74). We and others have demonstrated efficient uptake of PLGA microparticles by human peripheral blood monocyte-derived DCs (moDCs), murine immature bone-marrow derived DCs (BMDCs), as well as macrophages *in vitro* and by CD11c+ dendritic cells after subcutaneous immunization *in vivo* (75–77). The entrapped content in DCs is efficiently transported from peripheral tissue to the site of antigen-presentation in secondary lymphoid organs (SLOs) like spleen and liver, providing direct evidence for migration of immature, skin-resident DCs to draining lymph-nodes after PLGA MS uptake (78). This was experimentally confirmed by the presence of Quantum-Dot (QD) positive PLGA microspheres in CD169+ subcapsular sinus macrophages (SSM) in draining lymph nodes (dLN) after immunization with these fluorescent microspheres (79). In contrast to subcutaneous PLGA administration into dermis or epidermis, macrophages are the predominant cell type entrapping PLGA particles after i.p. administration (80, 81). PLGA MS uptake by human moDCs *in vitro* does not negatively influence biological properties, such as survival, cytokine secretion, antigen presentation or subsequent T cell stimulation (75, 82). Also, uptake of PLGA nanoparticles has been investigated using *in vitro* generated human and mouse DC population (83–85). Human moDCs, CD34+ stem cell-derived DCs and mouse BMDCs were able to engulf PLGA NP. Uptake of PLGA MS and NPs was prevented using cytochalasin B, which points to involvement of actin-polymerization during phagocytosis of PLGA particles

(86, 87). In fact, it was shown that PLGA nanoparticles are partly internalized via fluid phase pinocytosis but also through clathrin-dependent receptor mediated endocytosis, while uptake of PLGA microparticles by DCs was achieved by non-specific phagocytosis (88).

Present Challenges of PLGA Nanoparticle Mediated Cancer Vaccines

With respect to vaccine design, one must consider that nanoparticles with a size range of < 200 nm are able to directly enter the lymphatic vessel system from the interstitial space by diffusing through endothelial cell junctions. Additionally, NPs even can easily cross physiological barriers, such as the pulmonary tract, epithelial tight junctions or the blood-brain-barrier (BBB) without specific targeting. On the one hand, PLGA nanoparticles might facilitate stimulation of immune responses via direct delivery of antigens to lymph node (LN)-resident DCs and macrophages within hours after administration (82, 89). On the other hand, it has been established that premature antigen presentation may lead to induction of antigen tolerance. Furthermore, toxicity issues of unspecific uptake by other endocytic cells or non-specific distribution is still a problem of PLGA based nanoparticle-mediated vaccine delivery (90). In contrast, PLGA microspheres remain at the subcutaneous injection site in peripheral tissues and require active uptake by immature DCs resulting in proper activation of DCs and migration to skin-draining LNs where they efficiently present the processed antigens to naïve T cells. Additional toxicity concerns of nano-polymers have emerged, namely electrostatic interaction of positively charged nanoparticles with cell membranes, the recognition of hydrophobic NPs with cells of the reticuloendothelial system (RES) or aggregation of small cationic nanoparticles with serum proteins, potentially causing severe immunotoxicity by hemolysis or platelet aggregation ("nanotoxicology") (90). To improve directed targeting and to minimize safety issues of undesired biodistribution *in vivo*—a problem we are not facing with the use of PLGA microspheres–nanoparticles need to be either surface-modified by hydrophilic moieties like the non-ionic polymer poly ethylene glycol (PEG) or need to be decorated with anchoring endocytosis molecules such as mannose, fucose, N-acteylglucosamine directed against DC-specific surface receptors (e.g. DC-SIGN, mannose receptor, DEC-205) or with DC-specific antibodies such as anti-CD11c (91, 92). The attachment of DC targeting moieties on PLGA NP surfaces has resulted in enhanced vaccine efficacy due to selective cellular binding, facilitated receptor-mediated endocytosis, and subsequent increased antigen cross-presentation to CD8+ T cells (93, 94). Despite enhancing homing mechanisms, preclinical and clinical data over the last decade have unveiled that targeting optimizations did not increase intratumor delivery of NP, which is below 1% of the injected nanoparticle dose (95, 96).

Though present particle-based cancer vaccine strategies have been built upon the hypothesis of preferential uptake of nanoparticles (smaller than 200 nm) and subsequent superiority at priming of cytotoxic responses over microparticles (>1 μm) (97), the optimum particle size for eliciting maximum immune responses has been a challenging topic ever since. Particle size is an important but not the only factor for dictating cellular uptake and intracellular trafficking. In contrast, the induction of specific and potent immune responses depends on a vast array of parameters including physico-chemical properties of PLGA, polymer composition, molecular weight and preparation methods, as well as routes of administration and nature and content of the encapsulated material. We suggest that PLGA microspheres exhibit an ideal adjuvant particle size inducing consistent and very effective immune responses *in vivo* that encourages ongoing use and future optimization of PLGA microsphere-based anti-cancer vaccines (see **Figure 3**).

DC-MEDIATED ANTIGEN PRESENTATION FROM PLGA PARTICLES

Upon endocytic uptake of PLGA microspheres by iDCs, the particles are internalized into early endosomes. A combination of homogenous bulk polymer erosion and slow hydrolysis of microspheres leads to release of the micro-encapsulated antigens and molecules over a period of about 30–60 days, which elicits a low micro-environmental pH that further enhances PLGA hydrolysis (44). Inside the acidic endosomal compartment, lysosomal proteases, and peptidases cleave released antigens into peptides of 12–25 amino acids in length which normally enter classical endocytic pathway via MHC class II presentation for interaction with CD4+ T cells (98). Furthermore, release of the antigenic cargo, including TLR ligands with receptors located at the inner endosomal membrane, leads to endosomal acidification and maturation of the phagosome associated with TLR triggering (99). Reversion of the anionic particle surface charge (from negative to positive) in the acidic lysosomal compartment enables local interaction with endo-lysosomal membranes and facilitates escape from phagosomes into the cytoplasmic compartment. In fact, PLGA micro/nanoparticles rapidly escape the endo-lysosomal compartment within minutes (65, 76). Another possibility of endosomal escape has built upon the "proton-sponge mechanism." The influx of chloride and hydronium ions during endosomal acidification causes osmotic pressure and leads to rupture of the endosomal membrane and subsequent release of its content (25, 100). Cytosolic release of the encapsulated proteins leads to antigen degradation into 8–11 aa long peptides by the proteasome before loading of these peptide fragments onto MHC class I molecules in the ER, a process known as "cross-presentation" (101). MHC class I—peptide complexes are subsequently transported to the cell surface to be presented to CD8+ T cells, thereby inducing the differentiation of CTLs. PLGA encapsulated antigens can be cross-presented by either endosomal escape (phagosome-to-cytosol pathway) or even simultaneously via the vacuolar pathway in the endocytic compartment. Compared to that, other particulate antigen formulations are exclusively relying on the TAP/proteasome-dependent pathway (102). Via exploiting distinct pathways of antigen presentation, PLGA-based particles increase the peptide

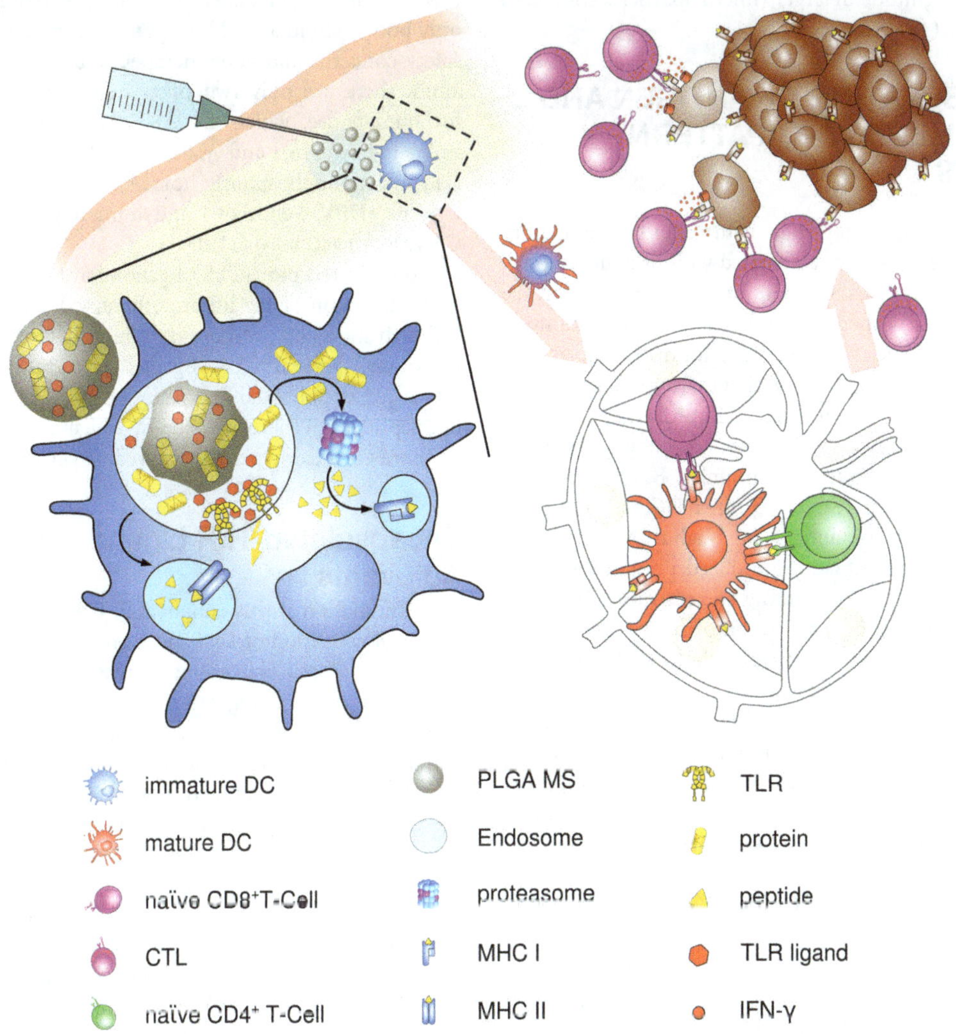

FIGURE 3 | Schematic description of PLGA microsphere mediated anti-tumor response. After subcutaneous immunization, PLGA microspheres are efficiently taken up by immature, skin-resident APCs, mainly DCs. Co-delivery of antigens and TLR ligands leads to enhanced DC activation and maturation by upregulation of co-stimulatory surface maturation marker and MHC class molecules I and II during migration to lymph nodes. In the draining lymph node, encapsulated cancer antigens are processed and presented on either MHC class II to naive CD4+ T helper cells or via cross presentation to CD8+ T cells. Priming and activation of CD8+ T cells leads to differentiation and proliferation of tumor antigen-specific effector CTLs. Clonal expansion and CTL infiltration into the tumor environment results in recognition and eradication of target tumor cells mediated via IFN-γ release and enhanced Th1 polarized immune functions.

pool that is presented on MHC class I and subsequently, the magnitude of the resulting CTL response. Furthermore, downregulation or loss of TAP activity is a major mechanism of tumor immune evasion (103). Thus, TAP deficiency in tumors won't necessarily hamper PLGA MS-mediated antigen cross-presentation by usage of the vacuolar pathway. Involvement of the cross-presentation pathway in processing of encapsulated protein and peptide antigens is further underlined by blockage of their presentation using proteasome inhibitors or brefeldin A (104). Cross-presentation is highly relevant for anti-tumor vaccines that rely on proper induction of tumor killing CTLs (25, 29, 38, 65, 79). Simultaneously, release of antigens into the cytosol may protect the antigenic content from further lysosomal degradation resulting in prolonged antigen presentation. Efficient presentation of PLGA MS delivered proteins and peptides onto MHC class I and II leads to development of a full-blown immune response, since activation of CD4+ T cells, particularly T helper 1 (Th1) cells, are central for activation and stimulation of antigen-specific CTLs through secretion of IFN-γ, IL-2, and IL-12. In addition to direct tumor cytolytic functions, IFN-γ secretion further recruits crucial mediators of the innate immune response, such as NK cells and macrophages thereby potentiating tumor cell killing or apoptotic tumor body clearance (105, 106). The only limitation of PLGA microparticles for use as anti-cancer vaccine is attributed to high initial burst due to dissolution of molecules that are adsorbed at the particle surface which may cause unintentional toxic side-effects (45). However, it has been demonstrated that the initial burst is of lower magnitude in larger (micro-)particles compared to smaller particles (46).

CO-ENCAPSULATION OF ANTIGEN AND IMMUNOSTIMULATORY PATTERN MOLECULES

Encapsulation of antigen together with immunomodulatory molecules overcomes obstacles associated with present adjuvant containing vaccines. For instance, an ameliorated safety profile of adjuvants is accomplished by dose reduction, thus limiting undesired toxicities due to systemic administration of the immune potentiators at non-targeted tissues. Immunogenicity of the encapsulated antigen can further be improved or increased using immunostimulatory adjuvants through providing cellular, humoral, and/or mucosal immunity. Besides ensuring efficient antigen presentation due to proper DC activation and maturation, co-delivery of antigen and adjuvants in PLGA MS/NPs may further potentiate the induced immune response through secretion of NK cell recruiting and activating cytokines by the stimulated DC. Hence, activation of both CTL and NK cell mediated anti-tumor responses are able to eliminate MHC class I positive as well as negative tumors.

The choice of the adjuvant critically determines the outcome and spectrum of the elicited immune response. Thus, addition of adjuvants improves the induction of immune responses of poorly immunogenic tumor self-antigens and potentially supports reduction of the required antigen amount.

Currently Used Adjuvant Agents in Vaccine Formulations

Delivery of both, the antigen and an appropriate DC maturation stimulus in physiological and temporal vicinity improves migratory capacity toward LNs and efficiently stimulates proper T cell responses. Indeed, T cell activation by single encapsulated antigens in the absence of costimulatory molecules or pro-inflammatory cytokines may induce Th2-associated unfavorable immune responses or may even result in tolerance induction against the antigen. The most common adjuvant which has been introduced for vaccination trials over 60 years ago is the water-in-oil emulsion incomplete Freund's adjuvants IFA (107), commonly used as Montanide™ ISA-51 in clinical trials of DC-based immunotherapy (108, 109). The adjuvant effect relies on formation of a local depot providing slow release and prolonged presentation of the antigen (110). Although, IFA is primarily known to induce Th2-biased responses and stimulating humoral responses of long-term IgG production, it can also stimulate CTL or Th1 immunity directed against the antigen that is emulsified in IFA (111). Due to emerging adverse effects such as local skin reactions, abscesses, inflammation or granulomas at the injection site, IFA is not allowed for routine immunotherapy (112). Aluminum salts (alum, and its derivate MF-59) were the first adjuvants approved by the FDA and EMA for clinical use in humans (113, 114) and are currently present in the composition of the majority of vaccines (115). Although generally well-tolerated, alum adjuvants skew immune responses toward humoral mediated and Th2-polarizing conditions and only poorly stimulate CTL responses (116), additional to critical safety concerns and poor therapeutic benefit (117). Apart from alum, there are only two other adjuvants clinically approved for human use, which are AS03 [used in the H5N1 vaccine Prepandrix®(118)] and AS04 (a combination of alum and TLR 4 ligand monophosphorly lipid A (MPL®) applied in hepatitis B virus (HBV, Fendrix®) and human papilloma virus (HPV, Cervarix®) vaccines) (119).

Toll-like receptor (TLR) ligands have been demonstrating a huge impact on cancer immunotherapy due to their capacities of DC activation and promotion of desired Th1 polarized immune responses. Several TLR ligands including oligonucleotides, single- or double-stranded RNA (ssRNA, dsRNA), flagellin or lipopeptides have already been investigated in clinical trials of a plethora of cancer types as reviewed in Temizoz et al. (120).

Encapsulated TLR Ligands as DC Priming Adjuvants

TLR stimulation greatly enhances PLGA vaccine efficacy through powerful activation of DCs including the three signals required for proper T cell activation: increased expression of peptide-MHC complexes, upregulation of co-stimulatory molecules and cytokine secretion (121, 122). Furthermore, TLR triggering enhances cross-presentation to CD8+ T cells and stimulates a Th1-polarized immune response (123). Co-encapsulation of the antigen with either TLR7 or TLR9 ligands into PLGA MS stimulates DC maturation as well as cytokine secretion, and facilitates cross-presentation *in vitro* as shown by Heit et al. (124). Encapsulation of other so-called pathogen recognition receptor (PRR) agonists such as NOD (nucleotide-binding oligomerization domain-like receptor) ligands into either PLGA NP or MS have resulted in similar improvement of vaccine efficiency through enhanced maturation and pro-inflammatory cytokine secretion of human moDCs (125, 126). A detailed list of studies demonstrating improved cellular responses elicited by PLGA particulate systems via association of TLR ligands compared to the antigen alone or over soluble counterparts was extensively reviewed by Silva et al. (20).

We have incorporated at least two TLR ligands into our PLGA MS regimen, which were chosen due to their described Th1 inducing immunomodulation and stimulation of both humoral and cellular immunity (127, 128), namely CG-rich unmethylated Oligodeoxynucleotides (CpG ODN) and the RNA virus associated danger signal polyI:C (polyinosinic:polycitidylic acid) (29, 71, 129, 130). Their receptors, TLR9 and TLR3 respectively, are localized in the membrane of the endosomal compartments of most APCs where PLGA MS are internalized after endocytic uptake (131). Importantly, actual expression pattern of the respective TLRs has to be considered for particle vaccine design and the preferred targeting cell type. While TLR9 expression is limited to plasmacytoid DCs (pDCs), B cells and keratinocytes, TLR3 is expressed more broadly (132). Co-encapsulation of the model antigen ovalbumin together with CpG ODNs or polyI:C into PLGA microspheres efficiently elicited potent antigen-specific CTL responses and

Thl differentiation in comparison with soluble antigen after a single subcutaneous PLGA MS immunization *in vivo* (71, 130). Mice immunized with PLGA MS OVA/CpG generated a 2-fold increase in antigen-specific CD4+ and CD8+ T cell proliferation and IFN-γ production compared to a mixture of MS loaded separately with either the antigen or the adjuvant (PLGA MS OVA + PLGA MS CpG) (71). Pulsing of DCs with empty PLGA microspheres did not induce DC maturation *in vitro* (130), nor did vaccination of mice with empty PLGA MS elicit undesirable T cell responses (36, 71, 79, 133) thus confirming antigen-specificity of immune responses induced with PLGA microspheres. In stark contrast to that, pro-inflammatory adjuvant properties of PLGA microparticles (in comparison to PLGA nanoparticles) have been observed in macrophages (134). Several other TLR agonists have proven strong potential of enhancing the immunogenicity and efficacy of PLGA particle mediated cancer therapy in preclinical settings such as the TLR4 ligand monophospholipid A (MPLA), a chemically modified derivative of the *S. minnesota* derived endotoxin lipid A (135). Indeed, co-administration of TLR agonists in protein and peptide based cancer vaccines have entered clinical phase such as the TLR3 ligand poly ICLC (Hiltonol®) demonstrating tumor regression of advanced facial rhabdomyosarcoma (136), or the TLR7 agonist Imiquimod which has been approved for treatment of basal cell carcinoma due to its ability of CTL-mediated tumor regression by DC and NK cell recruitment (137).

Enhancing PLGA Mediated Cancer Vaccines by Co-delivery of a Second TLR Ligand

Improvement of the PLGA MS system by adding a second TLR ligand, separately encapsulated has been shown to positively influence Th cell polarization to Th1—mediated immune response by targeted DCs (71, 129), suggesting that optimal DC activation depends on synergistic triggering of several TLR signaling pathways (138). Immunization of mice with PLGA MS OVA/CpG together with PLGA MS polyI:C resulted in greater number of KLRG1+ effector T cells (139) and increased cytotoxic effector functions of OVA-specific CD8+ CTLs, as demonstrated by IFN-γ production, oncolytic granzyme B and perforin secretion and increased CD107α expression (71). Several other groups have similarly demonstrated that concomitant delivery of antigen and adjuvant in the same endo-lysosomal compartment is required for proper activation of DCs and superior CTL induction *in vivo* (124). In any case, cross-presentation of the internalized antigen was enhanced with simultaneous co-encapsulation of either TLR3 or TLR9 ligands and the antigen (140, 141). The enhanced vaccine efficiency manifests in prolonged presentation of antigen derived epitopes and superior anti-tumor responses in mice (71, 124, 142). For example, co-delivery of PLGA NPs-OVA together with the TLR4 ligand MPLA (143) or the melanoma antigen TRP2 with another TLR4 ligand (7-acyl lipid A) (144) generated improved antigen-specific responses.

Surprisingly, other studies have come to the opposite conclusion, namely that co-administration of antigen and TLR ligand in different PLGA particles [PLGA NP OVA + PLGA NP (MPLA + R837)] yields better results compared to co-delivery of antigen and adjuvant in the same nanoparticle (PLGA NP OVA/MPLA/R837). Mentionable, these studies only focused on the humoral response and IgG1 and IgG2a production and have not analyzed cellular immunity. Of note, TLR7 (the receptor for R837) is not expressed in the cross-presenting CD8α+ splenic DC subset (145) which may cause inferior responsiveness toward imidazoquinolines. Moreover, the discrepancy between co-encapsulation and co-administration strategies probably depends on the particulate nature, the encapsulated antigen, the route of administration and the choice of adjuvant. Another possibility to enhance immunogenicity of PLGA MS mediated vaccine delivery system is co-encapsulation of multiple specific CTL epitopes. It was already demonstrated that administration of two OVA-derived epitopes into one PLGA microsphere elicited substantial IFN-γ secretion *in vivo* (146).

ANTI-TUMOR RESPONSES TO IMMUNOTHERAPY WITH PLGA PARTICLES

Co-delivery of antigen and adjuvant to DCs is required for PLGA MS-mediated anti-tumor immunotherapy. Reduction of tumor growth in various syngeneic tumor models in mice was better compared to the same antigen emulsion in IFA. Both, protective as well as therapeutic treatment with PLGA MS OVA/CpG + PLGA MS polyI:C elicited potent anti-tumor activity in subcutaneous tumor models as well as in lung metastasis models using EG-7 thymoma or the aggressive MO-5 melanoma tumor cells in mice (129). Remarkably, even a single administration of co-encapsulated OVA/CpG microspheres completely protected mice from tumor growth (129). Increased anti-tumor activity using PLGA associated nanoparticulate vaccines was shown by others as well. PLGA NP OVA/polyI:C or PLGA NP OVA/CpG exerted potent anti-tumor activity against subcutaneously implanted EG-7 tumor cells (147). Noticeably, Silva et al. demonstrated decreased growth of B16F10 melanoma in both therapeutic and prophylactic settings using MHC class I or II restricted melanoma peptides Melan-A and gp100 encapsulated into PLGA NP together with either one or both of the TLR3 and TLR9 ligands polyI:C and CpG (148). This study offered several distinct conclusions besides confirmation of the fact that co-encapsulation of antigens and adjuvants in PLGA particles improves antigen-specific anti-oncogenic immunity. First, the study shows synergistic effects of enhanced anti-tumor activity by co-encapsulation of the two immunopotentiators CpG and poly(I:C) into one particle. Second, mice were slightly more protected from tumor growth after immunization with nanoparticles containing two MHC class I-restricted melanoma epitopes simultaneously. Furthermore, the authors propose that co-administration of PLGA NPs with either an MHC class I or an additional MHC class II restricted epitope along with both TLR ligands induced almost complete blockage of tumor growth, suggesting the important activation of both CD8+ and CD4+ T cell responses for efficacy of anti-tumor immunity. IFN-γ secreting CD4+ T cells facilitate the differentiation of tumor antigen-specific CTLs and promote the recruitment of cells from the immune system participating in tumor cell containment (149). Further, tumor specific CD4+ T cells regulate the survival of CD8+ memory T cells (150). Combined TLR ligation on DCs triggering both MyD88 dependent and independent TLR mediated signaling pathways in parallel has already been demonstrated to promote broader activation of DCs. The marked increase in pro-inflammatory cytokine production and expression of co-stimulatory molecules resulted in enhanced T cell responses *in vivo* or even insensitivity to the immunosuppressive activity of Tregs at tumor sites (151–153). Additionally, tumor-induced immunosuppression of DCs is one of the main causes for ineffective anti-tumor responses (154). Thus, co-delivery of tumor antigens together with TLR ligands in PLGA MS not only targets the antigen to DCs, but might also rescue impaired DC function from tumor induced immunosuppression (155, 156).

Alternatives to TLR Ligands as Immunomodulatory Compounds

In addition to TLR ligands, it is possible to include lipid antigens (e.g. the extremely potent glycosphingplipid α-galactosyl-ceramide, α-GalCer), which activate natural killer T (NKT) cells by binding to the non-classical MHC CD1 molecules. This unique subset of the T cell lineage acts as a potent adjuvant in immune responses against cancer by downstream activation of both innate and adaptive immune responses (157). Although not directly killing tumor cells, NKT cells simulate the cross-priming of tumor antigens by DCs through rapid secretion of large amounts of IFN-γ, IL-12, and IP10 (IFN-γ inducible protein 10) and are able to induce further recruitment of NK cells, macrophages, DCs, CD4+ and CD8+ T cells to tumor sites (157). A combination of α-GalCer and the TLR4 agonist MPLA into PLGA microspheres markedly increased cellular immune responses (158). Moreover, co-encapsulation of the invariant NKT cell agonist, together with the TLR 7/8 agonist R848 (Resiquimod) and polyI:C into PLGA nanoparticles enhanced CD4+ and CD8+ mediated anti-tumor responses mainly dependent on DC condition via NKT cells (159). Interestingly, a non-glycosidic derivate of α-GalCer, threitolceramide (ThrCer) has already proven clinically effectiveness in human and mice (160).

Tumor Lysate as Antigen Source for Particulate PLGA Mediated Cancer Immunotherapy

As outlined above, endogenous and exogenous antigen supply in DC-mediated cancer immunotherapy has faced major limitations such as peptide degradation, rapid turnover of peptide/MHC complexes or dissociation of peptide from MHC during DC preparation/injection (161). This was likely attributed to the fact that only a limited number of peptides with few if any T helper peptides were used (162). Additionally, immunotherapy of solid malignancies is often hampered by low numbers of tumor-specific T cells due to inefficient antigen delivery of DC-based immunotherapy. Moreover, re-administered DCs displayed poor migratory capacity, thus limiting the amount of antigen presented to T lymphocytes in local dLN (163). The use of whole tumor lysates (TL) bypasses the limited potency of single antigen delivery thus broadening the repertoire of defined TAAs and neoantigens and thereby enhancing the probability of generating polyvalent, tumor-associated and antigen-specific CTL responses. Simultaneous stimulation of both CD8+ restricted CTL responses and CD4+ T helper cells is potentially complex enough to overcome the ability of tumors to down-regulate targeted antigens. PLGA MS co-encapsulating TRAMP-prostate derived tumor lysate and TLR ligands showed promising *ex vivo* cytotoxic T lymphocyte responses and achieved elimination of large tumor masses *in vivo* in TRAMP mice, a transgenic mouse model for prostate cancer (133). The anti-tumor efficacy of tumor lysate co-encapsulated with CpG ODNs in PLGA MS was also shown by Goforth et al. in a mouse model for melanoma (164). As well, a prime boost regimen of microspheres containing lysates of mammary gland tumor cells followed by a booster vaccination of bulk tumor lysate together with TLR ligands in liposome formulation was able to ameliorate tumor growth in a murine breast cancer model (165). Noticeably, patient-derived DCs loaded with PLGA NPs encapsulating lysed tumor tissue from patients with advanced head and neck squamous cell carcinoma (HNSSC) could efficiently induce IFN-γ production and could significantly reduce IL-10 secretion in autologous CD8+ T cells (166). Similar findings were made by Hanlon et al. demonstrating increased production of pro-inflammatory cytokines in healthy donor DCs that were pulsed with PLGA nanoparticles encapsulating tumor lysate of an ovarian cancer cell line (167). Malignant cells have developed prodigiously smart mechanisms to co-opt immune cells for tumor progression thereby creating an immunosuppressive microenvironment. Cancer cells are able to attract immunosuppressive cell types such as regulatory T cells (Tregs) and myeloid derived suppressor cells (MDSCs) and are known to drive TAM (tumor-associated macrophage) differentiation to the pro-tumorigenic M2 phenotype. PLGA MS mediated cancer therapy might be an ideal strategy to revert these immunosuppressive mechanisms by inducing factors that are essential for cytotoxicity against cancer cells such as intra-tumoral activated CD8+ T cell response and IFN-γ production as well as recruitment of NK cells. Moreover, upregulation and overexpression of immune checkpoints CTLA-4 (cytotoxic T lymphocyte associated antigen 4) or PD-L1 (programmed cell death protein ligand 1) on cancer cells induces T cell anergy and maintains Treg induced immunosuppression. Thus, it might also be interesting to combine PLGA microsphere-based immunotherapy with immune checkpoint inhibitors to restore T cell anti-tumor effector function.

Apart from generation of anti-tumor responses, we additionally could demonstrate the preeminence of PLGA MS in infectious diseases. PLGA MS encapsulated Influenza virus matrix M1 peptide together with CpG induced potent

TABLE 1 | Main advantages of PLGA microspheres as a DC-mediated particulate vaccine delivery system for cancer immunotherapy.

	Advantage	Rationale
General issues PLGA	Biodegradability and biocompatibility	Complete degradation into toxicologically safe metabolic products
	Approval for parenteral use by regulatory authorities	Improved safety; commercially available as cGMP product
	Versatile physico-chemical properties (e.g. MW, L:G ratio)	Adjustable drug release profile; tailoring of elicited responses
	Encapsulated material is protected from premature degradation	Preserving therapeutic activity
	Possibility of polymer surface modification	e.g. addition of targeting moieties
Spray Drying method	Long-term storage in powder form	Physical and chemical stability at 4°C without loss of biological activity
	Few processing parameters, short manufacturing time	Adjustable particle size and shape; ease of industrial scalability
	Low amount of residual organic solvent; no addition of stabilizers/emulsifiers needed	No adverse effects due to solvent impurities
	High reproducibility between spray-dried batches	Standardized and compendious protocols
	High drug loading and encapsulation efficiency	Reduced antigen/adjuvant doses minimize side effects or systemic immune activation by soluble immunomodulators
Boosting the immune response	Sustained and controlled release for extended time-period (≥30 days); depot effect at the injection site	Avoids risk of antigen tolerance; substitutes need for booster injections
	Particle sizes of 0.5–5 μm via spray-drying	Passive but facilitated internalization by APCs, particularly DCs
	Enhanced & prolonged antigen (cross-) presentation on MHC class I and II	Activation of adaptive and humoral immunity; cross-presentation of tumor antigens; stimulation of CTL and Th1 responses
	Concomitant delivery of antigens and adjuvant in the same PLGA microsphere	Enhanced, direct endolysosomal delivery in target cells, synergistic interaction of DC activation and T cell stimulation
	Induction of strong effector CTL responses	Increased immunogenicity of peptides or tumor antigens
	Single shot cancer vaccine	Reduction or complete protection of tumor growth; induction of long-term memory
	Microencapsulation of whole tumor lysate	Enhanced anti-tumor activity; possibility of personalized vaccination

anti-viral CTL responses and protected against Influenza A infection (168).

In relation to a potential use of PLGA MS in clinical application, sterilization of PLGA MS by γ-irradiation did not negatively affect T cell responses (133). The biggest advantage of spray-dried PLGA microspheres is the high reproducibility of the low-cost MS production meeting GMP requirements of efficacy, safety and stability of pharmaceuticals.

FUTURE PERSPECTIVES

PLGA microspheres have demonstrated great proficiency for potential use in cancer immunotherapy (see **Table 1**). They have overcome the major challenges of drug delivery systems, such as protection of encapsulated material from rapid degradation and clearance. PLGA MS exhibit ideal properties for facilitated and untargeted uptake of mainly DCs after subcutaneous injection. Concomitant delivery of antigens and adjuvants to the same APC leads to efficient DC activation and increased stimulation of CD4+ T cells as wells as of CD8+ T cells via cross-presentation by coordinate and synergistic pathways. PLGA MS mediated drug delivery allows particularly low doses of antigens and adjuvants–still inducing strong CTL responses but minimizing potential side-effects of unspecific activation of systemic immune responses. Reducing the doses of antigen or immunostimulants is generally desired regarding potential clinical application or approval by international regulatory agencies. Sustained and prolonged antigen release induces superior immune responses and CD8+ T cell memory while simultaneously avoiding the risk of tolerance induction. The depot effect created at the injection site substitutes the need for conventional booster injections to maintain immune responses. Co-encapsulation of antigens together with toll-like receptor ligands yields potent and long-lasting CTL and T helper cell responses *in vivo* leading to protective and therapeutic anti-tumor activity in several tumor mouse models.

Despite the mentioned advantages of PLGA particles, particulate cancer vaccines are not available for clinical application at present. By far, most *in vitro* and preclinical mouse studies have been performed with model antigens and model tumors. It is important to switch to clinically relevant antigens and autochthonous, transgenic or carcinogen-induced tumor models for more realistic efficacy assessments in the future. Moreover, the production of GMP-grade PLGA MS needs to be established and refined to get approval for clinical studies. Translation form bench-side into the clinic has always been challenging due to various aspects including characterization of all materials used, availability of cGMP products, the presence of residual organic solvent impurities, difficulties in controlling encapsulated drug release including high initial burst and incomplete release, variability in particle size or morphology between different batches and safety issues including effectiveness and ease of administration in human cancer patients. Increasing the implementation of process analytical technologies (PAT) will control manufacturing and development of PLGA particles to ensure reproducible, effective and safe vaccines and clinical transition. The spray drying process would overcome limits of applicability in larger clinical settings, since the production of PLGA MS is easy to scale-up, cost-effective and amenable to sterile manufacturing. Unlike vaccines for infectious diseases, cancer vaccines might need to be tailored for individual patients due to diverse gene mutations in cancer cells creating neo-antigens. Hence, the development of custom-designed whole tumor lysate encapsulated into personalized PLGA MS might introduce a very promising, rapid and potent cancer treatment approach. Tumor lysates provide a pool of tumor-associated antigens to trigger suitable CD8+ and CD4+ T cell mediated anti-tumor responses that overcome the infirmities of single peptide vaccinations. Currently we are investigating PLGA MS mediated immune responses of used immunostimulatory molecules in Vaccigrade™, GMP certified and endotoxin-free formulations as well as other adjuvant candidates.

In summary, concomitant delivery of antigens and immunomodulators in PLGA microparticles reveals a potent DC—centered therapeutic approach for inducing strong anti-tumor immunity in various cancer settings which might pave the way for PLGA microspheres to become a key member of current cancer vaccines.

AUTHOR CONTRIBUTIONS

JK wrote the manuscript. DH prepared the figures. MG supervised associated projects and corrected and refined the manuscript.

ACKNOWLEDGMENTS

The authors would like to thank Bruno Gander for advice and Ying Waeckerle-Men, Edith Uetz-von Allmen, Eva Schlosser, Marc Mueller, Valerie Herrmann, and Annette Sommershof for previous experimental work that contributed to this review.

REFERENCES

1. Sharma P, Hu-Lieskovan S, Wargo JA, Ribas A. Primary, adaptive, and acquired resistance to cancer immunotherapy. *Cell.* (2017) 168:707–23. doi: 10.1016/j.cell.2017.01.017
2. Seton-Rogers S. Immunotherapy: two antigens are better than one. *Nat Rev Cancer.* (2016) 16:128–9 doi: 10.1038/nrc.2016.17
3. Vlieghe P, Lisowski V, Martinez J, Khrestchatisky M. Synthetic therapeutic peptides: science and market. *Drug Discov Today.* (2010) 15:40–56. doi: 10.1016/j.drudis.2009.10.009
4. Schuler G, Schuler-Thurner B, Steinman RM. The use of dendritic cells in cancer immunotherapy. *Curr Opin Immunol.* (2003) 15:138–47. doi: 10.1016/S0952-7915(03)00015-3
5. Schuler G. Dendritic cells. *Cancer J.* (2011) 17:337–42. doi: 10.1097/PPO.0b013e3182350077
6. Nieda M, Nicol A, Kikuchi A, Kashiwase K, Taylor K, Suzuki K, et al. Dendritic cells stimulate the expansion of bcr-abl specific CD8+ T cells with cytotoxic activity against leukemic cells from patients with chronic myeloid leukemia. *Blood.* (1998) 91:977–83.
7. Kessler JH, Melief CJM. Identification of T-cell epitopes for cancer immunotherapy. *Leukemia.* (2007) 21:1859–74. doi: 10.1038/sj.leu.2404787
8. Thumann P, Moc I, Humrich J, Berger TG, Schultz ES, Schuler G, et al. Antigen loading of dendritic cells with whole tumor cell preparations. *J Immunol Methods.* (2003) 277:1–16. doi: 10.1016/S0022-1759(03)00102-9
9. Tjoa BA, Simmons SJ, Bowes VA, Ragde H, Rogers M, Elgamal A, et al. Evaluation of phase I/II clinical trials in prostate cancer with dendritic cells and PSMA peptides. *Prostate.* (1998) 36:39–44. doi: 10.1002/(SICI)1097-0045(19980615)36:1<39::AID-PROS6>3.0.CO;2-6
10. Schuler-Thurner B, Schultz ES, Berger TG, Weinlich G, Ebner S, Woerl P, et al. Rapid induction of tumor-specific type 1 T helper cells in metastatic melanoma patients by vaccination with mature, cryopreserved, peptide-loaded monocyte-derived dendritic cells. *J Exp Med.* (2002) 195:1279–88. doi: 10.1084/jem.20012100
11. Waeckerle-Men Y, Uetz-von Allmen E, Fopp M, von Moos R, Böhme C, Schmid H-P, et al. Dendritic cell-based multi-epitope immunotherapy of hormone-refractory prostate carcinoma. *Cancer Immunol Immunother.* (2006) 55:1524–33. doi: 10.1007/s00262-006-0157-3
12. Nestle FO, Alijagic S, Gilliet M, Sun Y, Grabbe S, Dummer R, et al. Vaccination of melanoma patients with peptide- or tumor lysate-pulsed dendritic cells. *Nat Med.* (1998) 4:328–32.
13. Thara E, Dorff TB, Pinski JK, Quinn DI. Vaccine therapy with sipuleucel-T (Provenge) for prostate cancer. *Maturitas.* (2011) 69:296–303. doi: 10.1016/j.maturitas.2011.04.012
14. Tacken PJ, de Vries IJM, Torensma R, Figdor CG. Dendritic-cell immunotherapy: from *ex vivo* loading to *in vivo* targeting. *Nat Rev Immunol.* (2007) 7:790–802. doi: 10.1038/nri2173
15. Gilboa E. DC-based cancer vaccines. *J Clin Invest.* (2007) 117:1195–203. doi: 10.1172/JCI31205
16. Schadendorf D, Ugurel S, Schuler-Thurner B, Nestles FO, Enk A, Bröcker EB, et al. Dacarbazine (DTIC) versus vaccination with autologous peptide-pulsed dendritic cells (DC) in first-line treatment of patients with metastatic melanoma: a randomized phase III trial of the DC study group of the DeCOG. *Ann Oncol.* (2006) 17:563–70. doi: 10.1093/annonc/mdj138
17. Brito LA, Malyala P, O'Hagan DT. Vaccine adjuvant formulations: a pharmaceutical perspective. *Semin Immunol.* (2013) 25:130–45. doi: 10.1016/j.smim.2013.05.007
18. Cruz LJ, Tacken PJ, Rueda F, Domingo JC, Albericio F, Figdor CG. Targeting nanoparticles to dendritic cells for immunotherapy. *Methods Enzymol.* (2012) 509:143–63. doi: 10.1016/B978-0-12-391858-1.00008-3
19. Danhier F, Ansorena E, Silva JM, Coco R, Le Breton A, Préat V. PLGA-based nanoparticles: an overview of biomedical applications. *J Control Release.* (2012) 161:505–22. doi: 10.1016/j.jconrel.2012.01.043
20. Silva JM, Videira M, Gaspar R, Préat V, Florindo HF. Immune system targeting by biodegradable nanoparticles for cancer vaccines. *J Control Release.* (2013) 168:179–99. doi: 10.1016/j.jconrel.2013.03.010
21. Akagi T, Baba M, Akashi M. Biodegradable nanoparticles as vaccine adjuvants and delivery systems: regulation of immune responses by nanoparticle-based vaccine. *Adv Polym Sci.* (2012) 28:3427–36. doi: 10.1007/12_2011_150
22. Pavot V, Berthet M, Rességuier J, Legaz S, Handké N, Gilbert SC, et al. Poly(lactic acid) and poly(lactic-co-glycolic acid) particles as versatile

carrier platforms for vaccine delivery. *Nanomedicine.* (2014) 9:2703–18. doi: 10.2217/nnm.14.156

23. Sahdev P, Ochyl LJ, Moon JJ. Biomaterials for nanoparticle vaccine delivery systems. *Pharm Res.* (2014) 31:2563–82. doi: 10.1007/s11095-014-1419-y
24. Nagavarma BVN, Yadav HKS, Ayaz A, Vasudha LS, Shivakumar HG. Different techniques for preparation of polymeric nanoparticles- a review. *Asian J Pharm Clin Res.* (2012) 26:1025–58.
25. Hamdy S, Haddadi A, Hung RW, Lavasanifar A. Targeting dendritic cells with nano-particulate PLGA cancer vaccine formulations. *Adv Drug Deliv Rev.* (2011) 63:943–55. doi: 10.1016/j.addr.2011.05.021
26. Vasir JK, Labhasetwar V. Biodegradable nanoparticles for cytosolic delivery of therapeutics. *Adv Drug Deliv Rev.* (2007) 59:718–28. doi: 10.1016/j.addr.2007.06.003
27. Jain A, Kunduru KR, Basu A, Mizrahi B, Domb AJ, Khan W. Injectable formulations of poly(lactic acid) and its copolymers in clinical use. *Adv Drug Deliv Rev.* (2016) 107:213–27. doi: 10.1016/j.addr.2016.07.002
28. Lee BK, Yun Y, Park K. PLA Micro-and nano-particles HHS public access. *Adv Drug Deliv Rev.* (2016) 107:176–91. doi: 10.1016/j.addr.2016.05.020
29. Waeckerle-Men Y, Allmen EU V, Gander B, Scandella E, Schlosser E, Schmidtke G, et al. Encapsulation of proteins and peptides into biodegradable poly(D,L-lactide-co-glycolide) microspheres prolongs and enhances antigen presentation by human dendritic cells. *Vaccine.* (2006) 24:1847–57. doi: 10.1016/j.vaccine.2005.10.032
30. Gander B. Trends in particulate antigen and DNA delivery systems for vaccines. *Adv Drug Deliv Rev.* (2005) 57:321–3. doi: 10.1016/j.addr.2004.10.002
31. Kazzaz J, Singh M, Ugozzoli M, Chesko J, Soenawan E, O'Hagan DT. Encapsulation of the immune potentiators MPL and RC529 in PLG microparticles enhances their potency. *J Control Release.* (2006) 110:566–73. doi: 10.1016/j.jconrel.2005.10.010
32. Uchida T, Yagi A, Oda Y, Goto S. Microencapsulation of ovalbumin in poly(lactide-co-glycolide) by an oil-in-oil (o/o) solvent evaporation method. *J Microencapsul.* (1996) 13:509–18. doi: 10.3109/02652049609026036
33. Alonso MJ, Gupta RK, Min C, Siber GR, Langer R. Biodegradable microspheres as controlled-release tetanus toxoid delivery systems. *Vaccine.* (1994) 12:299–306. doi: 10.1016/0264-410X(94)90092
34. Hunter SK, Andracki ME, Krieg a M. Biodegradable microspheres containing group B *Streptococcus* vaccine: immune response in mice. *Am J Obstet Gynecol.* (2001) 185:1174–9. doi: 10.1067/mob.2001.117658
35. Wang D, Robinson DR, Kwon GS, Samuel J. Encapsulation of plasmid DNA in biodegradable poly(D,L lactic-co-glycolic acid) microspheres as a novel approach for immunogene delivery. *J Control Release.* (1999) 57:9–18. doi: 10.1016/S0168-3659(98)00099-6
36. Herrmann VL, Wieland DE, Legler DF, Wittmann V, Groettrup M. The STEAP1(262-270) peptide encapsulated into PLGA microspheres elicits strong cytotoxic T cell immunity in HLA-A*0201 transgenic mice–A new approach to immunotherapy against prostate carcinoma. *Prostate.* (2016) 76:456–68. doi: 10.1002/pros.23136
37. Lu D, Garcia-Contreras L, Xu D, Kurtz SL, Liu J, Braunstein M, et al. Poly (lactide-co-glycolide) microspheres in respirable sizes enhance an in vitro T cell response to recombinant Mycobacterium tuberculosis antigen 85B. *Pharm Res.* (2007) 24:1834–43. doi: 10.1007/s11095-007-9302-8
38. Audran R, Peter K, Dannull J, Men Y, Scandella E, Groettrup M, et al. Encapsulation of peptides in biodegradable microspheres prolongs their MHC class-I presentation by dendritic cells and macrophages in vitro. *Vaccine.* (2003) 21:1250–5. doi: 10.1016/S0264-410X(02)00521-2
39. Demento SL, Cui W, Criscione JM, Stern E, Tulipan J, Kaech SM, et al. Role of sustained antigen release from nanoparticle vaccines in shaping the T cell memory phenotype. *Biomaterials.* (2012) 33:4957–64. doi: 10.1016/j.biomaterials.2012.03.041
40. Klose D, Siepmann F, Elkharraz K, Krenzlin S, Siepmann J. How porosity and size affect the drug release mechanisms from PLGA-based microparticles. *Int J Pharm.* (2006) 314:198–206. doi: 10.1016/j.ijpharm.2005.07.031
41. Ma W, Kaushal S, Bouvet M, Kruse C, Grotjahn D, Ichim T, et al. PLGA nanoparticle-mediated delivery of tumor antigenic peptides elicits effective immune responses. *Int J Nanomed.* (2012)1475–87. doi: 10.2147/IJN.S29506
42. Li S. Hydrolytic degradation characteristics of aliphatic polyesters derived from lactic and glycolic acids. *J Biomed Mater Res.* (1999) 48:342–53. doi: 10.1002/(SICI)1097-4636(1999)48:3<342::AID-JBM20>3.0.CO;2-7
43. Blanco MD, Sastre RL, Teijón C, Olmo R, Teijón JM. Degradation behaviour of microspheres prepared by spray-drying poly(d,l-lactide) and poly(d,l-lactide-co-glycolide) polymers. *Int J Pharm.* (2006) 326:139–47. doi: 10.1016/j.ijpharm.2006.07.030
44. Waeckerle-Men Y, Groettrup M. PLGA microspheres for improved antigen delivery to dendritic cells as cellular vaccines. *Adv Drug Deliv Rev.* (2005) 57:475–82. doi: 10.1016/j.addr.2004.09.007
45. Luan X, Skupin M, Siepmann J, Bodmeier R. Key parameters affecting the initial release (burst) and encapsulation efficiency of peptide-containing poly(lactide-co-glycolide) microparticles. *Int J Pharm.* (2006) 324:168–75. doi: 10.1016/j.ijpharm.2006.06.004
46. Wang J, Wang BM, Schwendeman SP. Characterization of the initial burst release of a model peptide from poly(D,L-lactide-co-glycolide) microspheres. *J Control Release.* (2002) 82:289–307. doi: 10.1016/S0168-3659(02)00137-2
47. Cohen S, Alonso MJ, Langer R. Novel approaches to controlled-release antigen delivery. *Int J Technol Assess Health Care.* (1994) 10:121–30. doi: 10.1017/S0266462300014045
48. Jiang W, Gupta RK, Deshpande MC, Schwendeman SP. Biodegradable poly(lactic-co-glycolic acid) microparticles for injectable delivery of vaccine antigens. *Adv Drug Deliv Rev.* (2005) 57:391–410. doi: 10.1016/j.addr.2004.09.003
49. Rao JP, Geckeler KE. Polymer nanoparticles: preparation techniques and size-control parameters. *Prog Polym Sci.* (2011) 219:536–47. doi: 10.1016/j.progpolymsci.2011.01.001
50. Schwendeman SP. Recent advances in the stabilization of proteins encapsulated in injectable PLGA delivery systems. *Crit Rev Ther Drug Carrier Syst.* (2002) 19:73–98. doi: 10.1615/CritRevTherDrugCarrierSyst.v19.i1.20
51. Ré MI. Microencapsulation by spray drying. *Int J.* (2007) 16: 1195–236. doi: 10.1080/07373939808917460
52. Patel RP, Patel MP, Suthar AM. Spray drying technology: an overview. *Indian J Sci Technol.* (2009) 8:63–78. doi: 10.17485/ijst/2009/v2i10/30719
53. Mosén K, Bäckström K, Thalberg K, Schaefer T, Kristensen HG, Axelsson A. Particle formation and capture during spray drying of inhalable particles. *Pharm Dev Technol.* (2004) 9:409–17. doi: 10.1081/PDT-200035795
54. Vehring R, Foss WR, Lechuga-Ballesteros D. Particle formation in spray drying. *J Aerosol Sci.* (2007) 38: 728–46. doi: 10.1016/j.jaerosci.2007.04.005
55. Mahapatro A, Singh DK. Biodegradable nanoparticles are excellent vehicle for site directed *in-vivo* delivery of drugs and vaccines. *J Nanobiotechnol.* (2011) 9:55. doi: 10.1186/1477-3155-9-55
56. Wan F, Yang M. Design of PLGA-based depot delivery systems for biopharmaceuticals prepared by spray drying. *Int J Pharm.* (2016) 498:82–95. doi: 10.1016/j.ijpharm.2015.12.025
57. Bodmeier R, Chen H. Preparation of biodegradable poly-lactide microparticles using a spray-drying technique. *J Pharm Pharmacol.* (1988) 40:754–7. doi: 10.1111/j.2042-7158.1988.tb05166.x
58. Baras B, Benoit M a, Gillard J. Influence of various technological parameters on the preparation of spray-dried poly(epsilon-caprolactone) microparticles containing a model antigen. *J Microencapsul.* (2000) 17:485–98. doi: 10.1080/026520400405732
59. Baras B, Benoit MA, Gillard J. Parameters influencing the antigen release from spray-dried poly(DL- lactide) microparticles. *Int J Pharm.* (2000) 200:133–45. doi: 10.1016/S0378-5173(00)00363-X
60. Haggag YA, Faheem AM. Evaluation of nano spray drying as a method for drying and formulation of therapeutic peptides and proteins. *Front Pharmacol.* (2015) 6:140. doi: 10.3389/fphar.2015.00140
61. Lee SH, Heng D, Ng WK, Chan HK, Tan RBH. Nano spray drying: a novel method for preparing protein nanoparticles for protein therapy. *Int J Pharm.* (2011) 403:192–200. doi: 10.1016/j.ijpharm.2010.10.012
62. Takada S, Uda Y, Toguchi H, Ogawa Y. Application of a spray drying technique in the production of TRH-containing injectable sustained-release microparticles of biodegradable polymers. *PDA J Pharm Sci Technol.* (1995) 49:180–4

63. Bitz C, Doelker E. Influence of the preparation method on residual solvents in biodegradable microspheres. *Int J Pharm.* (1996) 45:295–305. doi: 10.1016/0378-5173(95)04320-9
64. Shen Z, Reznikoff G, Dranoff G, Rock KL. Cloned dendritic cells can present exogenous antigens on both MHC class I and class II molecules. *J Immunol.* (1997) 158:2723–30.
65. Shen H, Ackerman AL, Cody V, Giodini A, Hinson ER, Cresswell P, et al. Enhanced and prolonged cross-presentation following endosomal escape of exogenous antigens encapsulated in biodegradable nanoparticles. *Immunology.* (2006) 117:78–88. doi: 10.1111/j.1365-2567.2005.02268.x
66. Li M, Davey GM, Sutherland RM, Kurts C, Lew AM, Hirst C, et al. Cell-associated ovalbumin is cross-presented much more efficiently than soluble ovalbumin *in vivo*. *J Immunol.* (2001) 166:6099–103. doi: 10.4049/jimmunol.166.10.6099
67. Gamvrellis A, Leong D, Hanley JC, Xiang SD, Mottram P, Plebanski M. Vaccines that facilitate antigen entry into dendritic cells. *Immunol Cell Biol.* (2004) 82:506–16. doi: 10.1111/j.0818-9641.2004.01271.x
68. Benne N, van Duijn J, Kuiper J, Jiskoot W, Slütter B. Orchestrating immune responses: how size, shape and rigidity affect the immunogenicity of particulate vaccines. *J Control Release.* (2016) 234:124–34. doi: 10.1016/j.jconrel.2016.05.033
69. Foged C, Brodin B, Frokjaer S, Sundblad A. Particle size and surface charge affect particle uptake by human dendritic cells in an *in vitro* model. *Int J Pharm.* (2005) 298:315–22. doi: 10.1016/j.ijpharm.2005.03.035
70. Joshi VB, Geary SM, Salem AK. Biodegradable particles as vaccine delivery systems: size matters. *AAPS J.* (2013) 15:85–94. doi: 10.1208/s12248-012-9418-6
71. Schlosser E, Mueller M, Fischer S, Basta S, Busch DH, Gander B, et al. TLR ligands and antigen need to be coencapsulated into the same biodegradable microsphere for the generation of potent cytotoxic T lymphocyte responses. *Vaccine.* (2008) 26:1626–37. doi: 10.1016/j.vaccine.2008.01.030
72. Kou L, Sun J, Zhai Y, He Z. The endocytosis and intracellular fate of nanomedicines: Implication for rational design. *Asian J Pharm Sci.* (2013) 9:2380–402. doi: 10.1016/j.ajps.2013.07.001
73. Akinc A, Battaglia G. Exploiting endocytosis for nanomedicines. *Cold Spring Harb Perspect Biol.* (2013) 5:a016980. doi: 10.1101/cshperspect.a016980
74. Gutierro I, Hernández RM, Igartua M, Gascón AR, Pedraz JL. Size dependent immune response after subcutaneous, oral and intranasal administration of BSA loaded nanospheres. *Vaccine.* (2002) 21:67–77. doi: 10.1016/S0264-410X(02)00435-8
75. Waeckerle-Men Y, Scandella E, Uetz-Von Allmen E, Ludewig B, Gillessen S, Merkle HP, et al. Phenotype and functional analysis of human monocyte-derived dendritic cells loaded with biodegradable poly(lactide-co-glycolide) microspheres for immunotherapy. *J Immunol Methods.* (2004) 287:109–24. doi: 10.1016/j.jim.2004.01.010
76. Schliehe CC, Schliehe CC, Thiry M, Tromsdorf UI, Hentschel J, Weller H, et al. Microencapsulation of inorganic nanocrystals into PLGA microsphere vaccines enables their intracellular localization in dendritic cells by electron and fluorescence microscopy. *J Control Release.* (2011) 151:278–85. doi: 10.1016/j.jconrel.2011.01.005
77. McDevitt TC, Angello JC, Whitney ML, Reinecke H, Hauschka SD, Murry CE, et al. Uptake of poly(D,L-lactic-co-glycolic acid) microspheres by antigen-presenting cells *in vivo*. *J Biomed Mater Res.* (2002) 60:480–6. doi: 10.1002/jbm.10019
78. Peyre M, Fleck R, Hockley D, Gander B, Sesardic D. *In vivo* uptake of an experimental microencapsulated diphtheria vaccine following sub-cutaneous immunisation. *Vaccine.* (2004) 22:2430–7. doi: 10.1016/j.vaccine.2003.11.068
79. Schliehe C, Redaelli C, Engelhardt S, Fehlings M, Mueller M, van Rooijen N, et al. CD8- Dendritic cells and macrophages cross-present poly(D,L-lactate-co-glycolate) acid microsphere-encapsulated antigen *in vivo*. *J Immunol.* (2011) 187:2112–21. doi: 10.4049/jimmunol.1002084
80. Brandhonneur N, Chevanne F, Vié V, Frisch B, Primault R, Le Potier MF, et al. Specific and non-specific phagocytosis of ligand-grafted PLGA microspheres by macrophages. *Eur J Pharm Sci.* (2009) 36:474–8. doi: 10.1016/j.ejps.2008.11.013
81. Pacheco P, White D, Sulchek T. Effects of microparticle size and Fc density on macrophage phagocytosis. *PLoS ONE.* (2013) 8:e60989. doi: 10.1371/journal.pone.0060989
82. Manolova V, Flace A, Bauer M, Schwarz K, Saudan P, Bachmann MF. Nanoparticles target distinct dendritic cell populations according to their size. *Eur J Immunol.* (2008) 38:1404–13. doi: 10.1002/eji.200737984
83. Elamanchili P, Diwan M, Cao M, Samuel J. Characterization of poly(D,L-lactic-co-glycolic acid) based nanoparticulate system for enhanced delivery of antigens to dendritic cells. *Vaccine.* (2004) 22:2406–12. doi: 10.1016/j.vaccine.2003.12.032
84. Lutsiak MEC, Robinson DR, Coester C, Kwon GS, Samuel J. Analysis of poly(D,L-lactic-co-glycolic acid) nanosphere uptake by human dendritic cells and macrophages *in vitro*. *Pharm Res.* (2002) 19:1480–7. doi: 10.1023/A:1020452531828
85. Diwan M, Elamanchili P, Lane H, Gainer A, Samuel J. Biodegradable nanoparticle mediated antigen delivery to human cord blood derived dendritic cells for induction of primary T cell responses. *J Drug Target.* (2003) 11:495–507. doi: 10.1080/10611860410001670026
86. Kumari A, Yadav SK, Yadav SC. Biodegradable polymeric nanoparticles based drug delivery systems. *Colloids Surfaces B Biointerfaces.* (2010) 75:1–18. doi: 10.1016/j.colsurfb.2009.09.001
87. Locatelli E, Franchini MC. Biodegradable PLGA-b-PEG polymeric nanoparticles: synthesis, properties, and nanomedical applications as drug delivery system. *J Nanoparticle Res.* (2012) 14:81. doi: 10.1007/s11051-012-1316-4
88. Cruz LJ, Tacken PJ, Fokkink R, Joosten B, Stuart MC, Albericio F, et al. Targeted PLGA nano- but not microparticles specifically deliver antigen to human dendritic cells via DC-SIGN *in vitro*. *J Control Release.* (2010) 144:118–26. doi: 10.1016/j.jconrel.2010.02.013
89. Rawat M, Singh D, Saraf S, Saraf S. Nanocarriers: promising vehicle for bioactive drugs. *Biol Pharm Bull.* (2006) 29:1790–8. doi: 10.1248/bpb.29.1790
90. Garnett MC, Kallinteri P. Nanomedicines and nanotoxicology: some physiological principles. *Occup Med.* (2006) 56:307–11. doi: 10.1093/occmed/kql052
91. Engering A, Geijtenbeek TBH, van Vliet SJ, Wijers M, van Liempt E, Demaurex N, et al. The dendritic cell-specific adhesion receptor DC-SIGN internalizes antigen for presentation to T cells. *J Immunol.* (2002) 168:2118–26. doi: 10.4049/jimmunol.168.5.2118
92. Joshi MD, Unger WJ, Storm G, Van Kooyk Y, Mastrobattista E. Targeting tumor antigens to dendritic cells using particulate carriers. *J Cont Release.* (2012) 161:25–37. doi: 10.1016/j.jconrel.2012.05.010
93. Zang X, Zhao X, Hu H, Qiao M, Deng Y, Chen D. Nanoparticles for tumor immunotherapy. *Eur J Pharm Biopharm.* (2017) 115:243–56. doi: 10.1016/j.ejpb.2017.03.013
94. Reddy ST, Swartz MA, Hubbell JA. Targeting dendritic cells with biomaterials: developing the next generation of vaccines. *Trends Immunol.* (2006) 27:573–9. doi: 10.1016/j.it.2006.10.005
95. Wilhelm S, Tavares AJ, Dai Q, Ohta S, Audet J, Dvorak HF, et al. Analysis of nanoparticle delivery to tumours. *Nat Rev Mater.* (2016) 9:151–8. doi: 10.1038/natrevmats.2016.14
96. Sengupta S. Cancer nanomedicine: lessons for immuno-oncology. *Trends Cancer.* (2017) 3:551–60. doi: 10.1016/j.trecan.2017.06.006
97. Slütter B, Jiskoot W. Sizing the optimal dimensions of a vaccine delivery system: a particulate matter. *Expert Opin Drug Deliv.* (2016) 13:167–70. doi: 10.1517/17425247.2016.1121989
98. Watts C. The exogenous pathway for antigen presentation on major histocompatibility complex class II and CD1 molecules. *Nat Immunol.* (2004) 5:685–92. doi: 10.1038/ni1088
99. Savina A, Jancic C, Hugues S, Guermonprez P, Vargas P, Moura IC, et al. NOX2 controls phagosomal pH to regulate antigen processing during crosspresentation by dendritic cells. *Cell.* (2006) 126:205–18. doi: 10.1016/j.cell.2006.05.035
100. Pack DW, Hoffman AS, Pun S, Stayton PS. Design and development of polymers for gene delivery. *Nat Rev Drug Discov.* (2005) 4:581–93. doi: 10.1038/nrd1775
101. Joffre OP, Segura E, Savina A, Amigorena S. Cross-presentation by dendritic cells. *Nat Rev Immunol.* (2012) 12:557–69. doi: 10.1038/nri3254

102. Shen L, Sigal LJ, Boes M, Rock KL. Important role of cathepsin S in generating peptides for TAP-independent MHC class I crosspresentation *in vivo*. *Immunity*. (2004) 21:155–65. doi: 10.1016/j.immuni.2004.07.004

103. Lankat-Buttgereit B, Tampé R. The Transporter associated with antigen processing: function and implications in human diseases. *Physiol Rev*. (2002) 82:187–204. doi: 10.1152/physrev.00025.2001

104. Guermonprez P, Amigorena S. Pathways for antigen cross presentation. *Springer Semin Immunopathol*. (2005) 26:257–71. doi: 10.1007/s00281-004-0176-0

105. Kim H-J, Cantor H. CD4 T-cell subsets and tumor immunity: the helpful and the not-so-helpful. *Cancer Immunol Res*. (2014) 2:91–8. doi: 10.1158/2326-6066.CIR-13-0216

106. Perez-Diez A, Joncker NT, Choi K, Chan WFN, Anderson CC, Lantz O, et al. CD4 cells can be more efficient at tumor rejection than CD8 cells. *Blood*. (2007) 109:5346–54. doi: 10.1182/blood-2006-10-051318

107. Freund J. The effect of paraffin oil and mycobacteria on antibody formation and sensitization; a review. *Am J Clin Pathol*. (1951) 21:645–56.

108. Toledo H, Baly A, Castro O, Resik S, Laferté J, Rolo F, et al. A phase I clinical trial of a multi-epitope polypeptide TAB9 combined with montanide ISA 720 adjuvant in non-HIV-1 infected human volunteers. *Vaccine*. (2001) 19:4328–36. doi: 10.1016/S0264-410X(01)00111-6

109. Berinstein NL. Enhancing cancer vaccines with immunomodulators. *Vaccine*. (2007) 25(Suppl 2):B72–88. doi: 10.1016/j.vaccine.2007.06.043

110. Jensen FC, Savary JR, Diveley JP, Chang JC. Adjuvant activity of incomplete Freund's adjuvant. *Adv Drug Deliv Rev*. (1998) 32:173–86.

111. Speiser DE, Liénard D, Rufer N, Rubio-Godoy V, Rimoldi D, Lejeune F, et al. Rapid and strong human CD8+ T cell responses to vaccination with peptide, IFA, and CpG oligodeoxynucleotide 7909. *J Clin Invest*. (2005) 115:739–46. doi: 10.1172/JCI200523373

112. Miller LH, Saul A, Mahanty S. Revisiting Freund's incomplete adjuvant for vaccines in the developing world. *Trends Parasitol*. (2005) 21:412–4. doi: 10.1016/j.pt.2005.07.005

113. Schultze V, D'Agosto V, Wack A, Novicki D, Zorn J, Hennig R. Safety of MF59 adjuvant. *Vaccine*. (2008) 26:3209–22. doi: 10.1016/j.vaccine.2008.03.093

114. Del Giudice G, Fragapane E, Bugarini R, Hora M, Henriksson T, Palla E, et al. Vaccines with the MF59 adjuvant do not stimulate antibody responses against squalene. *Clin Vaccine Immunol*. (2006) 24:3063–5. doi: 10.1128/CVI.00191-06

115. Baylor NW, Egan W, Richman P. Aluminum salts in vaccines—US perspective. *Vaccine*. (2002) 20:S18–23. doi: 10.1016/S0264-410X(02)00166-4

116. Seubert A, Monaci E, Pizza M, O'Hagan DT, Wack A. The adjuvants aluminum hydroxide and MF59 induce monocyte and granulocyte chemoattractants and enhance monocyte differentiation toward dendritic cells. *J Immunol*. (2008) 180:5402–12. doi: 10.4049/jimmunol.180.8.5402

117. Montomoli E, Piccirella S, Khadang B, Mennitto E, Camerini R, De Rosa A. Current adjuvants and new perspectives in vaccine formulation. *Expert Rev Vaccines*. (2011) 10:1053–61. doi: 10.1586/erv.11.48

118. Morel S, Didierlaurent A, Bourguignon P, Delhaye S, Baras B, Jacob V, et al. Adjuvant system AS03 containing α-tocopherol modulates innate immune response and leads to improved adaptive immunity. *Vaccine*. (2011) 29:2461–73. doi: 10.1016/j.vaccine.2011.01.011

119. Didierlaurent AM, Morel S, Lockman L, Giannini SL, Bisteau M, Carlsen H, et al. AS04, an aluminum salt- and TLR4 agonist-based adjuvant system, induces a transient localized innate immune response leading to enhanced adaptive immunity. *J Immunol*. (2009) 183:6186–97. doi: 10.4049/jimmunol.0901474

120. Temizoz B, Kuroda E, Ishii KJ. Vaccine adjuvants as potential cancer immunotherapeutics. *Int Immunol*. (2016) 28:329–38. doi: 10.1093/intimm/dxw015

121. Zhang W, Wang L, Yang T, Liu Y, Chen X, Liu Q, et al. Immunopotentiator-loaded polymeric microparticles as robust adjuvant to improve vaccine efficacy. *Pharm Res*. (2015) 32:2837–50. doi: 10.1007/s11095-015-1666-6

122. Celis E. Toll-like receptor ligands energize peptide vaccines through multiple paths. *Cancer Res*. (2007) 67:7945–7. doi: 10.1158/0008-5472.CAN-07-1652

123. Jelinek I, Leonard JN, Price GE, Brown KN, Meyer-Manlapat A, Goldsmith PK, et al. TLR3-Specific double-stranded RNA oligonucleotide adjuvants induce dendritic cell cross-presentation, CTL responses, and antiviral protection. *J Immunol*. (2011) 186:2422–9. doi: 10.4049/jimmunol.1002845

124. Heit A, Schmitz F, Haas T, Busch DH, Wagner H. Antigen co-encapsulated with adjuvants efficiently drive protective T cell immunity. *Eur J Immunol*. (2007) 37:2063–74. doi: 10.1002/eji.200737169

125. Mathew S, Roch T, Frentsch M, Lendlein A, Wischke C. Adjuvant effect of microencapsulated NOD ligands studied in a human phagocytic cell line. *J Appl Biomater Funct Mater*. (2012) 10:229–36. doi: 10.5301/JABFM.2012.10438

126. Wischke C, Mathew S, Roch T, Frentsch M, Lendlein A. Potential of NOD receptor ligands as immunomodulators in particulate vaccine carriers. *J Cont Release*. 164:299–306. doi: 10.1016/j.jconrel.2012.06.034

127. Jensen SS, Gad M. Differential induction of inflammatory cytokines by dendritic cells treated with novel TLR-agonist and cytokine based cocktails: targeting dendritic cells in autoimmunity. *J Inflamm*. (2010) 7:37. doi: 10.1186/1476-9255-7-37

128. Krutzik SR, Tan B, Li H, Ochoa MT, Liu PT, Sharfstein SE, et al. TLR activation triggers the rapid differentiation of monocytes into macrophages and dendritic cells. *Nat Med*. (2005) 11:653–60. doi: 10.1038/nm1246

129. Mueller M, Schlosser E, Gander B, Groettrup M. Tumor eradication by immunotherapy with biodegradable PLGA microspheres–an alternative to incomplete Freund's adjuvant. *Int J Cancer*. (2011) 129:407–16. doi: 10.1002/ijc.25914

130. Fischer S, Schlosser E, Mueller M, Csaba N, Merkle HP, Groettrup M, et al. Concomitant delivery of a CTL-restricted peptide antigen and CpG ODN by PLGA microparticles induces cellular immune response. *J Drug Target*. (2009) 17:652–61. doi: 10.1080/10611860903119656

131. Hafner AM, Corthésy B, Merkle HP. Particulate formulations for the delivery of poly(I:C) as vaccine adjuvant. *Adv Drug Deliv Rev*. (2013) 65:1386–99. doi: 10.1016/j.addr.2013.05.013

132. Kadowaki N, Ho S, Antonenko S, de Waal Malefyt R, Kastelein RA, Bazan F, et al. Subsets of human dendritic cell precursors express different toll-like receptors and respond to different microbial antigens. *J Exp Med*. (2001) 194:863–9. doi: 10.1084/jem.194.6.863

133. Mueller M, Reichardt W, Koerner J, Groettrup M. Coencapsulation of tumor lysate and CpG-ODN in PLGA-microspheres enables successful immunotherapy of prostate carcinoma in TRAMP mice. *J Control Release*. (2012) 162:159–66. doi: 10.1016/j.jconrel.2012.06.015

134. Nicolete R, Santos DF Dos, Faccioli LH. The uptake of PLGA micro or nanoparticles by macrophages provokes distinct *in vitro* inflammatory response. *Int Immunopharmacol*. (2011) 11:1557–63. doi: 10.1016/j.intimp.2011.05.014

135. Elamanchili P, Lutsiak CME, Hamdy S, Diwan M, Samuel J. "Pathogen-mimicking" nanoparticles for vaccine delivery to dendritic cells. *J Immunother*. (2007) 30:378–95. doi: 10.1097/CJI.0b013e31802cf3e3

136. Salazar AM, Erlich RB, Mark A, Bhardwaj N, Herberman RB. Therapeutic *In Situ* Autovaccination against solid cancers with intratumoral poly-ICLC: case report, hypothesis, and clinical trial. *Cancer Immunol Res*. (2014) 2:720–4. doi: 10.1158/2326-6066.CIR-14-0024

137. Williams HC, Bath-Hextall F, Ozolins M, Armstrong SJ, Colver GB, Perkins W, et al. Surgery versus 5% imiquimod for nodular and superficial basal cell carcinoma: 5-year results of the SINS randomized controlled trial. *J Invest Dermatol*. (2017) 15:96–105. doi: 10.1016/j.jid.2016.10.019

138. Napolitani G, Rinaldi A, Bertoni F, Sallusto F, Lanzavecchia A. Selected toll-like receptor agonist combinations synergistically trigger a T helper type 1-polarizing program in dendritic cells. *Nat Immunol*. (2005) 6:769–76. doi: 10.1038/ni1223

139. Sommershof A, Scheuermann L, Koerner J, Groettrup M. Brain, behavior, and immunity chronic stress suppresses anti-tumor T CD8 + responses and tumor regression following cancer immunotherapy in a mouse model of melanoma. *Brain Behav Immun*. (2017) 65:140–9. doi: 10.1016/j.bbi.2017.04.021

140. Walter E, Dreher D, Kok M, Thiele L, Kiama SG, Gehr P, et al. Hydrophilic poly(DL-lactide-co-glycolide) microspheres for the delivery of DNA to human-derived macrophages and dendritic cells. *J Control Release*. (2001) 76:149–68. doi: 10.1016/S0168-3659(01)00413-8

141. Zhang X-Q, Dahle CE, Weiner GJ, Salem AK. A comparative study of the antigen-specific immune response induced by co-delivery of CpG ODN and

antigen using fusion molecules or biodegradable microparticles. *J Pharm Sci.* (2007) 96:3283–92. doi: 10.1002/jps.20978
142. Blander JM, Medzhitov R. Toll-dependent selection of microbial antigens for presentation by dendritic cells. *Nature.* (2006) 440:808–12. doi: 10.1038/nature04596
143. Hamdy S, Elamanchili P, Alshamsan A, Molavi O, Satou T, Samuel J. Enhanced antigen-specific primary CD4+ and CD8+ responses by codelivery of ovalbumin and toll-like receptor ligand monophosphoryl lipid A in poly(D,L-lactic-co-glycolic acid) nanoparticles. *J Biomed Mater Res Part A.* (2007) 81:652–62. doi: 10.1002/jbm.a.31019
144. Hamdy S, Molavi O, Ma Z, Haddadi A, Alshamsan A, Gobti Z, et al. Co-delivery of cancer-associated antigen and Toll-like receptor 4 ligand in PLGA nanoparticles induces potent CD8+ T cell-mediated anti-tumor immunity. *Vaccine.* (2008) 26:5046–57. doi: 10.1016/j.vaccine.2008.07.035
145. Edwards AD, Diebold SS, Slack EMC, Tomizawa H, Hemmi H, Kaisho T, et al. Toll-like receptor expression in murine DC subsets: Lack of TLR7 expression of CD8α+DC correlates with unresponsiveness to imidazoquinolines. *Eur J Immunol.* (2003) 33:827–33. doi: 10.1002/eji.200323797
146. Rubsamen RM, Herst CV, Lloyd PM, Heckerman DE. Eliciting cytotoxic T-lymphocyte responses from synthetic vectors containing one or two epitopes in a C57BL/6 mouse model using peptide-containing biodegradable microspheres and adjuvants. *Vaccine.* (2014) 32:4111–6. doi: 10.1016/j.vaccine.2014.05.071
147. Lee Y-R, Lee Y-H, Kim K-H, Im S-A, Lee C-K. Induction of potent antigen-specific cytotoxic T cell response by PLGA-nanoparticles containing antigen and TLR agonist. *Immune Netw.* (2013) 13:30–3. doi: 10.4110/in.2013.13.1.30
148. Silva JM, Zupancic E, Vandermeulen G, Oliveira VG, Salgado A, Videira M, et al. *In vivo* delivery of peptides and Toll-like receptor ligands by mannose-functionalized polymeric nanoparticles induces prophylactic and therapeutic anti-tumor immune responses in a melanoma model. *J Control Release.* (2015) 198:91–103. doi: 10.1016/j.jconrel.2014.11.033
149. Bos R, Sherman LA. CD4+ T-cell help in the tumor milieu is required for recruitment and cytolytic function of CD8+ T lymphocytes. *Cancer Res.* (2010) 70:8368–77. doi: 10.1158/0008-5472.CAN-10-1322
150. Klebanoff CA, Gattinoni L, Restifo NP. CD8+ T-cell memory in tumor immunology and immunotherapy. *Immunol Rev.* (2006) 211:214–24. doi: 10.1111/j.0105-2896.2006.00391.x
151. Liu G, Zhang L, Zhao Y. Modulation of immune responses through direct activation of toll-like receptors to T cells. *Clin Exp Immunol.* (2010) 160:168–75. doi: 10.1111/j.1365-2249.2010.04091.x
152. Warger T, Osterloh P, Rechtsteiner G, Fassbender M, Heib V, Schmid B, et al. Synergistic activation of dendritic cells by combined Toll-like receptor ligation induces superior CTL responses *in vivo. Blood.* (2006) 108:544–50. doi: 10.1182/blood-2005-10-4015
153. Krumbiegel D, Zepp F, Meyer CU. Combined Toll-like receptor agonists synergistically increase production of inflammatory cytokines in human neonatal dendritic cells. *Hum Immunol.* (2007) 68:813–22. doi: 10.1016/j.humimm.2007.08.001
154. Verronèse E, Delgado A, Valladeau-Guilemond J, Garin G, Guillemaut S, Tredan O, et al. Immune cell dysfunctions in breast cancer patients detected through whole blood multi-parametric flow cytometry assay. *Oncoimmunology.* (2016) 5:e1100791. doi: 10.1080/2162402X.2015.1100791
155. Irvine DJ, Hanson MC, Rakhra K, Tokatlian T. Synthetic nanoparticles for vaccines and immunotherapy. *Chem Rev.* (2015) 115:11109–46. doi: 10.1021/acs.chemrev.5b00109
156. Emens LA, Ascierto PA, Darcy PK, Demaria S, Eggermont AMM, Redmond WL, et al. Cancer immunotherapy: opportunities and challenges in the rapidly evolving clinical landscape. *Eur J Cancer.* (2017) 81:116–29. doi: 10.1016/j.ejca.2017.01.035
157. Fujii S, Shimizu K, Okamoto Y, Kunii N, Nakayama T, Motohashi S, et al. NKT cells as an ideal anti-tumor immunotherapeutic. *Front Immunol.* (2013) 4:409.doi: 10.3389/fimmu.2013.00409
158. Salvador A, Igartua M, Hernández RM, Pedraz JL. Combination of immune stimulating adjuvants with poly(lactide-co-glycolide) microspheres enhances the immune response of vaccines. *Vaccine.* (2012) 30:589–96. doi: 10.1016/j.vaccine.2011.11.057
159. Dölen Y, Kreutz M, Gileadi U, Tel J, Vasaturo A, van Dinther EAW, et al. Co-delivery of PLGA encapsulated invariant NKT cell agonist with antigenic protein induce strong T cell-mediated antitumor immune responses. *Oncoimmunology.* (2016) 5:e1068493. doi: 10.1080/2162402X.2015.1068493
160. Jukes JP, Gileadi U, Ghadbane H, Yu TF, Shepherd D, Cox LR, et al. Non-glycosidic compounds can stimulate both human and mouse iNKT cells. *Eur J Immunol.* (2016) 46:12224–34. doi: 10.1002/eji.201546114
161. Wang HY, Wang R-F. Enhancing cancer immunotherapy by intracellular delivery of cell-penetrating peptides and stimulation of pattern-recognition receptor signaling. *Adv Immunol.* (2012) 114:151–76. doi: 10.1016/B978-0-12-396548-6.00006-8
162. Bijker MS, van den Eeden SJF, Franken KL, Melief CJM, van der Burg SH, Offringa R. Superior induction of anti-tumor CTL immunity by extended peptide vaccines involves prolonged, DC-focused antigen presentation. *Eur J Immunol.* (2008) 38:1033–42. doi: 10.1002/eji.200737995
163. Lesterhuis WJ, de Vries IJM, Schreibelt G, Lambeck AJ a, Aarntzen EHJG, Jacobs JFM, et al. Route of administration modulates the induction of dendritic cell vaccine-induced antigen-specific T cells in advanced melanoma patients. *Clin Cancer Res.* (2011) 17:5725–35. doi: 10.1158/1078-0432.CCR-11-1261
164. Goforth R, Salem AK, Zhu X, Miles S, Zhang X-QQ, Lee JH, et al. Immune stimulatory antigen loaded particles combined with depletion of regulatory T-cells induce potent tumor specific immunity in a mouse model of melanoma. *Cancer Immunol Immunother.* (2009) 58:517–30. doi: 10.1007/s00262-008-0574-6
165. Gross BP, Wongrakpanich A, Francis MB, Salem AK, Norian LA. A therapeutic microparticle-based tumor lysate vaccine reduces spontaneous metastases in murine breast cancer. *AAPS J.* (2014) 16:1194–203. doi: 10.1208/s12248-014-9662-z
166. Prasad S, Cody V, Saucier-Sawyer JK, Saltzman WM, Sasaki CT, Edelson RL, et al. Polymer nanoparticles containing tumor lysates as antigen delivery vehicles for dendritic cell–based antitumor immunotherapy. *Nanomed Nanotechnol Biol Med.* (2011) 7:1–10. doi: 10.1016/j.nano.2010.07.002
167. Hanlon DJ, Aldo PB, Devine L, Alvero AB, Engberg AK, Edelson R, et al. Enhanced stimulation of anti-ovarian cancer CD8+ T cells by dendritic cells loaded with nanoparticle encapsulated tumor antigen. *Am J Reprod Immunol.* (2011) 65:597–609. doi: 10.1111/j.1600-0897.2010.00968.x
168. Herrmann VL, Hartmayer C, Planz O, Groettrup M. Cytotoxic T cell vaccination with PLGA microspheres interferes with influenza a virus replication in the lung and suppresses the infectious disease. *J Control Release.* (2015) 216:121–31. doi: 10.1016/j.jconrel.2015.08.019

13

Are Conventional Type 1 Dendritic Cells Critical for Protective Antitumor Immunity and How?

Jean-Charles Cancel[†], Karine Crozat[†], Marc Dalod[*†] and Raphaël Mattiuz[†]*

CNRS, INSERM, Centre d'Immunologie de Marseille-Luminy, Turing Center for Living Systems, Aix Marseille University, Marseille, France

Correspondence:
Karine Crozat
crozat@ciml.univ-mrs.fr
Marc Dalod
dalod@ciml.univ-mrs.fr

[†]These authors have contributed equally to this work

Dendritic cells (DCs) are endowed with a unique potency to prime T cells, as well as to orchestrate their expansion, functional polarization and effector activity in non-lymphoid tissues or in their draining lymph nodes. The concept of harnessing DC immunogenicity to induce protective responses in cancer patients was put forward about 25 years ago and has led to a multitude of DC-based vaccine trials. However, until very recently, objective clinical responses were below expectations. Conventional type 1 DCs (cDC1) excel in the activation of cytotoxic lymphocytes including $CD8^+$ T cells (CTLs), natural killer (NK) cells, and NKT cells, which are all critical effector cell types in antitumor immunity. Efforts to investigate whether cDC1 might orchestrate immune defenses against cancer are ongoing, thanks to the recent blossoming of tools allowing their manipulation *in vivo*. Here we are reporting on these studies. We discuss the mouse models used to genetically deplete or manipulate cDC1, and their main caveats. We present current knowledge on the role of cDC1 in the spontaneous immune rejection of tumors engrafted in syngeneic mouse recipients, as a surrogate model to cancer immunosurveillance, and how this process is promoted by type I interferon (IFN-I) effects on cDC1. We also discuss cDC1 implication in promoting the protective effects of immunotherapies in mouse preclinical models, especially for adoptive cell transfer (ACT) and immune checkpoint blockers (ICB). We elaborate on how to improve this process by *in vivo* reprogramming of certain cDC1 functions with off-the-shelf compounds. We also summarize and discuss basic research and clinical data supporting the hypothesis that the protective antitumor functions of cDC1 inferred from mouse preclinical models are conserved in humans. This analysis supports potential applicability to cancer patients of the cDC1-targeting adjuvant immunotherapies showing promising results in mouse models. Nonetheless, further investigations on cDC1 and their implications in anti-cancer mechanisms are needed to determine whether they are the missing key that will ultimately help switching cold tumors into therapeutically responsive hot tumors, and how precisely they mediate their protective effects.

Keywords: conventional type 1 dendritic cells, tumor, type I IFN, $CD8^+$ T cells, NK cells, immunotherapy, cancer immunosurveillance, clinical trials

INTRODUCTION

Immune responses against cancer are sculpted by the tumor microenvironment, including its composition in terms of cell types and their physiological states. Indeed, tumors escape host immune defenses not only through decreasing their intrinsic immunogenicity but also by shaping a specific immunosuppressive microenvironment (1, 2). Exogenous factors such as the microbiota and its metabolites also modulate the tumor microenvironment and hence antitumor immune responses (3). According to their degree of infiltration by immune cells and to their capacity to activate antitumor immune responses, tumors have been classified as immunologically "Hot" or "Cold." "Hot" tumors are immunogenic, T cell-inflamed, and efficiently rejected by the immune system. They are characterized by the presence of activated $CD8^{+}$ cytotoxic T lymphocytes (CTLs), by the expression of T cell-attracting chemokines, and by a type I interferon (IFN-I) transcriptional signature (4). "Cold" tumors lack T cell infiltration, which is correlated with an absence of IFN-I signature and with a poor chemokine production (4). They are ignored by the immune system due to their poor immunogenicity and are very poorly responsive to immunotherapies. We propose to refine this bimodal classification through the addition of two other tumor states, which we called "Icy" and "Warm." We define as "Icy" the tumors that develop potent, active, mechanisms to prevent immune recognition and T cell activation, by inducing a highly immunosuppressive microenvironment very early on during their development. Hence, "Icy" tumors are even more refractory to immune control than "Cold" tumors. "Warm" tumors present an intermediate level of infiltration by "exhausted" CTLs, which have been functionally paralyzed by the local immunosuppressive environment that has been progressively shaped during tumor development. The exhaustion of CTLs is at least in part due to engagement of their immune checkpoint receptors by ligands expressed by the tumor cells themselves or by infiltrating antigen (Ag)-presenting cells. "Warm" tumors are more prone to be controlled by immune checkpoint blockade (ICB) treatments. These monoclonal antibody (mAb)-based immunotherapies have revolutionized cancer patient care, by significantly increasing not only overall survival rates but also very long-term remissions for tumor types previously difficult to treat. Despite this major advance, the majority of patients with difficult-to-treat cancers do not respond to ICB. To overcome this issue, it is critical to find additional means of manipulating the microenvironment of the "Cold" or "Warm" tumors unresponsive to ICB, in order to convert them into "Hot" tumors. It should be possible to achieve this by combining ICB with adjuvant immunotherapies able to counteract the other immune escape mechanisms established by these tumors, in order to (i) trigger *de novo* or enhance T cell infiltration, (ii) enhance cross-presentation of tumor-associated Ag, and (iii) promote a better induction or reactivation of CTL effector functions.

Dendritic cells (DCs) are the most potent Ag-presenting cells, with a unique efficacy for priming naïve T cells and inducing their functional polarization. They are more generally in charge of orchestrating the expansion and functions of T and natural killer (NK) cells in lymphoid and non-lymphoid tissues. Many clinical trials have been performed over the last 25 years to attempt harnessing DC functions for boosting protective antitumor CTL responses in cancer patients (5). Up to now, the results have been disappointingly far below expectations. These failures occurred at least in part because of the almost exclusive use of monocyte-derived DCs (MoDCs) for ACT in cancer patients. Indeed, later advancement of our basic understanding of the heterogeneity and functional plasticity of DCs suggested that other types than MoDCs should be better suited for this purpose (6–8). A relatively recent consensus has emerged on a universal and simplified classification of DC types both in mice and in humans, based on their ontogeny, gene expression programs, phenotype, functions and localization (9, 10). Five major types of DCs can be distinguished: plasmacytoid DC (pDCs), type 1 conventional DCs (cDC1), type 2 cDCs (cDC2), Langerhans cells and MoDCs. In mice, cDC1 encompass both the lymphoid tissue-resident $CD8\alpha^{+}$ cDCs as well as the $CD103^{+}CD11b^{-}$ cDCs that reside in the parenchyma of non-lymphoid tissues and, once matured upon activation, can migrate to the draining lymph nodes. In humans, cDC1 correspond to the CD141 $(BDCA3)^{high}$ $CD11b^{-/low}$ cDCs. Both mouse and human cDC1 express specifically the chemokine receptor XCR1 and selectively the C-type lectin endocytic receptor CLEC9A (11). cDC1 can directly enter tissues from the blood, or differentiate locally from a dedicated progenitor, the pre-cDC1 that has been characterized both in the mouse and the human (12, 13). Mouse cDC2 correspond to the $CD11b^{+}$ cDCs, and human cDC2 to the CD1c $(BDCA1)^{high}$ $CD11b^{+/high}$ cDCs. For a very long time, MoDCs were the only DC type that could be produced *in vitro*, in high numbers and under clinical-grade conditions (5, 6, 8). They were therefore used for most immunotherapeutic clinical trials based on adoptive cell transfer (ACT) of *in vitro* derived autologous DCs. However, MoDCs strikingly differ from cDC1 and cDC2 that are the major types of DCs residing in secondary lymphoid organs and orchestrating immune responses *in vivo* (14–16). For example, MoDCs do not migrate efficiently to lymph nodes and are particularly prone to develop immunosuppressive functions, whereas cDC1 excel in the activation of CTLs, which are critical effector cell types for antitumor immunity (17). Thus, major efforts have been conducted in the last 10 years to investigate whether cDC1 might be critical for defense against cancer, and how. Here, we are reporting on studies addressing this issue in mice, under experimental conditions of spontaneous immune rejection of tumor grafts in syngeneic recipients, or in preclinical models of immunotherapies. We also summarize human studies that mined large datasets of tumor gene expression profiles to investigate correlations between clinical outcome and digital deconvolution of the tumor immune infiltrate. We discuss how the knowledge generated by these studies can instruct innovative immunotherapeutic strategies to harness cDC1 functions for the benefits of cancer patients.

NO CURRENTLY AVAILABLE MUTANT MOUSE MODEL IS SPECIFICALLY TARGETING ONLY cDC1 *IN VIVO*

To determine whether and how a given type of immune cells plays a non-redundant role in antitumor immunity *in vivo*, it should be specifically and efficiently manipulated in mice. Different mutant mouse models have been generated to either deplete DCs, or inactivate candidate genes in DCs, as recently reviewed (18, 19). Here, we will specifically discuss the use of mutant mouse models to investigate the functions of cDC1 or their molecular regulation (**Table 1**) (14, 20–47). Mouse models expressing the Cre DNA recombinase under the control of the promoter of a gene selectively expressed in DCs have been generated to enable conditional deletion of candidate floxed genes in the targeted cells (e.g., *Itgax-Cre* targeting CD11c$^+$ cells and *Xcr1-Cre* targeting cDC1). Constitutive depletion models have been generated using two types of strategies. The first corresponds to the knock-out of a transcription factor shown to be crucial selectively for the development/homeostasis of cDCs (Zbtb46) or cDC1 (Batf3) (**Table 1**). The second consists in ectopic expression of the active subunit of the diphtheria toxin (*DTA*) selectively in DCs (e.g., *Xcr1-Cre;Rosa26-LSL-DTA* mice for cDC1, **Table 1**). Conditional depletion can be achieved upon diphtheria toxin administration in mutant animals engineered for ectopic expression of the gene encoding the human diphtheria toxin receptor (*hDTR*) selectively in DCs (e.g., *Karma-hDTR* or *Xcr1-hDTR* mice for cDC1).

One major caveat of using CD11c for targeting DCs is that the gene encoding this molecule, *Itgax*, is expressed by other immune cell types, including some that play critical roles in anti-tumor immunity, such as NK cells, effector memory CTLs, intraepithelial lymphocytes (IELs), plasmablasts, and subsets of monocytes or macrophages (32). Knock-in within the *Zbtb46* gene has been used to target all cDCs. However, this gene is also expressed by endothelial cells and committed erythroid progenitors (14, 32–34). Since angiogenesis critically affects solid tumor development, experiments should be performed using bone marrow chimera mice generated by engrafting mutant bone marrow cells into a wild type (WT) recipient animal. *Batf3*$^{-/-}$ mice have been the most frequently used model to investigate whether cDC1 play a critical role in physiological processes. However, even in this model, complementary strategies are needed before drawing final conclusions, because *Batf3* is also expressed in cDC2 and effector CD4$^+$ T cells, and because it represses *Foxp3* expression in CD4$^+$ T cells leading to increased numbers of regulatory T cells (Treg) in knock-out mice (35, 36). In addition, the impact of *Batf3* inactivation on cDC1 homeostasis is less efficient in the *C57BL6/J* genetic background than in the *129svEv* one. Under inflammatory settings, the knock-out of *Batf3* can be compensated for cDC1 development, by the induction in DC precursors of the paralog genes *Batf* and *Batf2* (37–39). We have engineered mutant mouse models for cDC1 targeting based on the knock-in of Cre (42) or hDTR (43) into the *Gpr141b* (alias *A530099j19rik* or *Karma)* gene, but these models also target mast cells (42). Finally, the *Xcr1* gene was targeted to generate mutant mouse models for specific, conditional or constitutive, cDC1 depletion, as well as for their genetic manipulation (42, 44, 46). The *Xcr1* gene is preserved in our models (42). In contrast, it is knocked-out in the other ones (46); hence, only heterozygous mice should be used for these models in order to avoid possible phenotypic effects due to a complete XCR1 deficiency. Besides cDC1, only a minute proportion of CD4$^+$ T cells are targeted in *Xcr1-Cre* mice (42). Although still imperfect, the mutant mouse models based on the manipulation of the *Xcr1* gene are the best to target cDC1 *in vivo*. In conclusion, none of the mutant mouse models used to date for cDC1 targeting are entirely specific and efficient, but some are better suited than others for this purpose. In any case, it is always important to use complementary methods to ensure that the phenotypes observed are only or mostly due to the manipulation of cDC1. For example, depleted mice should be replenished with wild-type cDC1 if possible. Alternately, results should be confirmed in other mutant models also targeting cDC1 but no other cell types in common.

THE ROLE OF cDC1 IN CANCER IMMUNOSURVEILLANCE HAS NOT YET BEEN INVESTIGATED

Cancer development is a multistep process consisting in the accumulation of genetic mutations within a cell leading to increased or deregulated proliferation and survival, with clonal selection of neoplastic progeny (48). There is a strong contribution of the host immune responses in this dynamical process of tumor selection, which has been described as the three E of cancer immunoediting: Elimination, Equilibrium and Escape of cancer cells (49). A failure of the immune system to eliminate all transformed cells early during their development is followed by an equilibrium state during which the immune system exerts a relentless pressure on surviving tumor cells, ultimately leading to tumor escape from the exhausted immune system. The initial elimination phase is therefore critical to restrict tumor growth very rapidly to prevent relapse or metastasis. Efficient recognition and elimination of transformed cells implies constant monitoring of the body by both the innate and adaptive immune systems, a process called cancer immunosurveillance. Upon monitoring spontaneous, carcinogen- or genetically-induced tumor development in mice bearing various immune deficiencies, critical roles in cancer immunosurveillance have been uncovered for αβ and γδ T cells, NKT cells and NK cells, as well as for the cytokines IFN-γ, IFN-I, IL-12 and for the cytotoxic effector molecules Perforin and TRAIL (50). The role of cDC1 in cancer immunosurveillance remains to be assessed. However, a wealth of data has accumulated on their role in the spontaneous immune rejection of tumor grafts in mice, a popular surrogate model for immunosurveillance (**Table 2**) (35, 51, 54–58).

TABLE 1 | Mouse models to deplete DCs, cDCs or cDC1 *in vivo*.

Mouse strain	Depleted cells	Gene also expressed in	Remarks	Expression profile references
CD11c-hDTR*	cDCs (pDCs?)	NK cells Effector/memory CTL Monocytes, macrophages Plasmablasts IELs	Off-target transgene expression leading to death upon multiple DT injections (Requiring to perform BM chimeras for prolonged depletion)	**(20)** (21–27) ImmGen Consortium
CD11c.DOG*	DCs	NK cells Effector/memory CTL Monocytes, Macrophages Plasmablasts IELs	hDTR expression only in CD11c$^+$ cells Prolonged DC depletion possible upon multiple DT injections Ovalbumin protein is expressed in DCs, resulting in extensive OT-I and OT-II proliferation after transfer	**(28)** (20–27) ImmGen Consortium
CD205-hDTR	cDC1 and LCs	Cortical thymic epithelium Tumor MoDC and cDC2	Death induced by DT injection Use of BM chimeras required to avoid death consecutive to depletion of radioresistant CD205$^+$ cells	**(29)** (30, 31)
Zbtb46-hDTR*	cDC1 and cDC2	Endothelial cells Committed erythroid progenitors	Death induced by a single DT injection Use of BM chimeras required	**(32)** (14, 33)
Zbtb46-LSL-hDTR*	cDC1 and cDC2	Endothelial cells Committed erythroid progenitors	Allows prolonged cDC depletion upon multiple DT injections (Need to cross with a Cre strain)	**(34)** (14, 32, 33)
Batf3$^{-/-}$	cDC1	cDC2 Eff (Th1) CD4$^+$ T cells Other T cells?	cDC1 depletion is effective in *129/SvEv* mice but less in *C57BL/6* animals Intracellular pathogens infections or IL-12 injection restore cDC1 development Higher differentiation in Treg of *Batf3$^{-/-}$* CD4$^+$ T cells	**(35)** (14, 36–40)
Clec9a-hDTR*	cDC1	pDCs	Half of the pDCs are depleted	**(41)**, (42)
Karma-hDTR*	cDC1	Skin and PC Mast cells	Mast cells are targeted in addition to cDC1	**(43)**, (42)
XCR1-hDTR* (Kaisho)	cDC1		Deletion of the endogenous *Xcr1* gene Requiring the use of heterozygous mice	**(44)**, (42)
XCR1-hDTR** (Dalod)	cDC1		Fate mapping of a minute proportion of CD4$^+$ T cells	(14, 43, 45), **(42)**
XCR1-DTA*** (Kaisho)	cDC1		Deletion of the endogenous *Xcr1* gene Requiring the use of heterozygous mice	(14, 43) **(46)**, (45)
XCR1-DTA*** (Dalod)	cDC1		Fate mapping of a minute proportion of CD4$^+$ T cells	(14, 43, 45), **(42)**

*Bold: First publication. *Mouse models expressing the Cre DNA recombinase under the same gene promoter have been generated. **Xcr1-Cre;Rosa26-LSL-hDTR mice; ***Xcr1-Cre;Rosa26-LSL-DTA mice.*

BATF3$^{-/-}$ MICE FAIL TO REJECT SYNGENEIC TUMOR GRAFTS, SUGGESTING A CRITICAL ROLE FOR cDC1 IN SPONTANEOUS ANTITUMOR IMMUNE DEFENSES

Most tumor cells are not able to directly prime naïve T cells, due to their low expression of MHC class I and co-stimulation molecules or to their acquisition of immunosuppressive functions such as high expression of ligands for immune checkpoint receptors. Thus, induction of CTL responses against most tumors requires accessory cells able to take-up, process and present exogenous tumor Ag in association with MHC-I molecules, a process known as cross-presentation. cDCs are highly efficient in initiating and globally orchestrating adaptive immunity, due to their professional capacities to simultaneously deliver all necessary signals to T cells, namely Ag presentation as signal 1, co-stimulation as signal 2, and cytokines as signal 3 (59). Mouse and human cDC1 excel at activating CTLs, due to their higher capacity to cross-present cellular Ag as compared to other types of Ag-presenting cells (11). It seemed therefore logical that cDC1 should play a critical role in anti-tumor immunity (**Table 2**). Kenneth Murphy's group was the first to confirm this hypothesis, by showing loss of spontaneous rejection of transplantable tumors in *Batf3$^{-/-}$* mice (35). Contrary to their WT counterparts, *Batf3$^{-/-}$* cDCs failed to induce proliferation of OT-I cells when co-cultured with cells loaded with the OVA protein, suggesting that cross-presentation of cellular Ag indeed constitutes one of the critical, non-redundant functions of cDC1. Several other studies have since reported similar results, altogether using a variety of transplantable tumors (**Table 2**). These studies strongly support a critical role for cDC1 in spontaneous antitumor immune defenses. However, a possible role of the loss of *Batf3* expression in cDC2 or in effector T cells has not been ruled out. In addition,

TABLE 2 | Tumor cell lines spontaneously rejected in immunocompetent hosts.

Tumor rejection	IFN-I-dependent	IFN-I-independent
Lost in $Batf3^{-/-}$ mice	1969 (51–53) 1773RS100 (35) B16.SIY (54) d38m2 (51) d42m1 (51) GAR4.GR1 (51) H31m1 (35, 51) ***Ptgs1/Ptgs2*** $^{-/-}$ **BRAF**$^{\mathbf{V600E}}$ (55, 56)	
ND	7835 (51) MC-57.SIY (54, 57, 58) P198 (51)	F515 (51)

Bold: NK cell dependent rejection. Underlined: NK cell independent rejection. Fibrosarcoma: 1969, 1773RS100, 7835, d38m2, d42m1, F515, GAR4.GR1, H31m1, MC-57.SIY. Melanoma: B16.SIY, Ptgs1/Ptgs2$^{-/-}$ *BRAF*^{V600E}*. Mastocytoma: P198. 129/SvEv background: 1773RS100, d38m2, d42m1, F515, GAR4.GR1, H31m1. C57BL6/J background: 1969, 7835, B16.SIY, MC-57.SIY, Ptgs1/Ptgs2* $^{-/-}$ *BRAF*^{V600E}*. DBA/2 background: P198.*

Batf3$^{-/-}$ mice can still achieve partial tumor control and mount tumor-specific CTL response under low-dose tumor challenge (35, 51, 54), which might be explained either by the incomplete cDC1 loss or by partial redundancy between cDC1 and other cell types for the cross-presentation of cellular Ag and the induction of antitumor adaptive immunity. Further studies are warranted to address these issues.

INSIGHTS INTO HOW cDC1 COULD PROMOTE PROTECTIVE SPONTANEOUS ANTITUMOR IMMUNITY

Cross-Presentation by cDC1 Is Necessary but Not Sufficient for Immune Control of a Regressor Fibrosarcoma

The importance of cross-presentation in cancer immunology has been extensively reviewed (60). Very recently, the WDFY4 molecule, a member of the BEACH (Beige and Chediak-Higashi) domain-containing family of proteins, was reported to be specifically required for cross-presentation of cell-associated Ag by cDC1, and for cDC1-dependant immune control of the highly immunogenic 1969 regressor fibrosarcoma (52). The demonstration of a cell-intrinsic requirement of WDFY4 in cDC1 for immunity against cancer was achieved by comparing tumor growth between *Wdfy4*$^{-/-}$:WT vs. *Wdfy4*$^{-/-}$:*Batf3*$^{-/-}$ mixed bone marrow chimera mice. Importantly, *Wdfy4*$^{-/-}$ cDC1 were not compromised in their abilities to produce IL-12 and to present Ag in association with MHC class II molecules for CD4^{+} T cell activation. *Wdfy4*-deficient cDC1 appeared to be selectively impaired in their ability to cross-present Ag but not in other functions also required for efficient CTL priming and expansion. To our knowledge, this study is the first to demonstrate that a specific defect in cDC1 cross-presentation *in vivo* leads to a failure of mice to control spontaneously tumor growth. Further studies are warranted to confirm these data and extend it to other preclinical tumor models. A major role of *Batf3* in cDC1 is to sustain their expression of *Irf8*. Consistent with this, the development of cDC1 and their ability to cross-present cell-associated Ag are rescued in *Batf3*$^{-/-}$ animals transgenic for *Irf8*. Nevertheless, these mice still fail to control the growth of a regressor fibrosarcoma, likewise to *Batf3*$^{-/-}$ animals. Thus, in addition to cross-presentation, other functions of cDC1 are also necessary for the promotion of protective antitumor immunity but remain to be identified (53). Moreover, both in mice and humans, cDC2 and pDCs can also perform cross-presentation of cell-associated Ag, under specific conditions of stimulation, less efficiently than cDC1 (11). Hence, we propose that cDC1 play a critical role in antitumor immunity not only due to their strong cross-presentation activity but rather because they uniquely combine several key features that are not simultaneously expressed together in other cell types, as detailed below (**Figure 1**).

Proposed Key Features Underlying cDC1 Non-redundant Role in Anti-tumor Immunity

First, the expression of XCR1 and CCR5 by cDC1 may enable their local recruitment by cytotoxic lymphocytes producing the ligands for these chemokine receptors, XCL1 and CCL4/5 (45, 55, 61–63). Second, reciprocally, cDC1 ability to produce high levels of CXCL9/10 may promote local recruitment of effector and memory CTLs expressing CXCR3 (43, 57, 64). Third, cDC1 can deliver positive co-stimulation signals. Fourth, cDC1 are a major source of IL-12, IFN-β, and IL-15, thereby promoting the survival and proper activation of NK, NKT cells and CTLs (43, 65–69). In a model of lung metastasis, cDC1 were the major source of IL-12, which was critical to control metastasis in a NK cell- and IFNγ-dependent manner (66). Fifth, cDC1 can promote Th1 induction (70–72) and favor CD4^{+} T cell help delivery to CTL through simultaneous presentation of Ag in association to MHC-I and MHC-II (73, 74). Depending on the cues that they receive during their activation at the time of Ag processing and presentation, DCs will polarize into different functions during their maturation (75, 76). At steady state, during their homeostatic activation, DCs acquire the ability to induce immune tolerance by causing the death, anergy or polarization into regulatory functions of self-reactive T cells, a process referred to as DC tolerogenic maturation. On the contrary, in proper activating contexts, DCs undergo an immunogenic maturation by acquiring the combined expression of activating co-stimulation molecules and cytokines leading to the induction of strong Ag-specific effector lymphocyte responses. The immunogenic maturation of cDC1 is promoted by IFN-I (51, 54, 68, 75), including through cross-talk with pDCs as a major source of these cytokines (77). Cell-intrinsic responses of cDC1 to IFN-I appear to be critical for spontaneous tumor rejection by enhancing their cross-presentation capacity (51, 54), and perhaps also their trans-presentation of IL-15 which promotes the proliferation and effector differentiation of CTLs

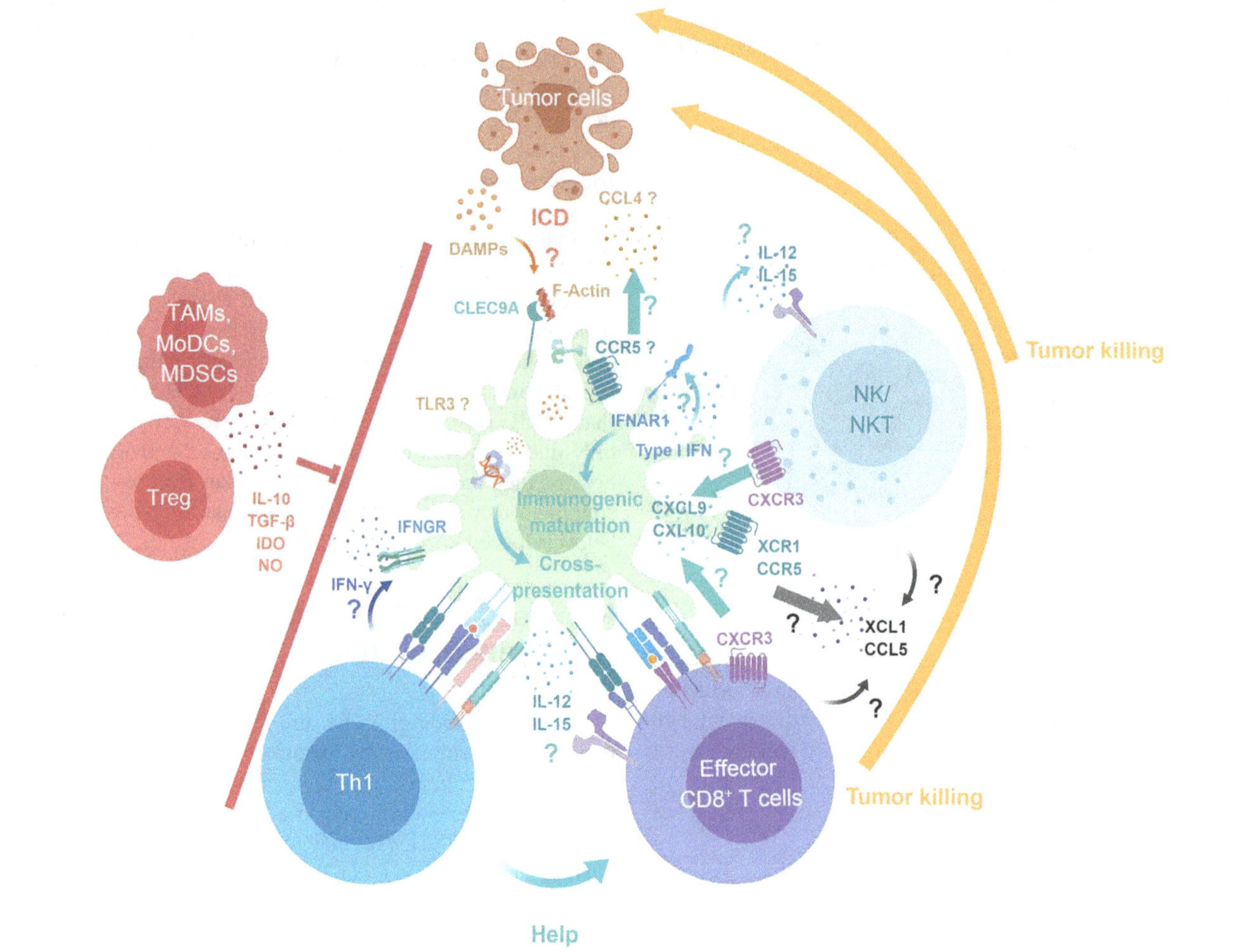

FIGURE 1 | cDC1 key functions in antitumor immunity. Tumor DAMPs and Ag are released upon immunogenic cell death. cDC1 selectively express Clec9A, which binds F-Actin exposed at the surface of necrotic cells, enabling intracellular trafficking of engulfed Ag into endosomes specialized in cross-presentation. cDC1 immunogenic maturation and cross-presentation is promoted by their cell-intrinsic responses to IFN-I. XCR1 and CCR5 expression by cDC1 may contribute to their recruitment by CTL/NK/NKT producing XCL1 and CCL4/5 and by tumor cells producing CCL4. Reciprocally, cDC1 produce CXCL9/10 for local recruitment of CTL/NK/NKT. cDC1 deliver positive co-stimulation and produce IL-12, IFN-β, and IL-15Rα/IL-15 promoting the survival and proper activation of NK and CTL. cDC1 promote Th1 induction and $CD4^+$ T cell help delivery to CTLs through simultaneous presentation of Ag in association to MHC-I and MHC-II. CTLs, NK, NKT cells can mediate tumor killing/cell death. Immunosuppressive cells infiltrating the tumor (TAMs, MoDCs, MDSCs, and Tregs) can dampen cDC1, Th1, CTLs, NK, and NKT antitumor immune responses. DAMPs, danger associated molecular patterns; F-Actin, filamentous actin; ICD, immunogenic cell death; MDSCs, Myeloid-derived suppressor cells; MoDCs, Monocyte-derived dendritic cells; TAMs, Tumor associated macrophages; Tregs, Regulatory T cells.

(68). However, cross-presentation was not totally abolished in *Ifnar1*$^{-/-}$ DCs (51, 54). Upon exposure to high doses of Ag *in vitro*, cross-presentation was even as efficient in *Ifnar1*$^{-/-}$ DCs as in WT DCs. Although, in spontaneously rejected tumor grafts, the cellular source of IFN-I was identified as expressing CD11c, IFN-β production was not altered in *Batf3*$^{-/-}$ mice. Further investigations are required to assess the roles of different types of DCs in CTL activation and in the production of, or responses to, IFN-I, during spontaneous tumor control. In summary, cDC1 constitute a versatile and efficient platform for CTL activation by uniquely bridging several components of innate and adaptive immune responses in a manner promoting mutually beneficial cross-talk (**Figure 1**). However, further studies are warranted to determine whether the different mechanisms detailed above are each critical for the protective antitumor functions of cDC1, as well as their respective importance.

When and Where Are cDC1 Functions Exerted During Cancer Immunosurveillance?

Intra-tumoral cDC1 have been suggested to be crucial for *in situ* maintenance of the effector functions of pre-activated CTLs (65). cDC1 promote memory CTL recall upon secondary infections (43). In an experimental model of established immune memory, only tumors that could be infiltrated by both cDC1 and CTLs were spontaneously controlled (57). While conditional cDC1 depletion was not performed in these settings to functionally confirm the importance of cDC1 for the reactivation of antitumor CTLs, this point was addressed in another study examining the reactivation of adoptively transferred antitumor central memory CTLs into WT vs. *Batf3*$^{-/-}$ recipient mice (78). In conclusion, cDC1 might not only be required for the initiation of adaptive immunity against intracellular pathogens or tumors but all along the life cycle of CTLs, including for their maintenance in the tumor as well as for the generation and recall of memory to prevent relapse or metastases.

Several studies have suggested that T cell priming in the tumor draining lymph node is required to mount anti-tumor immunity (79, 80) A study showed that tumor-associated cDC1 bearing intact tumor Ag traffic to the draining lymph node to prime naïve CTLs in a CCR7-dependent manner (80). However, *Ccr7* knock-out had little impact on tumor growth (80). Moreover, CTL priming, activation, proliferation and effector function acquisition in tumor was observed when T cell egress from lymph nodes was blocked (81) or in mice lacking lymph nodes (82). Although these experimental settings could alter cDC1 and lymphoid cell trafficking (83, 84), they nevertheless show that the activation of antitumor adaptive immunity can occur directly at the tumor site (82), possibly in tertiary lymphoid structures developing locally (85). In any case, for efficient tumor rejection without relapse or metastases, systemic immunity is likely important in addition to *in situ* responses, as recently appreciated in the context of immunotherapy (86).

Proposed Model of cDC1 Role in Antitumor Immunity

Based on the knowledge discussed in the previous sections, we propose a putative model of the mechanisms through which cDC1 promote the rejection of syngeneic tumor grafts in preclinical mouse models (**Table 2**) and may physiologically contribute to cancer immunosurveillance (**Figure 2**). cDC1 take up cell-associated Ag in the tumor after immunogenic cell death, undergo immunogenic maturation, and traffic to the tumor-draining lymph node. There, cDC1 prime naïve CTLs and polarize them toward protective effector functions. CTLs expand and migrate to tumor, where they can be attracted by chemokines secreted locally by cDC1. The tumor-associated cDC1 also sustain infiltrating CTL protective functions (expansion, maintenance and memory recall), and might also prime naïve CTLs *in situ*.

FAILURE OF IMMUNOSURVEILLANCE: ARE cDC1 DIRECT TARGETS OF TUMOR ESCAPE MECHANISMS?

We propose a classification of tumors (Hot/Warm/Cold/Icy) according to their immunogenicity, their cDC1 infiltration, maturation and phenotype, and the characteristics of the antitumor CTL response.

"Hot" tumors are characterized as strongly infiltrated by effector CTLs. They are spontaneously controlled by the immune system (**Figure 2**). They include the syngeneic cancer cell lines used to study spontaneous rejection of tumor grafts (**Table 2**).

"Warm" tumors express tumor neoAg and are infiltrated by cDC1 and CTLs (**Figure 3** Right). Experimental studies in mice suggest that the correlation between high CTL numbers and increased cDC infiltration in tumors is due to a positive feedback loop between these two cell types mutually promoting their local recruitment and survival. It is not clear how this process is initiated, i.e., which cell type is recruited first to the tumor site. This might depend on the combination of tumor type and host characteristics. "Warm" tumors are ultimately not controlled by the immune system, due to their late selection for harboring immune escape mechanisms, such as intrinsic impairment of Ag processing and presentation (87, 88) or induction of CTL exhaustion (89). In these tumors, cDC1 could have undergone immunogenic maturation but may present Ag to CTL in a manner contributing to their chronic activation and exhaustion, e.g., through engagement of checkpoint receptors such as PD-1 or CTLA4.

"Cold" tumors are weakly immunogenic and poorly infiltrated but induce some level of adaptive immunity (**Figure 3** Top). In such tumors, cDC1 could also be direct targets of immune escape mechanisms, such as local production of factors inhibiting DC differentiation or promoting tolerogenic over immunogenic maturation. Those factors include TGF-β, IL-10, IL-6, CSF-1, and VEGF (90). Although cDC1 are proposed to contribute to central and peripheral tolerance (75, 91, 92), whether they can be hijacked by tumors to promote local immunosuppression has not been rigorously investigated.

"Icy" tumors are not immunogenic *per se*, are not infiltrated by T cells and fail to induce immune responses (**Figure 3** Left). Those tumors have evaded or hijacked innate immunity in a manner preventing immune cell infiltration at very early stages of the cancer immunoediting process (87). cDC1 can be direct targets of these early immune escape mechanisms. In melanoma, the WNT/β-Catenin signaling pathway prevents the recruitment of cDC1 and CTLs into the tumor, at least in part by inhibiting the local production of CCL4 and CXCL9 (57, 93). CCL4 contributes to the recruitment of cDC1 through their CCR5 chemokine receptor (93). CXCL9 helps promoting the recruitment of both pre-cDC1 (94) and memory/effector T cells (57), through CXCR3. Another mechanism of evasion of innate immunity by melanoma is tumor-intrinsic elevated COX activity leading to PGE_2 production and downstream inhibition of NK cell, cDC1 and CTL infiltration (55, 56), by disrupting the XCL1/XCR1 and CCL5/CCR5 chemotactic axes. Impairment of CTL infiltration into the tumor is proposed to occur downstream of the failure of cDC1 recruitment (55, 56).

In brief, cDC1 are direct targets of tumor escape mechanisms since the tumor microenvironment can modulate all of the processes necessary to promote their protective antitumor functions. It can determine the tolerogenic vs. immunogenic nature of tumor cell death (95–97), control the expression of the growth factors and chemokines promoting local recruitment, differentiation, expansion and survival of cDC1 or their progenitors (55, 93, 98), dampen cDC1 production of activating

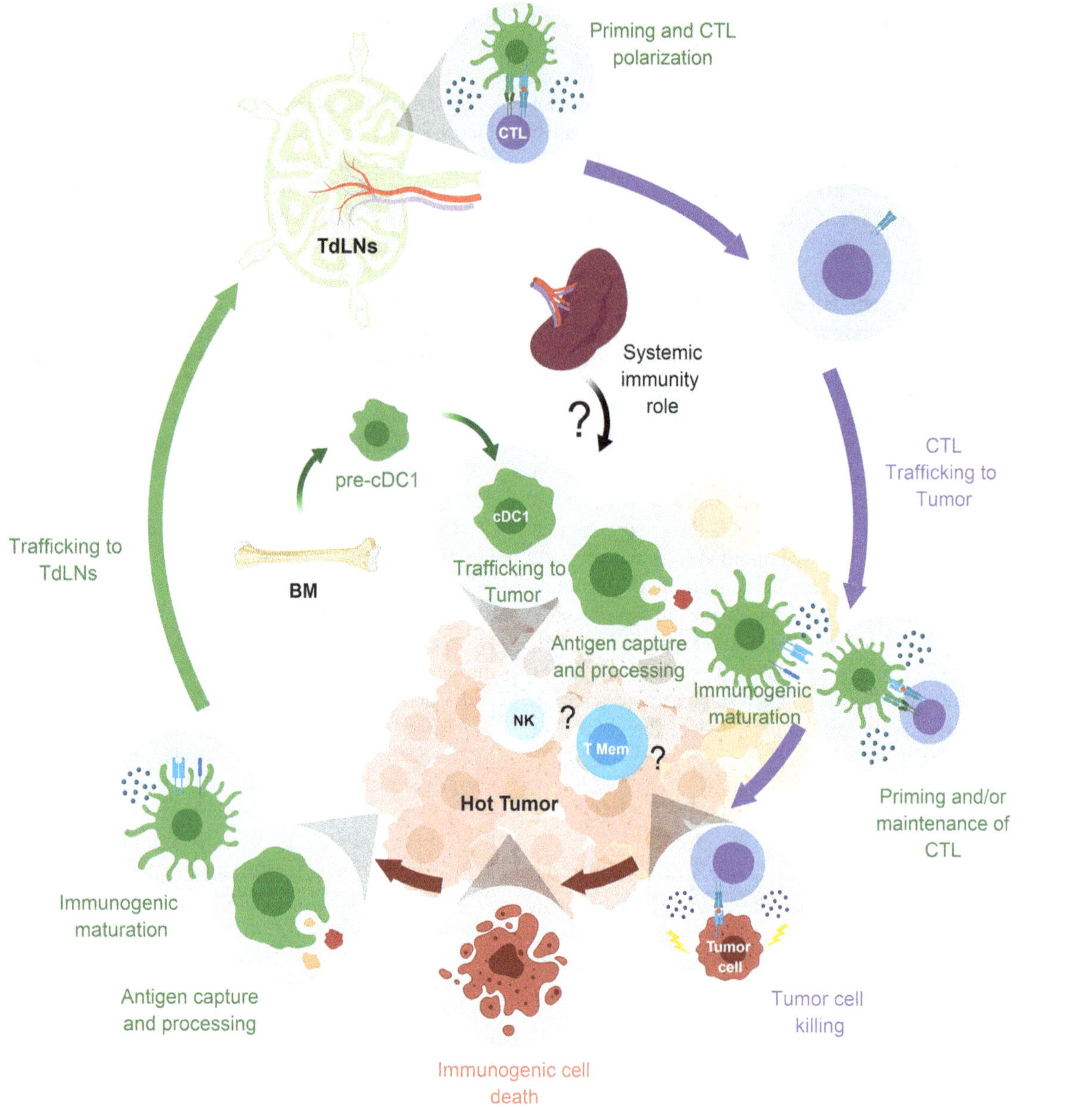

FIGURE 2 | cDC1 cancer immunosurveillance cycle. cDC1 traffic to hot tumor. They uptake cell-associated Ag in the tumor after immunogenic cell death, undergo immunogenic maturation, and traffic to the tumor-draining lymph node. cDC1 prime naïve CTLs and polarize them toward protective effector functions. CTLs expand and migrate to tumor where they can be attracted by chemokines secreted locally by cDC1. The tumor-associated cDC1 also sustain infiltrating CTL protective functions (expansion, maintenance, and memory recall). They might also prime naïve CTLs *in situ*. TdLN, Tumor draining lymph node.

cytokines (56, 67), and inhibit their maturation or even polarize it toward tolerance (99, 100).

STUDIES OF THE NATURAL ROLE OF cDC1 IN IMMUNOTHERAPIES

In the last two decades, cancer treatments have successfully shifted from only targeting the cancer itself to also manipulating the immune system, with the aim to boost or induce *de novo* protective antitumor cellular immune responses, mainly CTLs but also NK and NKT cells. These novel treatments called immunotherapies encompass different strategies. Here we will specifically discuss studies performed in experimental settings mirroring the two types of immunotherapies that have shown the best clinical benefits in cancer patients. First, we will focus on treatments providing exogenous effector cells through ACT of autologous antitumor CTLs, after their expansion and activation *in vitro* (eventually combined with genetic engineering for CAR T cells), i.e., CTL ACT. Second, we will discuss mAb

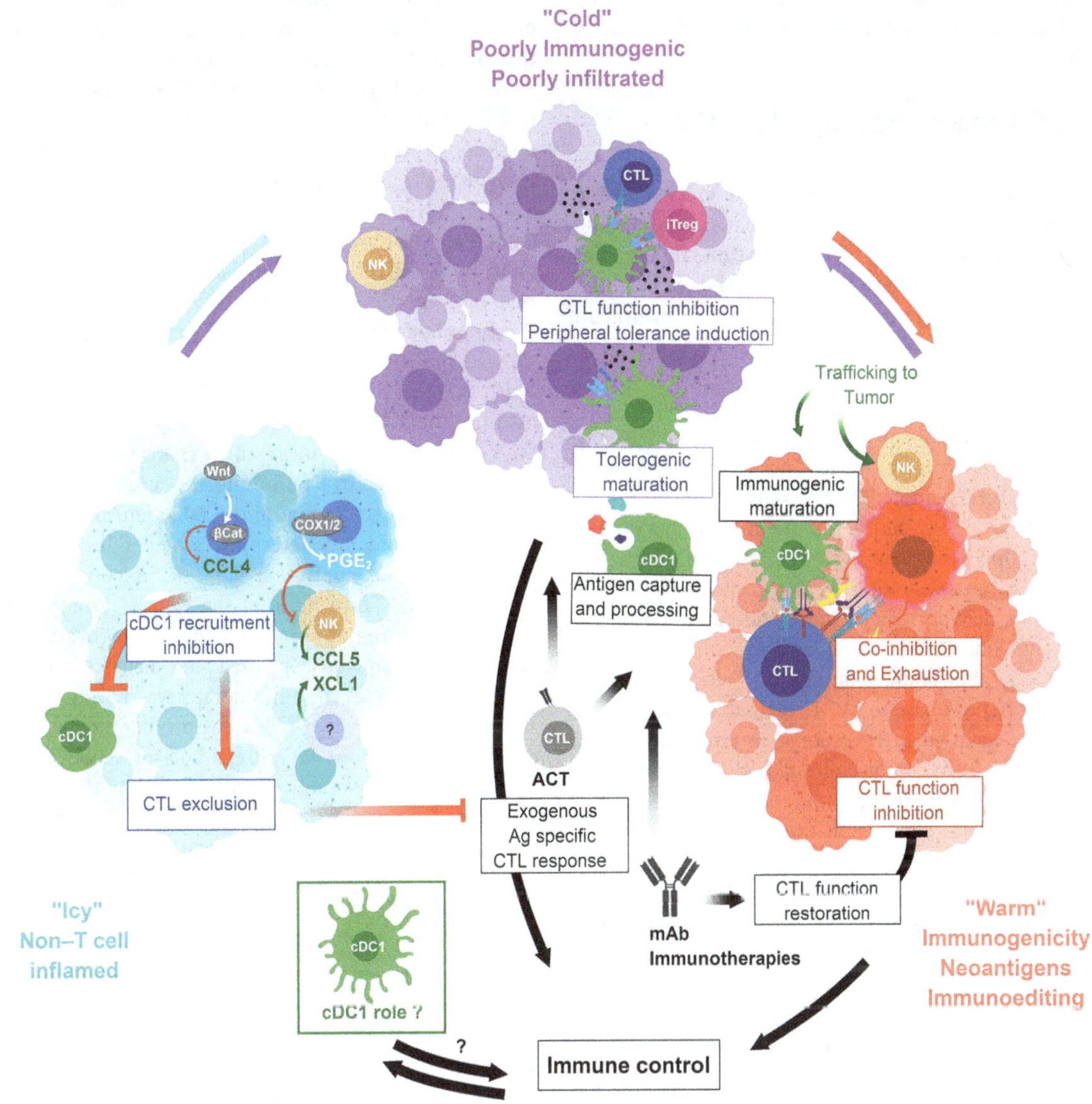

FIGURE 3 | Icy, Cold, and Warm tumors escape from cDC1 immunosurveillance. Icy tumors **(Left)** failed to induce adaptive immune responses. For example, tumors with WNT/β-Catenin signaling or COX elevated activity disrupt the chemokine axes required for local cDC1 recruitment. Impairment of CTL infiltration would occur downstream of the failure of cDC1 to infiltrate the tumor. Cold tumors **(top)** are poorly immunogenic and infiltrated but induce some level of adaptive immunity. Tumors product factors inhibiting cDC1 differentiation or promoting their tolerogenic over immunogenic maturation. This can potentially lead to CTL inhibition and induction of peripheral tolerance. Warm tumors **(Right)** express tumor neoAg and are infiltrated by cDC1 and CTLs but are ultimately not controlled. Cancer immunoediting leads to immune escape. cDC1 have undergone immunogenic maturation but contribute to CTL chronic activation and exhaustion. ACT or mAb immunotherapies could contribute to immune control in Cold and Warm tumors, and cDC1 could play a major role in these settings **(bottom)**. ACT, Adoptive cell transfer; β-Cat, β-Catenin; COX1/2, Cyclo-oxygenase 1/2; iTreg, induced regulatory T cell; mAb, monoclonal antibodies; PGE_2, Prostaglandin E2.

immunomodulation (mAIM) to block checkpoint receptors on CTLs or NK cells (101–106), i.e., ICB, which has proven more efficient than conventional chemotherapies or radiotherapies in several cancer types, with better overall responses, and, most strikingly, significantly increased long-term survival (107). ACT or ICB monotherapy promotes durable disease control only in 30% of the patients. While they dramatically improve the response rate in patients with metastatic melanoma, ICB bi-therapies cause significant adverse effects and toxicities, with high incidences of autoimmune manifestations (108, 109). Understanding the mechanisms controlling responsiveness to ACT or ICB is thus a prerequisite before complementing these immunotherapies by adjuvant treatments able to further improve the rate and duration of remission for cancer patients. One hypothesis to explain patient non-response to immunotherapies is an impairment of the accessory cells needed to promote CTL reactivation and to sustain their effector functions, rather than cell-intrinsic defects in the CTLs themselves. In this scenario, cDC1 are likely candidates, based on their critical role in promoting the spontaneous rejection of tumors in preclinical mouse models, and on their unique functional features endowing them with a high efficiency for nurturing cytotoxic cells all along their life cycle.

Role of cDC1 in Promoting CTL ACT Efficacy

The ACT procedure the most commonly used so far consists in isolating endogenous CTLs from a cancer patient, expanding them *in vitro* through tumor Ag-specific re-stimulation under conditions allowing reversal of exhaustion, and then re-infusing them into the host. By using autologous cells for the treatment, this strategy alleviates any side effects that could arise in allogenic settings. However, one major issue is that only few cancer types respond to this treatment. This might be due to immune escape mechanisms in the tumor limiting locally CTL access to the activating signals necessary to prevent their exhaustion and promote their proliferation, sustained activation and survival. Preclinical mouse models have been used to address this issue, aiming at determining whether professional Ag cross-presentation in the context of positive co-stimulation and delivery of specific cytokines is necessary for ACT efficacy. Since cDC1 excel at this combination of functions (**Figure 1**), they could promote ACT efficacy. Indeed, injection of diphtheria toxin in ACT recipient *Zbtb46-DTR* mice significantly decreased their response to immunotherapy. cDC1 but not cDC2 from tumor-engrafted control mice were shown to cross-present tumor Ag and produce IL-12 *ex vivo*. Thus, it was concluded that cDC1 are necessary for ACT efficacy in these experimental settings (65). However, opposite results were recently reported under similar experimental conditions, showing a lack of cDC requirement for ACT success (110). Differences between the experimental set-up of these two studies might explain their different conclusions, since only the second study used bone marrow chimera mice rather than directly Zbtb46-DTR animals, which is necessary to rule out any impact of loss of Zbtb46 expression in other cells than cDCs (33). Therefore, additional studies are necessary to determine whether cDCs are required for maximal ACT efficacy, and how. If those studies unravel specific pathways that can be potentiated, this could allow designing of a "DC adjuvant" therapy for ACT, which might broaden its success rate to more patients and for additional cancer types.

Role of cDC1 in Promoting Responses to mAIM

In the course of a normal immune response, Ag-presenting cells regulate their expression of ligands for T cell activating vs. inhibitory co-receptors. This contributes to fine tune the intensity and kinetics of the adaptive immune response, in order to balance efficient immune control of pathogens with the risk of developing an immunopathology due to an excessive T cell activation. Tumors can hijack this process by expressing ligands for T cell inhibitory receptors leading to premature termination/exhaustion of CTL responses (48, 107). This tumoral immune evasion strategy can be overcome by mAIM through infusion of mAbs capable of either inhibiting the engagement of T cell inhibitory co-receptors (i.e., ICB mAbs) or mimicking the engagement of T cell activating co-receptors (co-stimulation activating mAbs) [listed in (106)]. These mAbs can be used as monotherapy or bi-therapy. The ICB mAbs the most commonly used in clinics are directed against programmed cell death protein 1 (PD-1) and cytotoxic T-lymphocyte associated protein 4 (CTLA-4). Although their use has dramatically improved patient survival for different types of cancer, their precise mode of action is still a matter of debate. The mechanisms underlying lack of response in the majority of patients remain elusive. Preclinical mouse models have been used to address this issue and showed that treatment efficacy is abrogated in cDC1-deficient *Batf3*$^{-/-}$ animals (**Table 3**) (56, 57, 65, 69, 117, 118). This is the case for anti-CTLA4 (117) or anti-PD-L1 (79) monotherapies, for a bi-therapy combining anti-PD-1 and CTLA4 mAbs (69), and for a bi-therapy combining the anti-PD-1 mAb with the co-stimulation activating anti-CD137 mAb (118). However, these studies did not determine whether the lack of mAIM-dependent tumor control in *Batf3*$^{-/-}$ mice was due to a lack of antitumor CTL priming at the time of tumor engraftment, before immunotherapy, or to a failure of mAIM at inducing the reactivation of previously primed but exhausted antitumor CTLs, at the time when the immunotherapy was administered. Efficient activation of anti-tumor CTLs, for proliferation and acquisition of effector functions, requires cross-presentation of tumor-associated Ag, activating co-stimulation and delivery of specific cytokines from accessory cells. As described previously, cDC1 excel at simultaneously delivering all these signals (**Figure 1**). In particular, one of the critical functions of cDC1 during mAIM immunotherapies may be to deliver IL-12 (69). In addition, cDC1 may also be a major source of CXCL9/10 (43) for recruiting activated or memory CTLs into the tumors (57, 93) (**Figures 1, 2**).

Current Limitations, Controversies or Unknowns

Many of the conclusions drawn above are based on the use of *Batf3*$^{-/-}$ mice, or on the assumption that cDC1 are the main source of the cytokines or chemokines promoting response to mAIM therapies, without formal demonstration of this point by functional inactivation of candidate functions selectively in cDC1. Moreover, the respective importance of Ag cross-presentation vs. delivery of specific activating co-stimulation or cytokine signals by cDC1 has not been delineated yet under immunotherapies condition. Thus, further studies are required to confirm and extend these analyses, by using other mutant mouse models allowing specific cDC1 depletion or selective manipulation of each of their candidate functions.

HARNESSING cDC1 FUNCTIONS TO IMPROVE IMMUNOTHERAPIES AGAINST CANCER

In parallel of developing immunotherapies to directly boost lymphocyte effector responses against tumor cells, the

TABLE 3 | Studies in mouse preclinical cancer models investigating the impact of cDC1 depletion on the protective effects of various immunotherapies not designed to directly target these cells.

Model of cDC1 depletion	Tumor models	Therapy used	Outcome of cDC1 depletion	Remarks	References
CD11c-hDTR *Batf3*$^{-/-}$	B16gp100 (Melanoma)	Drug: Ad.*flagr170* MOA: Immune chaperone inducing NF-κB activity	Beneficial effect lost upon DT injection and in *Batf3*$^{-/-}$ mice	DT injection resulted in only a partial loss of protection	(111)
Batf3$^{-/-}$ CD11c-hDTR	B16-EGFR-SIY (Melanoma)	Drug: anti-EGFR-IFNβ MOA: IFN-I delivery to mAb resistant tumor enhance immune response	Beneficial effect lost upon DT injection but not in *Batf3*$^{-/-}$ mice		(112)
Batf3$^{-/-}$	Braf^{V600E} (Melanoma)	Drug: Aspirin/anti-PD-1 MOA: COX inhibition allows a more efficient mAIM therapy	Beneficial effect lost in *Batf3*$^{-/-}$ mice	CXCL9/10 source to be further investigated	(56)
Batf3$^{-/-}$	B16 (Melanoma) 4T1.2-Neu (Breast Cancer)	Drug: DC-targeted XBP1 plasmid/Tumor Ag MOA: XBP1 enhances DC cross-presenting capacity	Beneficial effect lost in *Batf3*$^{-/-}$ mice		(113)
Batf3$^{-/-}$	B16F10 (Melanoma)	Drug: IFN-α/TA99+FcIL-2 MOA: IFN-α given after Ag uptake by cDC1 promotes their immunogenic maturation	Beneficial effect lost in *Batf3*$^{-/-}$ mice		(114)
Batf3$^{-/-}$	B16 (Melanoma)	Drug: BRAFI/anti-PD-L1/poly(I:C) /Flt3-L MOA: Sequentially administered combination therapy targeting DC, CTL and the tumor itself	Beneficial effect lost in *Batf3*$^{-/-}$ mice	*Batf3*$^{-/-}$	(79)
Batf3$^{-/-}$	BP-SIY (Melanoma) BPC-SIY (Melanoma) MC-57.SIY (Fibrosarcoma)	Drug: Flt3-L-BM-DC/anti-CTLA-4/anti-PD-L1 MOA: Intratumoral injection of BM-DCs induce CTL recruitment	Beneficial effect lost in *Batf3*$^{-/-}$ mice	CXCL9/10 source to be further investigated	(57)
Batf3$^{-/-}$	B16-mCD20+ (Melanoma)	Drug: anti-Clec9A-IFNα2/TNF/Doxorubicin/anti-PD-L1/anti-CTLA-4/anti-OX40 MOA: IFN-I targeting to cDC1 through Clec9A mAb	Beneficial effect lost in *Batf3*$^{-/-}$ mice		(115)
Clec9a-hDTR *Batf3*$^{-/-}$ CD11c-hDTR	4T1 (Breast Cancer) B16F10 (Melanoma) B16-OVA (Melanoma)	Drug: poly(I:C) /MSU+M.*smeg* MOA: MSU+M*smeg* and poly(I:C) stimulate cDC1 immunogenic maturation through TLR3. poly(I:C) promotes MoDC recruitment	Poly(I:C) but no MSU+M.*smeg* beneficial effect preserved upon DT injection in *Batf3*$^{-/-}$ mice		(116)
Batf3$^{-/-}$	d42m1-T3 (Fibrosarcoma)	Drug : anti-CTLA-4 MOA : Injection of anti-CTLA-4 allowing tumor rejection	Beneficial effect lost in *Batf3*$^{-/-}$ mice		(117)
Batf3$^{-/-}$	B16F10 (Melanoma) MC-38 (Colon Carcinoma)	Drug: anti-PD-1/anti-CD137 MOA: Immunostimulatory mAbs used in combination enhance antitumor immunity	Beneficial effect lost in *Batf3*$^{-/-}$ mice	IL-12 source to be further investigated	(118)
Batf3$^{-/-}$	AT-3ovadim CD73+ (Breast Carcinoma)	Drug: anti-PD-1/anti-CTLA-4 MOA: Reactivation of endogenous CTLs and depletion of Treg	Beneficial effect lost in *Batf3*$^{-/-}$, *Il12p35*$^{-/-}$ and *Il12p40*$^{-/-}$ mice	IL-12 source to be further investigated	(69)
Zbtb46-hDTR	EG-7 (Thymoma)	Drug: *in vitro* pre-activated Ag specific CTL MOA: Ag-specific CTL infiltrate the tumor and delay its growth	Beneficial effect lost upon DT injection	These two studies drew diverging conclusion on cDC1 implication. Further studies are required.	(65)
Zbtb46-hDTR	B16-OVA (Melanoma)	Drug: *in vivo* pre-activated Ag specific CTL MOA: Ag-specific CTL delay the tumor growth	Beneficial effect preserved upon DT injection		(110)

MCA : Mode of action.

community has put much effort in trying to elaborate vaccines to ignite or reactivate endogenous antitumor immune responses in patients. Among all Ag presenting cells identified so far, cDC1 are the only ones to express selectively unique cell surface markers, such as CLEC9A or XCR1, which enables their specific targeting with mAb *in vivo*. Intratumor injection of bone marrow-derived DCs highly enriched in cDC1 increased local CTL infiltration and improved response to ICB (57). Therefore, in combination with other immunotherapies, cDC1 represent a very good candidate immune cell type to mobilize with off-the-shelf compounds for boosting patient antitumor immunity.

Specific Targeting of cDC1 for Vaccination Purposes

Many preclinical studies in various mouse models have demonstrated the efficacy of *in vivo* targeting of Ag specifically to cDC1 in combination with the administration of a proper adjuvant for priming or reactivating adaptive immunity, leading to a rapid yet long term immune protection against infections by intracellular pathogens or against tumors (119) (**Table S1**). Adjuvants used to induce a beneficial inflammation promoting an immunogenic environment to prevent or counterbalance tumor immunosuppressive functions include the Toll-Like-Receptor ligands LPS, Imiquimod, CpG or Poly(I:C). Other adjuvants include drugs which directly stimulate accessory lymphocytes, such as αGalCer for NKT cell activation (120, 121), or agonistic anti-CD40 antibodies which mimic the helper signal delivered by $CD4^+$ T cells to DCs for promoting their production of the lymphocyte activating cytokines IL-12 and IL-15/IL-15Rα (68, 122, 123). Vaccine formulation including naked DNA (124, 125), porous polymer matrices (126), or oil in water nano-emulsion (127) are intrinsically immunogenic. Vaccination based on macroporous polymer matrices encapsulating tumor lysates, GM-CSF and CpG, were quite effective in attenuating tumor growth (126), although not targeting specifically cDC1. DEC-205 has been by far the cell surface marker the most used to target cDC1 *in vivo* (**Table S1**). However, it is not specific of cDC1 since it is expressed on Langerhans cells in the epidermis, on all migratory DC in lymph nodes (128) and it is highly upregulated on various DC subsets in tumors (30). The same issue applies to CD40. This raises the question of the respective roles of cDC1 vs. other types of DC in the protection conferred by vaccines based on *in vivo* Ag delivery through DEC-205 or CD40. Indeed, tumor Ag delivery to pDCs or cDC2 by using anti-BST2 (129) or anti-DCIR2 mAb (130) respectively, or administration of tumor Ag-pulsed pDC (131), are highly efficient in conferring protection against cancer. This shows that not only cDC1 but also cDC2 or pDCs can induce protective antitumor immunity, providing that Ag is delivered to these cells through adequate endocytic receptors in the presence of proper maturation signals. Interestingly, immunization with tumor-associated exogenous cDC1 or cDC2 prior to tumor engraftment revealed complementary functions of these two DC types (30). In a model of challenge with Lewis Lung carcinoma, only cDC2 vaccination led to reduced tumor growth rate and weight, correlating with reduced tumor infiltration by myeloid-derived suppressor cells, functional polarization of tumor-associated macrophages toward a M1-like antitumor phenotype, and promotion of Th17 rather than Treg $CD4^+$ T cell responses (30). cDC1 were confirmed to be more efficient than cDC2 for the induction of antitumor CTL responses, which protected against a challenge with B16 melanoma (30).

In summary, even though other DC types can be successfully harnessed for cancer vaccines in mouse preclinical models, many studies showed that *in vivo* targeting of cDC1 is highly efficient for the activation of antitumor CTL responses able to induce complete tumor rejection in prophylactic settings and to delay significantly tumor progression or metastasis in therapeutic settings (**Table S1**). The efficacy of DC-targeted vaccines depends on three critical parameters: (i) the mode of delivery of the Ag, (ii) the nature of the Ag, and (iii) the nature of the adjuvant. Targeting Ag to cell surface receptors trafficking into late endosomes or lysosomes promotes more efficient cross-presentation by human cDC1 as compared to cDC2, whereas both cell types can mediate this function upon Ag delivery to early endosomes (132). The route of administration of the vaccine should be carefully determined depending on the necessity to induce mucosal and/or systemic immunity according to the type of cancer involved (86, 133). Once activated, tumor-associated DCs have the capacity to migrate to tumor-draining lymph nodes to prime T cells (80) and may rather favor a local antitumor immunity. There is also evidence that CTL priming can occur directly in the tumor (82). Hence, intra- or peri-tumoral administration of cDC1-targeted Ag for solid tumors may be the best way to enhance priming of CTLs both inside the tumor, and through migration of tumor-associated DCs to the draining lymph node. The tumor Ag should be well selected as the immune system can be almost irreversibly tolerized against certain self Ag (134). Some adjuvants are more efficient in promoting a beneficial inflammatory microenvironment in the tumor, linked to their ability to induce IFN-I. It might be desirable to include adjuvants that directly engage cDC1 since exposure to inflammatory mediators in the absence of direct signaling by pattern recognition receptors might not be sufficient to promote immunogenic DC maturation (135).

Mobilizing cDC1 Functions in Combination Immunotherapies

In most of the preclinical models discussed above, cDC1-targeting therapeutic vaccines delay tumor progression or metastasis, or even promote a better tumor control over a long time, but fail by themselves in inducing complete tumor rejection. However, combining strategies mobilizing cDC1 with current immunotherapies, in particular with ICB, should promote the induction of long lasting protective antitumor immunity in more patients, and should more generally improve the objective response rate, the response duration and the overall survival of patients. In preclinical mouse models of immunotherapies, the antitumor effects of various off-the-shelf treatments were shown to require cDC1 functions (**Table S1**), and a variety of strategies were specifically designed to harness cDC1 against cancer (**Table 4**). Hereafter, we discuss how these studies advanced our understanding of when, where and how to mobilize cDC1 functions in combination immunotherapies.

Upon immunotherapy, cDC1 are increased in the tumor very early after the beginning of the treatment, and have left the tumor in favor of cDC2 during the phase of immunotherapy-induced rejection of the tumor (86). Therefore, the location and timing of cDC1 booster administration in combination with immunotherapies are likely to be determinant for treatment success.

One way to attempt improving the response of cancer patients to immunotherapy is to boost the ability of their cDC1 to cross-present tumor Ag (60). Combined administration in mice of mAbs directed against tumor Ag with a stabilized form of IL-2 enhances antitumor immunity in a cDC1-dependent manner (**Table 4**) (114, 139). This is because antibody-dependent cell-mediated cytotoxicity provokes an immunogenic tumor cell death favoring the up-take and cross-presentation by cDC1 of tumor cell fragments. Indeed, tumor cell lysates or tumor plasma membrane vesicles may represent the best sources of Ag for cross-presentation, because they include a constellation of neoAg. Tumor Ag cross-presentation by cDC1 can also be triggered upon administration of tumor Ag coupled to mAb directed against cDC1 surface markers (**Table S1**).

Cross-presentation of tumor Ag by cDC1 must occur simultaneously to their immunogenic maturation such that they can deliver all of the signals required for the efficient priming of naïve CTLs or the reactivation of exhausted CTLs, including proper co-stimulation, activating cytokines, chemokines and $CD4^+$ T cell help, in the tumor bed or upon migration to the draining lymph node. This implies administrating the good adjuvant at the right time and in the proper place. TLR3, CpG, or STING agonist adjuvants promoting a strong production of IFN-I are especially efficient at promoting antitumor immunity, even more upon peritumoral rather than systemic delivery (79, 140–142). To further promote the beneficial anti-tumor activity of IFN-I and limit their deleterious side effects, a synthetic mutated IFNα2 has been engineered and coupled to anti-Clec9a mAb, allowing delivery of IFN-I activity specifically on cDC1. The administration of this cDC1-targeted adjuvant synergizes with mAIM, chemotherapy, or with low dose of TNF, resulting in a regression or a long-lasting protection against melanoma and breast carcinoma in the absence of toxic effects (115). Targeting IFN-I on tumor cells also improves the antitumor effects of mAIM (112, 114, 143), in part through direct effects on cDC1 and/or cDC2 (143) but also more generally by modulating the responses of many other immune cells in the tumor microenvironment. Importantly, to promote protective antitumor immunity, IFN-I must be delivered simultaneously to, or shortly after, the tumor Ag. Indeed, IFN-I-induced cDC1 maturation strongly decreases their phagocytic capacity and thus prevents their ability to cross-present if occurring before tumor Ag uptake (114).

IL-12 production by cDC1 is proposed to significantly contribute to their protective antitumor activity, at least in part by promoting Th1 response and activating IFN-γ production by NK cells and CTLs. Administration of recombinant IL-12 in combination or not with mAIM therapy displayed anti-metastatic (66) or immunotherapy-induced antitumor effect (118) in WT animals (**Table 4**). However, interestingly, these potentiating effect of the mAIM therapy was lost in *Batf3*$^{-/-}$ mice (118), showing that IL-12 administration is not sufficient to replace the antitumor functions of cDC1.

Another function of cDC1 that could be exploited for boosting current immunotherapies is their ability to respond to the chemoattractant XCL1, due to their specific expression of the chemokine receptor XCR1. At steady state, high levels of the *Xcl1* transcript are detected in NK cells, NKT cells and memory CTLs. Upon activation, *Xcl1* expression is further upregulated in these cells and induced in effector CTLs, which promotes the recruitment of cDC1 into inflamed tissues in close contact to XCL1-producing cells, leading to a cross-talk amplifying the responses of both cell types (77). Therefore, intra-tumoral delivery of XCL1 seemed a promising strategy to enhance local recruitment of cDC1 in order to harness their protective functions in combination immunotherapies. Certain types of melanoma or colon carcinoma tumors engineered to express high amount of XCL1 harbored a higher cDC1 infiltration and were rejected faster or grew more slowly in WT but not in *Batf3*$^{-/-}$ mice, as compared to control tumors. However, this process was inhibited in tumors producing PGE2, due in part to the ability of this molecule to decrease XCR1 expression in cDC1 (55). This study illustrates well the necessity not only to mobilize cDC1 in combination immunotherapies, but at the same time to dampen the immunosuppressive pathways targeting cDC1 functions in the tumor microenvironment. Hence, in addition to directly targeting CTL and cDC1 functions, combined immunotherapies should probably include means to counteract the tumor immunosuppressive pathways acting indirectly on these cells, such as inhibiting β-catenin, PGE_2 or adenosine receptor signaling (55, 57, 93, 144), or depleting/reprogramming the tumor-associated mononuclear phagocytes endowed with immunosuppressive functions including macrophages, MDSCs and pDCs (67, 145, 146).

Because cDC1 are the rarest subset of Ag presenting cells in tumors (30) and their numbers have been shown to decrease in the course of certain immunotherapies (86), strategies aiming at harnessing their functions for cancer treatment should include methods to promote their expansion *in vivo*. Tumor-infiltrating NK and T cells upregulate FLT3-L, which seems to contribute to the local expansion of tumor cDC1 (62), and most likely cDC2. Administration of recombinant FLT3-L to tumor-bearing mice as a supportive treatment to mAIM immunotherapy reinforces CTL infiltration and activation in the tumor (137), and the combined administration of FLT3-L and poly(I:C) which respectively support cDC1 expansion and activation significantly improved antitumor mAIM immunotherapy in mice (79, 118) (**Table 4**). Alternatively, large quantities of cDC1 could be injected peritumorally simultaneously to ICB administration, in order to further promote the priming of naïve CTLs toward neoAg or the reactivation of endogenous antitumor CTL responses. This should be achievable since recent studies showed that large numbers of fully functional cDC1 can be

TABLE 4 | Anti-tumor off-the shelf therapies relying on cDC1 functions.

Mode of action		Therapy	Putative "cDC1 booster" and protocol of administration	Type of tumors	Depend on	Does not depend on	Effects on cells	Impact of cDC1 depletion	References
Promoting maturation		Cytokine therapy (Fc-IL-2)	IFN-I delivery, 48h after induction of ADDC against tumor upon administration of an anti-tumor mAb	B16-F10 DD-Her2/neu breast cancer RM9 prostate cancer	CD8α+ cells CSF1R+ cells IFN-γ	IFN-γ-production by CTL is Batf3-independent	↑ CTL activation ↑ cDC1 maturation and tumor uptake Early influx of neutrophils ↑ production of chemokines	Delayed control in *Batf3*$^{-/-}$ mice	(114)
Blocking checkpoint inhibitors on cDC1 (and putatively on other cells)		Chemotherapy	anti-TIM3 antagonist mAb before chemotherapy	PPMTV-mCherry	IFN-I IL-12 IFN-γ CXCR3 CD8α+ cells	n.d.(*)	Potentiates CTL activation No effect on IL-12 production by cDC1 ↑ chemokine secretion by cDC	↑ growth in *Batf3*$^{-/-}$ and *Itgax-Cre; Irf8*$^{fl/fl}$ mice or in Zbtb46-hDTR BM chimera	(64)
		Chemotherapy	anti-galectin9 mAb before chemotherapy (Gal9 = Tim3 ligand)	PPMTV-mCherry	CXCR3 CD8β+ T cells	n.d.	n.d.	n.d.	(64)
Providing cytokine support for T cell reactivation and polarization		mAIM (Anti-CD137)	Recombinant IL-12 after mAIM (mimicking boosting of IL-12 production by cDC1)	MC38 s.c	n.d.	n.d.	↑ tumor control	no effect of IL-12 in *Batf3*$^{-/-}$ mice	(118)
Expansion of cDC	Promoting cytokine-production	mAIM (anti-PD-L1)	FLT3-L (for 9 consecutive days) + 2 inj. Poly(I:C)	B16 BRAF^{V600E}; PTEN melanoma	n.d.	n.d.	↑ CTL activation and infiltration in tumor	n.d.	(79)
		mAIM (anti-PD-1 or anti-CD137)	Hydrodynamically injected iv on the day of engraftment 1 inject. Poly(IC:LC) i.t. 7d after	B16-OVA s.c.	n.d.	n.d.	n.d.	↑ growth in *Batf3*$^{-/-}$ mice	(118)
		Radiation	Poly(I:C) 1 d before radiation	LLC-OVA s.c. (BALB/c)	CD8β+ T cells TNF (by improving ionizing radiation effect)	n.d.	↑ CTL activation in LN, spleen and tumor ↑ CXCL10 and IFN-β	↑ growth in *Batf3*$^{-/-}$ mice	(136)
		mAIM (anti-PD-L1 + anti-CTLA-4)	FLT3-L 1/week for 4 weeks	RCC Xenograft: Renca cells s.c. (BALB/c)	n.d.	n.d.	↑ CD103^{+} cell and CTL tumor infiltration ↑ CTL activation	n.d.	(137)

All tumor models were engrafted in C57BL/6J unless otherwise specified. LCC, Lewis Lung Carcinoma; RCC, Renal Cell Carcinoma; Fc, fragment, crystallizable region of murine immunoglobulin G2a (IgG2a); ↑increased; n.d., not determined.

**Of note: anti-TIM3 alone exerts its effect independently of CD11c+ cells (138).*

generated *in vitro* from hematopoietic progenitors cultured with FLT3-L on feeder cells expressing the Notch ligand Delta-like 1 (147, 148).

In summary, several studies have attempted to improve the response to cancer chemotherapies, radiotherapies or mAIM immunotherapies by combining these treatments with putative or known cDC1 boosters (**Table S1** and **Table 4**). In all cases, tumor progression was greatly dampened in parallel with enhanced CTL activation and sometimes with a documented increased maturation of cDC1. In many studies, this beneficial effect was shown to be abrogated in *Batf3*$^{-/-}$ mice. These studies in mouse preclinical models of combined immunotherapies strongly enforce the hypothesis that harnessing cDC1 functions in cancer patients should improve their response rate and long-term survival to already existing immunotherapies including ICB, and show how this could be achieved.

WHAT FUNCTIONAL SPECIFICITIES MAKE HUMAN cDC1 GOOD CANDIDATE AG-PRESENTING CELLS FOR THE PROMOTION OF PROTECTIVE ANTI-TUMOR IMMUNITY?

Comparative Genomics Established Overall Homology Between Mouse and Human cDC1

A striking overall homology between human and mouse cDC1 was established through cross-species comparative genomics of several immune cell types (14, 149–153). This provided a very strong incentive to investigate the role of human cDC1 in antitumor immunity, considering the body of evidence discussed above supporting a critical role of mouse cDC1 in promoting NK- and CTL-mediated tumor control in preclinical cancer models.

Conservation of Key Characteristics Proposed to Underlie Mouse cDC1 Protective Role Against Cancer

A number of shared and distinctive features of mouse and human cDC1 are summarized in **Table 5** (11, 14, 15, 61, 63, 79, 147–150, 154–162, 165–174), with their possible relevance for immune defense against cancer. Globally, the combination of features proposed to endow mouse cDC1 with their unique efficacy to promote protective anti-tumor immunity is well conserved in human cDC1. Differences in cross-presentation efficacy appear to be more subtle between human than mouse DC subsets (155, 175). Of note, however, a consensus has emerged from various studies that human cDC1 are more efficient than other DC types for the cross-presentation of cell-associated Ag (15, 45, 63, 155–157), likewise to the situation in the mouse. Human cDC1 were reported by several teams not to produce IL-12 (150, 167). However, other studies have shown that under optimal conditions of stimulation human cDC1 can produce this cytokine to levels equivalent or higher than those made by cDC2 or MoDCs (147, 156, 168, 169, 173, 174).

Current Limitations, Controversies or Unknowns

One study has recently reported that human cDC1 do not migrate efficiently from the parenchyma of non-lymphoid tissues to their draining lymph nodes (176). This bears important implications for vaccination or immunotherapies if it is confirmed.

The mechanisms that make human cDC1 especially efficient for cross-presentation of cell-associated Ag are still not understood. One of the main limitations to address this issue, and more generally to study the functions of human cDC1 and their molecular regulation, is their rarity and fragility.

WHAT EVIDENCES EXIST THAT HUMAN cDC1 CORRELATE WITH A BETTER OUTCOME IN CANCER PATIENTS AND WHAT CAN BE INFERRED FROM THESE STUDIES REGARDING THEIR PROTECTIVE MODE OF ACTION?

A Higher Expression of cDC1 Gene Signatures in Tumors Correlates With a Better Clinical Outcome

State-of-the-Art in Assessing cDC1 Infiltration From Whole Tumor Tissue Gene Expression Profiles

Several public datasets are available with gene expression profiles of whole tumor tissue from large cohorts of patients with well documented clinical characteristics. Increasing numbers of teams are querying this gold mine to test whether higher expression in tumors of gene signatures specific for various cell types or biological pathways are associated with a better or worse clinical outcome. Such analyses could allow high throughput testing of the possible relationship between overall survival and tumor infiltration by specific cell types in a given activation state. Such analyses would then allow focusing further studies on the most promising observations, to test whether they are confirmed by using immunohistofluorescence or flow cytometry to directly measure the frequency of specific combinations of immune cell types and activation states in the tumors. However, there is currently no consensus on which gene signatures are the most specific and robust for each immune cell type of interest. In particular, until very recently, to assess the prognostic value of DC infiltration into the tumors, the gene signatures used were those from *in vitro* derived MoDCs. The extent of DC infiltration into tumors as computationally inferred in these studies had no significant prognostic value for overall patient survival, or was even associated to an increased hazard risk (177–181). However, based on the known major differences between MoDCs and cDCs (14–16) and on the beneficial role of mouse cDC1 in antitumor immunity, further studies were needed to assess whether higher infiltration of human tumor by other DC types, in particular cDC1, could be associated with a better clinical outcome.

In the last four years, from the few studies performed to address this issue, a consensus has been emerging that

TABLE 5 | Shared and distinctive features of mouse and human cDC1.

Feature	Present in mouse cDC1	Present in human cDC1	Relevance to anti-tumor immunity	References
Dependency on IRF8 and NOTCH signaling for differentiation	YES	YES	Not applicable	(147, 148, 154)
High efficiency for cellular Ag cross-presentation	YES	YES	Cross-presentation of tumor-associated Ag	(15, 45, 63, 155–157)
Expression of CLEC9A	YES, shared with pDCs	YES	Intracellular routing of engulfed tumor Ag in endosomes specialized in cross-presentation	(158–160)
Higher efficacy for cytosolic export of engulfed proteins	YES, specific to cDC1	YES, shared with other DC types	Cross-presentation of tumor Ag	(155, 161)
Alkaline endosomes	YES, specific to cDC1	YES, shared with cDC2	Limits the degradation of endocytosed tumor Ag to favor their cross-presentation	(155, 162)
Selective high expression of *RAB11A*, *RAB7B*, *RAB43* and *SEPT3*	YES	YES	Small RAB GTPases with documented or putative role in promoting Ag cross-presentation	(14, 163–165)
GCSAM (*GCET2*), *CLNK*, *SNX22* and *WDFY4* expression	YES, Clnk expression shared with NK and mast cells	YES, CLNK expression specific to cDC1	WDFY4 involved in cross-presentation; other gene functions in cDC1 unknown	(11, 14, 52, 165)
CADM1 (IGSF4A) expression	YES	YES	CTL activation?	(166)
Specific expression of XCR1	YES	YES	Local recruitment of cDC1 by, or stabilization of their interactions with, NK cells and CTLs	(14, 45, 61, 63)
High TLR3 expression and specific production of IFN-βand IFN-λs upon TLR3 triggering	YES IL-12 induced as well	YES, high IL-12 production observed in some but not all studies	• Putative source of IFN-β/λs in tumors, promoting DC maturation and CTL activation? • Therapeutic target to promote immunogenic inflammation in combined immunotherapies	(15, 79, 147, 150, 156, 167–170)
TLR9 and TLR11 expression and production of IL-12 upon their triggering	YES, shared with other DC subsets for TLR9	NO, TLR9 not expressed in human cDC1, no TLR11 ortholog in humans	Not applicable in humans	(171, 172)
TLR8 expression and production of IL-12 upon its triggering	NO, loss of TLR8 ligand binding in mice	YES, under adequate conditions of stimulation	• Local recruitment and activation of CTL and NK cells • Therapeutic target to promote immunogenic inflammation in combined immunotherapies	(147, 173, 174)

higher expression of cDC1 transcriptomic fingerprints in various tumors correlates with a better clinical outcome (**Figure 4**, green cells, in the bold rectangle).

In the case for breast cancer (BRCA), a good prognosis of a higher tumor infiltration by cDC1 has been documented independently by 4 studies (55, 65, 66, 182), altogether interrogating three patient cohorts [TCGA, METABRIC, and the meta-cohort generated by Györffy et al. (183)]. A higher expression of the cDC1 transcriptomic signature in tumor was at least as powerful a predictor of prolonged patient survival to cancer as that of the CTL signature (55, 182). Transcriptomic fingerprints or genes associated to certain other immune cell types including cDC2, pDCs or monocytes/macrophages did not have a positive prognostic value (**Figure 4**, gray or red cells). This supports the hypothesis of a specific protective role of high infiltration of breast tumors by cDC1, rather than the alternate hypothesis that differential levels of cDC1 gene expression in tumors reflect differences in their overall leukocyte infiltration and lead recapitulates the known different clinical outcome of "Hot" or "Warm" vs. "Cold" or "Icy" tumors. However, more studies are warranted to address this issue. For triple negative breast cancer (TNBC), the positive prognostic value of higher cDC1 infiltration in tumors was even better than for all types of BRCA or for luminal BRCA. This was observed in three studies, encompassing altogether the analyses of two patient cohorts (55, 65, 66).

Similar analyses were performed for other types of cancer. For head and neck squamous cell carcinoma (HNSC) and lung adenocarcinoma (LUAD), a higher expression of the cDC1 transcriptomic signature in tumor was also associated to a better clinical outcome by at least two independent studies (55, 62, 80). This was also the case for skin cutaneous melanoma (SKCM) (**Figure 4**) (47, 72), on two distinct patient cohorts, TCGA and the cohort described by Boguvonic et al. (184). In addition, for metastatic melanoma, the specific positive prognostic value of high cDC1 infiltration in the

cancer types[1]	Inferred cell type infiltration, or gene high expression, prognostic value[2]																		# patients	cDC1, CD8 T cell, NK cell and other gene signature content[5]	study reference	dataset
	cDC1/other MNP[3]	cDC1 or cDC1e cells[4]	*CLEC9A*	cDC1-attracting chemokines	cDC2	pDC	Mono/Mac	CD8 T cells	NK cells	CD4 T cells	*FLT3LG*	*CCR7*	*CXCL9*	*LAMP3*	*GZMB*	*CD68*	*CD14*	*HAVCR2* (TIM3)				
12 different	+							+											3602	•cDC1: *KIT*, *CCR7*, *BATF3*, *FLT3*, *ZBTB46*, *IRF8*, *BTLA*, *MYCL1*, *CLEC9A*. •other MNP: 17 genes encompassing *ABCC3*, *C5AR1*, *LYVE1*, *MERTK*, *MRC1* (CD206), *SIGLEC1* (CD169), *STAB1*. •CD8 T cells: 222 genes encompassing *CCL5*, *CD3D*, *CD3E*, *CD3G*, *CD3Z*, *FLT3LG*, *GZMK*, *ITK*, *KLRB1*, *KLRG1*, *KLRK1*, *LCK*, *TRA*, *TRB* (see Palmer C. et al., BMC Genomics, 2006).	65	TCGA
BRCA	+							+											845			
HNSC	+							+											303			
LUAD	+							+											355			
BRCA		+	+	NS				NS	+							NS	NS		1098	•cDC1: *CLEC9A*, *XCR1*, *CLNK* and *BATF3*. •cDC1-specific gene: *CLEC9A*. •cDC1-attracting chemokines: *XCL1*, *XCL2* and *CCL5*. •CD8 T cell: *CD8A*, *CD8B* and *CD3E*. •NK cell: *NCR1*, *NCR3*, *KLRB1*, *CD160*, *PRF1*. •Mononuclear phagocyte-specific gene: *CD68*. •Mono/Mac-specific gene: *CD14*.	55	TCGA
HNSC		+	+	+				+	+							NS	NS		528			
LUAD		+	+	NS				+	+							NS	NS		585			
SKCM		+	+	+				+	+							NS	NS		470			
BRCA		+		NS					+										3953			183
BRCA, TNBC		++		+					+										255			
Melanoma, metastatic		+ and (AM)[6]			NS (AM)[6]	NS (AM)[6]	NS (AM)[6]	NS (AM)[6]	+ and (AM)[6]	+ (AM)[6]		+							38	•cDC1: *KIT*, *CCR7*, *BATF3*, *FLT3*, *ZBTB46*, *IRF8*, *BTLA*, *MYCL1*. •NK cell: *GNLY*, *KLRC3*, *KLRD1*, *KLRF1*, *NCR1*. •DC maturation & migration to draining lymph node: *CCR7*.	62, 8	184
Melanoma									+		+								454	•DC local differentiation/ survival factor: *FLT3LG*. •NK cell: *GNLY*, *KLRC3*, *KLRD1*, *KLRF1*, *NCR1*, each tested independently.	62	TCGA
BRCA, Luminal	+	+			+	+	-												1043	The Luminal BRCA cDC1e cell UP signature (signature of DAPI⁻CD45⁺Lin⁻CD11c⁺HLA-DR⁺CD14⁻CD1c⁻ cells isolated from the tumor bed and shown to be enriched in cDC1) includes 88 genes, encompassing 6 genes (7%) known to be selectively expressed in cDC1 (*CLNK*, *CLEC9A*, *XCR1*, *GCSAML*, *ENPP3*, *KIT*) and one gene (1%) known to be expressed in NK and/or T cells (*GNLY*).	182	METABRIC
BRCA, TNBC	NS	+			NS	NS	-												259	The TNBC cDC1e cell UP signature includes 24 genes, encompasses 2 genes (8%) known to be selectively expressed in cDC1 (*SNX22* and *CLEC9A*) and 10 genes (42%) known to be selectively expressed in NK / T cells (*IL2RB*, *SH2D1B*, *LAX1*, *SKAP1*, *PRF1*, *GZMK*, *ITK*, *LCK*, *AFAP1L2*, *CLEC2D*).		
BRCA		+							+			+								•cDC1: *IRF8*, *BATF3*, *ZBTB46*, *CCR7*, *IL12A* and *IL12B* each tested independently in BRCA; *IRF8*, *BATF3* and *CD103* each tested independently in TNBC; *IRF8* only in gastric cancer and LUAD. •NK cell: *NCR1*, *NKG2D*, *CD56*, *IFNG*, each tested independently.	65	TCGA
TNBC		+																				
Gastric cancer		+																				
LUAD		+																				
BRCA								+ (AM)[7]					+ (AM)[7]	+ (AM)[7]	+ (AM)[7]				379	•CD8⁺ T cells: *CD8A*. •Cytotoxic effector immune cells: *GZMB*. •mature immunogenic DCs: *LAMP3*, *CXCL9*. •Immune-checkpoint receptor expressed on cDC1 and other cells: *HAVCR2* (encoding TIM3).	64	GSE20194, GSE20271
BRCA, Luminal A								NS					NS	NS				-	1933			183
BRCA, Luminal B								+					NS	+				NS	1149			
BRCA, Her2+								+					+	+				NS	251			
BRCA, basal								+					+	+				+	618			

[1]BRCA, breast cancer; HNSC, head and neck squamous cell carcinoma; LUAD, lung adenocarcinoma; SKCM, skin cutaneous melanoma; TNBC, triple negative breast cancer.

[2]Unless alternative methods (AM) are mentioned Kaplan-Meier plots for overall survival were computed, comparing 2 patient groups parsed based on gene expression values or transcriptomic signature scores, at median value, or as upper versus lower quartile, or at 66% stringency threshold. Positive (+) prognostic values are highlighted in green, negative (-) ones in red, non significant (NS) ones in gray, and not determined ones in white.

[3]The "cDC1/other MNP" signature score was computed as z-score of the signature Log_2 Ratio. Log_2 Ratio=Log2(mean expression value across cDC1 genes/mean expression value across other MPN genes).
Z-score Ratio=[Log_2 Ratio - mean(Log_2 Ratio across patients)]/standard deviation(Log_2 Ratio across patients).
The cell population signature used were computed from healthy mouse spleen immune cell type gene expression profiling datasets and mouse gene symbols converted into those of their human orthologs.

[4]cDC1e cells are cells sorted from the tumors as DAPI⁻CD45⁺Lin⁻CD11c⁺HLA-DR⁺CD14⁻CD1c⁻ and shown to be enriched for cDC1 based on the comparaison on the expression of hallmark cell type genes between this cell population and the other cell populations isolated from the same tumors (pDCs, cDC2 and Mono/Mac).
Micro-bulk RNA sequencing was performed on each of these cell populations from several patients suffering from Luminal BRCA or TNBC. UP and DOWN specific transcriptomic signatures were derived for each of these cell populations and used for the Kaplan-Meier plot analyses on another, independent, cohort of Breast Cancer patient, applying the cell population signatures derived from one type of cancer onto the whole tumor gene expression profiles of patients suffering from the same type of cancer (e.g. TNBC cDC1e cell signature applied on the TNBC dataset, and Luminal BRCA cDC1e cell signature applied on the Luminal BRCA dataset).

[5]Genes that were used in at least two independent studies are shown in bold blue font when used for the same cell type and in bold orange font when used for different cell types or purposes.

[6]An alternative method (AM) was used to assess the prognostic value of the infiltration of the tumor by different immune cell types. Statistical analyses were performed between responder versus non-responder patients for the percent of the different types of mononuclear phagocytes within HLA-DR⁺ cells or for the percent of other myeloid cell types or of lymphocyte types within CD45⁺ cells.

[7]An alternative method (AM) was used to assess the prognostic value of higher expression of candidate genes in tumors. Chi-square was used to compute the significance of differences between frequencies of pathologic complete response between two groups of patients parsed by median expression for the candidate gene.

FIGURE 4 | Synthesis of various studies aiming at evaluating the prognosis value of the tumor infiltration by different immune cell types based on the analysis of the whole tumor gene expression profiles.

tumor bed was confirmed by flow cytometry analyses, whereas no significant prognostic value was observed for many other cell types including cDC2, pDCs, Mono/Mac and most surprisingly CTLs (62) (**Figure 4**). Finally, for LUAD, single cell RNA sequencing and paired CyTOF analyses of tumors and their neighboring normal lung tissue showed that cDC1 were significantly reduced in tumors, contrasting to increased numbers of macrophages in an immunosuppressive state and of cDC2/MoDCs (185). This study further supports the previously proposed hypothesis that the balance between cDC1 vs. cells of the monocyte/macrophage/neutrophil lineages in the tumor leukocyte infiltrate strongly determines the degree of local immunosuppression (65, 93).

Limitations, Controversies, or Unknowns

All of the above studies suggest that, in a variety of human cancers, intra-tumoral cDC1 abundance correlates with a better clinical outcome. However, further studies are required to confirm these results, to extend these types of analyses to other types of cancer, and to deepen our understanding of the underlying mechanisms.

A first issue that clearly stands out in **Figure 4** is the lack of a consensus definition of the transcriptomic fingerprints used for each immune cell type across studies, not only for cDC1 but even for CTLs or NK cells. Indeed, there is relatively little overlap between the gene signatures used for the same cell types across studies (blue names in **Figure 4**). Several genes used in some of the cDC1 transcriptomic fingerprints are known to have a promiscuous expression across many cell types (55). *CCR7* and *ITGAE* (CD103) are expressed on all mature DC types and on T cell subsets. *BATF3* and *ZBTB46* are shared with cDC2, and *FLT3* with cDC2, pDCs and hematopoietic progenitors. *IRF8* is highly expressed in pDCs and certain types of monocytes or macrophages. *THBD* (CD141/BDCA3) can be expressed on cDC2, pDCs, MoDCs and non-immune cell types. One study undertook the "tour de force" of profiling by microbulk RNAseq all the distinct mononuclear phagocyte types that they could identify in, and isolate from, BRCA or TNBC, in order to generate the cell-type specific transcriptomic signatures the most relevant to the cancer types studied (182). However, in this study, the TNBC gene signature of the cell population enriched in cDC1 (cDC1e) (182) encompasses only 8% of genes known to be selectively expressed in cDC1 but 42% of genes known to be expressed in NK cells. This raises the question of the interpretation of the positive prognostic value of that signature. It might not only reflect the infiltration of cDC1 but also that of NK cells, in consistency with other analyses in an independent study (55). Indeed, depending on individual samples, the cDC1e population encompassed 50–95% of other cells than cDC1. Using CD16 and CD56 for excluding NK cells from cDC1e cells might have been insufficient, since the strongly activated human NK cells expressing the highest levels of *XCL1* and *XCL2* express neither of these cell surface markers (55). More generally, it is likely that the much higher infiltration of TNBC by lymphocytes, as compared to luminal BRCA, led to major differences in the cell types other than cDC1 that were included in the cDC1e cell population between these two types of cancers. This could confound interpretation of the results of the enrichment analysis of these signatures.

There is a need to define better transcriptomic signatures for human immune cell types, allowing to more rigorously computationally deconvolute the extent of their infiltration in tumors and its eventual correlation with the clinical outcome. One strategy to achieve this aim is to select genes which show high selective expression in the targeted immune cell type across tissues and activation conditions, as well as between human and mouse (14, 45, 153). An alternative strategy could be to perform single cell RNA sequencing from tumor samples, in order to define the transcriptomic signatures specific to various combinations of relevant immune cell types and activation states in the most unbiased way. This strategy would also alleviate the potential confounding effect of cross-contamination between populations as can occur with microbulk gene expression profiling studies (11, 182). Moreover, it will generate transcriptomic signatures specific to the combination of the cell types and of the cancer studied. Indeed, it has been reported that using gene signatures derived from another tissue does not always work adequately to computationally deconvolute the immune cell type composition of tumors, due to differential imprinting of cells in distinct local microenvironments (181, 182).

A second issue is the necessity to include signatures of various types of immune cells, to ensure that the better prognostic value observed in the patients whose tumors harbor higher levels of the genes specific to the candidate immune cell type is not merely a reflect of a higher overall leukocyte infiltration. Indeed, the goal is not just to compare globally "Hot" or "Warm" vs. "Cold" tumors. Rather, it is to pinpoint which immune cell types specifically promote tumor control, or on the contrary contribute to local immunosuppression, in order to identify how to best manipulate the tumor infiltrate, for the benefits of cancer patients, through combined immunotherapies. Thus, the cell types considered to be functionally and/or developmentally the most closely related to the candidate one should be included, for example cDC2 or MoDCs for cDC1, NK cells and $\gamma\delta$ T cells for $\alpha\beta$ T cells. In addition, one should also include cell types expected to have no, or opposite, impact on tumor growth, for example neutrophils, macrophages and regulatory T cells which are considered as promoting immunosuppression.

A third issue is to deepen our understanding of when, where and how cDC1 promote tumor control. In several studies, the inferred higher cDC1 infiltration in tumors was correlated with higher inferred infiltrations of CTLs or NK cells, and with higher expression of *FLT3L, XCL1, XCL2, CCL4, CCL5, LAMP3, CCR7, CXCL9, CXCL10,* and *CXCL11* (**Figure 4**) (55, 57, 62, 64, 80, 93). These observations need further independent confirmation through the analysis of other cohorts of patients, and by using complementary methodologies including immunohistochemistry, CyTOF or single cell RNA sequencing to measure the correlation between cDC1 infiltration into the tumors and the status of antitumor

TABLE 6 | Completed clinical trials targeting cDC1.

Study start	Brief title	Condition	NCT identifier	Intervention	Phase	Results	References
2006	Peritumoral injection of CpG B with or without GM-CSF for treating patients with stage II Melanoma	Stage II melanoma, planned to undergo sentinel lymph node procedure	Not applicable	Preoperative local injection of either: • GM-CSF + CpG B • CpG B • saline around primary tumor excision site	II	Combined CpG/GM-CSF administration selectively increased cDC1 frequencies and cross-presenting capacity in SLN. cDC1 matured locally upon instruction by GM-CSF and pDCs type I IFN. CpG induced Th1 skewing and increased NK cell and antitumor CTL frequencies in SLN. Higher IL-10 production and Treg activity in SLN. Decreased metastasis in SLN from patients who received CpG.	(186, 187)
2009	A study of CDX-1401 (DEC205/NY-ESO-1) in patients with malignancies known to express NY-ESO-1	Advanced malignancies refractory to available therapies	NCT00948961	CDX-1401 + Resiquimod ± Poly(IC:LC)	I/II	Induction of humoral and cellular immunity to NY-ESO-1. Disease stabilization in 13 of 45 patients. Tumor regression in 2 patients. Objective tumor regression in 6 of 8 patients who received ICB after CDX-1401.	(185)
2014	CDX-1401 (DEC205/NY-ESO-1) and Poly(IC:LC) vaccine therapy with or without CDX-301 in treating patients with stage IIB–IV melanoma	Resected melanoma	NCT02129075	CDX-1401 + Poly(IC:LC) ± rhuFLT3-L (CDX-301) pre-treatment	II	Higher tumor-specific immune responses observed in subjects who received FLT3-L	(188, 189)

SLN, Sentinel lymph nodes.

NK and CTL responses. In any case, these studies support our proposed model of a critical positive cross talk between cDC1, cytotoxic lymphocytes and CD4$^+$ T cells for promoting effective antitumor immunity (**Figure 2**). Finally, it would be of utmost interest to extend to cohorts of patients benefiting from various types of immunotherapies these analyses aiming at deconvoluting the gene expression profiles of whole tumor tissue into immune cell type composition. This should help determining whether the clinical response can be predicted from cDC1 infiltration in the lesions, and to adapt the treatments accordingly for example by combining to ICB the use of drugs promoting cDC1 recruitment and activation into the tumors of patients when this process is defective (**Figure 3**).

Efficacy of Immunotherapeutic Protocols That May Preferentially Target/Harness Human cDC1

A few clinical trials have already been conducted using treatment protocols that have been proposed to preferentially target/harness human cDC1 (**Table 6**) (186, 187, 190). They gave encouraging results, which further supports the rationale of specifically targeting human cDC1 for the design of novel combined immunotherapies against cancer (189).

WHAT TOOLS ARE AVAILABLE TO STUDY AND MANIPULATE HUMAN cDC1 FOR THE BENEFITS OF CANCER PATIENTS?

Building on the conservation of cDC1 molecular makeup and functions between mouse and human, similar tools have been generated in both species to specifically target these cells for immunotherapy against cancer. This should accelerate translation from mouse preclinical studies to human clinical trials. Hence, most of the tools and approaches that have been detailed in the section on mouse experimental models (**Figure 3** and **Tables 3**, **4**) could be implemented in humans, as briefly summarized below.

Generation and Study of Novel *in vitro* Models of Human DC Types

To overcome the roadblock of the rarity of human cDC1 and of their fragility upon *ex vivo* isolation, we and others recently developed optimized *in vitro* culture systems to generate high numbers of cDC1, cDC2 and pDCs from CD34$^+$ hematopoietic progenitors (15, 147, 148). These novel *in vitro* models will allow rigorous comparison of the functions of the different human DC types, dissection of their molecular regulation, and better understanding of their cross talk. Further adaptations of these protocols are warranted to derive *in vitro* autologous cDC1 from the circulating $CD34^+$ cells of patients, load them with Ag and mature them, under conditions compatible for clinical use in vaccination or immunotherapy. It should be noted that encouraging results have been obtained with clinical trials of autologous ACT of *ex vivo* loaded and matured pDCs and cDC2 in melanoma patients, which seem superior to MoDCs to prime or boost endogenous CTL responses against the tumor. This emphasizes that, as in mice, cDC1 are not the only DC type that could be successfully harnessed for combined immunotherapy in cancer patients (6, 7, 191, 192).

Means to Specifically Deliver Ag and Maturation Signals to Human cDC1

Considering their conserved specific expression pattern on mouse and human cDC1, and the very encouraging results obtained in mouse preclinical models, the CLEC9A and XCR1 receptors are the best candidates for Ag, or Ag+adjuvant cargo, delivery to human cDC1, using recombinant ligands (193, 194) or monoclonal antibodies. A combination of TLR3- and TLR8-specific agonists is desirable to promote an immunogenic maturation associated with the production of both IL-12 and IFN-β/λ (**Table 6**) (195). Targeting delivery of IFN-I activity to cDC1 is another very promising adjuvant based on the proof-of-principle published in mice (**Tables 3, 5**). Additional means could be envisioned to favor the cross-talk between cDC1 and NK or NK T cells (196), e.g., use of NK cell immune checkpoint blockers (101–105) or targeted delivery to cDC1 of activating antigenic ligands for NK T cells (120).

Means to Promote cDC1 Differentiation, Survival and Local Recruitment in the Tumor Bed

Systemic injection of FLT3-L could promote cDC1 differentiation and survival (79). Local delivery of XCL1 could promote their recruitment in the tumor bed. In patients responding to checkpoint blockade inhibitors, these functions might be achieved upon local NK and CTL activation for FLT3-L, XCL1, and CCL4/5 production (55).

Blockade of cDC1 Checkpoint Inhibitors

A systematic analysis of immune factor checkpoint expression on human DC types is ongoing in order to investigate which ones could be reasonable candidates as components of combined immunotherapies targeting both CTLs and DCs (197).

CONCLUDING REMARKS

Lately, cDC1 have been in the spotlight of many studies investigating in mice the immune mechanisms driving tumor rejection, spontaneously or upon immunotherapy. All these studies converge toward a hub role of cDC1 in providing the initial priming, or in sustaining the activation, of antitumor T and NK cell responses. These advancements in our understanding of the role of cDC1 in antitumor immunity have been made possible by the recent blossoming of genetic tools allowing cDC1 manipulation. However, so far, most conclusions have been drawn from results obtained under experimental conditions that were not solely targeting cDC1, whether it was the use of genetically engineered mouse models or of mAb directing against cell surface markers. In fact, to be protective against immunosuppressive tumors such as those treated in the clinic, the immune response is necessarily complex and multi-parametric. More and more observations pinpoint that, in addition to cDC1, other DCs, type 1 $CD4^+$ T cells, and sometimes neutrophils are also central in promoting protective antitumor immunity, whereas Treg or type 17 $CD4^+$ T cells, monocytes and macrophages may rather play immunosuppressive roles. Further studies using models allowing conditional depletion of cDC1 will be critical in rigorously investigating whether cDC1 functions are instrumental at the time when immunotherapies are delivered. These studies will definitely settle the currently prevailing hypothesis that cDC1 functions, when specifically boosted, could provide great support to boost patient responses to currently used anticancer immunotherapies.

In human tumors, enrichment of genetic signatures described as cDC1-specific is associated with a good prognosis and a better clinical outcome in a several cancers, including luminal and TN breast cancer. These correlative analyses should be extended to additional types of cancer and to different patient treatment regimen. It is possible that the extent of cDC1 infiltration in the tumor fluctuates over time following the development or the suppression of an efficient antitumor immune response, as observed in mice during immunotherapy (86), and that cDC1 infiltration may not be protective against all types of cancer. Still, the perspective of exploiting cDC1 to improve current immunotherapies is extremely encouraging, and completion of cDC1-targeting vaccine clinical trials in human will surely help in gaining insight into their importance in cancer.

AUTHOR CONTRIBUTIONS

All authors wrote the manuscript, contributed to manuscript revision, read and approved the submitted version.

FUNDING

This work was supported by grants from the European Research Council under the European Community's Seventh Framework Program (FP7/2007–2013 grant agreement number 281225 to MD), from the Agence Nationale de la Recherche (ANR; XCR1-DirectingCells to KC), from the Fondation pour la Recherche Médicale (label Equipe FRM 2011, project number DEQ20110421284 to MD), from the Fondation ARC pour la recherche sur le cancer (to KC) and from the Institut National du Cancer (INCa PLBIO 2018-152). This work also benefited from institutional funding from CNRS and INSERM. J-CC was supported by doctoral fellowship from La Ligue Nationale Contre le Cancer. RM was supported by doctoral fellowships from the Biotrail Ph.D. program (Fondation A*MIDEX) and from Fondation ARC pour la recherche sur le cancer.

ACKNOWLEDGMENTS

Figures 1–3 have been created with BioRender (https://biorender.io/) under academic license.

REFERENCES

1. Quezada SA, Peggs KS, Simpson TR, Allison JP. Shifting the equilibrium in cancer immunoediting: from tumor tolerance to eradication. *Immunol Rev.* (2011) 241:104–18. doi: 10.1111/j.1600-065X.2011.01007.x
2. Schreiber RD, Old LJ, Smyth MJ. Cancer immunoediting: integrating immunity's roles in cancer suppression and promotion. *Science* (2011) 331:1565–70. doi: 10.1126/science.1203486
3. Zitvogel L, Ma Y, Raoult D, Kroemer G, Gajewski TF. The microbiome in cancer immunotherapy: Diagnostic tools and therapeutic strategies. *Science* (2018) 359:1366–70. doi: 10.1126/science.aar6918
4. Spranger S, Gajewski T. Rational combinations of immunotherapeutics that target discrete pathways. *J Immunother Cancer* (2013) 1:16. doi: 10.1186/2051-1426-1-16
5. Tacken PJ, de Vries IJM, Torensma R, Figdor CG. Dendritic-cell immunotherapy: from *ex vivo* loading to *in vivo* targeting. *Nat Rev Immunol.* (2007) 7:790–802. doi: 10.1038/nri2173
6. Wimmers F, Schreibelt G, Sköld AE, Figdor CG, De Vries IJM. Paradigm shift in dendritic cell-based immunotherapy: from *in vitro* generated monocyte-derived DCs to naturally circulating DC subsets. *Front Immunol.* (2014) 5:165. doi: 10.3389/fimmu.2014.00165
7. Bakdash G, Buschow SI, Gorris MAJ, Halilovic A, Hato SV, Sköld AE, et al. Expansion of a BDCA1+CD14+ myeloid cell population in melanoma patients may attenuate the efficacy of dendritic cell vaccines. *Cancer Res.* (2016) 76:4332–46. doi: 10.1158/0008-5472.CAN-15-1695
8. Garg AD, Coulie PG, Van den Eynde BJ, Agostinis P. Integrating next-generation dendritic cell vaccines into the current cancer immunotherapy landscape. *Trends Immunol.* (2017) 38:577–93. doi: 10.1016/j.it.2017.05.006
9. Guilliams M, Henri S, Tamoutounour S, Ardouin L, Schwartz-Cornil I, Dalod M, et al. From skin dendritic cells to a simplified classification of human and mouse dendritic cell subsets. *Eur J Immunol.* (2010) 40:2089–94. doi: 10.1002/eji.201040498
10. Guilliams M, Ginhoux F, Jakubzick C, Naik SH, Onai N, Schraml BU, et al. Dendritic cells, monocytes and macrophages: a unified nomenclature based on ontogeny. *Nat Rev Immunol.* (2014) 14:571–8. doi: 10.1038/nri3712
11. Vu Manh T-P, Bertho N, Hosmalin A, Schwartz-Cornil I, Dalod M. Investigating evolutionary conservation of dendritic cell subset identity and functions. *Front Immunol.* (2015) 6:260. doi: 10.3389/fimmu.2015.00260
12. Schlitzer A, Sivakamasundari V, Chen J, Sumatoh HRB, Schreuder J, Lum J, et al. Identification of cDC1- and cDC2-committed DC progenitors reveals early lineage priming at the common DC progenitor stage in the bone marrow. *Nat Immunol.* (2015) 16:718–28. doi: 10.1038/ni.3200
13. See P, Dutertre C-A, Chen J, Günther P, McGovern N, Irac SE, et al. Mapping the human DC lineage through the integration of high-dimensional techniques. *Science* (2017) 356:eaag3009. doi: 10.1126/science.aag3009
14. Robbins SH, Walzer T, Dembélé D, Thibault C, Defays A, Bessou G, et al. Novel insights into the relationships between dendritic cell subsets in human and mouse revealed by genome-wide expression profiling. *Genome Biol.* (2008) 9:R17. doi: 10.1186/gb-2008-9-1-r17
15. Balan S, Ollion V, Colletti N, Chelbi R, Montanana-Sanchis F, Liu H, et al. Human XCR1+ dendritic cells derived *in vitro* from CD34+ progenitors closely resemble blood dendritic cells, including their adjuvant responsiveness, contrary to monocyte-derived dendritic cells. *J Immunol.* (2014) 193:1622–35. doi: 10.4049/jimmunol.1401243
16. Alcántara-Hernández M, Leylek R, Wagar LE, Engleman EG, Keler T, Marinkovich MP, et al. High-Dimensional phenotypic mapping of human dendritic cells reveals interindividual variation and tissue specialization. *Immunity* (2017) 47:1037–50.e6. doi: 10.1016/j.immuni.2017.11.001
17. Fries A, Dalod M. "Dendritic Cells in Viral Infection," in *Encyclopedia of Immunobiology*, ed M. J. H. Ratcliffe (Oxford: Academic Press), 207–221.
18. van Blijswijk J, Schraml BU, Reis e Sousa C. Advantages and limitations of mouse models to deplete dendritic cells. *Eur J Immunol.* (2013) 43:22–6. doi: 10.1002/eji.201243022
19. Durai V, Murphy KM. Functions of murine dendritic cells. *Immunity* (2016) 45:719–36. doi: 10.1016/j.immuni.2016.10.010
20. Jung S, Unutmaz D, Wong P, Sano G-I, De los Santos K, Sparwasser T, et al. *In vivo* depletion of CD11c+ dendritic cells abrogates priming of CD8$^+$ T cells by exogenous cell-associated antigens. *Immunity* (2002) 17:211–20. doi: 10.1016/S1074-7613(02)00365-5
21. Sapoznikov A, Fischer JAA, Zaft T, Krauthgamer R, Dzionek A, Jung S. Organ-dependent *in vivo* priming of naive CD4+, but not CD8$^+$, T cells by plasmacytoid dendritic cells. *J Exp Med.* (2007) 204:1923–33. doi: 10.1084/jem.20062373
22. Probst HC, Tschannen K, Odermatt B, Schwendener R, Zinkernagel RM, Van Den Broek M. Histological analysis of CD11c-DTR/GFP mice after *in vivo* depletion of dendritic cells. *Clin Exp Immunol.* (2005) 141:398–404. doi: 10.1111/j.1365-2249.2005.02868.x
23. van Rijt LS, Jung S, Kleinjan A, Vos N, Willart M, Duez C, et al. *In vivo* depletion of lung CD11c+ dendritic cells during allergen challenge abrogates the characteristic features of asthma. *J Exp Med.* (2005) 201:981–91. doi: 10.1084/jem.20042311
24. Vallon-Eberhard A, Landsman L, Yogev N, Verrier B, Jung S. Transepithelial pathogen uptake into the small intestinal lamina propria. *J Immunol.* (2006) 176:2465–9. doi: 10.4049/jimmunol.176.4.2465
25. Huleatt JW, Lefrançois L. Antigen-driven induction of CD11c on intestinal intraepithelial lymphocytes and CD8$^+$ T cells *in vivo*. *J Immunol.* (1995) 154:5684–93.
26. Laouar Y, Sutterwala FS, Gorelik L, Flavell RA. Transforming growth factor-beta controls T helper type 1 cell development through regulation of natural killer cell interferon-gamma. *Nat Immunol.* (2005) 6:600–7. doi: 10.1038/ni1197
27. Hebel K, Griewank K, Inamine A, Chang H-D, Müller-Hilke B, Fillatreau S, Manz RA, Radbruch A, Jung S. Plasma cell differentiation in T-independent type 2 immune responses is independent of CD11c(high) dendritic cells. *Eur J Immunol.* (2006) 36:2912–9. doi: 10.1002/eji.200636356
28. Hochweller K, Striegler J, Hämmerling GJ, Garbi N. A novel CD11c.DTR transgenic mouse for depletion of dendritic cells reveals their requirement for homeostatic proliferation of natural killer cells. *Eur J Immunol.* (2008) 38:2776–83. doi: 10.1002/eji.200838659
29. Fukaya T, Murakami R, Takagi H, Sato K, Sato Y, Otsuka H, et al. Conditional ablation of CD205+ conventional dendritic cells impacts the regulation of T-cell immunity and homeostasis *in vivo*. *Proc Natl Acad Sci USA.* (2012) 109:11288–93. doi: 10.1073/pnas.1202208109
30. Laoui D, Keirsse J, Morias Y, Van Overmeire E, Geeraerts X, Elkrim Y, et al. The tumour microenvironment harbours ontogenically distinct dendritic cell populations with opposing effects on tumour immunity. *Nat Commun.* (2016) 7:13720. doi: 10.1038/ncomms13720
31. Fukaya T, Takagi H, Uto T, Arimura K, Sato K. Analysis of DC Functions Using CD205-DTR Knock-In Mice. *Methods Mol Biol.* (2016) 1423:291–308. doi: 10.1007/978-1-4939-3606-9_21
32. Satpathy AT, Kc W, Albring JC, Edelson BT, Kretzer NM, Bhattacharya D, et al. Zbtb46 expression distinguishes classical dendritic cells and their committed progenitors from other immune lineages. *J Exp Med.* (2012) 209:1135–52. doi: 10.1084/jem.20120030
33. Meredith MM, Liu K, Darrasse-Jeze G, Kamphorst AO, Schreiber HA, Guermonprez P, et al. Expression of the zinc finger transcription factor zDC (Zbtb46, Btbd4) defines the classical dendritic cell lineage. *J Exp Med.* (2012) 209:1153–65. doi: 10.1084/jem.20112675

34. Loschko J, Rieke GJ, Schreiber HA, Meredith MM, Yao K-H, Guermonprez P, et al. Inducible targeting of cDCs and their subsets *in vivo*. *J Immunol Methods* (2016) 434:32–8. doi: 10.1016/j.jim.2016.04.004
35. Hildner K, Edelson BT, Purtha WE, Diamond M, Matsushita H, Kohyama M, et al. Batf3 deficiency reveals a critical role for CD8alpha+ dendritic cells in cytotoxic T cell immunity. *Science* (2008) 322:1097–100. doi: 10.1126/science.1164206
36. Lee W, Kim HS, Hwang SS, Lee GR. The transcription factor Batf3 inhibits the differentiation of regulatory T cells in the periphery. *Exp Mol Med.* (2017) 49:e393. doi: 10.1038/emm.2017.157
37. Edelson BT, Bradstreet TR, Kc W, Hildner K, Herzog JW, Sim J, et al. Batf3-dependent CD11b(low/-) peripheral dendritic cells are GM-CSF-independent and are not required for Th cell priming after subcutaneous immunization. *PLoS ONE* (2011) 6:e25660. doi: 10.1371/journal.pone.0025660
38. Tussiwand R, Lee W-L, Murphy TL, Mashayekhi M, Kc W, Albring JC, et al. Compensatory dendritic cell development mediated by BATF-IRF interactions. *Nature* (2012) 490:502–7. doi: 10.1038/nature11531
39. Grajales-Reyes GE, Iwata A, Albring J, Wu X, Tussiwand R, Kc W, Kretzer NM, et al. Batf3 maintains autoactivation of Irf8 for commitment of a CD8α(+) conventional DC clonogenic progenitor. *Nat Immunol.* (2015) 16:708–17. doi: 10.1038/ni.3197
40. Iacobelli M, Wachsman W, McGuire KL. Repression of IL-2 promoter activity by the novel basic leucine zipper p21SNFT protein. *J Immunol.* (2000) 165:860–8. doi: 10.4049/jimmunol.165.2.860
41. Piva L, Tetlak P, Claser C, Karjalainen K, Renia L, Ruedl C. Cutting edge: Clec9A+ dendritic cells mediate the development of experimental cerebral malaria. *J Immunol.* (2012) 189:1128–32. doi: 10.4049/jimmunol.1201171
42. Mattiuz R, Wohn C, Ghilas S, Ambrosini M, Alexandre YO, Sanchez C, et al. Novel Cre-expressing mouse strains permitting to selectively track and edit type 1 conventional dendritic cells facilitate disentangling their complexity *in vivo*. *Front Immunol.* (2018) 9:2805 doi: 10.3389/fimmu.2018.02805
43. Alexandre YO, Ghilas S, Sanchez C, Le Bon A, Crozat K, Dalod M. XCR1$^+$ dendritic cells promote memory CD8$^+$ T cell recall upon secondary infections with *Listeria monocytogenes* or certain viruses. *J Exper Med.* (2016) 213:75–92. doi: 10.1084/jem.20142350
44. Yamazaki C, Sugiyama M, Ohta T, Hemmi H, Hamada E, Sasaki I, et al. Critical roles of a dendritic cell subset expressing a chemokine receptor, XCR1. *J Immunol.* (2013) 190:6071–82. doi: 10.4049/jimmunol.1202798
45. Crozat K, Guiton R, Contreras V, Feuillet V, Dutertre C-A, Ventre E, et al. The XC chemokine receptor 1 is a conserved selective marker of mammalian cells homologous to mouse CD8alpha+ dendritic cells. *J Exp Med.* (2010) 207:1283–92. doi: 10.1084/jem.20100223
46. Ohta T, Sugiyama M, Hemmi H, Yamazaki C, Okura S, Sasaki I, et al. Crucial roles of XCR1-expressing dendritic cells and the XCR1-XCL1 chemokine axis in intestinal immune homeostasis. *Sci Reports* (2016) 6:23505. doi: 10.1038/srep23505
47. Schraml BU, van Blijswijk J, Zelenay S, Whitney PG, Filby A, Acton SE, et al. Genetic tracing via DNGR-1 expression history defines dendritic cells as a hematopoietic lineage. *Cell* (2013) 154:843–58. doi: 10.1016/j.cell.2013.07.014
48. Hanahan D, Weinberg RA. Hallmarks of cancer: the next generation. *Cell* (2011) 144:646–74. doi: 10.1016/j.cell.2011.02.013
49. Dunn GP, Old LJ, Schreiber RD. The three Es of cancer immunoediting. *Annu Rev Immunol.* (2004) 22:329–60. doi: 10.1146/annurev.immunol.22.012703.104803
50. Vesely MD, Kershaw MH, Schreiber RD, Smyth MJ. Natural innate and adaptive immunity to cancer. *Annu Rev Immunol.* (2011) 29:235–71. doi: 10.1146/annurev-immunol-031210-101324
51. Diamond MS, Kinder M, Matsushita H, Mashayekhi M, Dunn GP, Archambault JM, et al. Type I interferon is selectively required by dendritic cells for immune rejection of tumors. *J Exp Med.* (2011) 208:1989–2003. doi: 10.1084/jem.20101158
52. Theisen DJ, Davidson JT, Briseño CG, Gargaro M, Lauron EJ, Wang Q, et al. WDFY4 is required for cross-presentation in response to viral and tumor antigens. *Science* (2018) 362:694–9. doi: 10.1126/science.aat5030
53. Theisen DJ, Ferris ST, Briseño CG, Kretzer N, Iwata A, Murphy KM, et al. BATF3-dependent genes control tumor rejection induced by dendritic cells independently of cross-presentation. *Cancer Immunol Res.* (2018). 7:29–39. doi: 10.1158/2326-6066.CIR-18-0138
54. Fuertes MB, Kacha AK, Kline J, Woo SR, Kranz DM, Murphy KM, et al. Host type I IFN signals are required for antitumor CD8$^+$ T cell responses through CD8{alpha}+ dendritic cells. *J Exper Med.* (2011) 208:2005–16. doi: 10.1084/jem.20101159
55. Bottcher JP, Bonavita E, Chakravarty P, Blees H, Cabeza-Cabrerizo M, Sammicheli S, Rogers NC, Sahai E, Zelenay S, Reis ESC. NK Cells Stimulate Recruitment of cDC1 into the Tumor Microenvironment Promoting Cancer Immune Control. *Cell* (2018) 172:1022-1037 e14. doi: 10.1016/j.cell.2018.01.004
56. Zelenay S, van der Veen AG, Bottcher JP, Snelgrove KJ, Rogers N, Acton SE, Chakravarty P, Girotti MR, Marais R, Quezada SA, et al. Cyclooxygenase-dependent tumor growth through evasion of immunity. *Cell* (2015) 162:1257–70. doi: 10.1016/j.cell.2015.08.015
57. Spranger S, Dai D, Horton B, Gajewski TF. Tumor-Residing Batf3 Dendritic Cells Are Required for Effector T Cell Trafficking and Adoptive T Cell Therapy. *Cancer cell* (2017) 31:711-723.e4. doi: 10.1016/j.ccell.2017.04.003
58. Iraolagoitia XLR, Spallanzani RG, Torres NI, Araya RE, Ziblat A, Domaica CI, et al. NK cells restrain spontaneous antitumor CD8$^+$ T cell priming through PD-1/PD-L1 interactions with dendritic cells. *J Immunol.* (2016) 197:953–961. doi: 10.4049/jimmunol.1502291
59. Steinman RM, Idoyaga J. Features of the dendritic cell lineage. *Immunol Rev.* (2010) 234:5–17. doi: 10.1111/j.0105-2896.2009.00888.x
60. Sanchez-Paulete AR, Teijeira A, Cueto FJ, Garasa S, Perez-Gracia JL, Sanchez-Arraez A, et al. Antigen cross-presentation and T-cell cross-priming in cancer immunology and immunotherapy. *Ann Oncol.* (2017) 28:xii44–55. doi: 10.1093/annonc/mdx237
61. Dorner BG, Dorner MB, Zhou X, Opitz C, Mora A, Guttler S, Hutloff A, et al. Selective expression of the chemokine receptor XCR1 on cross-presenting dendritic cells determines cooperation with CD8$^+$ T cells. *Immunity* (2009) 31:823–33. doi: 10.1016/j.immuni.2009.08.027
62. Barry KC, Hsu J, Broz ML, Cueto FJ, Binnewies M, Combes AJ, Nelson AE, et al. A natural killer–dendritic cell axis defines checkpoint therapy–responsive tumor microenvironments. *Nat Med.* (2018) 24:1178–91. doi: 10.1038/s41591-018-0085-8
63. Bachem A, Güttler S, Hartung E, Ebstein F, Schaefer M, Tannert A, et al. Superior antigen cross-presentation and XCR1 expression define human CD11c+CD141+ cells as homologues of mouse CD8$^+$ dendritic cells. *J Exp Med.* (2010) 207:1273–81. doi: 10.1084/jem.20100348
64. de Mingo Pulido A, Gardner A, Hiebler S, Soliman H, Rugo HS, Krummel MF, et al. TIM-3 Regulates CD103(+) Dendritic cell function and response to chemotherapy in breast cancer. *Cancer cell* (2018) 33:60–74.e6. doi: 10.1016/j.ccell.2017.11.019
65. Broz ML, Binnewies M, Boldajipour B, Nelson AE, Pollack JL, Erle DJ, et al. Dissecting the tumor myeloid compartment reveals rare activating antigen-presenting cells critical for T cell immunity. *Cancer Cell* (2014) 26:638–52. doi: 10.1016/j.ccell.2014.09.007
66. Mittal D, Vijayan D, Putz EM, Aguilera AR, Markey KA, Straube J, et al. Interleukin-12 from CD103(+) Batf3-dependent dendritic cells required for NK-Cell suppression of metastasis. *Cancer Immunol Res.* (2017) 5:1098–108. doi: 10.1158/2326-6066.CIR-17-0341
67. Ruffell B, Chang-Strachan D, Chan V, Rosenbusch A, Ho CM, Pryer N, et al. Macrophage IL-10 blocks CD8$^+$ T cell-dependent responses to chemotherapy by suppressing IL-12 expression in intratumoral dendritic cells. *Cancer Cell* (2014) 26:623–37. doi: 10.1016/j.ccell.2014.09.006
68. Greyer M, Whitney PG, Stock AT, Davey GM, Tebartz C, Bachem A, et al. T cell help amplifies innate signals in CD8(+) DCs for optimal CD8(+) T cell priming. *Cell Rep.* (2016) 14:586–97. doi: 10.1016/j.celrep.2015.12.058
69. Beavis PA, Henderson MA, Giuffrida L, Davenport AJ, Petley EV, House IG, et al. Dual PD-1 and CTLA-4 checkpoint blockade promotes antitumor immune responses through CD4$^+$ Foxp3$^-$ cell-mediated modulation of CD103 $^+$ dendritic cells. *Cancer Immunol Res.* (2018) 6:1069–81. doi: 10.1158/2326-6066.CIR-18-0291
70. Draheim M, Wlodarczyk MF, Crozat K, Saliou J-M, Alayi TD, Tomavo S, et al. Profiling MHC II immunopeptidome of blood-stage malaria reveals that cDC1 control the functionality of parasite-specific CD4 T cells. *EMBO Mol Med.* (2017) 9:1605–21. doi: 10.15252/emmm.201708123

71. Igyártó BZ, Haley K, Ortner D, Bobr A, Gerami-Nejad M, Edelson BT, et al. Skin-resident murine dendritic cell subsets promote distinct and opposing antigen-specific T helper cell responses. *Immunity* (2011) 35:260–72. doi: 10.1016/j.immuni.2011.06.005
72. Martínez-López M, Iborra S, Conde-Garrosa R, Sancho D. Batf3-dependent CD103+ dendritic cells are major producers of IL-12 that drive local Th1 immunity against Leishmania major infection in mice. *Eur J Immunol.* (2015) 45:119–29. doi: 10.1002/eji.201444651
73. Eickhoff S, Brewitz A, Gerner MY, Klauschen F, Komander K, Hemmi H, et al. Robust Anti-viral Immunity Requires Multiple Distinct T Cell-Dendritic Cell Interactions. *Cell* (2015) 162:1322–37. doi: 10.1016/j.cell.2015.08.004
74. Hor JL, Whitney PG, Zaid A, Brooks AG, Heath WR, Mueller SN. Spatiotemporally distinct interactions with dendritic cell subsets facilitates CD4+ and $CD8^+$ T cell activation to localized viral infection. *Immunity* (2015) 43:554–65. doi: 10.1016/j.immuni.2015.07.020
75. Ardouin L, Luche H, Chelbi R, Carpentier S, Shawket A, Montanana Sanchis F, et al. Broad and largely concordant molecular changes characterize tolerogenic and immunogenic dendritic cell maturation in thymus and periphery. *Immunity* (2016) 45:305–18. doi: 10.1016/j.immuni.2016.07.019
76. Dalod M, Chelbi R, Malissen B, Lawrence T. Dendritic cell maturation: functional specialization through signaling specificity and transcriptional programming. *EMBO J.* (2014) 33:1104–116. doi: 10.1002/embj.201 488027
77. Brewitz A, Eickhoff S, Dähling S, Quast T, Bedoui S, Kroczek RA, et al. $CD8^+$ T Cells Orchestrate pDC-XCR1+ dendritic cell spatial and functional cooperativity to optimize priming. *Immunity* (2017) 46:205–19. doi: 10.1016/j.immuni.2017.01.003
78. Enamorado M, Iborra S, Priego E, Cueto FJ, Quintana JA, Martinez-Cano S, et al. Enhanced anti-tumour immunity requires the interplay between resident and circulating memory CD8(+) T cells. *Nat Commun.* (2017) 8:16073. doi: 10.1038/ncomms16073
79. Salmon H, Idoyaga J, Rahman A, Leboeuf M, Remark R, Jordan S, et al. Expansion and activation of CD103(+) dendritic cell progenitors at the tumor site enhances tumor responses to therapeutic PD-L1 and BRAF inhibition. *Immunity* (2016) 44:924–38. doi: 10.1016/j.immuni.2016.03.012
80. Roberts EW, Broz ML, Binnewies M, Headley MB, Nelson AE, Wolf DM, et al. Critical role for CD103(+)/CD141(+) dendritic cells bearing CCR7 for tumor antigen trafficking and priming of T cell immunity in melanoma. *Cancer Cell* (2016) 30:324–36. doi: 10.1016/j.ccell.2016.06.003
81. Matloubian M, Lo CG, Cinamon G, Lesneski MJ, Xu Y, Brinkmann V, et al. Lymphocyte egress from thymus and peripheral lymphoid organs is dependent on S1P receptor 1. *Nature* (2004) 427:355–60. doi: 10.1038/nature02284
82. Thompson ED, Enriquez HL, Fu Y-X, Engelhard VH. Tumor masses support naive T cell infiltration, activation, and differentiation into effectors. *J Exper Med* (2010) 207:1791–804. doi: 10.1084/jem.20092454
83. Lan YY, De Creus A, Colvin BL, Abe M, Brinkmann V, Coates PTH, et al. The sphingosine-1-phosphate receptor agonist FTY720 modulates dendritic cell trafficking in vivo. *Am J Transp.* (2005) 5:2649–59. doi: 10.1111/j.1600-6143.2005.01085.x
84. Morris MA, Gibb DR, Picard F, Brinkmann V, Straume M, Ley K. Transient T cell accumulation in lymph nodes and sustained lymphopenia in mice treated with FTY720. *Eur J Immunol.* (2005) 35:3570–80. doi: 10.1002/eji.200526218
85. Dieu-Nosjean M-C, Giraldo NA, Kaplon H, Germain C, Fridman WH, Sautès-Fridman C. Tertiary lymphoid structures, drivers of the anti-tumor responses in human cancers. *Immunol Rev.* (2016) 271:260–75. doi: 10.1111/imr.12405
86. Spitzer MH, Carmi Y, Reticker-Flynn NE, Kwek SS, Madhireddy D, Martins MM, et al. Systemic immunity is required for effective cancer immunotherapy. *Cell* (2017) 168:487–502.e15. doi: 10.1016/j.cell.2016.12.022
87. Spranger S, Gajewski TF. Mechanisms of tumor cell–intrinsic immune evasion. *Ann Rev Cancer Biol.* (2018) 2:213–28. doi: 10.1146/annurev-cancerbio-030617-050606
88. Paulson KG, Voillet V, McAfee MS, Hunter DS, Wagener FD, Perdicchio M, et al. Acquired cancer resistance to combination immunotherapy from transcriptional loss of class I HLA. *Nat Commun.* (2018) 9:3868. doi: 10.1038/s41467-018-06300-3
89. Pauken KE, Wherry EJ. Overcoming T cell exhaustion in infection and cancer. *Trends Immunol.* (2015) 36:265–76. doi: 10.1016/j.it.2015.02.008
90. Zong J, Keskinov AA, Shurin GV, Shurin MR. Tumor-derived factors modulating dendritic cell function. *Cancer Immunol Immunother.* (2016) 65:821–33. doi: 10.1007/s00262-016-1820-y
91. Perry JSA, Lio C-WJ, Kau AL, Nutsch K, Yang Z, Gordon JI, et al. Distinct contributions of Aire and antigen-presenting-cell subsets to the generation of self-tolerance in the thymus. *Immunity* (2014) 41:414–26. doi: 10.1016/j.immuni.2014.08.007
92. Esterházy D, Loschko J, London M, Jove V, Oliveira TY, Mucida D. Classical dendritic cells are required for dietary antigen-mediated induction of peripheral T(reg) cells and tolerance. *Nat Immunol.* (2016) 17:545–55. doi: 10.1038/ni.3408
93. Spranger S, Bao R, Gajewski TF. Melanoma-intrinsic beta-catenin signalling prevents anti-tumour immunity. *Nature* (2015) 523:231–5. doi: 10.1038/nature14404
94. Cook SJ, Lee Q, Wong AC, Spann BC, Vincent JN, Wong JJ, et al. Differential chemokine receptor expression and usage by pre-cDC1 and pre-cDC2. *Immunol Cell Biol.* (2018) 96:1131–9 doi: 10.1111/imcb.12186
95. Fucikova J, Becht E, Iribarren K, Goc J, Remark R, Damotte D, et al. Calreticulin expression in human non-small cell lung cancers correlates with increased accumulation of antitumor immune cells and favorable prognosis. *Cancer Res.* (2016) 76:1746–56. doi: 10.1158/0008-5472.CAN-15-1142
96. Garg AD, Dudek AM, Ferreira GB, Verfaillie T, Vandenabeele P, Krysko DV, et al. ROS-induced autophagy in cancer cells assists in evasion from determinants of immunogenic cell death. *Autophagy* (2013) 9:1292–307. doi: 10.4161/auto.25399
97. Balogh KN, Templeton DJ, Cross JV. Macrophage Migration Inhibitory Factor protects cancer cells from immunogenic cell death and impairs anti-tumor immune responses. *PLoS ONE* (2018) 13:e0197702. doi: 10.1371/journal.pone.0197702
98. Meyer MA, Baer JM, Knolhoff BL, Nywening TM, Panni RZ, Su X, et al. Breast and pancreatic cancer interrupt IRF8-dependent dendritic cell development to overcome immune surveillance. *Nature Commun.* (2018) 9:1250. doi: 10.1038/s41467-018-03600-6
99. Veglia F, Tyurin VA, Mohammadyani D, Blasi M, Duperret EK, Donthireddy L, et al. Lipid bodies containing oxidatively truncated lipids block antigen cross-presentation by dendritic cells in cancer. *Nat Commun.* (2017) 8:2122. doi: 10.1038/s41467-017-02186-9
100. Kline DE, MacNabb BW, Chen X, Chan W-C, Fosco D, Kline J. CD8α+ dendritic cells dictate leukemia-specific $CD8^+$ T cell fates. *J Immunol.* (2018) 201:3759–69. doi: 10.4049/jimmunol.1801184
101. Hsu J, Hodgins JJ, Marathe M, Nicolai CJ, Bourgeois-Daigneault M-C, Trevino TN, et al. Contribution of NK cells to immunotherapy mediated by PD-1/PD-L1 blockade. *J Clin Invest.* (2018) 128:4654–68. doi: 10.1172/JCI99317
102. Zhang Q, Bi J, Zheng X, Chen Y, Wang H, Wu W, et al. Blockade of the checkpoint receptor TIGIT prevents NK cell exhaustion and elicits potent anti-tumor immunity. *Nat Immunol.* (2018) 19:723–32. doi: 10.1038/s41590-018-0132-0
103. Kohrt HE, Thielens A, Marabelle A, Sagiv-Barfi I, Sola C, Chanuc F, et al. Anti-KIR antibody enhancement of anti-lymphoma activity of natural killer cells as monotherapy and in combination with anti-CD20 antibodies. *Blood* (2014) 123:678–86. doi: 10.1182/blood-2013-08-519199
104. Sola C, André P, Lemmers C, Fuseri N, Bonnafous C, Bléry M, et al. Genetic and antibody-mediated reprogramming of natural killer cell missing-self recognition *in vivo*. *Proc Natl Acad Sci USA.* (2009) 106:12879–84. doi: 10.1073/pnas.0901653106
105. Chiossone L, Dumas P-Y, Vienne M, Vivier E. Natural killer cells and other innate lymphoid cells in cancer. *Nat Rev Immunol.* (2018) 18:671–88. doi: 10.1038/s41577-018-0061-z
106. Pardoll DM. The blockade of immune checkpoints in cancer immunotherapy. *Nat Rev Cancer* (2012) 12:252–64. doi: 10.1038/nrc3239
107. Farkona S, Diamandis EP, Blasutig IM. Cancer immunotherapy: the beginning of the end of cancer? *BMC Med.* (2016) 14:73. doi: 10.1186/s12916-016-0623-5

108. Larkin J, Chiarion-Sileni V, Gonzalez R, Grob JJ, Cowey CL, Lao CD, et al. Combined nivolumab and ipilimumab or monotherapy in untreated melanoma. *N Engl J Med.* (2015) 373:23–34. doi: 10.1056/NEJMoa1504030
109. Postow MA, Chesney J, Pavlick AC, Robert C, Grossmann K, McDermott D, et al. Nivolumab and Ipilimumab versus Ipilimumab in Untreated Melanoma. *N Engl J Med.* (2015) 372:2006–17. doi: 10.1056/NEJMoa1414428
110. Diao J, Gu H, Tang M, Zhao J, Cattral MS. Tumor dendritic cells (DCs) derived from precursors of conventional DCs are dispensable for intratumor CTL responses. *J Immunol* (2018) 201:1306–14. doi: 10.4049/jimmunol.1701514
111. Yu X, Guo C, Yi H, Qian J, Fisher PB, Subjeck JR, Wang XY. A multifunctional chimeric chaperone serves as a novel immune modulator inducing therapeutic antitumor immunity. *Cancer Res.* (2013) 73:2093–103. doi: 10.1158/0008-5472.can-12-1740
112. Yang X, Zhang X, Fu ML, Weichselbaum RR, Gajewski TF, Guo Y, et al. Targeting the tumor microenvironment with interferon-beta bridges innate and adaptive immune responses. *Cancer Cell* (2014) 25:37–48. doi: 10.1016/j.ccr.2013.12.004
113. Zhang Y, Chen G, Liu Z, Tian S, Zhang J, Carey CD, et al. Genetic vaccines to potentiate the effective CD103+ dendritic cell-mediated cross-priming of antitumor immunity. *J Immunol (Baltimore, Md: 1950)* (2015) 194:5937-47. doi: 10.4049/jimmunol.1500089
114. Tzeng A, Kauke MJ, Zhu EF, Moynihan KD, Opel CF, Yang NJ, et al. Temporally programmed CD8alpha(+) DC activation enhances combination cancer immunotherapy. *Cell Reports* (2016) 17:2503–11. doi: 10.1016/j.celrep.2016.11.020
115. Cauwels A, Van Lint S, Paul F, Garcin G, De Koker S, Van Parys A, et al. Delivering type I interferon to dendritic cells empowers tumor eradication and immune combination treatments. *Cancer Res.* (2018) 78:463–74. doi: 10.1158/0008-5472.CAN-17-1980
116. Gilfillan CB, Kuhn S, Baey C, Hyde EJ, Yang J, Ruedl C, et al. Clec9A^{+} dendritic cells are not essential for antitumor CD8^{+} T cell responses induced by Poly I:C immunotherapy. *J Immunol.* (2018) 200:2978–86. doi: 10.4049/jimmunol.1701593
117. Gubin MM, Zhang X, Schuster H, Caron E, Ward JP, Noguchi T, et al. Checkpoint blockade cancer immunotherapy targets tumour-specific mutant antigens. *Nature* (2014) 515:577–81. doi: 10.1038/nature13988
118. Sanchez-Paulete AR, Cueto FJ, Martinez-Lopez M, Labiano S, Morales-Kastresana A, Rodriguez-Ruiz ME, et al. Cancer immunotherapy with immunomodulatory Anti-CD137 and Anti-PD-1 monoclonal antibodies requires BATF3-dependent dendritic cells. *Cancer Disc.* (2016) 6:71–9. doi: 10.1158/2159-8290.cd-15-0510
119. Lehmann C, Heger L, Heidkamp G, Baranska A, Lühr J, Hoffmann A, et al. Direct delivery of antigens to dendritic cells via antibodies specific for endocytic receptors as a promising strategy for future therapies. *Vaccines* (2016) 4:8. doi: 10.3390/vaccines4020008
120. Ghinnagow R, Meester JD, Cruz LJ, Aspord C, Corgnac S, Macho-Fernandez E, et al. Co-delivery of the NKT agonist α-galactosylceramide and tumor antigens to cross-priming dendritic cells breaks tolerance to self-antigens and promotes antitumor responses. *OncoImmunology* (2017) 6:e1339855. doi: 10.1080/2162402X.2017.1339855
121. Macho-Fernandez E, Cruz LJ, Ghinnagow R, Fontaine J, Bialecki E, Frisch B, et al. Targeted delivery of α-Galactosylceramide to CD8α+ dendritic cells optimizes type I NKT cell–based antitumor responses. *J Immunol.* (2014) 193:961–9. doi: 10.4049/jimmunol.1303029
122. Filatenkov AA, Jacovetty EL, Fischer UB, Curtsinger JM, Mescher MF, Ingulli E. CD4 T cell-dependent conditioning of dendritic cells to produce IL-12 results in CD8-mediated graft rejection and avoidance of tolerance. *J Immunol.* (2005) 174:6909–17. doi: 10.4049/jimmunol.174.11.6909
123. Oh S, Perera LP, Terabe M, Ni L, Waldmann TA, Berzofsky JA. IL-15 as a mediator of CD4+ help for CD8^{+} T cell longevity and avoidance of TRAIL-mediated apoptosis. *Proc Natl Acad Sci USA.* (2008) 105:5201–6. doi: 10.1073/pnas.0801003105
124. Cao J, Jin Y, Li W, Zhang B, He Y, Liu H, et al. DNA vaccines targeting the encoded antigens to dendritic cells induce potent antitumor immunity in mice. *BMC Immunol.* (2013) 14:39. doi: 10.1186/1471-2172-14-39
125. Tenbusch M, Nchinda G, Storcksdieck genannt Bonsmann M, Temchura V, Überla K. Targeting the antigen encoded by adenoviral vectors to the DEC205 receptor modulates the cellular and humoral immune response. *Int Immunol.* (2013) 25:247–58. doi: 10.1093/intimm/dxs112
126. Ali OA, Verbeke C, Johnson C, Sands RW, Lewin SA, White D, et al. Identification of immune factors regulating antitumor immunity using polymeric vaccines with multiple adjuvants. *Cancer Res.* (2014) 74:1670–81. doi: 10.1158/0008-5472.can-13-0777
127. Zeng B, Middelberg AP, Gemiarto A, MacDonald K, Baxter AG, Talekar M, et al. Self-adjuvanting nanoemulsion targeting dendritic cell receptor Clec9A enables antigen-specific immunotherapy. *J Clin Invest* (2018) 128:1971–84. doi: 10.1172/JCI96791
128. Idoyaga J, Fiorese C, Zbytnuik L, Lubkin A, Miller J, Malissen B, et al. Specialized role of migratory dendritic cells in peripheral tolerance induction. *J Clin Investig.* (2013) 123:844–54. doi: 10.1172/JCI65260
129. Loschko J, Schlitzer A, Dudziak D, Drexler I, Sandholzer N, Bourquin C, et al. Antigen delivery to plasmacytoid dendritic cells via BST2 induces protective T cell-mediated immunity. *J Immunol.* (2011) 186:6718–25. doi: 10.4049/jimmunol.1004029
130. Neubert K, Lehmann CHK, Heger L, Baranska A, Staedtler AM, Buchholz VR, et al. Antigen delivery to CD11c+CD8- dendritic cells induces protective immune responses against experimental melanoma in mice *in vivo*. *J Immunol.* (2014) 192:5830–8. doi: 10.4049/jimmunol.1300975
131. Lou Y, Liu C, Kim GJ, Liu YJ, Hwu P, Wang G. Plasmacytoid dendritic cells synergize with myeloid dendritic cells in the induction of antigen-specific antitumor immune responses. *J Immunol.* (2007) 178:1534–41. doi: 10.4049/jimmunol.178.3.1534
132. Cohn L, Chatterjee B, Esselborn F, Smed-Sörensen A, Nakamura N, Chalouni C, et al. Antigen delivery to early endosomes eliminates the superiority of human blood BDCA3+ dendritic cells at cross presentation. *J Exp Med.* (2013) 210:1049–63. doi: 10.1084/jem.20121251
133. Sandoval F, Terme M, Nizard M, Badoual C, Bureau M-F, Freyburger L, et al. Mucosal imprinting of vaccine-induced CD8^{+} T cells is crucial to inhibit the growth of mucosal tumors. *Sci Transl Med.* (2013) 5:172ra20. doi: 10.1126/scitranslmed.3004888
134. Charalambous A, Oks M, Nchinda G, Yamazaki S, Steinman RM. Dendritic cell targeting of survivin protein in a xenogeneic form elicits strong CD4+ T cell immunity to mouse survivin. *J Immunol.* (2006) 177:8410–21. doi: 10.4049/jimmunol.177.12.8410
135. Kratky W, Reis e Sousa C, Oxenius A, Spörri R. Direct activation of antigen-presenting cells is required for CD8^{+} T-cell priming and tumor vaccination. *Proc Natl Acad Sci USA.* (2011) 108:17414–9. doi: 10.1073/pnas.1108945108
136. Yoshida S, Shime H, Takeda Y, Nam JM, Takashima K, Matsumoto M, et al. Toll-like receptor 3 signal augments radiation-induced tumor growth retardation in a murine model. *Cancer Sci.* (2018) 109:956–65. doi: 10.1111/cas.13543
137. Zhou J, Liu L, Yang T, Lu B. Prognostic and therapeutic value of CD103+ cells in renal cell carcinoma. *Exp Ther Med.* (2018) 15):4979–86. doi: 10.3892/etm.2018.6025
138. Ngiow SF, von Scheidt B, Akiba H, Yagita H, Teng MWL, Smyth MJ. Anti-TIM3 antibody promotes T cell IFN-γ-mediated antitumor immunity and suppresses established tumors. *Cancer Res.* (2011) 71:3540–51. doi: 10.1158/0008-5472.CAN-11-0096
139. Moynihan KD, Opel CF, Szeto GL, Tzeng A, Zhu EF, Engreitz JM, et al. Eradication of large established tumors in mice by combination immunotherapy that engages innate and adaptive immune responses. *Nat Med.* (2016) 22:1402–10. doi: 10.1038/nm.4200
140. Nierkens S, den Brok MH, Roelofsen T, Wagenaars JAL, Figdor CG, Ruers TJ, et al. Route of administration of the TLR9 agonist CpG critically determines the efficacy of cancer immunotherapy in mice. *PLoS ONE* (2009) 4:e8368. doi: 10.1371/journal.pone.0008368
141. Bald T, Landsberg J, Lopez-Ramos D, Renn M, Glodde N, Jansen P, et al. Immune cell–poor melanomas benefit from PD-1 blockade after targeted type I IFN activation. *Cancer Discov.* (2014) 4:674–87. doi: 10.1158/2159-8290.CD-13-0458
142. Corrales L, Glickman LH, McWhirter SM, Kanne DB, Sivick KE, Katibah GE, et al. Direct activation of STING in the tumor microenvironment leads

to potent and systemic tumor regression and immunity. *Cell Rep.* (2015) 11:1018–30. doi: 10.1016/j.celrep.2015.04.031

143. Cauwels A, Van Lint S, Garcin G, Bultinck J, Paul F, Gerlo S, et al. A safe and highly efficient tumor-targeted type I interferon immunotherapy depends on the tumor microenvironment. *Oncoimmunology* (2018) 7:e1398876. doi: 10.1080/2162402x.2017.1398876
144. Mittal D, Young A, Stannard K, Yong M, Teng MWL, Allard B, et al. Antimetastatic effects of blocking PD-1 and the adenosine A2A receptor. *Cancer Res.* (2014) 74:3652–8. doi: 10.1158/0008-5472.CAN-14-0957
145. Le Mercier I, Poujol D, Sanlaville A, Sisirak V, Gobert M, Durand I, et al. Tumor promotion by intratumoral plasmacytoid dendritic cells is reversed by TLR7 ligand treatment. *Cancer Res.* (2013) 73:4629–40. doi: 10.1158/0008-5472.CAN-12-3058
146. Georgoudaki A-M, Prokopec KE, Boura VF, Hellqvist E, Sohn S, Östling J, et al. Reprogramming tumor-associated macrophages by antibody targeting inhibits cancer progression and metastasis. *Cell Rep.* (2016) 15:2000–11. doi: 10.1016/j.celrep.2016.04.084
147. Balan S, Arnold-Schrauf C, Abbas A, Couespel N, Savoret J, Imperatore F, et al. Large-scale human dendritic cell differentiation revealing notch-dependent lineage bifurcation and heterogeneity. *Cell Reports* (2018) 24:1902–15.e6. doi: 10.1016/j.celrep.2018.07.033
148. Kirkling ME, Cytlak U, Lau CM, Lewis KL, Resteu A, Khodadadi-Jamayran A, et al. Notch signaling facilitates *in vitro* generation of cross-presenting classical dendritic cells. *Cell Rep.* (2018) 23:3658–72.e6. doi: 10.1016/j.celrep.2018.05.068
149. Crozat K, Guiton R, Guilliams M, Henri S, Baranek T, Schwartz-Cornil I, et al. Comparative genomics as a tool to reveal functional equivalences between human and mouse dendritic cell subsets. *Immunol Rev.* (2010) 234:177–98. doi: 10.1111/j.0105-2896.2009.00868.x
150. Haniffa M, Shin A, Bigley V, McGovern N, Teo P, See P, et al. Human tissues contain CD141hi cross-presenting dendritic cells with functional homology to mouse CD103+ nonlymphoid dendritic cells. *Immunity* (2012) 37:60–73. doi: 10.1016/j.immuni.2012.04.012
151. Schlitzer A, McGovern N, Teo P, Zelante T, Atarashi K, Low D, et al. IRF4 transcription factor-dependent CD11b+ dendritic cells in human and mouse control mucosal IL-17 cytokine responses. *Immunity* (2013) 38:970–83. doi: 10.1016/j.immuni.2013.04.011
152. Watchmaker PB, Lahl K, Lee M, Baumjohann D, Morton J, Kim SJ, et al. Comparative transcriptional and functional profiling defines conserved programs of intestinal DC differentiation in humans and mice. *Nat Immunol.* (2014) 15:98–108. doi: 10.1038/ni.2768
153. Carpentier S, Vu Manh T-P, Chelbi R, Henri S, Malissen B, Haniffa M, et al. Comparative genomics analysis of mononuclear phagocyte subsets confirms homology between lymphoid tissue-resident and dermal XCR1(+) DCs in mouse and human and distinguishes them from Langerhans cells. *J Immunol Methods* (2016) 432:35–49. doi: 10.1016/j.jim.2016.02.023
154. Bigley V, Maisuria S, Cytlak U, Jardine L, Care MA, Green K, et al. Biallelic interferon regulatory factor 8 mutation: a complex immunodeficiency syndrome with dendritic cell deficiency, monocytopenia, and immune dysregulation. *J Aller Clin Immunol.* (2018) 141:2234–48. doi: 10.1016/j.jaci.2017.08.044
155. Segura E, Durand M, Amigorena S. Similar antigen cross-presentation capacity and phagocytic functions in all freshly isolated human lymphoid organ-resident dendritic cells. *J Exp Med* (2013) 210:1035–47. doi: 10.1084/jem.20121103
156. Jongbloed SL, Kassianos AJ, McDonald KJ, Clark GJ, Ju X, Angel CE, et al. Human CD141+ (BDCA-3)+ dendritic cells (DCs) represent a unique myeloid DC subset that cross-presents necrotic cell antigens. *J Exp Med.* (2010) 207:1247–1260. doi: 10.1084/jem.20092140
157. Chiang M-C, Tullett KM, Lee YS, Idris A, Ding Y, McDonald KJ, et al. Differential uptake and cross-presentation of soluble and necrotic cell antigen by human DC subsets. *Eur J Immunol.* (2016) 46:329–39. doi: 10.1002/eji.201546023
158. Sancho D, Joffre OP, Keller AM, Rogers NC, Martinez D, Hernanz-Falcon P, Rosewell I, Reis e Sousa C. Identification of a dendritic cell receptor that couples sensing of necrosis to immunity. *Nature* (2009) 458:899–903. doi: 10.1038/nature07750
159. Huysamen C, Willment JA, Dennehy KM, Brown GD. CLEC9A is a novel activation C-type lectin-like receptor expressed on BDCA3+ dendritic cells and a subset of monocytes. *J Biol Chem.* (2008) 283:16693–701. doi: 10.1074/jbc.M709923200
160. Caminschi I, Proietto AI, Ahmet F, Kitsoulis S, Shin Teh J, Lo JCY, et al. The dendritic cell subtype-restricted C-type lectin Clec9A is a target for vaccine enhancement. *Blood* (2008) 112:3264–73. doi: 10.1182/blood-2008-05-155176
161. Lin ML, Zhan Y, Proietto AI, Prato S, Wu L, Heath WR, et al. Selective suicide of cross-presenting $CD8^+$ dendritic cells by cytochrome c injection shows functional heterogeneity within this subset. *Proc Natl Acad Sci USA.* (2008) 105:3029–34. doi: 10.1073/pnas.0712394105
162. Savina A, Peres A, Cebrian I, Carmo N, Moita C, Hacohen N, et al. The small GTPase Rac2 controls phagosomal alkalinization and antigen crosspresentation selectively in CD8(+) dendritic cells. *Immunity* (2009) 30:544–55. doi: 10.1016/j.immuni.2009.01.013
163. Nair-Gupta P, Baccarini A, Tung N, Seyffer F, Florey O, Huang Y, et al. TLR signals induce phagosomal MHC-I delivery from the endosomal recycling compartment to allow cross-presentation. *Cell* (2014) 158:506–21. doi: 10.1016/j.cell.2014.04.054
164. Kretzer NM, Theisen DJ, Tussiwand R, Briseño CG, Grajales-Reyes GE, Wu X, et al. RAB43 facilitates cross-presentation of cell-associated antigens by CD8α+ dendritic cells. *J Exp Med.* (2016) 213:2871–83. doi: 10.1084/jem.20160597
165. Crozat K, Tamoutounour S, Vu Manh T-P, Fossum E, Luche H, Ardouin L, et al. Cutting edge: expression of XCR1 defines mouse lymphoid-tissue resident and migratory dendritic cells of the CD8α+ type. *J Immunol.* (2011) 187:4411–5. doi: 10.4049/jimmunol.1101717
166. Galibert L, Diemer GS, Liu Z, Johnson RS, Smith JL, Walzer T, et al. Nectin-like protein 2 defines a subset of T-cell zone dendritic cells and is a ligand for class-I-restricted T-cell-associated molecule. *J Biol Chem.* (2005) 280:21955–64. doi: 10.1074/jbc.M502095200
167. Nizzoli G, Krietsch J, Weick A, Steinfelder S, Facciotti F, Gruarin P, et al. Human CD1c+ dendritic cells secrete high levels of IL-12 and potently prime cytotoxic T-cell responses. *Blood* (2013) 122:932–42. doi: 10.1182/blood-2013-04-495424
168. Hémont C, Neel A, Heslan M, Braudeau C, Josien R. Human blood mDC subsets exhibit distinct TLR repertoire and responsiveness. *J Leukoc Biol.* (2013) 93:599–609. doi: 10.1189/jlb.0912452
169. Lee J, Breton G, Oliveira TYK, Zhou YJ, Aljoufi A, Puhr S, et al. Restricted dendritic cell and monocyte progenitors in human cord blood and bone marrow. *J Exp Med.* (2015) 212:385–399. doi: 10.1084/jem.20141442
170. Lauterbach H, Bathke B, Gilles S, Traidl-Hoffmann C, Luber CA, Fejer G, et al. Mouse CD8alpha+ DCs and human BDCA3+ DCs are major producers of IFN-lambda in response to poly IC. *J Exp Med.* (2010) 207:2703–17. doi: 10.1084/jem.20092720
171. Yarovinsky F, Zhang D, Andersen JF, Bannenberg GL, Serhan CN, Hayden MS, et al. TLR11 activation of dendritic cells by a protozoan profilin-like protein. *Science* (2005) 308:1626–9. doi: 10.1126/science.1109893
172. Raetz M, Kibardin A, Sturge CR, Pifer R, Li H, Burstein E, et al. Cooperation of TLR12 and TLR11 in the IRF8-dependent IL-12 response to Toxoplasma gondii profilin. *J Immunol.* (2013) 191:4818–27. doi: 10.4049/jimmunol.1301301
173. Poulin LF, Salio M, Griessinger E, Anjos-Afonso F, Craciun L, Chen J-L, et al. Characterization of human DNGR-1+ BDCA3+ leukocytes as putative equivalents of mouse CD8alpha+ dendritic cells. *J Exp Med.* (2010) 207:1261–71. doi: 10.1084/jem.20092618
174. Sittig SP, Bakdash G, Weiden J, Sköld AE, Tel J, Figdor CG, et al. A comparative study of the T cell stimulatory and polarizing capacity of human primary blood dendritic cell subsets. *Med Inflamm.* (2016) 2016:3605643. doi: 10.1155/2016/3605643
175. Mittag D, Proietto AI, Loudovaris T, Mannering SI, Vremec D, Shortman K, et al. Human dendritic cell subsets from spleen and blood are similar in phenotype and function but modified by donor health status. *J Immunol.* (2011) 186:6207–17. doi: 10.4049/jimmunol.1002632
176. Granot T, Senda T, Carpenter DJ, Matsuoka N, Weiner J, Gordon CL, et al. Dendritic cells display subset and tissue-specific maturation dynamics over human life. *Immunity* (2017) 46:504–15. doi: 10.1016/j.immuni.2017.02.019

177. Gentles AJ, Newman AM, Liu CL, Bratman SV, Feng W, Kim D, et al. The prognostic landscape of genes and infiltrating immune cells across human cancers. *Nat Med.* (2015) 21:938–45. doi: 10.1038/nm.3909
178. Becht E, Giraldo NA, Lacroix L, Buttard B, Elarouci N, Petitprez F, et al. Estimating the population abundance of tissue-infiltrating immune and stromal cell populations using gene expression. *Genome Biol.* (2016) 17:218. doi: 10.1186/s13059-016-1070-5
179. Li B, Severson E, Pignon J-C, Zhao H, Li T, Novak J, et al. Comprehensive analyses of tumor immunity: implications for cancer immunotherapy. *Genome Biol.* (2016) 17:174. doi: 10.1186/s13059-016-1028-7
180. Charoentong P, Finotello F, Angelova M, Mayer C, Efremova M, Rieder D, et al. Pan-cancer immunogenomic analyses reveal genotype-immunophenotype relationships and predictors of response to checkpoint blockade. *Cell Rep.* (2017) 18:248–62. doi: 10.1016/j.celrep.2016.12.019
181. Schelker M, Feau S, Du J, Ranu N, Klipp E, MacBeath G, et al. Estimation of immune cell content in tumour tissue using single-cell RNA-seq data. *Nat Commun.* (2017) 8:2032. doi: 10.1038/s41467-017-02289-3
182. Michea P, Noël F, Zakine E, Czerwinska U, Sirven P, Abouzid O, et al. Adjustment of dendritic cells to the breast-cancer microenvironment is subset specific. *Nat Immunol.* (2018) 19:885–97. doi: 10.1038/s41590-018-0145-8
183. Győrffy B, Lanczky A, Eklund AC, Denkert C, Budczies J, Li Q, et al. An online survival analysis tool to rapidly assess the effect of 22,277 genes on breast cancer prognosis using microarray data of 1,809 patients. *Breast Cancer Res Treat.* (2010) 123:725–31. doi: 10.1007/s10549-009-0674-9
184. Bogunovic D, O'Neill DW, Belitskaya-Levy I, Vacic V, Yu Y-L, Adams S, et al. Immune profile and mitotic index of metastatic melanoma lesions enhance clinical staging in predicting patient survival. *Proc Natl Acad Sci USA.* (2009) 106:20429–34. doi: 10.1073/pnas.0905139106
185. Lavin Y, Kobayashi S, Leader A, Amir ED, Elefant N, Bigenwald C, et al. Innate immune landscape in early lung adenocarcinoma by paired single-cell analyses. *Cell* (2017) 169:750–765 e17. doi: 10.1016/j.cell.2017.04.014
186. Sluijter BJ, van den Hout MF, Koster BD, van Leeuwen PA, Schneiders FL, van de Ven R, et al. Arming the melanoma sentinel lymph node through local administration of CpG-B and GM-CSF: recruitment and activation of BDCA3/CD141(+) dendritic cells and enhanced cross-presentation. *Cancer Immunol Res.* (2015) 3:495–505. doi: 10.1158/2326-6066.CIR-14-0165
187. van den Hout MFCM, Sluijter BJR, Santegoets SJAM, van Leeuwen PAM, van den Tol MP, van den Eertwegh AJM, et al. Local delivery of CpG-B and GM-CSF induces concerted activation of effector and regulatory T cells in the human melanoma sentinel lymph node. *Cancer Immunol Immunother.* (2016) 65:405–15. doi: 10.1007/s00262-016-1811-z
188. Bhardwaj N. *Treatment of Solid Tumors With Intratumoral Hiltonol® (Poly-ICLC)-Full Text View - ClinicalTrials.gov.* Available online at: https://clinicaltrials.gov/ct2/show/NCT01984892 (Accessed Dec 9, 2018).
189. Saxena M, Bhardwaj N. Re-emergence of dendritic cell vaccines for cancer treatment. *Trends Can.* (2018) 4:119–37. doi: 10.1016/j.trecan.2017.12.007
190. Dhodapkar MV, Sznol M, Zhao B, Wang D, Carvajal RD, Keohan ML, et al. Induction of antigen-specific immunity with a vaccine targeting NY-ESO-1 to the dendritic cell receptor DEC-205. *Sci Transl Med.* (2014) 6:232ra51. doi: 10.1126/scitranslmed.3008068
191. Tel J, Aarntzen EHJG, Baba T, Schreibelt G, Schulte BM, Benitez-Ribas D, et al. Natural human plasmacytoid dendritic cells induce antigen-specific T-cell responses in melanoma patients. *Cancer Res.* (2013) 73:1063–75. doi: 10.1158/0008-5472.CAN-12-2583
192. Schreibelt G, Bol KF, Westdorp H, Wimmers F, Aarntzen EHJG, Duiveman-de Boer T, et al. Effective clinical responses in metastatic melanoma patients after vaccination with primary myeloid dendritic cells. *Clin Cancer Res.* (2016) 22:2155–66. doi: 10.1158/1078-0432.CCR-15-2205
193. Terhorst D, Fossum E, Baranska A, Tamoutounour S, Malosse C, Garbani M, et al. Laser-assisted intradermal delivery of adjuvant-free vaccines targeting XCR1+ dendritic cells induces potent antitumoral responses. *J Immunol.* (2015) 194:5895–902. doi: 10.4049/jimmunol.1500564
194. Yan Z, Wu Y, Du J, Li G, Wang S, Cao W, et al. A novel peptide targeting Clec9a on dendritic cell for cancer immunotherapy. *Oncotarget* (2016) 7:40437–50. doi: 10.18632/oncotarget.9624
195. Pearson FE, Chang K, Minoda Y, Rojas IML, Haigh OL, Daraj G, et al. Activation of human CD141+ and CD1c+ dendritic cells *in vivo* with combined TLR3 and TLR7/8 ligation. *Immunol Cell Biol.* (2018) 96:390–400. doi: 10.1111/imcb.12009
196. Deauvieau F, Ollion V, Doffin A-C, Achard C, Fonteneau J-F, Verronese E, et al. Human natural killer cells promote cross-presentation of tumor cell-derived antigens by dendritic cells. *Int J Can.* (2015) 136:1085–94. doi: 10.1002/ijc.29087
197. Saxena M, Balan S, Roudko V, Bhardwaj N. Towards superior dendritic-cell vaccines for cancer therapy. *Nat Biomed Eng.* (2018) 2:341–6. doi: 10.1038/s41551-018-0250-x
198. Wang B, Zaidi N, He L-Z, Zhang L, Kuroiwa JM, Keler T, et al. Targeting of the non-mutated tumor antigen HER2/neu to mature dendritic cells induces an integrated immune response that protects against breast cancer in mice. *Breast Cancer Res.* (2012) 14:R39. doi: 10.1186/bcr3135
199. Mahnke K, Qian Y, Fondel S, Brueck J, Becker C, Enk AH. Targeting of antigens to activated dendritic cells *in vivo* cures metastatic melanoma in mice. *Cancer Res.* (2005) 65:7007–12. doi: 10.1158/0008-5472.CAN-05-0938
200. Hartung E, Becker M, Bachem A, Reeg N, Jäkel A, Hutloff A, et al. Induction of potent CD8 T cell cytotoxicity by specific targeting of antigen to cross-presenting dendritic cells *in vivo* via murine or human XCR1. *J Immunol.* (2015) 194:1069–79. doi: 10.4049/jimmunol.1401903
201. Sancho D, Mourão-Sá D, Joffre OP, Schulz O, Rogers NC, Pennington DJ, et al. Tumor therapy in mice via antigen targeting to a novel, DC-restricted C-type lectin. *J Clin Investig.* (2008) 118:2098–110. doi: 10.1172/JCI34584
202. Sartorius R, Bettua C, D'Apice L, Caivano A, Trovato M, Russo D, et al. Vaccination with filamentous bacteriophages targeting DEC-205 induces DC maturation and potent anti-tumor T-cell responses in the absence of adjuvants. *Eur J Immunol.* (2011) 41:2573–84. doi: 10.1002/eji.201141526
203. Broekhoven CL van, Parish CR, Demangel C, Britton WJ, Altin JG. Targeting dendritic cells with antigen-containing liposomes: a highly effective procedure for induction of antitumor immunity and for tumor immunotherapy. *Cancer Res.* (2004) 64:4357–65. doi: 10.1158/0008-5472.CAN-04-0138
204. Picco G, Beatson R, Taylor-Papadimitriou J, Burchell JM. Targeting DNGR-1 (CLEC9A) with antibody/MUC1 peptide conjugates as a vaccine for carcinomas. *Euro J Immunol.* (2014) 44:1947–55. doi: 10.1002/eji.201344076
205. Kreutz M, Giquel B, Hu Q, Abuknesha R, Uematsu S, Akira S, et al. Antibody-antigen-adjuvant conjugates enable co-delivery of antigen and adjuvant to dendritic cells in cis but only have partial targeting specificity. *PLoS ONE* (2012) 7:e40208. doi: 10.1371/journal.pone.0040208
206. Flacher V, Tripp CH, Mairhofer DG, Steinman RM, Stoitzner P, Idoyaga J, et al. Murine Langerin+ dermal dendritic cells prime CD8$^+$ T cells while Langerhans cells induce cross-tolerance. *EMBO Mol Med.* (2014) 6:1191–204. doi: 10.15252/emmm.201303283
207. Bonifaz LC, Bonnyay DP, Charalambous A, Darguste DI, Fujii S-I, Soares H, et al. *In vivo* targeting of antigens to maturing dendritic cells via the DEC-205 receptor improves T cell vaccination. *J Exp Med.* (2004) 199:815–24. doi: 10.1084/jem.20032220

14

Human Dendritic Cells: Their Heterogeneity and Clinical Application Potential in Cancer Immunotherapy

Thiago A. Patente [1], *Mariana P. Pinho* [1], *Aline A. Oliveira* [1], *Gabriela C. M. Evangelista* [1], *Patrícia C. Bergami-Santos* [1] *and José A. M. Barbuto* [1,2]*

[1] *Laboratory of Tumor Immunology, Department of Immunology, Institute of Biomedical Sciences, University of São Paulo, São Paulo, Brazil,* [2] *Discipline of Molecular Medicine, Department of Medicine, Faculty of Medicine, University of São Paulo, São Paulo, Brazil*

***Correspondence:**
José A. M. Barbuto
jbarbuto@icb.usp.br

Dendritic cells (DC) are professional antigen presenting cells, uniquely able to induce naïve T cell activation and effector differentiation. They are, likewise, involved in the induction and maintenance of immune tolerance in homeostatic conditions. Their phenotypic and functional heterogeneity points to their great plasticity and ability to modulate, according to their microenvironment, the acquired immune response and, at the same time, makes their precise classification complex and frequently subject to reviews and improvement. This review will present general aspects of the DC physiology and classification and will address their potential and actual uses in the management of human disease, more specifically cancer, as therapeutic and monitoring tools. New combination treatments with the participation of DC will be also discussed.

Keywords: human dendritic cells, DC, monocyte-derived dendritic cells, mo-DC, cancer vaccines, cancer combination therapies

INTRODUCTION

Identified in mouse spleen for their peculiar shape and capacity to activate naïve lymphocytes (1–3), dendritic cells (DC) are considered the most efficient antigen presenting cells (APC) (3, 4), uniquely able to initiate, coordinate, and regulate adaptive immune responses. Though their ability to capture, process and present antigens is considered their main characteristic, their phenotypic heterogeneity is striking and very different consequences can come from their action. This review will present an overview of the main subpopulations of human DC described and will focus on their potential translational use.

OVERVIEW OF DENDRITIC CELLS IN THE IMMUNE SYSTEM PHYSIOLOGY

Human DC are identified by their high expression of major histocompatibility complex (MHC) class II molecules (MHC-II) and of CD11c, both of which are found on other cells, like lymphocytes, monocytes and macrophages (5–12). DC express many other molecules which allow their classification into various subtypes (**Table 1**). Although some of the DC subtypes were originally described as macrophages, DC and macrophages have distinct characteristics (13–15) and ontogeny, so that, currently, little doubt remains that they belong to distinct lineages (16–24).

DC can be found in practically all tissues, where they detect homeostatic imbalances and process antigens for presentation to T cells, establishing a link between innate and adaptive immune responses. Furthermore, DC can secrete cytokines and growth factors (25) that modify ongoing immune responses, and are influenced by their interactions with other immune cells, like natural killer (26–28) and innate lymphoid cells (ILCs) (29).

DC are found in two different functional states, "mature" and "immature". These are distinguished by many features, but the ability to activate antigen-specific naïve T cells in secondary lymphoid organs is the hallmark of mature DC (30–32). DC maturation is triggered by tissue homeostasis disturbances, detected by the recognition of pathogen-associated molecular patterns (PAMP) or damage-associated molecular patterns (DAMP) (33, 34) (**Figure 1**). Maturation turns on metabolic, cellular, and gene transcription programs allowing DC to migrate from peripheral tissues to T-dependent areas in secondary lymphoid organs, where T lymphocyte-activating antigen presentation may occur (35–40).

During maturation, DC lose adhesive structures, reorganize the cytoskeleton and increase their motility (41). DC maturation also leads to a decrease in their endocytic activity but increased expression of MHC-II and co-stimulatory molecules (42–44). Mature DC express higher levels of the chemokine receptor, CCR7 (45–48) and secrete cytokines, essential for T-cell activation (42, 49–52). Thus, the interaction between mature DC and antigen-specific T cells is the trigger of antigen-specific immune responses (53, 54). When interacting with CD4+ T cells, DC may induce their differentiation into different T helper (Th) subsets (52) such as Th1 (55–60), Th2 (56, 57, 61, 62), Th17 (63–65), or other CD4+ T cell subtypes (66) (**Figure 2**). T cell differentiation in each subtype is a complex phenomenon, that can be influenced by the cytokines in the DC tissue of origin (67), their maturation state (42) and cause of tissue imbalance (68). However, this process is not completely elucidated, as, for example, the source of IL-4 during Th2 responses, which is discussed extensively elsewhere (69).

DC present a unique characteristic: the ability to perform cross-presentation (70–74). This phenomenon was described in 1976, by Bevan (75) and is defined as the presentation, in the context of class I MHC molecules (MHC-I), of antigens captured from the extracellular milieu. This feature allows DC to trigger responses against intracellular antigens from other cell types, thus providing means for the system to deal with threats that avoid professional APC (70, 76, 77) and, even, to prime CD8+ lymphocytes in the absence of CD4+ T cells (78, 79). Cross-presentation is involved also in the induction of tolerance to intracellular self-antigens that are not expressed by APC and, then, called, cross-tolerance (80, 81).

Before receiving maturation stimuli, DC are said to be in an "immature state." Immature DC are poor inducers of naïve lymphocyte effector responses, since they have low surface expression of co-stimulatory molecules, low expression of chemokine receptors, and do not release immunostimulatory cytokines (44, 82). These "immature" cells, though, are very efficient in antigen capture due to their high endocytic capacity, via receptor-mediated endocytosis, including lectin- (83–85);

TABLE 1 | Main surface markers of human and mouse DC subtypes.

DC subtype	Human	Mouse
cDC1	CD141/CLEC9A/XCR1	CD8a/CD103/XCR1
cDC2	CD1c/CD172a	CD11b/CD172a
pDC	CD123/CD303/CD304	B220/SiglecH
LC	Langerin/CD1a	Langerin/CD24

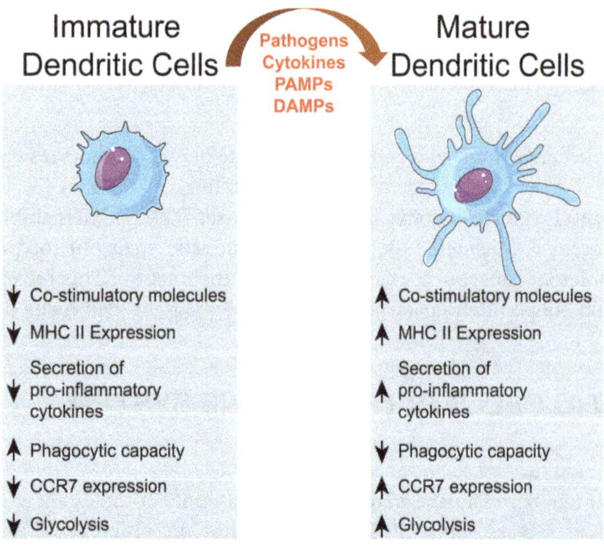

FIGURE 1 | Dendritic cells activation. Extracellular signals, such as PAMPs or DAMPs, trigger alterations on immature DCs culminating on significant changes on surface proteins, intracellular pathways and metabolic activity.

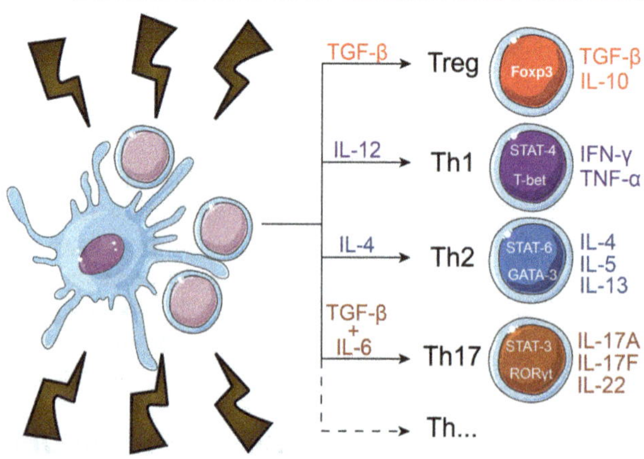

FIGURE 2 | CD4+ T cell fate induced by dendritic cells. When in contact with DC, naïve CD4+ T cells can differentiate into a number of subtypes. Among them, are regulatory T cells (Treg) and T helper (Th) subsets, which include Th1, Th2, and Th17 cells. Each subtype expresses different transcription factors, which regulate the function and cytokine secretion pattern of the cells. The T cell fate decision is a complex phenomenon that heavily depends on the interaction of DC with the T cells and the cytokines present in the microenvironment.

Toll-like- (86–88), FC- and complement receptors (89) and macropinocytosis (84). Thus, immature DC act, indeed, as sentinels against invading pathogens (32, 90), but also as tissue scavengers, capturing apoptotic and necrotic cells (91).

This latter feature confers to immature DC an essential role in the induction and maintenance of immune tolerance (31, 92–95). Apoptotic cells that arise in consequence of natural tissue turnover (96, 97) are internalized by DC but do not induce their maturation (31, 98–100). Thus, their antigens are presented to T cells without the activating co-stimulatory signals that a mature DC would deliver, resulting in T cell apoptosis (80, 101), anergy (102, 103) or development into regulatory T cells (104, 105).

These "tolerogenic DC" express less co-stimulatory molecules and proinflammatory cytokines, but upregulate the expression of inhibitory molecules (like PD-L1 and CTLA-4), secrete anti-inflammatory cytokines (IL-10, for example) (102, 106–108) and are essential to prevent responses against healthy tissues (30, 31, 109–112). However, in some contexts, immature DC can be harmful to the body. It is known that DC that are unable to induce lymphocyte effector responses may contribute to the immune system's failure to fight infections (113, 114) or tumors (115–120). In these situations, DC, even after recognition of pathogens or other changes in microenvironment, fail to increase the co-stimulatory molecules required to activate T cells, thus allowing the disease to "escape" immune control.

Although many factors are recognized as contributing to drive DC maturation (100, 121, 122), the full set of such factors is not precisely defined, but involves a long series of transcriptional adaptations (119, 121, 123–125). The complexity and heterogeneity of these adaptations allows DC to translate effectively (most of the times) the pattern of homeostatic disturbance to interacting T lymphocytes, thus establishing DC as the main connector between innate and acquired mechanisms of immunity (43, 126).

HUMAN DENDRITIC CELL SUBPOPULATIONS AND MONOCYTE-DERIVED DENDRITIC CELLS

Dendritic cells can be divided into resident lymphoid tissue DC and migratory non-lymphoid tissue DC (16). Both are heterogeneous cell populations with different subsets that can be distinguished by phenotypic markers and genetic profile. The first identification of different DC subsets arose from the observation that CD8 expression occurred on some, but not all, mouse resident splenic and thymic DCs (127). While the identification of mouse DC subpopulations is well advanced (128, 129), mostly due to tissue accessibility, the same is not true for human DC, where most studies were performed only in peripheral blood or skin, in spite of recent data characterizing DC subpopulations in human lung (130) and intestine (131).

Recent efforts have been addressed to understand the ontogeny and function of human DC subsets, attempting to correlate well-defined murine subpopulations with those found in human peripheral blood (16, 128, 132). DC arise from a CD34$^+$ hematopoietic precursor that gives rise to myeloid (MP) and lymphoid (LP) precursors (**Figure 3**). MP differentiate into monocyte, macrophage and DC precursors (MDP), which will give rise to monocytes and to the common DC precursors (CDP). CDP can differentiate into plasmacytoid DC (pDC) or the preclassical DC (pre-cDC). Pre-cDC are the progenitors of the two major cDC subpopulations named cDC1 and cDC2 (14), which will be further discussed latter. Recent technologies, such as single cell RNAseq, are allowing a better characterization of DC ontogeny and the identification of DC subset precursors in peripheral blood (133), demonstrating that the commitment with a DC subset may be an early event, both in mice (134) and humans (135).

Curiously, in lymphohematopoietic tissue, such as spleen, thymus and blood, DC commitment to a subpopulation is mainly defined by ontogeny, while in non-lymphohematopoietic tissue, such as lung and skin, DC subpopulations are more influenced by signals derived from the microenvironment. This, once again, confirms that DC are a very plastic cell population that can shape its phenotype to the microenvironment and to homeostatic state of the tissue where it is located (136).

In blood, DC constitute a rare cell population that can be broadly divided into two subtypes (**Figure 4**): CD123$^+$CD11c$^-$ DC, called plasmacytoid DC (pDC), and CD123$^-$CD11c$^+$ cells, called classical DC or myeloid DC (cDC) (25, 128, 137). Dzionek et al. (138) identified three antigens called BDCA-2, BDCA-3, and BDCA-4 (Blood Dendritic Cell Antigens), which, together with BDCA-1 (CD1c), allowed the further discrimination of human blood DC subsets. cDC can be separated into cDC1 and cDC2 (139): cDC1 are characterized by the expression of BDCA-3 (CD141) and Clec9A, while cDC2 express CD1c. BDCA-2 (CD303) and–4 (CD304), on the other hand, together with CD123, characterize pDC.

It is noteworthy that recent genomic studies, with emphasis on the subpopulations of monocytes and DC, made it possible to align CD141$^+$ DC (cDC1) and CD1c$^+$ (cDC2) from human peripheral blood with the mouse CD8α$^+$/CD103$^+$ and CD11b$^+$DC, respectively (140, 141). This will allow the confirmation, or not, of the roles played by these subsets in murine immune responses also in humans.

cDC1

The human cDC1 subpopulation is present in blood and in lymphoid and non-lymphoid tissues (142). This subpopulation is characterized by the expression of CD141, the chemokine receptor XCR1, C-type lectin CLEC9A, the cell adhesion molecule CADM1, and is the counterpart of mouse CD8α$^+$/CD103$^+$ cross-presenting DC subset (132, 142). cDC1 can be generated *in vitro* from CD34$^+$ progenitors after 21 days of culture with fms-like tyrosine kinase 3 ligand (Flt3L) and thrombopoietin (TPO) (143) or with Flt3L and murine bone marrow stromal cell lines (144). As mentioned above, this subpopulation of DC seems to be specially adapted to perform cross-presentation, a phenomenon that is associated with the expression of the chemokine receptor XCR1 (145). The main transcription factors (TF) shown to be essential for the generation of cDC1 are the basic leucine zipper transcriptional factor ATF-like 3 (BATF3) (146) and IFN-regulatory factor 8

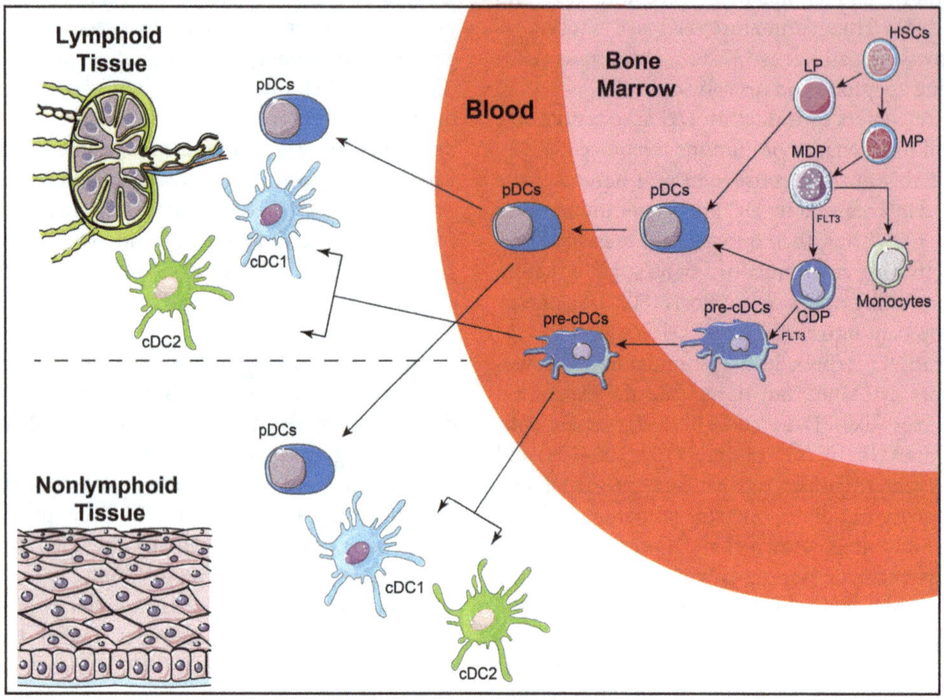

FIGURE 3 | Simplified scheme of DC ontogeny. DC arise from HSC that give rise to MP and LP. MP are further differentiated into MDP that can differentiate into CDP and monocytes. CDP differentiate further into pDC or pre-cDC. LP can also give rise to pDC, although this ontogenic pathway is not completely elucidated. Once in the blood, pre-cDC give rise to two of the main DC subtypes: cDC1 and cDC2. Both pDC and cDC can migrate from the blood to lymphoid and non-lymphoid tissues. HSC, hematopoietic stem cell; MP, myeloid precursors; LP, lymphoid precursors; MDP, macrophage-DC precursors; CDP, common DC precursors; pre-cDC, pre-classical dendritic cells; pDC, plasmacytoid dendritic cells; cDCs, conventional dendritic cells; FLT3, Fms-Related Tyrosine Kinase 3.

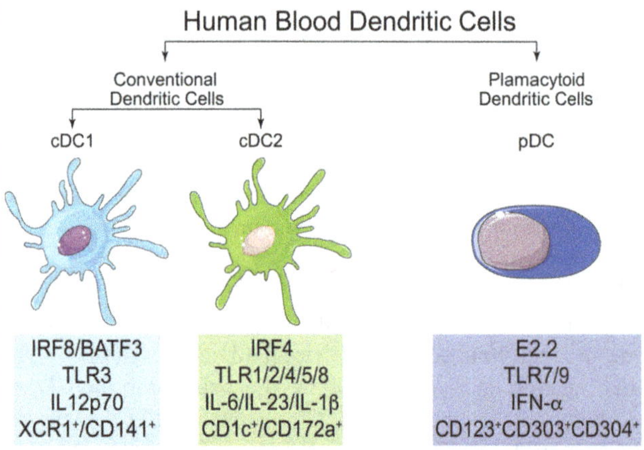

FIGURE 4 | Main characteristics and differences of cDC1, cDC2, and pDC. In human blood, it is possible to find two main populations of DC, named conventional DC (cDC) and plasmacytoid DC (pDC). cDC can be further subdivided in cDC1 and cDC2. All three subtypes of DC can be differentiated by their signature transcription factors and also by the expression of specific surface markers.

(IRF8) (130). In mice, besides BATF3 (147) and IRF8 (148), gene knockout models pointed out to the role of two other TF: DNA binding protein inhibitor ID2 (149) and nuclear factor interleukin-3-regulated protein (NFIL3) (150), whose participation in the generation of human cDC1 needs yet to be demonstrated.

cDC1 prime $CD8^+$ T cells efficiently, what is important in anti-tumor and anti-virus immunity. However, the induction and modulation of an immune response is a very complex phenomenon that involves many cell interactions, including interactions among different DC subsets, as recently demonstrated in mice infected with modified vaccinia virus Ankara (MVA) (151). In this model, activated $CD8^+$ T cells recruit both pDC (via CCL3/CCL4) and cDC1 (via XCL1); type I interferons, (IFN-I) produced by pDC, act on cDC1 optimizing their maturation, costimulatory capacity and ability to cross-present viral antigens, thus leading to an effective anti-virus response. cDC1 were also shown to be important for the antitumor activity induced by heat-inactivated MVA in murine melanoma and colon cancer models (152). Furthermore, both in mice and humans, cDC1 are found sparsely distributed along tumor margins (competing with tumor associated macrophages–TAM-for tumor antigens?) and their presence was important for the success of adoptively transferred cytotoxic T cells (CTL) (153) and for the delivery of tumor antigens to the draining lymph nodes, in a CCR7 dependent manner (154).

cDC2

cDC2 constitute a heterogeneous subset of DC that can be found in blood, lymphoid and non-lymphoid tissue (16, 142).

SIRPα (CD172a) is expressed by cDC2 (both in humans and mice) (130) and, along with CD1c (humans) and CD11b (mice), characterizes this subpopulation (25, 132). Coherently with its heterogeneity, other markers are expressed by cDC2, according to their localization, as for example, CD1a in dermal and CD103 in gut cDC2 (25, 141). Like cDC1, cDC2 can also be differentiated from $CD34^+$ progenitors, after 21 days of culture with Flt3L and TPO (143) or with Flt3L and murine bone marrow stromal cell lines (144). More than one transcription factor is involved in cDC2 differentiation and IRF4 seems to be the master transcription factor (155), but other transcription factors are required. In mice, PU.1 (156), RelB (157) and recombining binding protein suppressor of hairless (RBP/J) (158) were shown to be associated with the differentiation of cDC2, and in humans, IRF8 (159).

Again, in accordance with their heterogeneity and innate plasticity (132), cDC2 have been show to induce Th1, Th2, and Th17 responses (160, 161). The puzzling heterogeneity of these cells is further illustrated by the recent description of two novel DC subtypes within the $CD1c^+$ subpopulation: DC2 and DC3. These two subpopulations diverged by the expression of CD32B and CD163/CD36. Functional experiments showed that both these cDC2 subtypes were potent stimulators of naïve T cell proliferation, but show a different pattern of cytokine secretion after stimulation with a series of toll like receptors (TLR) agonists (162).

In the immune system physiology, cDC2 seem to have many, but frequently, regulatory roles. These cells have been described as potent inducers of regulatory T cells in intestine (141), and as responsible for maintaining tolerance in the liver (163). Also, cDC2 have been described as the only DC subset able to produce retinoic acid upon stimulation with vitamin D3, thus stimulating $CD4^+$ naïve T cells to express gut-homing molecules and to produce Th2 cytokines (164).

Plasmacytoid DC (pDC)

The pDC subpopulation is a subset of DC distinct from cDC, that arises directly from the CDP (while cDC arise from pre-DC precursor) (14). These cells are characterized by the secretion of high levels of IFN-α/β upon TLR7/9 stimulation, and are extremely important in viral infections (165). This subset of DC is phenotypically distinct in mice and humans. In mice, it is characterized as $CD11c^{int}CD11b^-B220^+SiglecH^+CD317^+$ while in humans it is characterized by the absence of expression of CD11c and the expression of CD123, CD303, and CD304 (25, 128, 132). In terms of transcription factors, on the other hand, both mouse and human pDC seem to depend on the same master transcription factor, E2.2 (25, 132, 166).

Since the secretion of IFN-α/β is the main feature of pDC, their association with viral infections is not surprising. The secretion of IFN-α/β by pDCs can be a consequence of direct viral infection [like in HIV infection, where the virus infects pDC via CD4, CCR5 and CXCR4 (167)], or from external stimuli. Indeed, human pDC were shown to secrete high levels of IFN-α/β in *Aspergilus fumigatus* infection in a Dectin-2-dependent manner (168).

In keeping with the other DC subpopulations heterogeneity, human pDC may be subdivided into two subpopulations, distinguished by the expression of CD2 (169). Both pDC subsets secrete IFN-α/β efficiently, but only the $CD2^{hi}$ subset secretes IL-12p40 and induces $CD4^+$ T cell proliferation. These data, however, may be in need of a second look. As mentioned before, single cell RNAseq analysis is providing new data and allowing better characterization of DC subpopulations. When this approach was used to study pDC subpopulations, a "contaminant" putative precursor of cDC (pre-cDC), characterized as $CD123^+CD33^+CD303^+CD304^+CD2^+$, was identified. When these putative pre-cDC and "pure" pDC populations (characterized by the absence of CD2 and CD33 expression) were separated and stimulated, only pre-cDC were able to induce $CD4^+$ T cell proliferation and secrete IL-12p40 (135). This raises the possibility that many of the observed attributes of pDC, such as their ability to induce Th1 responses (170), to perform cross-presentation (171), to exhibit naïve T cell allostimulatory capacity (169) and expression of co-stimulatory (172) molecules might reflect the activity of this contaminating pre-cDC population.

Puzzling, as these data may seem, they illustrate quite well the plasticity of the cells "clustered" under the name of DC. They further suggest that attempts to classify strictly these cells may lead to more confusion than it is necessary to understand their role in responding to microenvironmental challenges, in shaping immune response patterns in the body and, eventually, in driving the immune response toward therapeutic goals in humans.

Monocyte-Derived DC (mo-DC)

Much of the knowledge acquired in the past years about human DC biology was possible due to the methodology of *in vitro* deriving DC from $CD34^+$ precursors (stimulated with GM-CSF and TNF-α) (173) or from monocytes (stimulated with GM-CSF and IL-4) (174). Like cDC2, mo-DC depend on IRF4 for their differentiation (175). However, they do not seem to be an equivalent population, since they arise from different precursors (14).

In mice, the precursors used for *in vitro* generation of DC are extracted from the bone marrow. In the presence of GM-CSF, these precursors give rise to large number of cells that resemble tissue DC and are called bone marrow-derived dendritic cells (BMDC) (176). Helft et al. showed that BMDC comprise a heterogeneous population expressing both CD11c and MHCII. A $CD11c^+MHCII^{int}$ population seems to be more closely related to macrophages (hence, called GM-Macs), while the $CD11c^+MHCII^{high}$ population resembles DC and is, thus, called GM-DC. Addition of IL-4 to these cultures limits, but does not eliminate, the generation of GM-Macs (177). The heterogeneity of precursors and cell populations obtained *in vitro* fuels a vivid and complex discussion about the biological relevance of these cells (178–180).

It is still unclear to which subpopulation of DC, mo-DC are more closely related, but DC ontogeny data suggest that mo-DC are similar to the inflammatory DC (132). Not surprisingly, inflammatory DC is the designation of another heterogeneous subpopulation of DC, typically $CD11c^{hi}MHCII^{hi}$. One of the first reports of inflammatory DCs described a population of DC characterized by the production of TNF and iNOS, named Tip-DCs (181). Another study identified inflammatory DC in the skin of atopic dermatitis patients and named these cells inflammatory epidermal dendritic cells (IDECs), which were characterized by the expression of CD11c, CD206, CD1a, CD11b, CD209, FcεRI (182). Recently, another inflammatory DC population was described in the synovial fluid of rheumatoid arthritis patients and in the inflammatory ascites of untreated cancer patients. In this study, inflammatory DC were characterized as $CD14^+CD1c^+SIRP\alpha^+CD206^+Fc\varepsilon RI^+$ and their gene signature (when compared to *in vitro* generated mo-DC, macrophages, cDC2, $CD16^+$ monocytes and $CD14^+$ monocytes) was more closely related to that of mo-DC, suggesting that inflammatory DC could be, indeed, the *in vivo* counterparts of mo-DC (183).

MO-DC AS A "WINDOW" TO IMMUNE SYSTEM EVALUATION IN CANCER PATIENTS

It has been known for a while that established tumors affect their microenvironment in ways that facilitate their persistence and progression. These local modifications include zones of hypoxia, altered pH, induction of angiogenesis (184), alterations of pre-mRNA splicing in surrounding cells (185) and the recruitment of cells that facilitate tumor progression, such as tumor-associated macrophages (TAM) (186), immature DC (115), myeloid-derived suppressor cells (MDSC) (187) and regulatory T cells (188). However, mechanisms to avoid immune system surveillance and tumor progression (189) are not limited to the tumor site and, today, it is recognized that individuals with cancer present also systemic modifications to that effect as well (190). As discussed before, DC are a plastic and heterogeneous population and it should be expected that, among these systemic adaptations, some affect the various DC subpopulations, including mo-DC.

Described Alterations in mo-DC of Cancer Patients

Various publications have described phenotypic and functional alterations in mo-DC from patients with different tumors (191–193). Our group demonstrated that mo-DC from breast cancer patients are poor stimulators of allogeneic T lymphocytes proliferation but are good inducers of regulatory T cells. These characteristics were observed both in immature and mature mo-DC and the regulatory T cell bias, though decreased by blocking of TGF-β, was not completely inhibited (192). Similar phenomena were also observed in patients with CLL, whose mo-DC expressed reduced levels of important molecules involved in antigen presentation and lymphocyte activation, such as HLA-DR, CD80, CD86, CD83, and CD40, and, coherently, were less effective in inducing proliferation of both $CD4^+$ and $CD8^+$ T cells. Furthermore, $CD4^+$ T lymphocytes co-cultivated with mo-DC from CLL patients presented reduced IFN-γ and IL-4 production, when compared to healthy donors (193). Further similar results were also observed in chronic myeloid leukemia (194), colorectal cancer (195), and cervical neoplasia (196). It is worth noting that dysfunctional and apoptosis prone mo-DC were also obtained from healthy donors, when their monocytes were exposed to tumor culture supernatants (197).

Although detected in cancer patients, the altered phenotype and functions of mo-DC could precede the emergence of the tumor and reflect an individual constitutional characteristic of the patients, which might be related or not to their disease. The follow up of cancer patients that present such alterations, however, suggests otherwise and indicate that, indeed, it is the presence of the tumor that affects the cells.

In a study of a chromophobe renal carcinoma patient, mo-DC obtained before surgery induced less allogeneic T cell proliferation and more regulatory T cells when compared to cells from healthy donors. Three months after surgery, yet, mo-DC from the patient exhibited functional properties similar to that of healthy controls, suggesting that the presence of the tumor was the cause of the biased mo-DC function in the patient (198). Another example of the transitory and, possibly, in this case, tumor-dependent functional bias of circulating cells has been described in a study with patients with obstructive jaundice. Monocytes from 53 patients with obstructive jaundice (44 due to cancer and 9 due to non-neoplastic diseases) were obtained before surgery and found unable to release H_2O_2 upon stimulation, but this was progressively reversed after surgery (199). Yet, in another paper we described a patient with type 2-papillary renal cell carcinoma, whose mo-DC also presented functional biases. Though after the tumor was surgically removed, the patient's mo-DC already regained some activity, their T lymphocyte-stimulating activity reached healthy controls' levels only after the patient was submitted to treatment with a dendritic cell-based cancer vaccine (200).

Altogether, these data point out to the fact that circulating monocytes may reflect systemic effects of tumors in such a manner that their functional evaluation could become an effective tool to monitor disease progression and/or response to therapy.

Alterations in Circulating Subpopulations of DC in Cancer Patients

Circulating subsets of DC are also affected in cancer patients. Diminished numbers of total DC have been observed in melanoma patients; this was more intense in stage IV patients and, though it was more pronounced in the pDCs, it also occurred among cDC (201). In breast cancer patients, reductions in total circulating DC and in DC IL-12 production was also described. However, in these patients cDC were the culprit and not pDC (117). Circulating DC isolated from patients with CLL showed decreased expression of co-stimulatory molecules, lower ability to stimulate allogeneic T lymphocytes and did not secrete IL-12, but retained the ability to secrete IL-10 (202). A recent publication, evaluating the effects of different TLR-L in cDC1, cDC2, pDC, and monocytes from breast cancer patients showed that, upon stimulation with IFN-α, cDC2 and non-classical monocytes ($CD14^-CD16^+$) exhibited reduced secretion of TNF-α (203).

These observations point out to systemic effects induced by tumors upon the immune-hematopoietic system and suggest that circulating cells are influenced and, possibly functionally handicapped to fight the tumor, even before actually infiltrating the tumor mass. These phenomena, added to our view and understanding of tumor biology, should allow the design of improved therapeutic approaches, even for those that do not specifically target the immune system.

Possible Mechanisms

It is quite evident, thus, that tumors promote local and systemic alterations in immune cells and substantial efforts have been made to identify possible mechanisms of how tumors promote these alterations and, most importantly, how to correct them.

Signal Transducer and Activator of Transcription 6 (STAT6) is an important molecule, induced by IL-4, in the process of mo-DC differentiation. STAT6 is naturally inhibited by the Suppressor Of Cytokine Signaling 5 (SOCS5), which, in turn, is up regulated by phosphorylated STAT3 in monocytes. In CLL patients, IL-10 induces the phosphorylation of STAT3, thus up regulating the expression of SOCS5. As a consequence, monocytes of CLL patients have impaired phosphorylation of STAT6 and its downstream genes, blocking their differentiation and maturation into functional mo-DC (193). However, mo-DC from healthy donors differentiated in the presence of lung cancer patients' sera, showed decreased STAT3 phosphorylation (204). Although apparently contradictory, these findings might reflect a difference in the monocytes of patients and healthy donors or a difference in the moment of analysis. If monocytes from patients and healthy donors differ, it would not be surprising that they would respond differently to the same stimuli. Likewise, the moment when STAT3 phosphorylation is analyzed may show quite different results. When monocytes from healthy donors were pre-treated with IL-10 and then stimulated with IL-4, an initial increase in STAT3 phosphorylation occurred during the first 72 h, but with the increasing SOCS5 expression, STAT3 (and STAT6) phosphorylation was downregulated (193).

The STAT3 pathway is activated also by IL-6, which, like IL-10, is found in higher concentration in patients sera (205). The impaired functions of DC have been, thus, also attributed to upregulation of IL-6-induced STAT3 activity, both in animal models (206) and humans (207)- these data were recently reviewed by Kitamura et al. (208). Offering a potential solution to these hard to reconcile data is the fact that STAT3 signaling induced by IL-6 seems to be modulated by SOCS in a different way than the IL-10-induced signaling, at least in human macrophages (209).

Undeniably, the available data, though suggesting possible pathways are not enough to elucidate the complex molecular mechanisms underlying DC dysfunction in patients.

DENDRITIC CELLS AS THERAPEUTIC INSTRUMENTS

The key concept of the cancer immunotherapy is that the manipulation of the immune system can achieve cancer control and, ideally, cure. The possibility of cancer immunotherapy was first shown by Coley, who used a mixture of bacterial toxins to treat patients with inoperable sarcomas (210). Since then, many studies have shown clinical benefit when using general immune system activators, such as bacterial products (211) and TLR agonists (212). The antitumor activity of these approaches, when it occurs, is attributed to the ability of these compounds to activate the immune system that, in turn, acquires the ability to kill tumor cells. Much of this effect was shown to be due to DC activation followed by the generation of T cell responses (213). Dendritic cells, as key activators of the adaptive immune response, would be expected to have a central role in inducing antitumor immune responses and the many functional deviations these cells show in cancer patients emphasize the relevant role they may, indeed, play in anti-tumor immune responses. In face of these data, it would be intuitive to exploit the immune activating potential of DC to induce antitumor responses in cancer patients. However, because of the difficulty of obtaining large numbers of these cells by non-invasive methods, therapeutic approaches using DC became possible only after methods for the *in vitro* generation of these cells were described (174).

Use of Monocyte-Derived Dendritic Cells

mo-DC are able to present antigens in the context of both MHC class I (91) and class II molecules (214) and, hence, can be used to generate therapeutic cancer vaccines. When injected in humans, mo-DC can prime CD4+ and CD8+ T cells (215) and expand antigen-specific cytotoxic T cells, which can lead to regression of metastatic lesions in patients (216). Nevertheless, some argue that mo-DC, possibly due to a limited migration potential, might be insufficient to consistently induce effective immune responses *in vivo* (217). Contrastingly, Kuhn and co-workers have shown that successful therapy using immune-activating compounds was followed by the appearance of mo-DC in the draining lymph nodes of treated mice (218) and these cells were essential for the priming of CD8+ T cells and antitumor immunity (219).

Nonetheless, to be used as therapeutic instruments, mo-DC must be properly differentiated *in vitro*, induced to mature, loaded with tumor antigens, and, finally, administered to the patient (**Figure 5**). It is easy, thus, to realize the challenges that face the development of mo-DC-based vaccines. What are the markers of a "properly activated" DC? What is the "proper" response to be induced? What are the relevant tumor antigens? What is the best pathway for these cells to reach secondary lymphoid organs, where they should encounter tumor-specific T lymphocytes? Not surprisingly, each of the aforementioned steps diverges among the various clinical reported protocols, adding much complexity to the evaluation of the approach, but also a possible explanation for the large diversity in the reported efficiencies of such treatments.

To differentiate monocytes into dendritic cells, the cytokines IL-4 and GM-CSF are classically used (174). Most approaches use this protocol to obtain mo-DC, but other ways to differentiate monocytes into dendritic cells have been described and tested. mo-DC differentiated in the presence of GM-CSF and IFN-α, for example, secrete large amounts of pro-inflammatory cytokines, induce a IL-12p70-independent Th1 response (220) and have

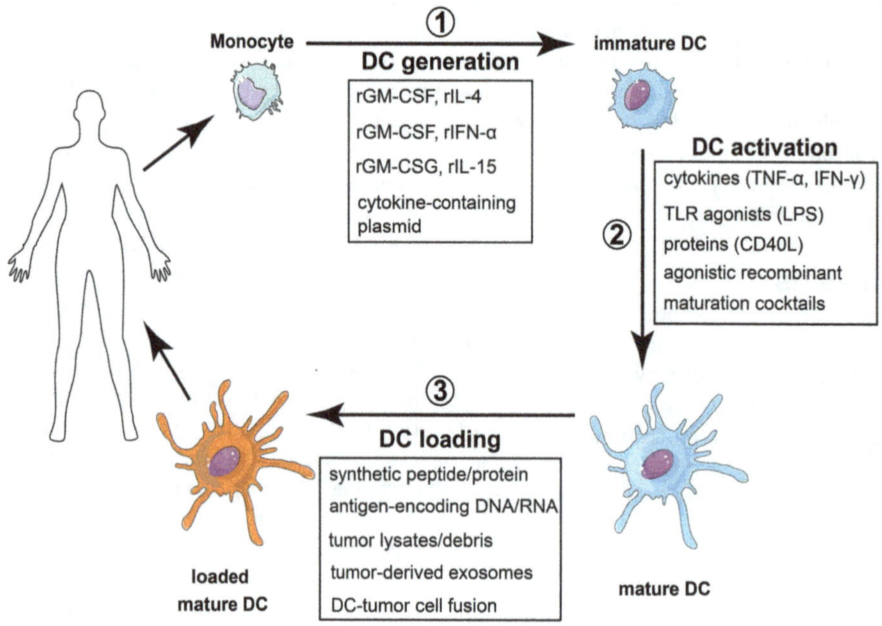

FIGURE 5 | Vaccination strategy with monocyte derived dendritic cells. (1) Monocytes are obtained from peripheral blood and differentiated into dendritic cells. This differentiation can be achieved by using different recombinant cytokines, with rGMCSF + rIL-4 as the most common combination, or by transfecting monocytes with plasmids encoding the cytokines. (2) Once differentiated, DC activation can be accomplished by using different stimuli, most of them associated with tissue damage, inflammation or the presence of a pathogen. (3) The last step is to load the DC with selected or total tumor antigens. Finally, the cells are injected in the patient, expecting them to induce a tumor-specific adaptive immune response able to eradicate the tumor.

given rise to cancer-specific CD8 responses, in phase I/II clinical trials (221). mo-DC differentiated in the presence of GM-CSF and IL-15, on the other hand, were better inducers of Th17 responses (222).

The lengthy culture time to achieve the differentiation of mo-DC (usually 5–7 days) is a limitation of the wide clinical use of these protocols. Thus, alternative protocols for mo-DC differentiation were developed. Dauer et al. have shown that monocytes cultured for 48-hours with IL-4 and GM-CSF already have characteristics of immature DC (223) and these, so called FastDC, prime tumor-antigen specific CD8 T cells as efficiently as conventional mo-DC (224). Another strategy is the transduction of monocytes with plasmids containing the genes of the cytokines, which, constitutively expressed, will lead to their differentiation into DC (225). The FDA-approved cancer vaccine, Sipuleucel-T (PROVENGE®) uses a similar approach for mo-DC generation, in a protocol that only requires 3 days for manufacturing (226). This vaccine is approved for castration-resistant prostate cancer and consists of autologous PBMC incubated with a fusion protein containing both GM-CSF and PAP, a prostate-specific cancer-associated antigen (227).

The second step in vaccines generation consists of mo-DC activation, since differentiation generates immature cells. The maturation stimulus can come from a variety of molecules, including cytokines (TNF-α, IFN-γ), TLR agonists (LPS), agonistic recombinant proteins (CD40L) or maturation cocktails (228). However, the best conditions for mo-DC activation are still unclear. Activation with TNF-α, for example, has been implicated in the induction of mo-DC with impaired ability to secrete pro-inflammatory cytokines, which could even protect mice from autoimmunity (229). On the other hand, combinations of TLR agonists synergize to promote Th1 responses (230). Vopenkova et al. made a direct *in vitro* comparison of different maturation stimuli to induce tumor-specific T cells, showing that the highest response was achieved with the combination of IFN-γ and LPS (231). However, clinical effectiveness comparisons of different mo-DC formulations are still lacking.

Next, mo-DC need to be loaded with tumor antigens. For this, bulk tumor products or selected tumor antigens have been used. Tumor associated antigens (TAAs), recognized by T cells, are found in several tumors (232). Immunodominant synthetic peptides derived from TAAs have been tested and were able to induce clinical and immunological responses of the vaccinated patients (233). Also DNA molecules encoding TAA genes can be employed to load mo-DC, in which case, viral vectors, intrinsically able to activate DC (234), bring further advantage. It is noteworthy that, for all these methods, there is no need of tumor samples from the patient, which may be scarce. However, the use of single antigens has its drawback. Due to the cellular heterogeneity of tumors, they can escape from the immune response generated by the vaccine, through the selection of cells that do not express the immunizing antigens (235). Strategies that involve the induction of a poly-antigenic response can be used to avoid this resistance, especially in melanoma, where this effect is frequently observed. Bulk tumor products may be used as a broad source of tumor antigens.

In addition to tumor lysates, living tumor cells, necrotic debris, apoptotic bodies and tumor-derived exosomes have been used (236). The type of antigenic source used, however, can interfere with the type of immune response obtained and it is impossible, today, to predict which would be the most appropriate antigenic source. For example, in mice, dendritic cells loaded with apoptotic tumor cells were show to induce better responses than tumor lysates, peptides or RNA (237), a finding that contradicts the many data showing that apoptotic cells captured by DC constitute a mechanism of immune tolerance induction.

Although several protocols of vaccination with mo-DC have been tested in clinical trials, only a few obtained relevant clinical responses, and most of them failed to reach the expected results (238). The lack of success in these approaches could be attributed to the functional alterations found in cancer patients mo-DC (239). The use of allogeneic mo-DC obtained from healthy histocompatible donors would be a strategy to bypass this problem, although limited by the need of a MHC-matched donor. Another approach is the use of dendritic cell-tumor cell hybrids. These fused cells express MHC molecules from both tumor and DC origin, forsaking the need of a MHC-matched donor to generate the mo-DC (240). They are also superior than the mixture of these cells, induce antitumor responses and clinical response in patients with advanced metastatic tumors (241). Regardless of the strategy, however, clinical responses to mo-DC-based vaccines are still beyond the desired. This suggests that it may be not enough to have an efficient antigen presentation to induce tumor regression, once it is established. Other compromises between the tumor and the immune system might still prevent an effective tumor-clearing immune response requiring the design of new approaches and, very likely, the combined targeting of different immunological pathways.

Targeting DC Subsets *in vivo*

More recently, a new modality of DC-based immunotherapy strategy is under development. With the better DC subsets characterization and the identification of specific surface markers for these subsets, it became possible to design strategies to deliver different molecules or "packages" to these cells *in vivo* (242). This would allow the selective delivery of antigens and/or immunostimulatory molecules to defined cell subtypes *in vivo*, preventing the costly and laborious *ex vivo* mo-DC generation.

Among the most studied DC-targeting antibodies are those specific for DEC205, CLEC9A, and CLEC12A. These C-type lectin receptors are expressed, in mice, by cDC1 and, the last two, also by pDC (243). Due to their cross-presentation ability, targeting to cDC1 seems to be a reasonable choice, which would favor a higher CD8+ T cell response.

Indeed, experimental settings targeting these molecules were able to induce T cell responses (244, 245) and regression of metastatic melanoma in mice (246). Interesting and well designed as this strategy may be, in humans this strategy is still restricted to *in vitro* studies (247) and awaits, urgently, translational research.

STRATEGIES TO IMPROVE THE CLINICAL EFFECTIVENESS OF MO-DC-BASED THERAPIES

Before specifically addressing the many current pathways for the improved translation of our knowledge of DC biology into clinical applications, it is worth mentioning that, though most of this effort is concentrated into the use of these cells to induce effector immune responses, it is only a matter of time till it becomes feasible to delineate DC-based strategies to treat conditions where the immune system went rogue and is causing autoimmunity, or where medical interventions require the limitation of immune responses, like organ transplantations.

That said, let us consider the strategies that may lead to enhanced immunogenic effects of mo-DC-based treatments.

Approaches for the Improvement of DC-Based Treatments

Since mo-DC show deviant phenotypes in cancer (192) and are susceptible to negative modulation by different drugs, for example STAT5 inhibitors (248), the converse is also true and various approaches are under development to achieve the generation of "better" mo-DC.

The chemokine CXCL-4 is a powerful chemoattractant to monocytes and an important immunoregulator that has been shown to enhance the expression of MHC, CD86, and CD83 molecules by mo-DC of healthy donors, leading to more efficient antigen presentation, induction of $CD4^+$ and $CD8^+$ T cells proliferation and production of IFN-γ (249).

As mentioned before, IL-6 through the activation of STAT3 interferes with proper DC maturation and, indeed, in patients with colorectal cancer has been associated with poor $CD4^+$ T cells responses (207). Coherently, a phase-I study in ovarian cancer patients showed that, combined with chemotherapy, IL-6 blockade was safe and induced a series of positive modifications in immune parameters of the treated patients, including increases in IL-12, IL-1β, TNF-α, and IFN-γ secretion (250).

Besides targeting the negative regulators of DC activation, it is possible to overcome this phenomenon by changing the activating signals delivered to these cells. Following this line of research, a cocktail of inflammatory cytokines (TNF-α, IL-1β, poly I:C, IFN-α, and IFN-γ) has been tested for mo-DC maturation and was shown to increase their IL-12 production and their ability to prime melanoma-antigens-specific T cells *in vitro* (251). This mo-DC activating cocktail, in a vaccination study of 22 recurrent glioma patients, was associated with increases in serum type 1 cytokines and chemokines, tumor-associated antigens-specific T cell responses and clinical benefit in 9 patients (252).

Another approach is based on the use of adjuvants to boost the immune response. Among these, GM-CSF used in vaccines as GVAX (253) and STINGVAX (254) and, even TLR agonists (255), may be more effective for cell maturation. Other adjuvants could be listed, as for example, aluminum salts (256) (an inflammasome activator), and montanide (257) (an equivalent to incomplete Freund's adjuvant). Those adjuvants may boost responses due to physical effects upon antigens and cells, but also enhance DC activation. Nonetheless, the consideration of such a heterogeneous group of substances is enough to realize that adjuvant research is a rich field that may broaden the applicability and enhance the effectiveness of DC-based vaccination (258).

A different pathway to improve the effectiveness of DC-based therapy focuses on the selection of the immunizing antigens. In cancer, the mapping of a patient's set of neoantigens and use thereof would represent the epitome of personalized medicine. Though very tempting, this approach would still have its drawbacks, a significant one being the fact that not all tumors express immunogenic neoantigens (259), not to mention the cost that such strategy would impose on any health care system. Nevertheless, its feasibility and efficacy has already been demonstrated in an elegant study (260) where personalized vaccines were prepared for 6 melanoma patients. Whole-exome sequencing of their tumors allowed the identification of the mutated antigens from which a set of peptides was selected and synthesized so that they would be presented in the context of MHC-I. Four patients presented complete clinical responses to the vaccine alone and the other two, who had progressive disease after the vaccination, experienced complete responses after treatment with anti-PD-1. Curiously, in spite of the selection of MHC-I selective peptides, both CD4+ and CD8+ antigen-specific T cells were stimulated, with a predominance of CD4+ T cell responses. This observation illustrates very well how much "real life" immune responses still differ from our predictions.

Another ingenious strategy bypasses many of the known hurdles to exploit the immunogenic potential of DC. This approach aims to deliver RNA-containing nanoparticles systemically, which due to their lipid composition would be preferentially captured by DC and, then, release the RNA encoding the selected antigen(s) to be synthesized and presented. In a murine model, this approach lead, indeed, to DC maturation, IFN-α production and strong antigen-specific immune responses, which were effective in a series of tumor models (261). Accordingly, this strategy is under investigation in a clinical trial (NCT02410733) for patients with advanced melanoma.

Combination Treatments Including mo-DC

Chemotherapy and radiotherapy, together with surgery, still remain as the main pillars of cancer therapy. Since chemotherapy in general was formerly considered immunosuppressive, little attention was given to the fact that this is not always true. Indeed, some drugs might potentiate the anti-tumor immune response, by inducing the now recognized "immunogenic cell death" (262, 263). However, due to the frequently observed cancer patients' DC dysfunctions, the simple immunogenic death may not be enough to disrupt the tumor-favoring status of the immune response in patients. To achieve that, active immune interventions may be necessary to take advantage of the phenomenon. Indeed, a series of studies, both experimental and in humans, has been addressing this issue with promising results (264–266).

Radiation may also favor the induction of anti-tumor immune responses and, as with chemotherapy, there are plenty of data indicating a beneficial effect of its combination with cancer vaccines or other immune-stimulating strategies in different settings, including hepatocellular carcinoma (267), prostate cancer (268), lymphoma (269), and glioblastoma (270). Currently, the potential of such combinations are under scrutiny in a series of clinical trials for patients with such disparate diseases as anal (NCT01671488), lung (NCT01579188) and pancreatic cancer (NCT01072981) (271).

The disparity of the diseases mentioned at the previous paragraphs is a good indicator of the contrast between therapeutic strategies directed against the tumor cell and those targeting the immune system. Those that aim at the tumor cell will differ significantly from one tumor to the other, since each tumor has its own set of genetic changes and will respond differently to a given treatment. On the other hand, strategies that target the immune system, though still dealing with a very complex set of interactions, will face, very frequently, standard responses of the immune system to the perturbations caused by the presence of the tumor, regardless of the tumor's set of genetic mutations.

Actually, the realization of this scenario and the better understanding of the immune system and its interactions with tumors opened the way to a very attractive and successful approach for cancer immunotherapy: instead of targeting directly the tumor, one could target the immune regulatory mechanisms that allow a frequently immunogenic tumor to grow in an otherwise immunocompetent host. With this, the "checkpoint inhibitors era" started and achieved unprecedented good clinical results (272), leading to this 2018's award of the Nobel Prize in Medicine for James Allison and Tasuku Honjo for their work in this area.

However, after the initial excitement and even after the inclusion of other checkpoint inhibitors among the available armamentarium against cancer, it is necessary to appreciate that not all patients will respond to this approach, since it needs an existing response, kept in check and "waiting" to be released by the treatment. On the other hand, it is quite possible that the frequently unsatisfactory response to cancer vaccines is caused by the pre-existence or vaccine-induced activation of these same regulatory circuits. Hence, a coherent path to achieve better clinical results would be the combination of both immune modulating strategies. Indeed, experimental (273) and clinical data (274) suggest that this may be true. In the aforementioned clinical study, patients with advanced melanoma were treated with a combination of MART-1-peptide pulsed-DC and anti-CTLA-4 and the results indicated that the combination might be, indeed, more effective than either approach alone. Likewise, also in the PD-1/PD-L1-PD-L2 pathway (275, 276) the combination of DC vaccination with checkpoint inhibition may offer, at least theoretical, advantages.

A different set of combination treatments has been targeting immune modulatory enzymes. The enzyme indoleamine 2,3-dioxygenase (IDO) catalyzes the degradation of tryptophan contributing to tolerance induction by favoring regulatory T cell differentiation and reducing DC activity (277). IDO expression by DC is induced by inflammatory stimuli (278), but also by CTLA-4 and PD-1 (279). Accordingly, IDO inhibition has shown positive effects in murine models of pancreatic cancer (280) and a study combining IDO inhibitors with DC vaccines for breast cancer patients has completed recruitment (NCT01042535). Similarly, an inhibitor of BCR-ABL, SRC, c-KIT, PDGFR, and ephrin tyrosine kinases has shown synergistic effects with a DC vaccine in a mouse melanoma model (281) and this combination is the object of ongoing clinical trials in patients with melanoma (NCT01876212) and metastatic renal cells carcinoma (NCT02432846 phase II e NCT01582672 phase III). Arginase-1, an enzyme that regulates cell proliferation and is constitutively expressed by myeloid-derived suppressor cells (MDSC) (282) and cyclooxygenase-2 (COX2), are other two enzyme whose inhibition might have positive interactions with immunotherapeutic approaches, including those that exploit DC.

CONCLUDING REMARKS

Dendritic cells have a central role in the immune system homeostasis and are directly involved in defining the patterns of response the system develops when facing an antigenic challenge. Their normal function warrants protection against infections, possibly cancer, but also against autoimmunity and hypersensitivity reactions. The more is uncovered of the mechanisms that drive these cells to modulate the response in one way or another, the more tools will be available to direct the immune system to desired therapeutic outcomes. Today, much of the efforts and clinical results are focused into harnessing these cells to induce effector responses, mainly, but not only, in cancer. With the advancement of the understanding of their physiology and regulatory pathways, it is possible to predict their effective use in such opposing conditions as cancer and diabetes, with less untoward and more durable effects.

AUTHOR CONTRIBUTIONS

TP, MP, AO, and GE reviewed the literature and wrote the manuscript. PB-S revised the literature and the manuscript and JB designed, wrote and revised the manuscript.

REFERENCES

1. Steinman RM, Cohn ZA. Identification of a novel cell type in peripheral lymphoid organs of mice. I. Morphology, quantitation, tissue distribution. *J Exp Med.* (1973) 137:1142–62.
2. Steinman RM, Idoyaga J. Features of the dendritic cell lineage. *Immunol Rev.* (2010) 234:5–17. doi: 10.1111/j.0105-2896.2009.00888.x
3. Steinman RM, Witmer MD. Lymphoid dendritic cells are potent stimulators of the primary mixed leukocyte reaction in mice. *Proc Natl Acad Sci USA.* (1978) 75:5132–6.
4. Banchereau J, Briere F, Caux C, Davoust J, Lebecque S, Liu YJ, et al. Immunobiology of dendritic cells. *Annu Rev Immunol.* (2000) 18:767–811. doi: 10.1146/annurev.immunol.18.1.767
5. Carlens J, Wahl B, Ballmaier M, Bulfone-Paus S, Förster R, Pabst O. Common γ-chain-dependent signals confer selective survival of eosinophils in the murine small intestine. *J Immunol.* (2009) 183:5600–7. doi: 10.4049/jimmunol.0801581
6. Drutman SB, Kendall JC, Trombetta ES. Inflammatory spleen monocytes can upregulate CD11c expression without converting into dendritic cells. *J Immunol.* (2012) 188:3603–10. doi: 10.4049/jimmunol.1102741
7. Hebel K, Griewank K, Inamine A, Chang HD, Hilke BM, Fillatreau S, et al. Plasma cell differentiation in T-independent type 2 immune responses is independent of CD11chigh dendritic cells. *Eur J Immunol.* (2006) 36:2912–9. doi: 10.1002/eji.200636356
8. Hochweller K, Striegler J, Hämmerling GJ, Garbi N. A novel CD11c.DTR transgenic mouse for depletion of dendritic cells reveals their requirement for homeostatic proliferation of natural killer cells. *Eur J Immunol.* (2008) 38:2776–83. doi: 10.1002/eji.200838659
9. Huleatt JW, Lefrançois L. Antigen-driven induction of CD11c on intestinal intraepithelial lymphocytes and CD8+ T cells *in vivo*. *J Immunol.* (1995) 154:5684–93.
10. Rubtsov AV, Rubtsova K, Fischer A, Meehan RT, Gillis JZ, Kappler JW, et al. Toll-like receptor 7 (TLR7)–driven accumulation of a novel CD11c+ B-cell population is important for the development of autoimmunity. *Blood* (2011) 118:1305–15. doi: 10.1182/blood-2011-01-331462
11. Probst HC, Tschannen K, Odermatt B, Schwendener R, Zinkernagel RM, Van Den Broek M. Histological analysis of CD11c-DTR/GFP mice after *in vivo* depletion of dendritic cells. *Clin Exp Immunol.* (2005) 141:398–404. doi: 10.1111/j.1365-2249.2005.02868.x
12. Vermaelen K, Pauwels R. Accurate and simple discrimination of mouse pulmonary dendritic cell and macrophage populations by flow cytometry: methodology and new insights. *Cytometry* (2004) 61A:170–7. doi: 10.1002/cyto.a.20064
13. Delamarre L, Pack M, Chang H, Mellman I, Trombetta ES. Differential lysosomal proteolysis in antigen-presenting cells determines antigen fate. *Science* (2005) 307:1630–4. doi: 10.1126/science.1108003
14. Geissmann F, Manz MG, Jung S, Sieweke MH. Development of monocytes, macrophages, and dendritic cells. *Science* (2010) 327:656–61. doi: 10.1126/science.1178331
15. van Montfoort N, Camps MG, Khan S, Filippov DV, Weterings JJ, Griffith JM, et al. Antigen storage compartments in mature dendritic cells facilitate prolonged cytotoxic T lymphocyte cross-priming capacity. *Proc Natl Acad Sci USA.* (2009) 106:6730–5. doi: 10.1073/pnas.0900969106
16. Haniffa M, Collin M, Ginhoux F. Ontogeny and functional specialization of dendritic cells in human and mouse. (2013) 120:1–49. doi: 10.1016/B978-0-12-417028-5.00001-6
17. Hashimoto D, Chow A, Noizat C, Teo P, Beasley MB, Leboeuf M, et al. Tissue-resident macrophages self-maintain locally throughout adult life with minimal contribution from circulating monocytes. *Immunity* (2013) 38:792–804. doi: 10.1016/j.immuni.2013.04.004
18. Hettinger J, Richards DM, Hansson J, Barra MM, Joschko A-C, Krijgsveld J, et al. Origin of monocytes and macrophages in a committed progenitor. *Nat Immunol.* (2013) 14:821–30. doi: 10.1038/ni.2638
19. McGovern N, Schlitzer A, Gunawan M, Jardine L, Shin A, Poyner E, et al. Human dermal CD14? cells are a transient population

of monocyte-derived macrophages. *Immunity* (2014) 41:465–77. doi: 10.1016/j.immuni.2014.08.006

20. Naik SH, Perié L, Swart E, Gerlach C, van Rooij N, de Boer RJ, et al. Diverse and heritable lineage imprinting of early haematopoietic progenitors. *Nature Publish Group* (2013) 496:229–32. doi: 10.1038/nature12013
21. Schulz C, Gomez Perdiguero E, Chorro L, Szabo-Rogers H, Cagnard N, Kierdorf K, et al. A lineage of myeloid cells independent of Myb and hematopoietic stem cells. *Science* (2012) 336:86–90. doi: 10.1126/science.1219179
22. Schraml BU, van Blijswijk J, Zelenay S, Whitney PG, Filby A, Acton SE, et al. Genetic tracing via DNGR-1 expression history defines dendritic cells as a hematopoietic lineage. *Cell* (2013) 154:843–58. doi: 10.1016/j.cell.2013.07.014
23. Wang J, Dai X, Hsu C, Ming C, He Y, Zhang J, Wei L, et al. Discrimination of the heterogeneity of bone marrow-derived dendritic cells. *Mol Med Rep.* (2017) 16:6787–93. doi: 10.3892/mmr.2017.7448
24. Yona S, Kim K-W, Wolf Y, Mildner A, Varol D, Breker M, et al. Fate mapping reveals origins and dynamics of monocytes and tissue macrophages under homeostasis. *Immunity* (2013) 38:79–91. doi: 10.1016/j.immuni.2012.12.001
25. O'Keeffe M, Mok WH, Radford KJ. Human dendritic cell subsets and function in health and disease. *Cell Mol Life Sci.* (2015) 72:1–17. doi: 10.1007/s00018-015-2005-0
26. Hermans IF, Silk JD, Gileadi U, Salio M, Mathew B, Ritter G, et al. NKT cells enhance CD4+ and CD8+ T cell responses to soluble antigen *in vivo* through direct interaction with dendritic cells. *J Immunol.* (2003) 171:5140–7. doi: 10.4049/jimmunol.171.10.5140
27. Münz C, Steinman RM, Fujii S-I. Dendritic cell maturation by innate lymphocytes: coordinated stimulation of innate and adaptive immunity. *J Exp Med.* (2005) 202:203–7. doi: 10.1084/jem.20050810
28. Smyth MJ, Crowe NY, Hayakawa Y, Takeda K, Yagita H, Godfrey DI. NKT cells - conductors of tumor immunity? *Curr Opin Immunol.* (2002) 14:165–71. doi: 10.1016/S0952-7915(02)00316-3
29. Halim TYF, Hwang YY, Scanlon ST, Zaghouani H, Garbi N, Fallon PG, et al. Group 2 innate lymphoid cells license dendritic cells to potentiate memory TH2 cell responses. *Nat Immunol.* (2016) 17:57–64. doi: 10.1038/ni.3294
30. Hawiger D, Inaba K, Dorsett Y, Guo M, Mahnke K, Rivera M, et al. Dendritic cells induce peripheral T cell unresponsiveness under steady state conditions *in vivo*. *J Exp Med.* (2001) 194:769–79. doi: 10.1084/jem.194.6.769
31. Steinman RM, Hawiger D, Liu K, Bonifaz L, Bonnyay D, Mahnke K, et al. Dendritic cell function *in vivo* during the steady state: a role in peripheral tolerance. *Ann NY Acad Sci.* (2003) 987:15–25. doi: 10.1111/j.1749-6632.2003.tb06029.x
32. Worbs T, Hammerschmidt SI, Förster R. Dendritic cell migration in health and disease. *Nat Rev Immunol.* (2017) 17:30–48. doi: 10.1038/nri.2016.116
33. Hemmi H, Akira S. TLR signalling and the function of dendritic cells. *Chem Immunol Aller.* (2005) 86:120–135. doi: 10.1159/000086657
34. Cerboni S, Gentili M, Manel N. Diversity of pathogen sensors in dendritic cells. *Adv Immunol.* (2013) 120:211–237. doi: 10.1016/B978-0-12-417028-5.00008-9
35. Alvarez D, Vollmann EH, Andrian von UH. Mechanisms and consequences of dendritic cell migration. *Immunity* (2008) 29:325–42. doi: 10.1016/j.immuni.2008.08.006
36. Dong H, Bullock TNJ. Metabolic influences that regulate dendritic cell function in tumors. *Front Immunol.* (2014) 5:24. doi: 10.3389/fimmu.2014.00024
37. Friedl P, Gunzer M. Interaction of T cells with APCs: the serial encounter model. *Trends Immunol.* (2001) 22:187–91. doi: 10.1016/S1471-4906(01)01869-5
38. Henderson RA, Watkins SC, Flynn JL. Activation of human dendritic cells following infection with *Mycobacterium tuberculosis*. *J Immunol.* (1997) 159:635–43.
39. Randolph GJ, Angeli V, Swartz MA. Dendritic-cell trafficking to lymph nodes through lymphatic vessels. *Nature Rev Immunol.* (2005) 5:617–28. doi: 10.1038/nri1670
40. Imai Y, Yamakawa M, Kasajima T. The lymphocyte-dendritic cell system. *Histol Histopathol.* (1998) 13:469–510.
41. Winzler C, Rovere P, Rescigno M, Granucci F, Penna G, Adorini L, et al. Maturation stages of mouse dendritic cells in growth factor-dependent long-term cultures. *J Exp Med.* (1997) 185:317–28.
42. Reis e Sousa C. Dendritic cells in a mature age. *Nature Rev Immunol.* (2006) 6:476–83. doi: 10.1038/nri1845
43. Steinman RM. Decisions about dendritic cells: past, present, and future. *Annu Rev Immunol.* (2012) 30:1–22. doi: 10.1146/annurev-immunol-100311-102839
44. Trombetta ES, Mellman I. Cell biology of antigen processing *in vitro* and *in vivo*. *Annu Rev Immunol.* (2005) 23:975–1028. doi: 10.1146/annurev.immunol.22.012703.104538
45. Förster R, Schubel A, Breitfeld D, Kremmer E, Renner-Müller I, Wolf E, et al. CCR7 coordinates the primary immune response by establishing functional microenvironments in secondary lymphoid organs. *Cell* (1999) 99:23–33.
46. Ohl L, Mohaupt M, Czeloth N, Hintzen G, Kiafard Z, Zwirner J, et al. CCR7 governs skin dendritic cell migration under inflammatory and steady-state conditions. *Immunity* (2004) 21:279–88. doi: 10.1016/j.immuni.2004.06.014
47. Sallusto F, Schaerli P, Loetscher P, Schaniel C, Lenig D, Mackay CR, et al. Rapid and coordinated switch in chemokine receptor expression during dendritic cell maturation. *Eur J Immunol.* (1998) 28:2760–9. doi: 10.1002/(SICI)1521-4141(199809)28:09<2760::AID-IMMU2760>3.0.CO;2-N
48. Steinman RM. The control of immunity and tolerance by dendritic cell. *Pathol Biol.* (2003) 51:59–60. doi: 10.1016/S0369-8114(03)00096-8
49. Caux C, Massacrier C, Vanbervliet B, Dubois B, Van Kooten C, Durand I, et al. Activation of human dendritic cells through CD40 cross-linking. *J Exp Med.* (1994) 180:1263–72.
50. Jensen SS, Gad M. Differential induction of inflammatory cytokines by dendritic cells treated with novel TLR-agonist and cytokine based cocktails: targeting dendritic cells in autoimmunity. *J Inflamm (Lond)* (2010) 7:37. doi: 10.1186/1476-9255-7-37
51. Tan JKH, O'Neill HC. Maturation requirements for dendritic cells in T cell stimulation leading to tolerance versus immunity. *J Leukocyte Biol.* (2005) 78:319–324. doi: 10.1189/jlb.1104664
52. Iwasaki A, Medzhitov R. Control of adaptive immunity by the innate immune system. *Nat Immunol.* (2015) 16:343–353. doi: 10.1038/ni.3123
53. Luft T, Rodionova E, Maraskovsky E, Kirsch M, Hess M, Buchholtz C, et al. Adaptive functional differentiation of dendritic cells: integrating the network of extra- and intracellular signals. *Blood* (2006) 107:4763–9. doi: 10.1182/blood-2005-04-1501
54. Jonuleit H, Knop J, Enk AH. Cytokines and their effects on maturation, differentiation and migration of dendritic cells. *Arch Dermatol Res.* (1996) 289:1–8.
55. Amsen D, Blander JM, Lee GR, Tanigaki K, Honjo T, Flavell RA. Instruction of distinct CD4 T helper cell fates by different notch ligands on antigen-presenting cells. *Cell* (2004) 117:515–26. doi: 10.1038/nri1402
56. Constant S, Pfeiffer C, Woodard A, Pasqualini T, Bottomly K. Extent of T cell receptor ligation can determine the functional differentiation of naive CD4+ T cells. *J Exp Med* (1995) 182:1591–6.
57. Hosken NA, Shibuya K, Heath AW, Murphy KM, O'Garra A. The effect of antigen dose on CD4+ T helper cell phenotype development in a T cell receptor-alpha beta-transgenic model. *J Exp Med.* (1995) 182:1579–84.
58. Kadowaki N. Dendritic cells: a conductor of T cell differentiation. *Allergol Int.* (2007) 56:193–9. doi: 10.2332/allergolint.R-07-146
59. Maekawa Y, Tsukumo S-I, Chiba S, Hirai H, Hayashi Y, Okada H, et al. Delta1-Notch3 interactions bias the functional differentiation of activated CD4+ T cells. *Immunity* (2003) 19:549–59. doi: 10.1016/S1074-7613(03)00270-X
60. Pulendran B, Smith JL, Caspary G, Brasel K, Pettit D, Maraskovsky E, et al. Distinct dendritic cell subsets differentially regulate the class of immune response *in vivo*. *Proc Natl Acad Sci USA.* (1999) 96:1036–41.
61. Jenkins SJ, Perona-Wright G, Worsley AGF, Ishii N, MacDonald AS. Dendritic cell expression of OX40 ligand acts as a costimulatory, not polarizing, signal for optimal Th2 priming and memory induction *in vivo*. *J Immunol.* (2007) 179:3515–23. doi: 10.4049/jimmunol.179.6.3515
62. Soumelis V, Reche PA, Kanzler H, Yuan W, Edward G, Homey B, et al. Human epithelial cells trigger dendritic cell mediated allergic inflammation by producing TSLP. *Nat Immunol.* (2002) 3:673–680. doi: 10.1038/ni805

63. Bailey SL, Schreiner B, McMahon EJ, Miller SD. CNS myeloid DCs presenting endogenous myelin peptides "preferentially" polarize CD4+ T(H)-17 cells in relapsing EAE. *Nat Immunol.* (2007) 8:172–80. doi: 10.1038/ni1430
64. Iezzi G, Sonderegger I, Ampenberger F, Schmitz N, Marsland BJ, Kopf M. CD40-CD40L cross-talk integrates strong antigenic signals and microbial stimuli to induce development of IL-17-producing CD4+ T cells. *Proc Natl Acad Sci USA.* (2009) 106:876–81. doi: 10.1073/pnas.08107 69106
65. Huang G, Wang Y, Chi H. Regulation of TH17 cell differentiation by innate immune signals. *Cell Mol Immunol.* (2012) 9:287–95. doi: 10.1038/cmi.2012.10
66. Levings MK, Gregori S, Tresoldi E, Cazzaniga S, Bonini C, Roncarolo MG. Differentiation of Tr1 cells by immature dendritic cells requires IL-10 but not CD25+CD4+ Tr cells. *Blood* (2005) 105:1162–9. doi: 10.1182/blood-2004-03-1211
67. Rescigno M. Dendritic cell-epithelial cell crosstalk in the gut. *Immunol Rev.* (2014) 260:118–28. doi: 10.1111/imr.12181
68. Vega-Ramos J, Roquilly A, Asehnoune K, Villadangos JA. Modulation of dendritic cell antigen presentation by pathogens, tissue damage and secondary inflammatory signals. *Curr Opin Pharmacol.* (2014) 17:64–70. doi: 10.1016/j.coph.2014.07.013
69. Na H, Cho M, Chung Y. Regulation of Th2 cell immunity by dendritic cells. *Immune Netw.* (2016) 16:1–12. doi: 10.4110/in.2016.16.1.1
70. Coulon P-G, Richetta C, Rouers A, Blanchet FP, Urrutia A, Guerbois M, et al. HIV-infected dendritic cells present endogenous MHC class II-restricted antigens to HIV-specific CD4+ T cells. *J Immunol.* (2016) 197:517–32. doi: 10.4049/jimmunol.1600286
71. Delamarre L, Mellman I. Harnessing dendritic cells for immunotherapy. *Semin Immunol.* (2011) 23:2–11. doi: 10.1016/j.smim.2011.02.001
72. Jung S, Unutmaz D, Wong P, Sano G-I, De los Santos K, Sparwasser T, et al. *In vivo* depletion of CD11c+ dendritic cells abrogates priming of CD8+ T cells by exogenous cell-associated antigens. *Immunity* (2002) 17:211–20. doi: 10.1016/S1074-7613(02)00365-5
73. Segura E, Amigorena S. Cross-presentation in mouse and human dendritic cells. *Adv Immunol.* (2015) 127:1–31. doi: 10.1016/bs.ai.2015.03.002
74. Segura E, Villadangos JA. Antigen presentation by dendritic cells *in vivo*. *Curr Opin Immunol.* (2009) 21:105–110. doi: 10.1016/j.coi.2009.03.011
75. Bevan MJ. Cross-priming for a secondary cytotoxic response to minor H antigens with H-2 congenic cells which do not cross-react in the cytotoxic assay. *J Exp Med.* (1976) 143:1283–8.
76. Bevan MJ. Cross-priming for a secondary cytotoxic response to minor H antigens with H-2 congenic cells which do not cross-react in the cytotoxic assay. *J Exp Med.* (1976) 143:1283–8.
77. Sánchez-Paulete AR, Teijeira A, Cueto FJ, Garasa S, Pérez-Gracia JL, et al. Antigen cross-presentation and T-cell cross-priming in cancer immunology and immunotherapy. *Ann Oncol.* (2017) 28:xii74. doi: 10.1093/annonc/mdx727
78. McCoy KD, Hermans IF, Fraser JH, Le Gros G, Ronchese F. Cytotoxic T lymphocyte-associated antigen 4 (CTLA-4) can regulate dendritic cell-induced activation and cytotoxicity of CD8(+) T cells independently of CD4(+) T cell help. *J Exp Med.* (1999) 189:1157–62.
79. Young JW, Steinman RM. Dendritic cells stimulate primary human cytolytic lymphocyte responses in the absence of CD4+ helper T cells. *J Exp Med.* (1990) 171:1315–32.
80. Kurts C, Kosaka H, Carbone FR, Miller JF, Heath WR. Class I-restricted cross-presentation of exogenous self-antigens leads to deletion of autoreactive CD8(+) T cells. *J Exp Med.* (1997) 186:239–45.
81. Rock KL, Shen L. Cross-presentation: underlying mechanisms and role in immune surveillance. *Immunol Rev.* (2005) 207:166–83. doi: 10.1111/j.0105-2896.2005.00301.x
82. Steinman RM, Swanson J. The endocytic activity of dendritic cells. *J Exp Med.* (1995) 182:283–8.
83. Geijtenbeek TB, Torensma R, van Vliet SJ, van Duijnhoven GC, Adema GJ, van Kooyk Y, et al. Identification of DC-SIGN, a novel dendritic cell-specific ICAM-3 receptor that supports primary immune responses. *Cell* (2000) 100:575–585. doi: 10.1016/S0092-8674(00)80693-5
84. Sallusto F, Cella M, Danieli C, Lanzavecchia A. Dendritic cells use macropinocytosis and the mannose receptor to concentrate macromolecules in the major histocompatibility complex class II compartment: downregulation by cytokines and bacterial products. *J Exp Med.* (1995) 182:389–400.
85. Valladeau J, Ravel O, Dezutter-Dambuyant C, Moore K, Kleijmeer M, Liu Y, et al. Langerin, a novel C-type lectin specific to Langerhans cells, is an endocytic receptor that induces the formation of Birbeck granules. *Immunity* (2000) 12:71–81. doi: 10.1016/S1074-7613(00)80160-0
86. Keller R, Gehri R, Keist R. Macrophage response to viruses, protozoa, and fungi: secretory and cellular activities induced in resting unprimed bone marrow-derived mononuclear phagocytes. *Cell Immunol.* (1994) 159:323–30. doi: 10.1006/cimm.1994.1318
87. Medzhitov R, Preston-Hurlburt P, Janeway CA. A human homologue of the Drosophila Toll protein signals activation of adaptive immunity. *Nature* (1997) 388:394–7. doi: 10.1038/41131
88. Muzio M, Bosisio D, Polentarutti N, D'amico G, Stoppacciaro A, Mancinelli R, et al. Differential expression and regulation of toll-like receptors (TLR) in human leukocytes: selective expression of TLR3 in dendritic cells. *J Immunol.* (2000) 164:5998–6004. doi: 10.4049/jimmunol.164.11.5998
89. Rescigno M, Granucci F, Ricciardi-Castagnoli P. Molecular events of bacterial-induced maturation of dendritic cells. *J Clin Immunol* (2000) 20:161–166. doi: 10.1023/A:1006629328178
90. Wilson NS, El-Sukkari D, Villadangos JA. Dendritic cells constitutively present self antigens in their immature state *in vivo* and regulate antigen presentation by controlling the rates of MHC class II synthesis and endocytosis. *Blood* (2004) 103:2187–95. doi: 10.1182/blood-2003-08-2729
91. Albert ML, Sauter B, Bhardwaj N. Dendritic cells acquire antigen from apoptotic cells and induce class I-restricted CTLs. *Nature* (1998) 392:86–9. doi: 10.1038/32183
92. Castellano G, Woltman AM, Schena FP, Roos A, Daha MR, van Kooten C. Dendritic cells and complement: at the cross road of innate and adaptive immunity. *Mol Immunol.* (2004) 41:133–40. doi: 10.1016/j.molimm.2004.03.018
93. Deluce-Kakwata-Nkor N, Lamendour L, Chabot V, Héraud A, Ivanovic Z, Halary F, et al. Differentiation of human dendritic cell subsets for immune tolerance induction. *Transfus Clin Biol.* (2018) 25:90–5. doi: 10.1016/j.tracli.2017.08.002
94. Liu J, Cao X. Regulatory dendritic cells in autoimmunity: a comprehensive review. *J Autoimmun.* (2015) 63:1–12. doi: 10.1016/j.jaut.2015.07.011
95. Shiokawa A, Kotaki R, Takano T, Nakajima-Adachi H, Hachimura S. Mesenteric lymph node CD11b- CD103+ PD-L1High dendritic cells highly induce regulatory T cells. *Immunology* (2017) 152:52–64. doi: 10.1111/imm.12747
96. Huang FP, Platt N, Wykes M, Major JR, Powell TJ, Jenkins CD, et al. A discrete subpopulation of dendritic cells transports apoptotic intestinal epithelial cells to T cell areas of mesenteric lymph nodes. *J Exp Med.* (2000) 191:435–44. doi: 10.1084/jem.191.3.435
97. Steinman RM, Turley S, Mellman I, Inaba K. The induction of tolerance by dendritic cells that have captured apoptotic cells. *J Exp Med.* (2000) 191:411–416. doi: 10.1084/jem.191.3.411
98. Liu K, Iyoda T, Saternus M, Kimura Y, Inaba K, Steinman RM. Immune tolerance after delivery of dying cells to dendritic cells *in situ*. *J Exp Med.* (2002) 196:1091–1097. doi: 10.1084/jem.20021215
99. Stuart LM, Lucas M, Simpson C, Lamb J, Savill J, Lacy-Hulbert A. Inhibitory effects of apoptotic cell ingestion upon endotoxin-driven myeloid dendritic cell maturation. *J Immunol.* (2002) 168:1627–35. doi: 10.4049/jimmunol.168.4.1627
100. Wallet MA, Sen P, Flores RR, Wang Y, Yi Z, Huang Y, et al. MerTK is required for apoptotic cell-induced T cell tolerance. *J Exper Med.* (2008) 205:219–32. doi: 10.1084/jem.20062293
101. Hong J, Gu X-D, Xiang J-B, Zhang Z, Zang Y-W, Zhang Q-H, et al. Recipient dendritic cells modified by RNA interference targeting CD80 and CD86 elicit T cell hyporesponsiveness via enhanced T cell apoptosis. *Chin Med J.* (2013) 126:2139–44.
102. Manicassamy S, Pulendran B. Dendritic cell control of tolerogenic responses. *Immunol Rev.* (2011) 241:206–27. doi: 10.1111/j.1600-065X.2011.01015.x

103. Zhu H-C, Qiu T, Liu X-H, Dong W-C, Weng X-D, Hu C-H, et al. Tolerogenic dendritic cells generated by RelB silencing using shRNA prevent acute rejection. *Cell Immunol.* (2012) 274:12–8. doi: 10.1016/j.cellimm.2012.02.012
104. Saito M, Nagasawa M, Takada H, Hara T, Tsuchiya S, Agematsu K, et al. Defective IL-10 signaling in hyper-IgE syndrome results in impaired generation of tolerogenic dendritic cells and induced regulatory T cells. *J Exper Med.* (2011) 208:235–49. doi: 10.1084/jem.20100799
105. Sela U, Park CG, Park A, Olds P, Wang S, Steinman RM, et al. Dendritic cells induce a subpopulation of IL-12Rβ2-Expressing treg that specifically consumes IL-12 to control Th1 responses. *PLoS ONE* (2016) 11:e0146412. doi: 10.1371/journal.pone.0146412
106. Grohmann U, Orabona C, Fallarino F, Vacca C, Calcinaro F, Falorni A, et al. CTLA-4-Ig regulates tryptophan catabolism *in vivo*. *Nat Immunol.* (2002) 3:1097–101. doi: 10.1038/ni846
107. Morelli AE, Thomson AW. Tolerogenic dendritic cells and the quest for transplant tolerance. *Nature Rev Immunol.* (2007) 7:610–21. doi: 10.1038/nri2132
108. Sakaguchi S, Miyara M, Costantino CM, Hafler DA. FOXP3+ regulatory T cells in the human immune system. *Nat Rev Immunol.* (2010) 10:490–500. doi: 10.1038/nri2785
109. Idoyaga J, Fiorese C, Zbytnuik L, Lubkin A, Miller J, Malissen B, et al. Specialized role of migratory dendritic cells in peripheral tolerance induction. *J Clin Invest.* (2013) 123:844–54. doi: 10.1172/JCI65260
110. Mahnke K, Qian Y, Knop J, Enk AH. Induction of CD4+/CD25+ regulatory T cells by targeting of antigens to immature dendritic cells. *Blood* (2003) 101:4862–9. doi: 10.1182/blood-2002-10-3229
111. Yates SF, Paterson AM, Nolan KF, Cobbold SP, Saunders NJ, Waldmann H, et al. Induction of regulatory T cells and dominant tolerance by dendritic cells incapable of full activation. *J Immunol* (2007) 179:967–76. doi: 10.4049/jimmunol.179.2.967
112. Yogev N, Frommer F, Lukas D, Kautz-Neu K, Karram K, Ielo D, et al. Dendritic cells ameliorate autoimmunity in the CNS by controlling the homeostasis of PD-1 receptor(+) regulatory T cells. *Immunity* (2012) 37:264–75. doi: 10.1016/j.immuni.2012.05.025
113. Campanelli AP, Roselino AM, Cavassani KA, Pereira MSF, Mortara RA, Brodskyn CI, et al. CD4+CD25+ T cells in skin lesions of patients with cutaneous leishmaniasis exhibit phenotypic and functional characteristics of natural regulatory T cells. *J Infect Dis.* (2006) 193:1313–22. doi: 10.1086/502980
114. Montagnoli C, Bacci A, Bozza S, Gaziano R, Mosci P, Sharpe AH, et al. B7/CD28-dependent CD4+CD25+ regulatory T cells are essential components of the memory-protective immunity to *Candida albicans*. *J Immunol.* (2002) 169:6298–308. doi: 10.4049/jimmunol.169.11.6298
115. Baleeiro RB, Anselmo LB, Soares FA, Pinto CAL, Ramos O, Gross JL, et al. High frequency of immature dendritic cells and altered in situ production of interleukin-4 and tumor necrosis factor-α in lung cancer. *Cancer Immunol Immunother* (2008) 57:1335–45. doi: 10.1007/s00262-008-0468-7
116. Almand B, Resser JR, Lindman B, Nadaf S, Clark JI, Kwon ED, et al. Clinical significance of defective dendritic cell differentiation in cancer. *Clin Cancer Res.* (2000) 6:1755–66.
117. Bella SD, Gennaro M, Vaccari M, Ferraris C, Nicola S, Riva A, et al. Altered maturation of peripheral blood dendritic cells in patients with breast cancer. *Br J Cancer* (2003) 89:1463–72. doi: 10.1038/sj.bjc.6601243
118. Dunn GP, Old LJ, Schreiber RD. The immunobiology of cancer immunosurveillance and immunoediting. *Immunity* (2004) 21:137–48. doi: 10.1016/j.immuni.2004.07.017
119. Johnson DJ, Ohashi PS. Molecular programming of steady-state dendritic cells: impact on autoimmunity and tumor immune surveillance. *Anna NY Acad Sci.* (2013) 1284:46–51. doi: 10.1111/nyas.12114
120. Vicari AP, Caux C, Trinchieri G. Tumour escape from immune surveillance through dendritic cell inactivation. *Semin Cancer Biol.* (2002) 12:33–42. doi: 10.1006/scbi.2001.0400
121. Ardouin L, Luche H, Chelbi R, Carpentier S, Shawket A, Montanana Sanchis F, et al. Broad and largely concordant molecular changes characterize tolerogenic and immunogenic dendritic cell maturation in thymus and periphery. *Immunity* (2016) 45:305–18. doi: 10.1016/j.immuni.2016.07.019
122. George TC, Bilsborough J, Viney JL, Norment AM. High antigen dose and activated dendritic cells enable Th cells to escape regulatory T cell-mediated suppression *in vitro*. *Eur J Immunol.* (2003) 33:502–11. doi: 10.1002/immu.200310026
123. Gon Y, Asai Y, Hashimoto S, Mizumura K, Jibiki I, Machino T, et al. A20 inhibits toll-like receptor 2- and 4-mediated interleukin-8 synthesis in airway epithelial cells. *Am J Respir Cell Mol Biol.* (2004) 31:330–6. doi: 10.1165/rcmb.2003-0438OC
124. Hammer GE, Turer EE, Taylor KE, Fang CJ, Advincula R, Oshima S, et al. Expression of A20 by dendritic cells preserves immune homeostasis and prevents colitis and spondyloarthritis. *Nat Immunol.* (2011) 12:1184–93. doi: 10.1038/ni.2135
125. Kool M, van Loo G, Waelput W, De Prijck S, Muskens F, Sze M, et al. The ubiquitin-editing protein A20 prevents dendritic cell activation, recognition of apoptotic cells, and systemic autoimmunity. *Immunity* (2011) 35:82–96. doi: 10.1016/j.immuni.2011.05.013
126. Steinman RM. Dendritic cells and the control of immunity. *Nature* (1998) 392:245–52. doi: 10.1038/32588
127. Vremec D. The surface phenotype of dendritic cells purified from mouse thymus and spleen: investigation of the CD8 expression by a subpopulation of dendritic cells. *J Exp Med.* (1992) 176:47–58. doi: 10.1084/jem.176.1.47
128. Merad M, Sathe P, Helft J, Miller J, Mortha A. The dendritic cell lineage: ontogeny and function of dendritic cells and their subsets in the steady state and the inflamed setting. *Annu Rev Immunol.* (2013) 31:563–604. doi: 10.1146/annurev-immunol-020711-074950
129. Mildner A, Jung S. Development and function of dendritic cell subsets. *Immunity* (2014) 40:642–56. doi: 10.1016/j.immuni.2014.04.016
130. Guilliams M, Dutertre C-A, Scott CL, McGovern N, Sichien D, Chakarov S, et al. Unsupervised high-dimensional analysis aligns dendritic cells across tissues and species. *Immunity* (2016) 45:669–84. doi: 10.1016/j.immuni.2016.08.015
131. Granot T, Senda T, Carpenter DJ, Matsuoka N, Weiner J, Gordon CL, et al. Dendritic cells display subset and tissue-specific maturation dynamics over human life. *Immunity* (2017) 46:504–15. doi: 10.1016/j.immuni.2017.02.019
132. Reynolds G, Haniffa M. Human and mouse mononuclear phagocyte networks: a tale of two species? *Front Immunol.* (2015) 6:330. doi: 10.3389/fimmu.2015.00330
133. Breton G, Lee J, Zhou YJ, Schreiber JJ, Keler T, Puhr S, et al. Circulating precursors of human CD1c+ and CD141+ dendritic cells. *J Exp Med.* (2015) 212:401–13. doi: 10.1084/jem.20141441
134. Schlitzer A, Sivakamasundari V, Chen J, Bin Sumatoh HR, Schreuder J, Lum J, et al. Identification of cDC1- and cDC2-committed DC progenitors reveals early lineage priming at the common DC progenitor stage in the bone marrow. *Nat Immunol.* (2015) 16:1–13. doi: 10.1038/ni.3200
135. See P, Dutertre C-A, Chen J, Günther P, McGovern N, Irac SE, et al. Mapping the human DC lineage through the integration of high-dimensional techniques. *Science* (2017) 66:eaag3009. doi: 10.1126/science.aag3009
136. Heidkamp GF, Sander J, Lehmann CHK, Heger L, Eissing N, Baranska A, et al. Human lymphoid organ dendritic cell identity is predominantly dictated by ontogeny, not tissue microenvironment. *Sci Immunol.* (2016) 1:eaai7677. doi: 10.1126/sciimmunol.aai7677
137. Boltjes A, van Wijk F. Human dendritic cell functional specialization in steady-state and inflammation. *Front Immunol.* (2014) 5:131. doi: 10.3389/fimmu.2014.00131
138. Dzionek A, Fuchs A, Schmidt P, Cremer S, Zysk M, Miltenyi S, et al. BDCA-2, BDCA-3, and BDCA-4: three markers for distinct subsets of dendritic cells in human peripheral blood. *J Immunol.* (2000) 165:6037–46. doi: 10.4049/jimmunol.165.11.6037
139. Guilliams M, Ginhoux F, Jakubzick C, Naik SH, Onai N, Schraml BU, et al. Dendritic cells, monocytes and macrophages: a unified nomenclature based on ontogeny. *Nat Rev Immunol.* (2014) 14:571–8. doi: 10.1038/nri3712
140. Robbins SH, Walzer T, Dembélé D, Thibault C, Defays A, Bessou G, et al. Novel insights into the relationships between dendritic cell subsets in human and mouse revealed by genome-wide expression profiling. *Genome Biol.* (2008) 9:R17. doi: 10.1186/gb-2008-9-1-r17
141. Watchmaker PB, Lahl K, Lee M, Baumjohann D, Morton J, Kim SJ, et al. Comparative transcriptional and functional profiling defines conserved

programs of intestinal DC differentiation in humans and mice. *Nat Immunol.* (2013) 15:98–108. doi: 10.1038/ni.2768

142. Haniffa M, Shin A, Bigley V, McGovern N, Teo P, See P, et al. Human tissues contain CD141hi cross-presenting dendritic cells with functional homology to mouse CD103+ nonlymphoid dendritic cells. *Immunity* (2012) 37:60–73. doi: 10.1016/j.immuni.2012.04.012
143. Proietto AI, Mittag D, Roberts AW, Sprigg N, Wu L. The equivalents of human blood and spleen dendritic cell subtypes can be generated *in vitro* from human CD34+ stem cells in the presence of fms-like tyrosine kinase 3 ligand and thrombopoietin. *Cell Mol Immunol.* (2012) 9:446–54. doi: 10.1038/cmi.2012.48
144. Lee J, Breton G, Aljoufi A, Zhou YJ, Puhr S, Nussenzweig MC, et al. Clonal analysis of human dendritic cell progenitor using a stromal cell culture. *J Immunol Methods* (2015) 425:21–6. doi: 10.1016/j.jim.2015.06.004
145. Bachem A, Güttler S, Hartung E, Ebstein F, Schaefer M, Tannert A, et al. Superior antigen cross-presentation and XCR1 expression define human CD11c +CD141 +cells as homologues of mouse CD8 +dendritic cells. *J Exp Med.* (2010) 207:1273–81. doi: 10.1084/jem.20100348
146. Poulin LF, Reyal Y, Uronen-Hansson H, Schraml BU, Sancho D, Murphy KM, et al. DNGR-1 is a specific and universal marker of mouse and human Batf3-dependent dendritic cells in lymphoid and nonlymphoid tissues. *Blood* (2012) 119:6052–62. doi: 10.1182/blood-2012-01-406967
147. Hildner K, Edelson BT, Purtha WE, Diamond M, Matsushita H, Kohyama M, et al. Batf3 deficiency reveals a critical role for CD8alpha+ dendritic cells in cytotoxic T cell immunity. *Science* (2008) 322:1097–100. doi: 10.1126/science.1164206
148. Schiavoni G, Mattei F, Sestili P, Borghi P, Venditti M, Morse HC III, et al. ICSBP is essential for the development of mouse Type I interferon-producing cells and for the generation and activation of CD8α +Dendritic Cells. *J Exp Med.* (2002) 196:1415–25. doi: 10.1084/jem.20021263
149. Hacker C, Kirsch RD, Ju X-S, Hieronymus T, Gust TC, Kuhl C, et al. Transcriptional profiling identifies Id2 function in dendritic cell development. *Nat Immunol.* (2003) 4:380–6. doi: 10.1038/ni903
150. Kashiwada M, Pham N-LL, Pewe LL, Harty JT, Rothman PB. NFIL3/E4BP4 is a key transcription factor for CD8α? dendritic cell development. *Blood* (2011) 117:6193–97. doi: 10.1182/blood-2010-07-295873
151. Brewitz A, Eickhoff S, Dähling S, Quast T, Bedoui S, Kroczek RA, et al. CD8+ T cells orchestrate pDC-XCR1+ dendritic cell spatial and functional cooperativity to optimize priming. *Immunity* (2017) 46:205–19. doi: 10.1016/j.immuni.2017.01.003
152. Dai P, Wang W, Yang N, Serna-Tamayo C, Ricca JM, Zamarin D, et al. Intratumoral delivery of inactivated modified vaccinia virus Ankara (iMVA) induces systemic antitumor immunity via STING and Batf3-dependent dendritic cells. *Sci Immunol.* (2017) 2:eaal1713. doi: 10.1126/sciimmunol.aal1713
153. Broz ML, Binnewies M, Boldajipour B, Nelson AE, Pollack JL, Erle DJ, et al. Dissecting the tumor myeloid compartment reveals rare activating antigen-presenting cells critical for T cell immunity. *Cancer Cell* (2014) 26:638–52. doi: 10.1016/j.ccell.2014.09.007
154. Roberts EW, Broz ML, Binnewies M, Headley MB, Nelson AE, Wolf DM, et al. Critical Role for CD103+/CD141+ Dendritic Cells Bearing CCR7 for Tumor Antigen Trafficking and Priming of T Cell Immunity in Melanoma. *Cancer Cell* (2016) 30:324–36. doi: 10.1016/j.ccell.2016.06.003
155. Schlitzer A, McGovern N, Teo P, Zelante T, Atarashi K, Low D, et al. IRF4 Transcription factor-dependent CD11b+ dendritic cells in human and mouse control mucosal IL-17 cytokine responses. *Immunity* (2013) 38:970–83. doi: 10.1016/j.immuni.2013.04.011
156. Guerriero A, Langmuir PB, Spain LM, Scott EW. PU.1 is required for myeloid-derived but not lymphoid-derived dendritic cells. *Blood* (2000) 95:879–85.
157. Wu L, D'Amico A, Winkel KD, Suter M, Lo D, Shortman K. RelB is essential for the development of myeloid-related CD8alpha- dendritic cells but not of lymphoid-related CD8alpha+ dendritic cells. *Immunity* (1998) 9:839–47.
158. Caton ML, Smith-Raska MR, Reizis B. Notch–RBP-J signaling controls the homeostasis of CD8 –dendritic cells in the spleen. *J Exp Med.* (2007) 204:1653–64. doi: 10.1084/jem.20062648
159. Hambleton S, Salem S, Bustamante J, Bigley V, Boisson-Dupuis S, Azevedo J, et al. IRF8 mutations and human dendritic-cell immunodeficiency. *N Engl J Med.* (2011) 365:127–38. doi: 10.1056/NEJMoa1100066
160. Segura E, Valladeau-Guilemond J, Donnadieu M-H, Sastre-Garau X, Soumelis V, Amigorena S. Characterization of resident and migratory dendritic cells in human lymph nodes. *J Exp Med.* (2012) 209:653–60. doi: 10.1084/jem.20111457
161. Leal Rojas IM, Mok WH, Pearson FE, Minoda Y, Kenna TJ, Barnard RT, et al. Human blood CD1c+ dendritic cells promote Th1 and Th17 effector function in memory CD4+ T Cells. *Front Immunol.* (2017) 8:563–11. doi: 10.3389/fimmu.2017.00971
162. Villani A-C, Satija R, Reynolds G, Sarkizova S, Shekhar K, Fletcher J, et al. Single-cell RNA-seq reveals new types of human blood dendritic cells, monocytes, and progenitors. *Science* (2017) 356:eaah4573–14. doi: 10.1126/science.aah4573
163. Bamboat ZM, Stableford JA, Plitas G, Burt BM, Nguyen HM, Welles AP, et al. Human Liver Dendritic Cells Promote T Cell Hyporesponsiveness. *J Immunol.* (2009) 182:1901–11. doi: 10.4049/jimmunol.0803404
164. Sato T, Kitawaki T, Fujita H, Iwata M, Iyoda T, Inaba K, et al. Human CD1c+ myeloid dendritic cells acquire a high level of retinoic acid-producing capacity in response to vitamin D3. *J Immunol.* (2013) 191:3152–60. doi: 10.4049/jimmunol.1203517
165. Reizis B, Bunin A, Ghosh HS, Lewis KL, Sisirak V. Plasmacytoid dendritic cells: recent progress and open questions. *Annu Rev Immunol.* (2011) 29:163–83. doi: 10.1146/annurev-immunol-031210-101345
166. Swiecki M, Colonna M. The multifaceted biology of plasmacytoid dendritic cells. *Nat Rev Immunol.* (2015) 15:471–85. doi: 10.1038/nri3865
167. Evans VA, Lal L, Akkina R, Solomon A, Wright E, Lewin SR, et al. Thymic plasmacytoid dendritic cells are susceptible to productive HIV-1 infection and efficiently transfer R5 HIV-1 to thymocytes *in vitro*. *Retrovirology* (2011) 8:43. doi: 10.1186/1742-4690-8-43
168. Loures FV, Röhm M, Lee CK, Santos E, Wang JP, Specht CA, et al. Recognition of *Aspergillus fumigatus* hyphae by human plasmacytoid dendritic cells is mediated by dectin-2 and results in formation of extracellular traps. *PLoS Pathog.* (2015) 11:e1004643–23. doi: 10.1371/journal.ppat.1004643
169. Matsui T, Connolly JE, Michnevitz M, Chaussabel D, Yu CI, Glaser C, et al. CD2 distinguishes two subsets of human plasmacytoid dendritic cells with distinct phenotype and functions. *J Immunol.* (2009) 182:6815–23. doi: 10.4049/jimmunol.0802008
170. Cella M, Facchetti F, Lanzavecchia A, Colonna M. Plasmacytoid dendritic cells activated by influenza virus and CD40L drive a potent TH1 polarization. *Nat Immunol.* (2000) 1:305–10. doi: 10.1038/79747
171. Hoeffel G, Ripoche A-C, Matheoud D, Nascimbeni M, Escriou N, Lebon P, et al. Antigen crosspresentation by human plasmacytoid dendritic cells. *Immunity* (2007) 27:481–92. doi: 10.1016/j.immuni.2007.07.021
172. Krug A, Towarowski A, Britsch S, Rothenfusser S, Hornung V, Bals R, et al. Toll-like receptor expression reveals CpG DNA as a unique microbial stimulus for plasmacytoid dendritic cells which synergizes with CD40 ligand to induce high amounts of IL-12. *Eur J Immunol.* (2001) 31:3026–37. doi: 10.1002/1521-4141(2001010)31:10<3026::AID-IMMU3026>3.0.CO;2-H
173. Caux C, Dezutter-Dambuyant C, Schmitt D. GM-CSF and TNF- cooperate in the generation of dendritic Langerhans cells. *Nature* (1992) 360:258–61.
174. Sallusto F, Lanzavecchia A. Efficient presentation of soluble antigen by cultured human dendritic cells is maintained by granulocyte/macrophage colony-stimulating factor plus interleukin 4 and downregulated by tumor necrosis factor alpha. *J Exp Med.* (1994) 179:1109–18. doi: 10.1084/jem.179.4.1109
175. Lehtonen A, Veckman V, Nikula T, Lahesmaa R, Kinnunen L, Matikainen S, et al. Differential expression of IFN regulatory factor 4 gene in human monocyte-derived dendritic cells and macrophages. *J Immunol.* (2005) 175:6570–9. doi: 10.4049/jimmunol.175.10.6570
176. Inaba K, Inaba M, Romani N, Aya H, Deguchi M, Ikehara S, et al. Generation of large numbers of dendritic cells from mouse bone marrow cultures supplemented with granulocyte/macrophage colony-stimulating factor. *J Exp Med.* (1992) 176:1693–702.
177. Helft J, Böttcher J, Chakravarty P, Zelenay S, Huotari J, Schraml BU, et al. GM-CSF mouse bone marrow cultures comprise a heterogeneous population

of CD11c(+)MHCII(+) macrophages and dendritic cells. *Immunity* (2015) 42:1197–211. doi: 10.1016/j.immuni.2015.05.018
178. Guilliams M, Malissen B. A death notice for *in-vitro*-Generated GM-CSF dendritic cells? *Immunity* (2015) 42:988–90. doi: 10.1016/j.immuni.2015.05.020
179. Lutz MB, Inaba K, Schuler G, Romani N. Still alive and kicking: *in-vitro*-generated GM-CSF dendritic cells! *Immunity* (2016) 44:1–2. doi: 10.1016/j.immuni.2015.12.013
180. Helft J, Böttcher JP, Chakravarty P, Zelenay S, Huotari J, Schraml BU, et al. Alive but confused: heterogeneity of CD11c+ MHC class II+ cells in GM-CSF mouse bone marrow cultures. *Immunity* (2016) 44:3–4. doi: 10.1016/j.immuni.2015.12.014
181. Serbina NV, Salazar-Mather TP, Biron CA, Kuziel WA, Pamer EG. TNF/iNOS-producing dendritic cells mediate innate immune defense against bacterial infection. *Immunity* (2003) 19:59–70. doi: 10.1016/S1074-7613(03)00171-7
182. Wollenberg A, Kraft S, Hanau D, Bieber T. Immunomorphological and ultrastructural characterization of langerhans cells and a novel, inflammatory dendritic epidermal cell (IDEC) population in lesional skin of atopic eczema. *J Invest Dermatol.* (1996) 106:446–53. doi: 10.1111/1523-1747.ep12343596
183. Segura E, Touzot M, Bohineust A, Cappuccio A, Chiocchia G, Hosmalin A, et al. Human inflammatory dendritic cells induce Th17 cell differentiation. *Immunity* (2013) 38:336–48. doi: 10.1016/j.immuni.2012.10.018
184. Quail DF, Joyce JA. Microenvironmental regulation of tumor progression and metastasis. *Nat Med.* (2013) 19:1423–37. doi: 10.1038/nm.3394
185. Brosseau JP, Lucier JF, Nwilati H, Thibault P, Garneau D, Gendron D, et al. Tumor microenvironment-associated modifications of alternative splicing. *RNA* (2014) 20:189–201. doi: 10.1261/rna.042168.113
186. Bingle L, Brown NJ, Lewis CE. The role of tumour-associated macrophages in tumour progression: implications for new anticancer therapies. *J Pathol.* (2002) 196:254–65. doi: 10.1002/path.1027
187. Nagaraj S, Gabrilovich DI. Myeloid-derived suppressor cells in human cancer. *Cancer J.* (2010) 16:348–53. doi: 10.1097/PPO.0b013e3181eb3358
188. Ichihara F, Kono K, Takahashi A, Kawaida H, Sugai H, Fujii H. Increased populations of regulatory T cells in peripheral blood and tumor-infiltrating lymphocytes in patients with gastric and esophageal cancers. *Clin Cancer Res.* (2003) 9:4404–8.
189. Hanahan D, Weinberg RA. Hallmarks of Cancer: the next generation. *Cell* (2011) 144:646–74. doi: 10.1016/j.cell.2011.02.013
190. McAllister SS, Weinberg RA. The tumour-induced systemic environment as a critical regulator of cancer progression and metastasis. *Nat Cell Biol.* (2014) 16:717–27. doi: 10.1038/ncb3015
191. Alvarez KLF, Beldi M, Sarmanho F, Rossetti RAM, Silveira CRF, Mota GR, et al. Local and systemic immunomodulatory mechanisms triggered by Human Papillomavirus transformed cells: a potential role for G-CSF and neutrophils. *Sci Rep.* (2017) 7:1–16. doi: 10.1038/s41598-017-09079-3
192. Ramos RN, Chin LS, Santos Dos APSA, Bergami-Santos PC, Laginha F, Barbuto JAM. Monocyte-derived dendritic cells from breast cancer patients are biased to induce CD4+CD25+Foxp3+ regulatory T cells. *J Leukoc Biol.* (2012) 92:673–82. doi: 10.1189/jlb.0112048
193. Toniolo PA, Liu S, Yeh JE, Ye DQ, Barbuto JAM, Frank DA. Deregulation of SOCS5 suppresses dendritic cell function in chronic lymphocytic leukemia. *Oncotarget* (2016) 7:46301–14. doi: 10.18632/oncotarget.10093
194. Brown S, Hutchinson CV, Aspinall-O'Dea M, Whetton AD, Johnson SM, Rees-Unwin K, et al. Monocyte-derived dendritic cells from chronic myeloid leukaemia have abnormal maturation and cytoskeletal function that is associated with defective localisation and signalling by normal ABL1 protein. *Eur J Haematol.* (2014) 93:96–102. doi: 10.1111/ejh.12306
195. Orsini G, Legitimo A, Failli A, Ferrari P, Nicolini A, Spisni R, et al. Defective generation and maturation of dendritic cells from monocytes in colorectal cancer patients during the course of disease. *IJMS* (2013) 14:22022–41. doi: 10.3390/ijms141122022
196. Lopes A, Michelin MR, Murta E. Monocyte-derived dendritic cells from patients with cervical intraepithelial lesions. *Oncol Lett.* (2017) 13:1456–62. doi: 10.3892/ol.2017.5595
197. Kiertscher SM, Luo J, Dubinett SM, Roth MD. Tumors promote altered maturation and early apoptosis of monocyte-derived dendritic cells. *J Immunol.* (2000) 164:1269–76. doi: 10.4049/jimmunol.164.3.1269
198. Clavijo-Salomon MA, Ramos RN, Crippa A, Pizzo CR, Bergami-Santos PC, Barbuto JAM. Monocyte-derived dendritic cells reflect the immune functional status of a chromophobe renal cell carcinoma patient: could it be a general phenomenon? *Cancer Immunol Immunother* (2015) 64:161–71. doi: 10.1007/s00262-014-1625-9
199. Lago MT-D, Jukemura J, Machado MCC, Da Cunha JEM, Barbuto JAM. Phagocytosis and production of H_2O_2 by human peripheral blood mononuclear cells from patients with obstructive jaundice. *Pancreatology* (2006) 6:273–8. doi: 10.1159/000092688
200. Clavijo-Salomon MA, Bergami-Santos PC, M Barbuto JA. Immunomonitoring reveals interruption of anergy after vaccination in a case of type-2-papillary renal cell carcinoma. *Immunotherapy* (2017) 9:319–29. doi: 10.2217/imt-2016-0145
201. Failli A, Legitimo A, Orsini G, Romanini A, Consolini R. Numerical defect of circulating dendritic cell subsets and defective dendritic cell generation from monocytes of patients with advanced melanoma. *Cancer Lett.* (2013) 337:1–9. doi: 10.1016/j.canlet.2013.05.013
202. Orsini E, Guarini A, Chiaretti S, Mauro FR, Foa R. The circulating dendritic cell compartment in patients with chronic lymphocytic leukemia is severely defective and unable to stimulate an effective T-cell response. *Cancer Res.* (2003) 63:4497–506.
203. Verronèse E, Delgado A, Valladeau-Guilemond J, Garin G, Guillemaut S, Tredan O, et al. Immune cell dysfunctions in breast cancer patients detected through whole blood multi- parametric flow cytometry assay. *OncoImmunology* (2016) 5:1–15. doi: 10.1080/2162402X.2015.1100791
204. Li R, Fang F, Jiang M, Wang C, Ma J, Kang W, et al. STAT3 and NF-κB are simultaneously suppressed in dendritic cells in lung cancer. *Sci Rep.* (2017) 7:1–11. doi: 10.1038/srep45395
205. Fayad L, Keating MJ, Reuben JM, O'Brien S, Lee BN, Lerner S, et al. Interleukin-6 and interleukin-10 levels in chronic lymphocytic leukemia: correlation with phenotypic characteristics and outcome. *Blood* (2001) 97:256–63. doi: 10.1182/blood.V97.1.256
206. Park SJ, Nakagawa T, Kitamura H, Atsumi T, Kamon H, Sawa SI, et al. IL-6 Regulates *in vivo* dendritic cell differentiation through STAT3 activation. *J Immunol.* (2004) 173:3844–54. doi: 10.4049/jimmunol.173.6.3844
207. Ohno Y, Kitamura H, Takahashi N, Ohtake J, Kaneumi S, Sumida K, et al. IL-6 down-regulates HLA class II expression and IL-12 production of human dendritic cells to impair activation of antigen-specific CD4+ T cells. *Cancer Immunol. Immunother* (2016) 65:1–12. doi: 10.1007/s00262-015-1791-4
208. Kitamura H, Ohno Y, Toyoshima Y, Ohtake J, Homma S, Kawamura H, et al. Interleukin-6/STAT3 signaling as a promising target to improve the efficacy of cancer immunotherapy. *Cancer Sci.* (2017) 108:1947–52. doi: 10.1111/cas.13332
209. Niemand C, Nimmesgern A, Haan S, Fischer P, Schaper F, Rossaint R, et al. Activation of STAT3 by IL-6 and IL-10 in primary human macrophages is differentially modulated by suppressor of cytokine signaling 3. *J Immunol.* (2003) 170:3263–72. doi: 10.4049/jimmunol.170.6.3263
210. Coley WB. The Treatment of inoperable sarcoma by bacterial toxins (the mixed toxins of the *Streptococcus erysipelas* and the *Bacillus prodigiosus*). *Proc R Soc Med.* (1910) 3:1–48.
211. Bernardes N, Seruca R, Chakrabarty AM, Fialho AM. Microbial-based therapy of cancer: current progress and future prospects. *Bioeng. Bugs* (2010) 1:178–90. doi: 10.4161/bbug.1.3.10903
212. Adams S. Toll-like receptor agonists in cancer therapy. *Immunotherapy* (2009) 1:949–64. doi: 10.2217/imt.09.70
213. Burns EM, Yusuf N. Toll-like receptors and skin cancer. *Front Immunol.* (2014) 5:135. doi: 10.3389/fimmu.2014.00135
214. Tanaka H, Demeure CE, Rubio M, Delespesse G, Sarfati M. Human monocyte-derived dendritic cells induce naive T cell differentiation into T helper cell type 2 (Th2) or Th1/Th2 effectors. Role of stimulator/responder ratio. *J Exp Med.* (2000) 192:405–12. doi: 10.1084/jem.192.3.405
215. Dhodapkar MV, Steinman RM, Sapp M, Desai H, Fossella C, Krasovsky J, et al. Rapid generation of broad T-cell immunity in humans after a single injection of mature dendritic cells. *J Clin Invest.* (1999) 104:173–80. doi: 10.1172/JCI6909

216. Thurner B, Haendle I, Röder C, Dieckmann D, Keikavoussi P, Jonuleit H, et al. Vaccination with mage-3A1 peptide-pulsed mature, monocyte-derived dendritic cells expands specific cytotoxic T cells and induces regression of some metastases in advanced stage IV melanoma. *J Exp Med.* (1999) 190:1669–78.
217. Soruri A, Zwirner J. Dendritic cells: limited potential in immunotherapy. *Int J Biochem Cell Biol.* (2005) 37:241–5. doi: 10.1016/j.biocel.2004.07.003
218. Kuhn S, Hyde EJ, Yang J, Rich FJ, Harper JL, Kirman JR, et al. Increased numbers of monocyte-derived dendritic cells during successful tumor immunotherapy with immune-activating agents. *J Immunol.* (2013) 191:1984–92. doi: 10.4049/jimmunol.1301135
219. Kuhn S, Yang J, Ronchese F. Monocyte-derived dendritic cells are essential for CD8(+) T cell activation and antitumor responses after local immunotherapy. *Front Immunol.* (2015) 6:584. doi: 10.3389/fimmu.2015.00584
220. Mohty M, Vialle-Castellano A, Nunes JA, Isnardon D, Olive D, Gaugler B. IFN-alpha skews monocyte differentiation into Toll-like receptor 7-expressing dendritic cells with potent functional activities. *J Immunol.* (2003) 171:3385–93. doi: 10.4049/jimmunol.171.7.3385
221. Farkas A, Kemény L. Interferon-α in the generation of monocyte-derived dendritic cells: recent advances and implications for dermatology. *Br J Dermatol.* (2011) 165:247–54. doi: 10.1111/j.1365-2133.2011.10301.x
222. Harris KM. Monocytes differentiated with GM-CSF and IL-15 initiate Th17 and Th1 responses that are contact-dependent and mediated by IL-15. *J Leukoc Biol.* (2011) 90:727–34. doi: 10.1189/jlb.0311132
223. Dauer M, Obermaier B, Herten J, Haerle C, Pohl K, Rothenfusser S, et al. Mature dendritic cells derived from human monocytes within 48 hours: a novel strategy for dendritic cell differentiation from blood precursors. *J Immunol* (2003) 170:4069–76. doi: 10.4049/jimmunol.170.8.4069
224. Dauer M, Schad K, Herten J, Junkmann J, Bauer C, Kiefl R, et al. FastDC derived from human monocytes within 48 h effectively prime tumor antigen-specific cytotoxic T cells. *J Immunol Methods* (2005) 302:145–55. doi: 10.1016/j.jim.2005.05.010
225. Sundarasetty BS, Singh VK, Salguero G, Geffers R, Rickmann M, Macke L, et al. Lentivirus-induced dendritic cells for immunization against high-risk WT1(+) acute myeloid leukemia. *Hum Gene Ther.* (2013) 24:220–37. doi: 10.1089/hum.2012.128
226. Anassi E, Ndefo UA. Sipuleucel-T (provenge) injection: the first immunotherapy agent (vaccine) for hormone-refractory prostate cancer. *PT* (2011) 36:197–202.
227. Sims RB. Development of sipuleucel-T: autologous cellular immunotherapy for the treatment of metastatic castrate resistant prostate cancer. *Vaccine* (2012) 30:4394–7. doi: 10.1016/j.vaccine.2011.11.058
228. Castiello L, Sabatino M, Jin P, Clayberger C, Marincola FM, Krensky AM, et al. Monocyte-derived DC maturation strategies and related pathways: a transcriptional view. *Cancer Immunol Immunother* (2011) 60:457–66. doi: 10.1007/s00262-010-0954-6
229. Menges M, Rößner S, Voigtländer C, Schindler H, Kukutsch NA, Bogdan C, et al. Repetitive injections of dendritic cells matured with tumor necrosis factor alpha induce antigen-specific protection of mice from autoimmunity. *J Exp Med.* (2002) 195:15–21. doi: 10.1084/jem.20011341
230. Napolitani G, Rinaldi A, Bertoni F, Sallusto F, Lanzavecchia A. Selected Toll-like receptor agonist combinations synergistically trigger a T helper type 1-polarizing program in dendritic cells. *Nat Immunol.* (2005) 6:769–76. doi: 10.1038/ni1223
231. Vopenkova K, Mollova K, Buresova I, Michalek J. Complex evaluation of human monocyte-derived dendritic cells for cancer immunotherapy. *J Cell Mol Med.* (2012) 16:2827–37. doi: 10.1111/j.1582-4934.2012.01614.x
232. Coulie PG, Van den Eynde BJ, van der Bruggen P, Boon T. Tumour antigens recognized by T lymphocytes: at the core of cancer immunotherapy. *Nat Rev Cancer* (2014) 14:135–46. doi: 10.1038/nrc3670
233. Brossart P, Wirths S, Stuhler G, Reichardt VL, Kanz L, Brugger W. Induction of cytotoxic T-lymphocyte responses *in vivo* after vaccinations with peptide-pulsed dendritic cells. *Blood* (2000) 96:3102–8.
234. Jenne L, Schuler G, Steinkasserer A. Viral vectors for dendritic cell-based immunotherapy. *Trends Immunol.* (2001) 22:102–7. doi: 10.1016/S1471-4906(00)01813-5
235. Slingluff CL. The present and future of peptide vaccines for cancer: single or multiple, long or short, alone or in combination? *Cancer J.* (2011) 17:343–50. doi: 10.1097/PPO.0b013e318233e5b2
236. Mosca PJ, Clay TM, Morse MA, Lyerly HK. Dendritic cell vaccines. *Front Biosci.* (2007) 12:4050–60.
237. Fry TJ, Shand JL, Milliron M, Tasian SK, Mackall CL. Antigen loading of DCs with irradiated apoptotic tumor cells induces improved anti-tumor immunity compared to other approaches. *Cancer Immunol Immunother* (2009) 58:1257–64. doi: 10.1007/s00262-008-0638-7
238. Kalinski P, Urban J, Narang R, Berk E, Wieckowski E, Muthuswamy R. Dendritic cell-based therapeutic cancer vaccines: what we have and what we need. *Future Oncol.* (2009) 5:379–90. doi: 10.2217/fon.09.6
239. Barbuto JAM. Are dysfunctional monocyte-derived dendritic cells in cancer an explanation for cancer vaccine failures? *Immunotherapy* (2013) 5:105–7. doi: 10.2217/imt.12.153
240. Pinho MP, Sundarasetty BS, Bergami-Santos PC, Steponavicius-Cruz K, Ferreira AK, Stripecke R, et al. Dendritic-tumor cell hybrids induce tumor-specific immune responses more effectively than the simple mixture of dendritic and tumor cells. *Cytotherapy* (2016) 18:570–80. doi: 10.1016/j.jcyt.2016.01.005
241. Barbuto JAM, Ensina LFC, Neves AR, Bergami-Santos P, Leite KRM, Marques R, et al. Dendritic cell-tumor cell hybrid vaccination for metastatic cancer. *Cancer Immunol Immunother* (2004) 53:1111–8. doi: 10.1007/s00262-004-0551-7
242. Tacken PJ, de Vries IJM, Torensma R, Figdor CG. Dendritic-cell immunotherapy: from *ex vivo* loading to *in vivo* targeting. *Nat Rev Immunol.* (2007) 7:790–802. doi: 10.1038/nri2173
243. van Dinther D, Stolk DA, van de Ven R, van Kooyk Y, de Gruijl TD, Haan den JMM. Targeting C-type lectin receptors: a high-carbohydrate diet for dendritic cells to improve cancer vaccines. *J Leukoc Biol.* (2017) 102:1017–34. doi: 10.1189/jlb.5MR0217-059RR
244. Caminschi I, Maraskovsky E, Heath WR. Targeting Dendritic Cells *in vivo* for cancer therapy. *Front Immunol.* (2012) 3:13. doi: 10.3389/fimmu.2012.00013
245. Macri C, Dumont C, Johnston AP, Mintern JD. Targeting dendritic cells: a promising strategy to improve vaccine effectiveness. *Clin Trans Immunol.* (2016) 5:e66. doi: 10.1038/cti.2016.6
246. Mahnke K, Qian Y, Fondel S, Brueck J, Becker C, Enk AH. Targeting of antigens to activated dendritic cells *in vivo* cures metastatic melanoma in mice. *Cancer Res.* (2005) 65:7007–12. doi: 10.1158/0008-5472.CAN-05-0938
247. Tullett KM, Leal Rojas IM, Minoda Y, Tan PS, Zhang J-G, Smith C, et al. Targeting CLEC9A delivers antigen to human CD141+ DC for CD4+ and CD8+T cell recognition. *JCI Insight* (2016) 1:e87102. doi: 10.1172/jci.insight.87102
248. Toniolo PA, Liu S, Yeh JE, Moraes-Vieira PM, Walker SR, Vafaizadeh V, et al. Inhibiting STAT5 by the BET bromodomain inhibitor JQ1 disrupts human dendritic cell maturation. *J Immunol.* (2015) 194:3180–90. doi: 10.4049/jimmunol.1401635
249. Silva-Cardoso SC, Affandi AJ, Spel L, Cossu M, van Roon JAG, Boes M, et al. CXCL4 Exposure Potentiates TLR-Driven polarization of human monocyte-derived dendritic cells and increases stimulation of T Cells. *J Immunol.* (2017) 199:253–62. doi: 10.4049/jimmunol.1602020
250. Dijkgraaf EM, Santegoets SJAM, Reyners AKL, Goedemans R, Wouters MCA, Kenter GG, et al. A phase I trial combining carboplatin/doxorubicin with tocilizumab, an anti-IL-6R monoclonal antibody, and interferon-α2b in patients with recurrent epithelial ovarian cancer. *Ann Oncol.* (2015) 26:2141–9. doi: 10.1093/annonc/mdv309
251. Mailliard RB, Wankowicz-Kalinska A, Cai Q, Wesa A, Hilkens CM, Kapsenberg ML, et al. alpha-type-1 polarized dendritic cells: a novel immunization tool with optimized CTL-inducing activity. *Cancer Res.* (2004) 64:5934–7. doi: 10.1158/0008-5472.CAN-04-1261
252. Okada H, Kalinski P, Ueda R, Hoji A, Kohanbash G, Donegan TE, et al. Induction of CD8+ T-cell responses against novel glioma-associated antigen peptides and clinical activity by vaccinations with {alpha}-type 1 polarized dendritic cells and polyinosinic-polycytidylic acid stabilized by lysine and carboxymethylcellulose in patients with recurrent malignant glioma. *J Clin Oncol.* (2011) 29:330–6. doi: 10.1200/JCO.2010.30.7744

253. Sakamoto C, Kohara H, Inoue H, Narusawa M, Ogawa Y, Hirose-Yotsuya L, et al. Therapeutic vaccination based on side population cells transduced by the granulocyte-macrophage colony-stimulating factor gene elicits potent antitumor immunity. *Cancer Gene Ther.* (2017) 24:165–74. doi: 10.1038/cgt.2016.80
254. Fu J, Kanne DB, Leong M, Glickman LH, McWhirter SM, Lemmens E, et al. STING agonist formulated cancer vaccines can cure established tumors resistant to PD-1 blockade. *Sci Transl Med.* (2015) 7:283ra52. doi: 10.1126/scitranslmed.aaa4306
255. Gonzalez-Gugel E, Saxena M, Bhardwaj N. Modulation of innate immunity in the tumor microenvironment. *Cancer Immunol Immunother* (2016) 65:1261–8. doi: 10.1007/s00262-016-1859-9
256. Oleszycka E, Lavelle EC. Immunomodulatory properties of the vaccine adjuvant alum. *Curr Opin Immunol.* (2014) 28:1–5. doi: 10.1016/j.coi.2013.12.007
257. van Doorn E, Liu H, Huckriede A, Hak E. Safety and tolerability evaluation of the use of Montanide ISA^{TM}51 as vaccine adjuvant: a systematic review. *Hum Vaccin Immunotherapeut.* (2016) 12:159–69. doi: 10.1080/21645515.2015.1071455
258. Saxena M, Bhardwaj N. ScienceDirect Turbocharging vaccines: emerging adjuvants for dendritic cell based therapeutic cancer vaccines. *Curr Opin Immunol.* (2017) 47:35–43. doi: 10.1016/j.coi.2017.06.003
259. Yarchoan M, Johnson BA, Lutz ER, Laheru DA, Jaffee EM. Targeting neoantigens to augment antitumour immunity. *Nat Rev Cancer* (2017) 17:209–222. doi: 10.1038/nrc.2016.154
260. Ott PA, Hu Z, Keskin DB, Shukla SA, Sun J, Bozym DJ, et al. An immunogenic personal neoantigen vaccine for patients with melanoma. *Nature Publish. Group* (2017) 547:217–21. doi: 10.1038/nature22991
261. Kranz LM, Diken M, Haas H, Kreiter S, Loquai C, Reuter KC, et al. Systemic RNA delivery to dendritic cells exploits antiviral defence for cancer immunotherapy. *Nature* (2016) 534:1–16. doi: 10.1038/nature18300
262. Marzbani E, Inatsuka C, Lu H, Disis ML. The invisible arm of immunity in common cancer chemoprevention agents. *Cancer Prev Res.* (2013) 6:764–73. doi: 10.1158/1940-6207.CAPR-13-0036
263. Fecek RJ, Storkus WJ. Combination strategies to enhance the potency of monocyte-derived dendritic cell-based cancer vaccines. *Immunotherapy* (2016) 8:1205–18. doi: 10.2217/imt-2016-0071
264. Ouyang M, White EE, Ren H, Guo Q, Zhang I, Gao H, et al. Metronomic doses of temozolomide enhance the efficacy of carbon nanotube CpG immunotherapy in an invasive glioma model. *PLoS ONE* (2016) 11:e0148139. doi: 10.1371/journal.pone.0148139
265. Noguchi M, Moriya F, Koga N, Matsueda S, Sasada T, Yamada A, et al. A randomized phase II clinical trial of personalized peptide vaccination with metronomic low-dose cyclophosphamide in patients with metastatic castration-resistant prostate cancer. *Cancer Immunol Immunother* (2016) 65:151–60. doi: 10.1007/s00262-015-1781-6
266. Tseng C-W, Hung C-F, Alvarez RD, Trimble C, Huh WK, Kim D, et al. Pretreatment with cisplatin enhances E7-specific CD8+ T-Cell-mediated antitumor immunity induced by DNA vaccination. *Clin Cancer Res.* (2008) 14:3185–92. doi: 10.1158/1078-0432.CCR-08-0037
267. Shen J, Wang L-F, Zou Z-Y, Kong W-W, Yan J, Meng F-Y, et al. Phase I clinical study of personalized peptide vaccination combined with radiotherapy for advanced hepatocellular carcinoma. *World J Gastroenterol.* (2017) 23:5395–404. doi: 10.3748/wjg.v23.i29.5395
268. Gulley JL, Arlen PM, Bastian A, Morin S, Marte J, Beetham P, et al. Combining a recombinant cancer vaccine with standard definitive radiotherapy in patients with localized prostate cancer. *Clin Cancer Res.* (2005) 11:3353–62. doi: 10.1158/1078-0432.CCR-04-2062
269. Brody JD, Ai WZ, Czerwinski DK, Torchia JA, Levy M, Advani RH, et al. In situ vaccination with a TLR9 agonist induces systemic lymphoma regression: a phase I/II study. *J Clin Oncol.* (2010) 28:4324–32. doi: 10.1200/JCO.2010.28.9793
270. Inogés S, Tejada S, de Cerio AL-D, Gállego Pérez-Larraya J, Espinós J, Idoate MA, et al. A phase II trial of autologous dendritic cell vaccination and radiochemotherapy following fluorescence-guided surgery in newly diagnosed glioblastoma patients. *J Transl Med.* (2017) 15:104. doi: 10.1186/s12967-017-1202-z
271. Loi M, Desideri I, Greto D, Mangoni M, Sottili M, Meattini I, et al. Radiotherapy in the age of cancer immunology: Current concepts and future developments. *Crit Rev Oncol Hematol.* (2017) 112:1–10. doi: 10.1016/j.critrevonc.2017.02.002
272. Raval RR, Sharabi AB, Walker AJ, Drake CG, Sharma P. Tumor immunology and cancer immunotherapy: summary of the 2013 SITC primer. *J Immunother Cancer* (2014) 2:14. doi: 10.1186/2051-1426-2-14
273. Son C-H, Bae J-H, Shin D-Y, Lee H-R, Choi Y-J, Jo W-S. CTLA-4 blockade enhances antitumor immunity of intratumoral injection of immature dendritic cells into irradiated tumor in a mouse colon cancer model. *J Immunother* (2014) 37:1–7. doi: 10.1097/CJI.0000000000000007
274. Ribas A, Comin-Anduix B, Chmielowski B, Jalil J, la Rocha de P, McCannel TA, et al. Dendritic cell vaccination combined with CTLA4 blockade in patients with metastatic melanoma. *Clin Cancer Res.* (2009) 15:6267–76. doi: 10.1158/1078-0432.CCR-09-1254
275. Freeman GJ, Long AJ, Iwai Y, Bourque K, Chernova T, Nishimura H, et al. Engagement of the PD-1 immunoinhibitory receptor by a novel B7 family member leads to negative regulation of lymphocyte activation. *J Exp Med.* (2000) 192:1027–34. doi: 10.1084/jem.192.7.1027
276. Latchman Y, Wood CR, Chernova T, Chaudhary D, Borde M, Chernova I, et al. PD-L2 is a second ligand for PD-1 and inhibits T cell activation. *Nat Immunol.* (2001) 2:261–8. doi: 10.1038/85330
277. Munn DH, Mellor AL. Indoleamine 2,3 dioxygenase and metabolic control of immune responses. *Trends Immunol.* (2013) 34:137–43. doi: 10.1016/j.it.2012.10.001
278. Grohmann U, Fallarino F, Bianchi R, Orabona C, Vacca C, Fioretti MC, et al. A Defect in tryptophan catabolism impairs tolerance in nonobese diabetic mice. *J Exp Med.* (2003) 198:153–60. doi: 10.1084/jem.20030633
279. Baban B, Chandler PR, Johnson BA, Huang L, Li M, Sharpe ML, et al. Physiologic Control of IDO Competence in Splenic Dendritic Cells. *J Immunol.* (2011) 187:2329–35. doi: 10.4049/jimmunol.1100276
280. Liu X, Shin N, Koblish HK, Yang G, Wang Q, Wang K, et al. Selective inhibition of IDO1 effectively regulates mediators of antitumor immunity. *Blood* (2010) 115:3520–30. doi: 10.1182/blood-2009-09-246124
281. Lowe DB, Bose A, Taylor JL, Tawbi H, Lin Y, Kirkwood JM, et al. Dasatinib promotes the expansion of a therapeutically superior T-cell repertoire in response to dendritic cell vaccination against melanoma. *OncoImmunology* (2014) 3:e27589. doi: 10.4161/onci.27589
282. Bronte V, Zanovello P. Regulation of immune responses by L-arginine metabolism. *Nature Rev Immunol.* (2005) 5:641–654. doi: 10.1038/nri1668

15

Current Concepts on 6-sulfo LacNAc Expressing Monocytes (slanMo)

Fareed Ahmad[1], Thomas Döbel[1,2], Marc Schmitz[3,4] and Knut Schäkel[1*]

[1] Department of Dermatology, Heidelberg University Hospital, Heidelberg, Germany, [2] Dermatology Branch, National Institute of Arthritis and Musculoskeletal and Skin Diseases, Bethesda, MD, United States, [3] Institute of Immunology, Faculty of Medicine Carl Gustav Carus, Technische Universtät Dresden, Dresden, Germany, [4] Partner Site Dresden, National Center for Tumor Diseases (NCT), Dresden, Germany

***Correspondence:**
Knut Schäkel
knut.schaekel@med.uni-heidelberg.de

The human mononuclear phagocytes system consists of dendritic cells (DCs), monocytes, and macrophages having different functions in bridging innate and adaptive immunity. Among the heterogeneous population of monocytes the cell surface marker slan (6-sulfo LacNAc) identifies a specific subset of human $CD14^-$ $CD16^+$ non-classical monocytes, called $slan^+$ monocytes (slanMo). In this review we discuss the identity and functions of slanMo, their contributions to immune surveillance by pro-inflammatory cytokine production, and cross talk with T cells and NK cells. We also consider the role of slanMo in the regulation of chronic inflammatory diseases and cancer. Finally, we highlight unresolved questions that should be the focus of future research.

Keywords: $slan^+$ monocytes, slanMo, non-classical monocytes, inflammation, autoimmunity, cancer, infection, psoriasis

$CD16^+$ MONOCYTES

Monocytes are important regulatory cells in innate and adaptive immunity (1, 2). Studies on blood leukocytes showed that monocytes are a heterogeneous cell population that can be roughly separated into three populations: classical monocytes $CD14^+CD16^-$, intermediate monocytes $CD14^+CD16^+$, and non-classical monocytes $CD14^-CD16^+$ (1, 3–5). The murine counter part of non-classical monocytes was identified as $Ly6C^{low}CCR2^-CX3CR1^{hi}$ cells (4, 6, 7). So far the most distinctive and best-studied function of mouse non-classical monocytes is their migration independent of the direction of blood flow along the luminal side of the vascular endothelium (8–10). There, they function in immune surveillance of the vasculature and exert both anti-inflammatory and pro-inflammatory functions. Therefore, they are also called patrolling monocytes (8). Patrolling behavior is a common feature of both murine and human non-classical monocytes (8, 9, 11, 12). However, murine non-classical monocytes are currently considered to be cells of vascular homeostasis, while the majority of studies describe an overall pro-inflammatory function of human non-classical monocytes (9, 11, 13, 14). The pro-inflammatory function of human non-classical monocytes is mainly attributed to the production of TNF-α and IL-12 (6, 11, 15–17). Concerning the origin of non-classical monocytes, there is now evidence from studies in mice and humans that classical monocytes give rise to non-classical monocytes (18, 19). The transcription factor Nur77 (NR4A1) is upregulated in human and murine non-classical monocytes (17, 19, 20). Mice, having a deletion in the NR4A1 super enhancer, lack non-classical monocytes and serve as a model to study their function *in vivo* (10).

In the absence of specific markers, studies on human $CD16^+$ monocytes are largely descriptive, and rely on CD14/CD16-gating strategies with no clear-cut definition. Numbers of intermediate monocytes and non-classical monocytes in blood were found altered under various conditions (15, 21–25). These studies are confined to blood leukocytes, as there is no stable expression of CD14 and CD16 on non-classical monocytes entering into tissues or differentiating into macrophages and DCs.

Within human $CD14^-CD16^+$ non-classical monocytes, our group defined a 6-sulfo LacNAc (slan) expressing cell population (slanMo) in peripheral blood (16, 26, 27). Subsequently, slan expressing cells have been identified in tissues (16, 28–31). Therefore, the stably expressed slan antigen provides a unique opportunity to study these cells in different organs.

IDENTITY OF slanMo EXPRESSING CELLS

slanMo research began in 1998 when a $CD16^+$ cell population accounting for 50% of non-classical monocytes was defined by the mAb M-DC8 (32, 33). The mAb M-DC8 (IgM) was generated by immunizing mice with peripheral blood mononuclear cells (PBMCs), depleted of $CD14^+$ monocytes, T cells and B cells (33). DD1 and DD2 (IgM, generated by immunization with slanMo) are additional slan-specific mAbs that allowed for the detection of $slan^+$ cells in paraffin-embedded tissue sections (30, 31, 34). slanMo specifically express the eponymous "slan" antigen (6-sulfo LacNAc), an O-linked glycosylated variant of P-selectin glycoprotein ligand-1 (PSGL-1) (25, 30). At the molecular level, the slan-antigen is a non-sialylated and non-fucosylated 6-sulfated N-acetyllactosamine (LacNAc) (26). This is in contrast to the cutaneous lymphocyte-associated antigen (CLA, also known as sialyl 6-sulfo Lewis X), which is a sialylated and fucosylated variant of 6-sulfo LacNAc. While CLA binds to E-selectin and thereby facilitates skin homing of T cells, slan was shown to be devoid of binding to E- and -L-selectin (35). The exact function and the binding partners of slan are unknown. However, sulfated terminal glycotopes as found in the slan-antigen were shown to serve as ligands for lectins other than E- and–L-selectin, including members of the galectins and siglec families (36–41).

Transcriptomic studies on blood leukocytes clearly identified $slan^+$ cells as a subset of monocytes and accordingly they were called slanMo (4, 11, 42, 43). While being of monocyte origin, slanMo may either rapidly acquire dendritic cell functions (4, 42, 44) or differentiate into macrophages (29, 45). Their initial recognition as dendritic cells (DCs) (33) was based on their DC-like phenotype with very low or undetectable levels of the classical monocytes markers CCR2, CD14, CD62L, CD11b, and CD36 as well as their function as professional antigen presenting cells as revealed by T cell stimulatory experiments (16, 30). Similarly, in skin tissue of psoriasis patients, $slan^+$ cells showed a DC-like phenotype ($CD14^-$, $CD163^-$) and function ($IL\text{-}23p19^+$) (30).

slanMo purified from human tonsil tissue resembled DCs by morphology and function (28). They co-localized with T cells in tonsils and induced their proliferation several times more efficient than macrophages and similar to bona fide DCs (DC1, DC2, and pDC). In addition, peripheral blood slanMo cultured in tonsil-derived condition medium acquired the phenotype of slanMo in tonsils (28). $slan^+$ cells in lymph nodes of patients with diffuse large B-cell lymphoma, exhibited a phenotype of either immature DCs ($CD163^{low}/CD14^{low}/CD64^{low}/CD16^{low}$) or macrophages ($CD163^{hi}/CD14^{hi}/CD64^{hi}/CD16^{hi}$) (29). Furthermore, *in vitro* studies revealed that GM-CSF and IL-4-treated slanMo can differentiate into cells with a DC-like phenotype, while IL-34-treated slanMo revealed a macrophage-like phenotype (28). Thus, slanMo may be considered as a type of circulating and tissue myeloid cell population with remarkable plasticity (28, 29, 46).

Recently, Hamers et al. defined heterogeneity within human monocytes (**Table 1**) using mass cytometry combined with single cell sequencing data (47). slanMo, but not slan-negative non-classical monocytes, were shown to express CXCR6, which facilitated chemotactic migration toward CXCL16 (47, 48). Interestingly, CXCL16 was previously shown to be upregulated in psoriasis, lupus nephritis as well as in cardiovascular disease (47, 49–52). In line with this study describing slanMo as having phenotype and functions distinct from other non-classical monocytes, Hofer et al. reported on a selective depletion of slan-negative $CD16^+$ cells in patients with sarcoidosis (53). Furthermore, they demonstrated a 5-fold depletion of slan-positive monocytes in patients with hereditary diffuse leukoencephalopathy with axonal spheroids (HDLS), a disease caused by macrophage colony-stimulating factor (M-CSF) receptor mutations.

FUNCTION OF slanMo

The selective slan-marker opened the possibility for functional studies (**Figures 1, 2**) after mAb-directed purification of slanMo. In blood, slanMo circulate as cells with low-level expression of HLA-DR and co-stimulatory molecules (26, 30, 47). They express a broad range of toll-like receptors (TLRs) but lack TLR3 and TLR9 (46). Stimulation of freshly isolated or immature slanMo with lipopolysaccharide (LPS) or CD40 ligand resulted in high-level TNF-α production (16, 26, 54). TNF-α-producing slanMo were identified in psoriasis, lupus skin lesions, glomerular capillaries of lupus nephritis, and tumor draining lymph nodes (30, 31, 43, 46). Stimulating freshly isolated slanMo did not induce IL-12 or IL-23 production (11, 26, 42) however, slanMo revealed an outstanding capacity to produce IL-12 and IL-23 compared to blood monocytes and DCs, when stimulated after a brief culture period of 6 h (16, 31, 44). This functional maturation occurred when slanMo were left unseparated as in whole PBMC cultures and also after their purification by slan-directed magnetic cell sorting. The phenotypic maturation was reflected by upregulation of CD83, CD80, and HLA-DR, while CD16 was shed from the surface by activation of a disintegrin and metalloproteinase domain-containing protein 17 (ADAM17) (16). During this maturation process, expression of the slan antigen remained stable. Interestingly, maturation of slanMo could be completely prevented when erythrocytes were added to *in vitro* cultures of already purified slanMo. Therefore, in peripheral blood, maturation of slanMo may be tightly controlled by circulating erythrocytes (16). mAb-directed blocking experiment revealed

Abbreviations: PSGL1, P selectin glycoprotein ligand 1; slanMo, 6-sulfo LacNAc expressing monocytes; DCs, Dendritic cells; Ly, Lymphocyte antigen; ROS, Reactive oxygen species; HO-1, Heme oxygenase 1; PD-L1, Programmed death-ligand 1; TLR, Toll like receptor; NR4A1, Nuclear receptor transcription factor 4A1; G-CSF, Granulocyte-colony stimulating factor; LPS, Lipopolysaccharides; PBMCs, Peripheral blood mononuclear cells; COPD, Chronic Obstructive Pulmonary Diseases; HGF, Hepatocyte Growth Factor.

TABLE 1 | Human monocyte heterogeneity.

Name	Non-classical monocytes (slanMo)	Intermeditate monocytes	Classical monocytes
Distinctive phenotype	slan⁺ CXCR6⁺; CD9⁻ / CD9⁺; *	*	*; FcεRI⁺ CD1c⁺ TIM3⁺; TREM-1⁺; *
General phenotype	CD14⁻ CD16⁺ HLA-DR⁺; CD16⁺ CX3CR1⁺ CD45RA⁺ LFA-1⁺	CD14⁺ CD16⁺ HLA-DR⁺⁺	CD14⁺ CD16⁻ HLA-DR⁺; CD14⁺ CD11b⁺ CD33⁺ CD36⁺ CD38⁺ CCR2⁺ CD45RO⁺ CD62L⁺ CD136⁺ CD64⁺ CD63⁺ CD163⁺ CD82⁺ CD93⁺ CD61⁺ CD41⁺
Cytokine production	IL-23, IL-12, TNF-α, IL-1β		IL-10

Defined by a rather complex set of differentially expressed molecules (47). The table summarizes phenotypic and functional aspects of human monocyte heterogeneity. According to previous work and the recent study, 4 classical, 1 intermediate, and 3 non-classical monocyte populations can be defined (represented by different color code) (47). The 3 non-classical monocyte populations are identified by the differential expression of slan and CD9. General differences in phenotype and cytokine production are depicted as well. Intensity of color represent the expression level of surface marker and cytokines production from non-classical monocytes to classical monocytes and vice-versa.

that the inhibitory effect of erythrocytes depended on the expression of CD47 on erythrocytes and its binding to signal-regulatory protein α (SIRPα) on slanMo (16). The *in vitro* findings of slanMo producing TNF-α and IL-23 are mirrored by studies on psoriasis skin lesions where 85% of dermal slanMo were found to express IL-23p19 and 50% of the cells expressed TNF-α (31). Conditioning slanMo with IFN-γ for 6 h before stimulation with LPS or R848 increased (10-fold) their IL-12 secretion acknowledging the relevance of a positive feedback loop with IFN-γ producers such as Th1 cells and NK cells (55). slanMo revealed a strong response to TLR7 and TLR8 ligands with high IL-12 and IL-23 production (31, 54). Interestingly, IL-23 production required autocrine signaling by TNF-α and IL-1β (56, 57). The responsiveness to TLR7 and TLR8 stimulation is relevant for the activation of slanMo in autoimmune diseases and psoriasis where single stranded RNA motives are either contained within autoimmune complexes or being complexed by the antimicrobial peptide LL37 as in psoriasis (31, 46).

Leeuwen-Kerkhoff et al. and Cros et al. reported a low IL-12 production and Th1 programming capacity of slanMo (11, 42). In these studies, the short maturation step through which slanMo gain their outstanding IL-12 and IL-23 producing capacity was not taken into account. In addition, some groups rely on staining of CD16 in addition to slan for the isolation of slanMo. However, CD16 cross-linking can induce an inhibitory signal (inhibitory ITAM signaling, ITAMi), reducing pro-inflammatory cytokine production (58, 59). In addition, we realized that slanMo are sensitive to flow cytometric cell sorting as they rapidly undergo apoptosis thereafter. In summary, studies revealed that slanMo circulate in blood as immature cells that readily produce TNF-α and acquire the capacity to produce IL-12 and IL-23.

IMMUNE CROSS-TALK OF slanMo WITH OTHER CELLS

T Lymphocytes

Mononuclear phagocytes largely differ in their function to regulate adaptive immune responses by directing the quality and magnitude of T cell responses (**Figure 1**). Different studies assessed the function of slanMo to stimulate T cell proliferation and direct the production of T cell derived cytokines (16, 31, 60–62). slanMo revealed a better capacity to stimulate the proliferation of allogeneic CD4$^+$ T cells than CD14$^+$ monocytes (16, 26, 31). In contrast to CD14$^+$ monocytes, slanMo efficiently primed T cells for the neoantigen keyhole limpet hemocyanin (KLH), and induced allo-antigen specific CD8$^+$ cytotoxic T cells (33). Similar to CD1c$^+$ DCs (DC2), slanMo primed naïve allogenic cord blood T cells (26). Further, slanMo demonstrated a stronger programming of Th1 cells as compared to DC2 when cultured for 6 h before stimulation with LPS and then co-culture with cord blood T cells (26, 45). This is in line with the superior IL-12 production of slanMo when compared with DC2 after 6 h of spontaneous maturation (54). Another study assessed the Th17 programming capacity using allogenic naïve T cells. Here again a higher capacity of slanMo to induce Th17/Th1 T cells was observed in cultures stimulated with slanMo instead of DC2 (31). The strong T cell stimulatory capacity of slanMo may be relevant for recall responses in peripheral tissues as well as for the priming of naïve T cells in lymphoid tissue (46).

Natural Killer Cells

The interaction of mononuclear phagocytes and natural killer (NK) cells is well known. The main mechanisms by which mononuclear phagocytes can activate NK cells are soluble mediators as well as through direct cell-to-cell contacts.

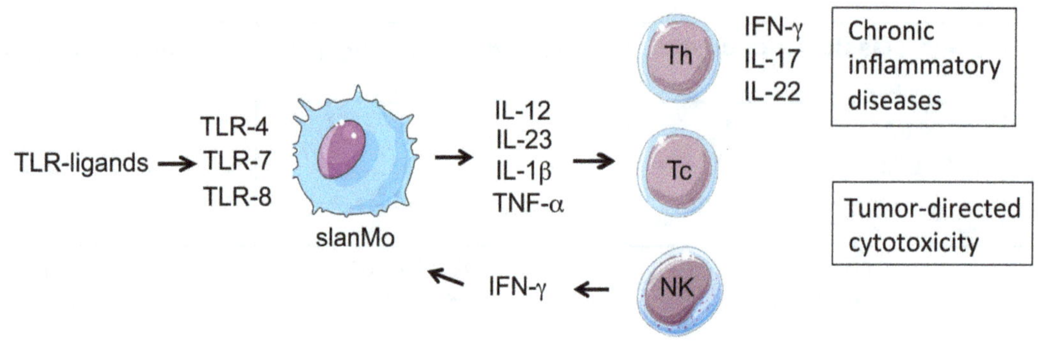

FIGURE 1 | Immune regulatory function of slanMo: slanMo are activated via TLR stimulation to produce pro-inflammatory cytokines, thereby programming and enhancing Th1 and Th17 T cell responses, which play a major role in chronic inflammatory diseases. Activated slanMo also promote cytotoxic CD8 and NK cell-mediated anti-tumor responses. In a positive forward feedback loop slanMo producing IL-12 stimulate NK cells for early production of IFN-γ, which amplifies IL-12 production by slanMo.

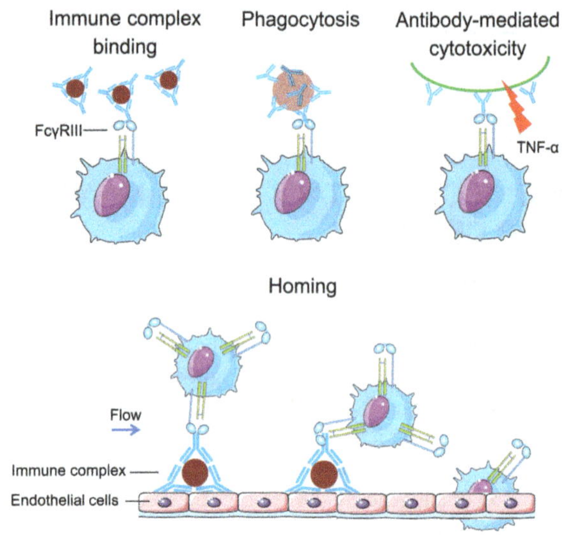

FIGURE 2 | CD16 equips slanMo with a strong capacity to handle complexed IgG: slanMo can bind to IgG immune complexes through CD16. They can also phagocytose and mediate antibody-mediated cellular cytotoxicity (ADCC) after binding of CD16 to antibody (IgG)- coated cells. This is in difference to monocytes expressing CD32 for engaging immune complexes. Moreover, slanMo in the blood flow can home to immobilized vascular immune complexes via CD16.

Co-culture of slanMo with NK cells promotes mutual activation (63, 64). Stimulation of slanMo with LPS induced an IL-12 production that stimulated NK cells to produce IFN-γ, which in a positive forward feedback loop potentiated the IL-12 production of slanMo and the IFN-γ production of NK cells. This resulted in an increased NK cell activation (CD69, NKp30, NKp44, NKG2D) as well as an increased tumor-directed cytotoxicity against chronic myeloid leukemia (CML) blasts and the leukemia cell line K562 compared to those NK cells stimulated without slanMo (63, 65). This cross talk of slanMo and NK cells also improved the slanMo-mediated differentiation of näive $CD4^+$ T cells into IFN-γ producing Th1 cells (66).

Optimal reciprocal activation of slanMo and NK cells required direct cellular contact. Tufa et al. identified a cellular communication circuit through transmembrane TNF-α expressed by slanMo and its interaction with upregulated TNFR2 on NK cells leading to higher secretion of GM-CSF by NK cells (65). Similarly, ICAM-1 expressed by slanMo bound to LFA-1 on NK cells thereby promoting an enhanced IL-1β secretion by slanMo (63). Stimulation of slanMo with TLR7/8 ligands resulted in a pronounced production of TNF-α, IL-1β, IL-12, and IL-6 allowing for an improved tumor directed cytotoxicity of slanMo and NK cells (67).

Neutrophils

Human neutrophils were shown to directly interact with both NK cells and slanMo *in vitro*, which eventually enhanced the activity of both cell types—NK cells and slanMo—after LPS, IL-12 or IL-12/IL-18 stimulation (64). Neutrophils engaged with slanMo via CD18 (integrin ß2) and intracellular adhesion molecule 1 (ICAM-1) that boosted the release of IL-12 by slanMo, which further stimulated activated NK cells to produce IFN-γ. Neutrophils were also shown to interact with NK cells via CD18 and ICAM-3 thereby augmenting IFN-γ production by NK cells (68). Co-localization of slanMo, NK cell, and neutrophils in inflamed tissue of psoriasis and Crohn's disease provided evidence for cooperation between these cells in which neutrophils may function as amplifiers of immune responses mediated by slanMo and NK cells.

Mesenchymal Stem Cells

Mesenchymal stem cells (MSCs) are well known for their immunomodulatory properties. Results from therapeutic studies are encouraging and there is hope that the application of MSCs open new options for the therapy of immune-related diseases (69). slanMo were found in increased numbers in tissues affected by chronic inflammatory diseases such as Crohn's disease, multiple sclerosis, rheumatoid arthritis, and lupus erythematosus. Treatment with MSCs was regarded successful in these diseases. Co-culture of slanMo with MSCs resulted in a reduced production of TNF-α, IL-6, and IL-12, while production of the immunosuppressive cytokine IL-10 was enhanced in response to LPS stimulation (70). MSCs also inhibited slanMo-induced proliferation of allogeneic CD4$^+$ and CD8$^+$ T cells and dampened the polarization of naïve CD4$^+$ T lymphocytes into Th1 cells (70). In these experiments prostaglandin E2 (PGE2) was identified as a main MSC-derived immune regulatory molecule. These findings fit well with the overall function of MSCs. Other MSC-derived immunoregulatory molecules are IL-10, IL-4, TGF-β, HGF, and PDL-1, all of which act by inhibiting differentiation of autoreactive CD4$^+$ T cells into pathogenic Th1 cells by stimulating their differentiation into Th2 and Treg lymphocytes (69). These data suggest that MSCs considerably impair the immunostimulatory properties of inflammatory slanMo.

slanMo *IN VIVO*

In healthy individuals, roughly 1% of PBMCs stain positive for the slan marker (71). In healthy stem cell donors treated with granulocyte-colony stimulating factor (G-CSF), the frequency of slanMo increased from 14.9×10^6/L to 64.0×10^6/L. G-CSF was described to increase the numbers of tolerogenic DCs and T cells among mobilized blood leukocytes in the graft (72). In contrast, slanMo mobilized by G-CSF retained their capacity to produce IL-12 and TNF-α (73). Furthermore, G-CSF–mobilized slanMo programmed the differentiation of Th1 cells and displayed a strong capacity to stimulate the proliferation of naïve allogeneic cord blood T cells (73). Thus, slanMo transfused into recipients of allogeneic peripheral blood stem cell (PBSC) transplants are functionally fully capable and may support graft-vs. -host disease as well as graft- vs. -leukemia effects.

During the first month after allogeneic stem cell transplantation slanMo showed slow reconstitution in blood compared to cDCs and pDCs (74), however, a steady increase in the frequency of slanMo has been observed in the 2nd and 3rd month after post-transplantation (75, 76). The slow reconstitution of slanMo after bone marrow transplantation as observed in this study is reflected by reports on non-classical monocytes demonstrating the same slow reconstitution in blood (18). Whether these findings argue for slanMo to develop from classical monocytes, as described for non-classical monocytes has not been addressed and requires further studies.

slanMo IN DISEASES

The contribution of slanMo to the immune pathogenesis of different diseases has been studied (**Table 2**) and will be discussed in the following chapter.

Psoriasis

Psoriasis is a chronic inflammatory skin disease with an immune response steered by IL-23 and TNF-α producing antigen presenting cells (16, 31, 80–82), thereby stimulating T cells to produce IL-17, a cytokine that is now identified to be of chief importance for inducing skin inflammation in psoriasis (83). Therapeutic responses to antibody mediated neutralization of IL-17, IL-23, and TNF-α (84, 85) underscore the role of these cytokines as predominant drivers of the disease.

slanMo have been found at increased frequencies in psoriasis skin lesions and these numbers rapidly normalized with clinically effective anti-TNF therapy (31, 84, 85). In parallel to the reduced numbers of slanMo in skin lesions their frequency in blood increased. Interestingly, these cells showed a decrease in their expression of HLA-DR (76, 85). Lesional slanMo expressed IL-23, TNF-α as well as inducible nitric oxide synthase (iNOS). The phenotype (CD1c$^-$ and CD11c$^+$) and function (IL23$^+$, TNF-α$^+$, iNOS$^+$) of slanMo in active psoriasis skin lesions corresponded to TNF-α-producing iNOS expressing (TIP)-DCs, that were earlier defined by Lowes et al. (82). *In vitro* slanMo demonstrated the capacity to program T cells producing IFN-γ, IL-17, IL-22 but not IL-10 (16, 31, 81). These data lend additional support to the role of slanMo as relevant stimulatory cells in psoriasis.

Autocrine TNF-α stimulation of slanMo allows for high level production of IL-12, IL-23, IL-1ß, and IL-6 (56). In accord with the general role of TNF-α as a stimulatory cytokine, treatment with the potent TNF-α-inhibitor infliximab rapidly reduced IL-12, IL-1β, and CCL20 mRNA expression in psoriasis patients (84). The migration of slanMo from the peripheral blood into psoriasis skin lesions may be facilitated by the local expression of the anaphylatoxin C5a, fractalkine (CX3CL1), and CXCL12 for which the respective receptors are expressed by slanMo (C5aR, CX3CR1, and CXCR4) (31). Self-nucleic acid complexed to the antimicrobial peptide cathelicidin (LL37) is the best-studied autologous immune stimulus in psoriasis. Stimulating slanMo with LL37-RNA-complexes induced TNF-α production at higher levels compared to DC2 (31). The cytokine production clearly places these cells on center stage for orchestrating Th17-mediated immune responses in psoriasis. As there are other slan-negative antigen presenting cells producing IL-23 and TNF-α in psoriasis skin lesions, it remains to be elucidated whether slanMo have a unique and non-redundant stimulatory role in psoriasis skin inflammation. Given the selective expression of the slan on a pro-inflammatory cell type in psoriasis and other diseases, an antibody-directed targeting approach of slanMo has been developed (29, 31, 81, 86) that may have potential of serving as a new treatment option in psoriasis and other inflammatory diseases.

Atopic Dermatitis

Atopic dermatitis (AD) is a chronic relapsing inflammatory skin disease affecting 15–25% of children and 1–3% of adults (87, 88). The changes within the mononuclear phagocyte system in AD are complex. Inflammatory epidermal dendritic cells (IDECs) (CD1a$^+$, Langerin$^-$, FcεRI$^+$) are believed to enhance local inflammation and eczema severity in AD patients (89). Higher frequencies of dermal mononuclear phagocytes expressing CD11c, CD1a, CD206, and DC-SIGN have been identified in AD patients (90). Similar to psoriasis, a higher frequency of slanMo is also reported in the dermis of active skin lesions of AD patients. These slanMo lacked expression of FcεRI, CD1a, CD14, and CD163, thereby displaying a phenotype different from already described mononuclear phagocytes in AD patients (54). Peripheral blood slanMo of these patients retained their capacity to produce inflammatory cytokines and produced more TNF-α and IL-12 than myeloid DCs or classical monocytes

TABLE 2 | The observed location and potential role of slanMo in different diseases.

Diseases	Presence	Function	Ref.
Psoriasis	Higher frequency in skin lesions	Local expression of TNF-α, iNOS and IL-23	(31)
Atopic dermatitis	Higher frequency in skin lesions	Highly responsive to TLR4 or TLR7/8 ligands	(54)
Lupus nephritis (type III)	Selective accumulation in glomeruli with immune complex deposition	Local secretion of TNF-α and activation of endothelial cells	(43)
Lupus erythematosus	Higher frequency in skin lesions	Highly responsive to TLR7/TLR8 stimulation	(46)
Multiple sclerosis	Accumulation in highly inflamatory brain lesions	Local expression of TNF-α	(77)
Crohn 's disease	Abundent in inflamed ilial mucosa and mesentric lymphnodes	Local secretion of TNF-α and IL-1β	(78)
HIV	Higher frequency detected in peripheral blood	Secretion of TNF-α and IL-1β in peripheral blood	(71, 79)
Carcinoma	Presence in metastatic tumor draining lymphnodes	Efficient phagocytosis of tumor cells	(30)
Renal cell carcinoma	Increased frequency in ccRCC tissues	Higher frequency of slanMo associated with poor prognosis of ccRCC patients	(45)
Diffuse large B- cell lymphoma	Increased frequency in peripheral blood	Effector of antibody mediated cellular cytotoxicity	(29)

iNOS- Inducible nitric oxide synthase, TLR- Toll-like receptors. ccRCC- clear cell renal cell carcinoma Ref.- References.

after LPS or R848 stimulation (54). Mental stress is a well-known factor to trigger flares of AD (91). A standardized mental stress test in patients with AD induced an instant mobilization of slanMo into the blood circulation. Testing for their TNF-α-production showed their unchanged capacity to do so (54). The mobilization of CD16$^+$ monocytes was previously shown for psoriasis patients (92). Whether this mobilization includes all CD16$^+$ monocytes or applies preferentially to slanMo has not been addressed. Non-classical monocytes are known to function as patrolling monocytes along endothelial cells. Therefore, the observed stress induced mobilization may reflect detachment of slanMo from the vasculature into blood circulation. This process was shown to be induced by a transient rise of catecholamines induced by mental stress (54).

Cytokine production of slanMo is not a fixed condition and can be modulated by micro environmental factors relevant to AD and allergic diseases. Histamine is an important regulator of allergic inflammation that modulates pro-inflammatory functions of slanMo. Different histamine receptors are expressed by slanMo, particularly the recently identified histamine H4 receptor (H4R). Histamine effectively blunted TNF-α and IL-12 production of slanMo, a reduction mediated via the H4R and the combined action of H2R and H4R (93). Hence, H4R agonists might have therapeutic potential to down-regulate immune reactions, e.g., in allergic inflammatory skin diseases (93, 94). Birch pollen contains antigens potentially inducing allergic IgE-mediated sensitization. Pollen also contain immunomodulatory substances. In this context, pollen-associated E1-phytoprostanes (PPE1) were shown to license human monocyte-derived dendritic cell for T-helper type 2 (Th2) polarization of naïve T cells (95). Aqueous birch pollen extracts inhibited IL-12 production by slanMo in a dose-dependent manner, while the levels of IL-6 remained unaffected. PPE1 inhibited secretion of both IL-12p70 and IL-6. slanMo exposed to aqueous pollen extracts were impaired in eliciting an IFN-γ response in naïve CD4$^+$ T cells (95). These data demonstrated that slanMo having a constitutively high potency to induce Th1 responses, are susceptible to the Th2 polarizing effect of low molecular weight, non-protein factors derived from pollen.

Lupus Erythematosus

Lupus erythematosus is an autoimmune disease in which genetic and environmental factors lead to autoantibody production and induction of inflammation manifesting to multiple organs (96). The autoantibodies in lupus erythematosus patients are directed against nuclear antigens and form immune complexes containing double-stranded DNA (dsDNA) and single-stranded RNA (ssRNA) that activate DCs and drive pathogenic T cell responses (97–99). In response to ssRNA and dsDNA, plasmacytoid dendritic cells (pDCs) produce IFN-α, a critical immunoregulatory cytokine in lupus erythematosus (100, 101). slanMo were shown to lack IFN-α production but may contribute to the disease progression through high TNF-α production (46). Immunohistochemistry showed an increased frequency of slanMo in skin lesions of patients with cutaneous and systemic lupus erythematosus (46). slanMo were found scattered in the dermis where they locally expressed TNF-α. They appeared to cluster in lymph follicle-like structures where they co-localized with T cells. Incubating slanMo with serum from lupus erythematosus patients induced production of TNF-α (46). The stimulatory components of the lupus erythematosus sera are autoimmune complexes containing single-stranded RNA (ssRNA) binding to TLR7 and TLR8 or double stranded DNA binding to TLR9 (11). slanMo lack the DNA-sensor TLR9, but instead express TLR7 and TLR8 (46). In fact, ssRNA or selective TLR7 and TLR8 ligands induce TNF-α and IL-12 production in slanMo at higher levels compared to conventional dendritic cells (cDCs) or plasmacytoid dendritic cells (pDCs) (26, 31, 54).

Immune complexes binding to the vasculature frequently causes vasculitis in lupus patients (102, 103). In lupus nephritis, intracapillary accumulation of immune complexes can prime the activation of Fc receptor-bearing myeloid cells (99, 104, 105). The observation that slanMo have a CD16-mediated capacity to bind IgG-ICs (34) and to be present in lupus skin lesions (46) made us to investigate the role of IgG-ICs for the direct recruitment and activation of slanMo from the blood flow in lupus nephritis (34). Among the different types of lupus nephritis, intracapillary IC deposition and accumulation of monocytes are hallmarks of diffuse proliferative lupus nephritis class III and IV frequently leading to end stage renal disease (22, 106). The relevance of intracapillary IgG-ICs in terms of monocytes recruitment and activation, as well as the nature and function of these monocytes were not well understood. For the early focal form of lupus nephritis (class III) we demonstrated a selective accumulation of slanMo, which locally expressed TNF-α (43). *In vitro* and *in vivo* mouse studies showed that immobilized IgG-ICs induced a direct recruitment of slanMo from the microcirculation via interaction with FcγRIIIA (CD16) (43). Intravenous immunoglobulins block CD16 and completely prevented slanMo recruitment (34). Engagement of immobilized IgG-ICs by slanMo induced the production of neutrophil-attracting chemokine CXCL2 as well as TNF-α, which in a forward feedback loop stimulated endothelial cells to produce the slanMo-recruiting chemokine CX3CL1 (fractalkine) (43). These studies demonstrated that expression of CD16 equips slanMo with a capacity to orchestrate early IC-induced inflammatory responses in glomeruli and identified slanMo as a pathogenic cell type in lupus nephritis.

Multiple Sclerosis (MS)

Multiple sclerosis is a chronic inflammatory disease of the central nervous system characterized by injury to the myelin sheath and axonal loss (107). Discussions of MS pathophysiology frequently put cells of the adaptive immune response in the spotlight. However, dendritic cells, monocytes, macrophages, and microglia, collectively referred to as mononuclear phagocytes, appear to have prominent roles in MS pathogenesis. These populations of mononuclear phagocytes function as antigen presenting effector cells in neuroinflammation (108–110). In a study on MS, slanMo were found in the patient's cerebrospinal fluid and accumulated in inflammatory brain lesions. The degree of local inflammation positively correlated with the number of slanMo (77). Recruitment of CXCR4 expressing slanMo to brain lesions may be induced by CXCL12, which was found elevated in MS patients (111, 112).

Crohn's Disease

Crohn's disease is characterized by patchy inflammatory lesions and affects the entire gastrointestinal tract (113, 114). In humans, intestinal lamina propria, a subset of myeloid cells HLA-DR^{high} Lin^{-} CD14^{+} CD163^{low}, have been identified that can enhance immunity and differentiation of Th17 cells (62). A study on slanMo revealed an increased frequency of IL-1β and TNF-α-producing slanMo in the mesenteric lymph nodes of Crohn's disease patients. slanMo accumulated in inflamed colons of Crohn's disease but not in ulcerative colitis patients (78). In parallel to the presence of slanMo in peripheral tissues, their frequency in blood circulation was reduced. Thus, slanMo may contribute to the immunopathogenesis of Crohn's disease.

HIV Infection

Chronic immune activation and a breakdown of the gastrointestinal mucosal barrier allow translocation of microbial products (e.g., LPS) from gut associated lymphoid tissue into the circulation (115). LPS activates monocytes and DCs that produced pro-inflammatory cytokines such as TNF-α and IL-1β (71). Increased serum TNF-α has been reported for HIV-infected individuals and is known to promote viral replication in infected CD4^{+} T lymphocytes (116, 117). Therefore, the potential role of slanMo in fueling chronic immune activation during HIV-1 infection has been evaluated (71, 79). Dutertre et al. investigated the role of slanMo (referred to as mAb M-DC8^{+} monocytes) in peripheral blood of HIV infected individuals (79). Specifically, they addressed chronic immune hyperactivation caused by production of TNF-α. Viremic HIV patients showed an increase in CD16^{+} monocytes and a marked increase in slanMo (M-DC8^{+} cells). PBMCs of viremic patients displayed an overproduction of TNF-α in response to LPS that was mostly attributed to slanMo (79). Tufa et al. reported higher relative and absolute numbers of slanMo in peripheral blood of untreated HIV infected individuals, which were activated and secrete increased amounts of IL-1β, TNF-α and IL-12 compared to healthy controls. Furthermore, the frequency of IL-1β^{+} slanMo directly correlated with TNF-α^{+} slanMo and viral load, suggesting virus-driven immune activation of slanMo in HIV-infected individuals (71). These data are in support of a role of slanMo in the maintenance of chronic immune activation and HIV disease progression.

slanMo IN CANCER

Recently, slanMo have been implicated in a novel type of immune surveillance in cancer (45). Vermi et al. demonstrated that slanMo are recruited to metastatic tumor-draining lymph nodes (M-TDLN) where they are aligned along the tumor tissue (30). The recruitment of slanMo depended on the arrival of cancer cells to M-TDLN, as slanMo were absent in unaffected lymphnodes and at primary carcinoma sites. Within M-TDLN, slanMo were found adjacent to dead cells where they phagocytosed tumor cells (30). These slanMo expressed HLA-DR, CD40 and TNF-α. More importantly, unlike pDCs from the same patient cohort, circulating slanMo from patients with advanced colorectal cancer remained substantially intact in terms of numbers, cytokine production (TNF-α and IL-12p70) and induction of T-cell proliferation (62). Thus, in contrast to other mononuclear phagocytes these data suggested that circulating slanMo are not developmentally or functionally hijacked or converted into immunosuppressive cells by growing tumors.

A study on diffuse large B cell lymphoma highlighted slanMo as prominent effectors of antibody-mediated tumor cell targeting (29). slanMo from these patients showed an effective rituximab-mediated antibody dependent cell-mediated cellular cytotoxicity (ADCC) slightly lower when compared with the one displayed by NK cells. Moreover, slanMo acquired a macrophage-like phenotype and became very efficient in rituximab-mediated antibody dependent cellular phagocytosis (29). Previous studies identified the critical role of CD16 in slanMo mediated ADCC (118).

In multiple myeloma, numbers of circulating slanMo significantly reduced compared to healthy controls (119). Stimulation of bone marrow or peripheral blood from multiple myeloma patients with TLR7/8 ligand (R848) showed a reduced IL-12 production by slanMo. Further co-culture of slanMo with a multiple myeloma cell line or cells isolated from patients revealed a phenotypic shift of slanMo toward intermediate monocytes and these cells demonstrated a reduced capacity to induce T cell immune responses (119). In the tumor tissue of renal cell carcinoma, an increased number of slanMo have been reported, where they produced IL-10 and revealed a macrophage like phenotype (45).

Taken together, these studies identify different roles for slanMo in cancer. slanMo may be helpful by stimulating tumor specific T cells responses (32) and by conducting a tumor-directed cytotoxicity (ADCC) (29). On the other hand, slanMo can differentiate into cells that are part of a tolerogenic immune response (29, 30, 46). Thus, in cancer slanMo seem to display a remarkable functional plasticity.

CONTROLLING THE PRO-INFLAMMATORY FUNCTION OF slanMo

In this chapter, we discuss studies investigating how the immune related function of slanMo is modulated by several common therapeutics that are applied for the treatment of chronic inflammatory diseases or cancer.

PDE4-Inhibitor

A new option for the treatment of psoriasis and psoriasis arthritis is the phosphodiesterase 4 (PDE4)-inhibitor apremilast. PDE4-inhibitors increase intracellular cAMP levels and were shown to attenuate pro-inflammatory functions in different cell types and diseases (120, 121). Apremilast is currently tested in a phase III trial in Behçet's disease and is under study in a number of other inflammatory diseases (122, 123). Previous studies demonstrated that apremilast could reduce the production of GM-CSF, IL-12p70, TNF-α, and IFN-γ while increasing the production of IL-10 and IL-6 in LPS-stimulated PBMCs (124). Studies on ultraviolet B-irradiated keratinocytes showed a reduced production of TNF-α when cultured in the presence of apremilast while skin fibroblasts exhibited a reduced migratory capacity (125). Inhibition of PDE4 in slanMo reduced IL-12 and TNF-α production while this treatment enhanced their IL-23 production. As a consequence, apremilast-treated slanMo showed a reduced induction of Th1 cells while at the same time sustaining Th17 responses. A strong Th17-promoting effect of a drug that is effective in the treatment of an IL-17-mediated disease is unexpected. The enhanced IL-23p19 production in response to PDE4-inhibition can be explained by cAMP-dependent activation of protein kinase A and subsequent phosphorylation of the cAMP-response element binding protein (CREB) (126). Recently, the PDE4 inhibitor roflumilast licensed for the treatment of COPD was studied in mouse DCs generated *in vitro* from bone marrow precursor cells (127). In line with our study, these authors also demonstrated a PDE-4-inhibitor induced production of IL-23 in DCs and of IL-17 in T cells. Therefore, PDE4-inhibitors possibly exert their good therapeutic effects through modulation of functions on other immune and non-immune cells.

Dimethylfumarate

Dimethylfumarate (DMF) is a small molecule licensed for the treatment of psoriasis and multiple sclerosis (128). Skin lesions of psoriasis patients treated with DMF (in combination with monomethylfumarate—fumaderm®) showed a reduced frequency of slanMo. Studying the function of slanMo in the presence of DMF demonstrated an inhibition of CX3CL1- and C5a-induced migration of slanMo. Both, CX3CL1- as well as C5a are expressed in psoriasis plaques. DMF also attenuated the rapid spontaneous phenotypic maturation of slanMo, as judged by reduced expression of CD80, CD86, CD83, and HLA-DR (124). In addition, slanMo showed a DMF-dependent decrease in the production of IL-23, IL-12, TNF-α, and IL-10, and a reduced capacity to stimulate Th17/Th1 responses. At the level of intracellular signaling, DMF-treated slanMo showed an increased expression of heme oxygenase 1 (HO-1) (124). HO-1 is an enzyme with import antioxidant, anti-inflammatory, and cytoprotective functions. Treatment of slanMo with DMF also inhibited phosphorylation of NFκB p65. This may directly affect IL-12p70 transcription as NFκB p65 binding sites were found within the IL-23p19 promoter (124). Moreover, the observed DMF-dependent reduction in STAT1 phosphorylation would explain the reduced IL-12/IL-23 production of DMF-treated slanMo, as STAT1 signaling is essential in this respect (124, 129). Collectively, these findings demonstrated that slanMo found in psoriasis as well as in MS are a relevant target for the therapeutic immunomodulatory effects of DMF.

Chemotherapeutic Agent

Treatment of cancer with chemotherapeutic agents remains a challenge for immunological researcher. An ideal therapy should target the proliferation of cancer cells and leave the function of tumor-directed immune responses intact. In a study, comparing different chemotherapeutic agents for their *in vitro* capacity to modulate the function of slanMo, mitomycin-c, methotrexate, and paclitaxel have no influence on the ability of slanMo to secrete pro-inflammatory cytokines. The ability of treated slanMo to activate T lymphocytes and NK cells also remained intact (130). These observations provided arguments of slanMo contributing to tumor cell elimination in patients treated with respective drugs. However, in this context, doxorubicin and vinblastine significantly impaired production of TNF-α, IL-12, and IL-6 by slanMo (130). Both drugs also inhibited slanMo-mediated T cell proliferation and suppressed their ability to stimulate NK cells.

Bortezomib is an efficient targeted form of chemotherapy for treatment of multiple myeloma (131). The anti-tumor activity of bortezomib is mediated by proteasome inhibition, leading to NFκB inhibition, decreased cell proliferation and induction of apoptosis (132). Bortezomib mediated proteasome inhibition efficiently impaired *in vitro* maturation of slanMo as well as release of TNF-α and IL-12 upon LPS stimulation. In addition, it also inhibited slanMo-mediated proliferation and differentiation of $CD4^+$ T cells. Furthermore, bortezomib impaired the ability of slanMo to stimulate IFN-γ secretion and tumor-directed cytotoxicity of NK cells (133).

CONCLUSIONS AND PERSPECTIVES

Many studies have contributed to the current understanding of slanMo as cells with a pronounced potential to stimulate innate and adaptive immune responses. slanMo appear similar but not identical to non-classical monocytes with some genes such as CXCR6 being differentially expressed. In the case of the most obvious difference, namely the selective expression of the slan-antigen, the function remains to be determined. Other open questions regard the precursor cells of slanMo and the signals guiding their development.

In regard to their likely function as patrolling monocytes, slanMo may play an unexplored role in immune surveillance of the vasculature. Our recent study in immune complex induced lupus nephritis would be in line with this task. Here slanMo were shown to play an important role for the initiation of the immune complex induced immune response in the glomerular capillaries. Whether this early stimulatory function during the beginning of an immune response holds true also for other inflammatory diseases such as psoriasis is an open question. Additional investigations to the function of slanMo in cancer are to be awaited and appear relevant as *in vitro* studies demonstrated their effective tumor-directed cytotoxicity and stimulation of tumor-directed immune responses.

Overall, there is a high interest in gaining a better understanding of the function of slanMo and slan-negative non-classical monocytes. Further in-depth studies of slanMo can be highly informative for understanding immunopathology and provide an attractive target for therapeutic intervention.

ACKNOWLEDGMENTS

We thank to Steffi Oehrl, Ramona Geske, Lukas Freund, Felix Funck, and Hao Zhang for their suggestions and critical discussion. This work was funded by the Deutsche Forschungsgemeinschaft (DFG, German Research Foundation) to KS—SFB TRR 156, SCHA 1693/1-1, and project number 259332240/RTG 2099.

REFERENCES

1. Guilliams M, Mildner A, Yona S. Developmental and functional heterogeneity of monocytes. *Immunity.* (2018) 49:595–613. doi: 10.1016/j.immuni.2018.10.005
2. Zhao Y, Zou W, Du J, Zhao Y. The origins and homeostasis of monocytes and tissue-resident macrophages in physiological situation. *J Cell Physiol.* (2018) 233:6125–39. doi: 10.1002/jcp.26461
3. Passlick B, Flieger D, Ziegler-Heitbrock HW. Identification and characterization of a novel monocyte subpopulation in human peripheral blood. *Blood.* (1989) 74:2527–34.
4. Ziegler-Heitbrock L, Ancuta P, Crowe S, Dalod M, Grau V, Hart DN, et al. Nomenclature of monocytes and dendritic cells in blood. *Blood.* (2010) 116:e74-80. doi: 10.1182/blood-2010-02-258558
5. Auffray C, Sieweke MH, Geissmann F. Blood monocytes: development, heterogeneity, and relationship with dendritic cells. *Annu Rev Immunol.* (2009) 27:669–92. doi: 10.1146/annurev.immunol.021908.132557
6. Ingersoll MA, Spanbroek R, Lottaz C, Gautier EL, Frankenberger M, Hoffmann R, et al. Comparison of gene expression profiles between human and mouse monocyte subsets. *Blood.* (2010) 115:e10-9. doi: 10.1182/blood-2009-07-235028
7. Imhof BA, Jemelin S, Ballet R, Vesin C, Schapira M, Karaca M, et al. CCN1/CYR61-mediated meticulous patrolling by Ly6Clow monocytes fuels vascular inflammation. *Proc Natl Acad Sci USA.* (2016) 113:E4847–56. doi: 10.1073/pnas.1607710113
8. Thomas G, Tacke R, Hedrick CC, Hanna RN. Nonclassical patrolling monocyte function in the vasculature. *Arterioscler Thromb Vasc Biol.* (2015) 35:1306–16. doi: 10.1161/ATVBAHA.114.304650
9. Auffray C, Fogg D, Garfa M, Elain G, Join-Lambert O, Kayal S, et al. Monitoring of blood vessels and tissues by a population of monocytes with patrolling behavior. *Science.* (2007) 317:666–70. doi: 10.1126/science.1142883
10. Hanna RN, Cekic C, Sag D, Tacke R, Thomas GD, Nowyhed H, et al. Patrolling monocytes control tumor metastasis to the lung. *Science.* (2015) 350:985–90. doi: 10.1126/science.aac9407
11. Cros J, Cagnard N, Woollard K, Patey N, Zhang SY, Senechal B, et al. Human CD14dim monocytes patrol and sense nucleic acids and viruses via TLR7 and TLR8 receptors. *Immunity.* (2010) 33:375–86. doi: 10.1016/j.immuni.2010.08.012
12. Buscher K, Marcovecchio P, Hedrick CC, Ley K. Patrolling mechanics of non-classical monocytes in vascular inflammation. *Front Cardiovasc Med.* (2017) 4:80. doi: 10.3389/fcvm.2017.00080
13. Finsterbusch M, Hall P, Li A, Devi S, Westhorpe CL, Kitching AR, et al. Patrolling monocytes promote intravascular neutrophil activation and glomerular injury in the acutely inflamed glomerulus. *Proc Natl Acad Sci USA.* (2016) 113:E5172–81. doi: 10.1073/pnas.1606253113
14. Anbazhagan K, Duroux-Richard I, Jorgensen C, Apparailly F. Transcriptomic network support distinct roles of classical and non-classical monocytes in human. *Int Rev Immunol.* (2014) 33:470–89. doi: 10.3109/08830185.2014.902453
15. Stansfield BK, Ingram DA. Clinical significance of monocyte heterogeneity. *Clin Transl Med.* (2015) 4:5. doi: 10.1186/s40169-014-0040-3
16. Schakel K, von Kietzell M, Hansel A, Ebling A, Schulze L, Haase M, et al. Human 6-sulfo LacNAc-expressing dendritic cells are principal producers of early interleukin-12 and are controlled by erythrocytes. *Immunity.* (2006) 24:767–77. doi: 10.1016/j.immuni.2006.03.020
17. Hilgendorf I, Gerhardt LM, Tan TC, Winter C, Holderried TA, Chousterman BG, et al. Ly-6Chigh monocytes depend on Nr4a1 to balance both inflammatory and reparative phases in the infarcted myocardium. *Circ Res.* (2014) 114:1611–22. doi: 10.1161/CIRCRESAHA.114.303204
18. Patel AA, Zhang Y, Fullerton JN, Boelen L, Rongvaux A, Maini AA, et al. The fate and lifespan of human monocyte subsets in steady state and systemic inflammation. *J Exp Med.* (2017) 214:1913–23. doi: 10.1084/jem.20170355
19. Hanna RN, Carlin LM, Hubbeling HG, Nackiewicz D, Green AM, Punt JA, et al. The transcription factor NR4A1 (Nur77) controls bone marrow differentiation and the survival of Ly6C- monocytes. *Nat Immunol.* (2011) 12:778–85. doi: 10.1038/ni.2063
20. Carlin LM, Stamatiades EG, Auffray C, Hanna RN, Glover L, Vizcay-Barrena G, et al. Nr4a1-dependent Ly6C(low) monocytes monitor endothelial cells and orchestrate their disposal. *Cell.* (2013) 153:362–75. doi: 10.1016/j.cell.2013.03.010
21. Zhong H, Bao W, Li X, Miller A, Seery C, Haq N, et al. CD16+ monocytes control T-cell subset development in immune thrombocytopenia. *Blood.* (2012) 120:3326–35. doi: 10.1182/blood-2012-06-434605

22. Yoshimoto S, Nakatani K, Iwano M, Asai O, Samejima K, Sakan H, et al. Elevated levels of fractalkine expression and accumulation of CD16+ monocytes in glomeruli of active lupus nephritis. *Am J Kidney Dis.* (2007) 50:47–58. doi: 10.1053/j.ajkd.2007.04.012
23. Wong KL, Yeap WH, Tai JJ, Ong SM, Dang TM, Wong SC. The three human monocyte subsets: implications for health and disease. *Immunol Res.* (2012) 53:41–57. doi: 10.1007/s12026-012-8297-3
24. Kowal K, Moniuszko M, Dabrowska M, Bodzenta-Lukaszyk A. Allergen challenge differentially affects the number of circulating monocyte subsets. *Scand J Immunol.* (2012) 75:531–9. doi: 10.1111/j.1365-3083.2012.02685.x
25. Ziegler-Heitbrock L, Hofer TP. Toward a refined definition of monocyte subsets. *Front Immunol.* (2013) 4:23. doi: 10.3389/fimmu.2013.00023
26. Schakel K, Kannagi R, Kniep B, Goto Y, Mitsuoka C, Zwirner J, et al. 6-Sulfo LacNAc, a novel carbohydrate modification of PSGL-1, defines an inflammatory type of human dendritic cells. *Immunity.* (2002) 17:289–301. doi: 10.1016/S1074-7613(02)00393-X
27. Siedlar M, Frankenberger M, Ziegler-Heitbrock LH, Belge KU. The M-DC8-positive leukocytes are a subpopulation of the CD14+ CD16+ monocytes. *Immunobiology.* (2000) 202:11–7. doi: 10.1016/S0171-2985(00)80047-9
28. Micheletti A, Finotti G, Calzetti F, Lonardi S, Zoratti E, Bugatti M, et al. slan/M-DC8+ cells constitute a distinct subset of dendritic cells in human tonsils. *Oncotarget.* (2016) 7:161–75. doi: 10.18632/oncotarget.6660
29. Vermi W, Micheletti A, Finotti G, Tecchio C, Calzetti F, Costa S, et al. slan+ monocytes and macrophages mediate CD20-dependent B cell lymphoma elimination via ADCC and ADCP. *Cancer Res.* (2018) 78:3544–59. doi: 10.1158/0008-5472.CAN-17-2344
30. Vermi W, Micheletti A, Lonardi S, Costantini C, Calzetti F, Nascimbeni R, et al. slanDCs selectively accumulate in carcinoma-draining lymph nodes and marginate metastatic cells. *Nat Commun.* (2014) 5:3029. doi: 10.1038/ncomms4029
31. Hansel A, Gunther C, Ingwersen J, Starke J, Schmitz M, Bachmann M, et al. Human slan (6-sulfo LacNAc) dendritic cells are inflammatory dermal dendritic cells in psoriasis and drive strong TH17/TH1 T-cell responses. *J Allergy Clin Immunol.* (2011) 127:787-94 e1-9. doi: 10.1016/j.jaci.2010.12.009
32. Schakel K, Mayer E, Federle C, Schmitz M, Riethmuller G, Rieber EP. A novel dendritic cell population in human blood: one-step immunomagnetic isolation by a specific mAb (M-DC8) and *in vitro* priming of cytotoxic T lymphocytes. *Eur J Immunol.* (1998) 28:4084–93. doi: 10.1002/(SICI)1521-4141(199812)28:12<4084::AID-IMMU4084>3.0.CO;2-4
33. Schakel K, Poppe C, Mayer E, Federle C, Riethmuller G, Rieber EP. M-DC8+ leukocytes–a novel human dendritic cell population. *Pathobiology.* (1999) 67:287–90. doi: 10.1159/000028081
34. Dobel T, Kunze A, Babatz J, Trankner K, Ludwig A, Schmitz M, et al. FcgammaRIII (CD16) equips immature 6-sulfo LacNAc-expressing dendritic cells (slanDCs) with a unique capacity to handle IgG-complexed antigens. *Blood.* (2013) 121:3609–18. doi: 10.1182/blood-2012-08-447045
35. Yu SY, Hsiao CT, Izawa M, Yusa A, Ishida H, Nakamura S, et al. Distinct substrate specificities of human GlcNAc-6-sulfotransferases revealed by mass spectrometry-based sulfoglycomic analysis. *J Biol Chem.* (2018) 293:15163–77. doi: 10.1074/jbc.RA118.001937
36. Bochner BS, Alvarez RA, Mehta P, Bovin NV, Blixt O, White JR, et al. Glycan array screening reveals a candidate ligand for Siglec-8. *J Biol Chem.* (2005) 280:4307–12. doi: 10.1074/jbc.M412378200
37. Campanero-Rhodes MA, Childs RA, Kiso M, Komba S, Le Narvor C, Warren J, et al. Carbohydrate microarrays reveal sulphation as a modulator of siglec binding. *Biochem Biophys Res Commun.* (2006) 344:1141–6. doi: 10.1016/j.bbrc.2006.03.223
38. Carlsson S, Oberg CT, Carlsson MC, Sundin A, Nilsson UJ, Smith D, et al. Affinity of galectin-8 and its carbohydrate recognition domains for ligands in solution and at the cell surface. *Glycobiology.* (2007) 17:663–76. doi: 10.1093/glycob/cwm026
39. Tateno H, Ohnishi K, Yabe R, Hayatsu N, Sato T, Takeya M, et al. Dual specificity of Langerin to sulfated and mannosylated glycans via a single C-type carbohydrate recognition domain. *J Biol Chem.* (2010) 285:6390–400. doi: 10.1074/jbc.M109.041863
40. Ideo H, Matsuzaka T, Nonaka T, Seko A, Yamashita K. Galectin-8-N-domain recognition mechanism for sialylated and sulfated glycans. *J Biol Chem.* (2011) 286:11346–55. doi: 10.1074/jbc.M110.195925
41. Kletter D, Singh S, Bern M, Haab BB. Global comparisons of lectin-glycan interactions using a database of analyzed glycan array data. *Mol Cell Proteomics.* (2013) 12:1026–35. doi: 10.1074/mcp.M112.026641
42. van Leeuwen-Kerkhoff N, Lundberg K, Westers TM, Kordasti S, Bontkes HJ, de Gruijl TD, et al. Transcriptional profiling reveals functional dichotomy between human slan(+) non-classical monocytes and myeloid dendritic cells. *J Leukoc Biol.* (2017) 102:1055–68. doi: 10.1189/jlb.3MA0117-037R
43. Olaru F, Dobel T, Lonsdorf AS, Oehrl S, Maas M, Enk AH, et al. Intracapillary immune complexes recruit and activate slan-expressing CD16+ monocytes in human lupus nephritis. *JCI Insight.* (2018) 3:96942. doi: 10.1172/jci.insight.96492
44. Calzetti F, Tamassia N, Micheletti A, Finotti G, Bianchetto-Aguilera F, Cassatella MA. Human dendritic cell subset 4 (DC4) correlates to a subset of CD14(dim/-)CD16(++) monocytes. *J Allergy Clin Immunol.* (2018) 141:2276–9.e3. doi: 10.1016/j.jaci.2017.12.988
45. Toma M, Wehner R, Kloss A, Hubner L, Fodelianaki G, Erdmann K, et al. Accumulation of tolerogenic human 6-sulfo LacNAc dendritic cells in renal cell carcinoma is associated with poor prognosis. *Oncoimmunology.* (2015) 4:e1008342. doi: 10.1080/2162402X.2015.1008342
46. Hansel A, Gunther C, Baran W, Bidier M, Lorenz HM, Schmitz M, et al. Human 6-sulfo LacNAc (slan) dendritic cells have molecular and functional features of an important pro-inflammatory cell type in lupus erythematosus. *J Autoimmun.* (2013) 40:1–8. doi: 10.1016/j.jaut.2012.07.005
47. Hamers AAJ, Dinh HQ, Thomas GD, Marcovecchio P, Blatchley A, Nakao CS, et al. Human monocyte heterogeneity as revealed by high-dimensional mass cytometry. *Arterioscler Thromb Vasc Biol.* (2019) 39:25–36. doi: 10.1161/ATVBAHA.118.311022
48. Hofnagel O, Engel T, Severs NJ, Robenek H, Buers I. SR-PSOX at sites predisposed to atherosclerotic lesion formation mediates monocyte-endothelial cell adhesion. *Atherosclerosis.* (2011) 217:371–8. doi: 10.1016/j.atherosclerosis.2011.04.021
49. Gunther C, Carballido-Perrig N, Kaesler S, Carballido JM, Biedermann T. CXCL16 and CXCR6 are upregulated in psoriasis and mediate cutaneous recruitment of human CD8+ T cells. *J Invest Dermatol.* (2012) 132:626–34. doi: 10.1038/jid.2011.371
50. Qin M, Guo Y, Jiang L, Wang X. Elevated levels of serum sCXCL16 in systemic lupus erythematosus; potential involvement in cutaneous and renal manifestations. *Clin Rheumatol.* (2014) 33:1595–601. doi: 10.1007/s10067-014-2741-9
51. Gutwein P, Abdel-Bakky MS, Schramme A, Doberstein K, Kampfer-Kolb N, Amann K, et al. CXCL16 is expressed in podocytes and acts as a scavenger receptor for oxidized low-density lipoprotein. *Am J Pathol.* (2009) 174:2061–72. doi: 10.2353/ajpath.2009.080960
52. Dahl CP, Husberg C, Gullestad L, Waehre A, Damas JK, Vinge LE, et al. Increased production of CXCL16 in experimental and clinical heart failure: a possible role in extracellular matrix remodeling. *Circ Heart Fail.* (2009) 2:624–32. doi: 10.1161/CIRCHEARTFAILURE.108.821074
53. Hofer TP, Zawada AM, Frankenberger M, Skokann K, Satzl AA, Gesierich W, et al. slan-defined subsets of CD16-positive monocytes: impact of granulomatous inflammation and M-CSF receptor mutation. *Blood.* (2015) 126:2601–10. doi: 10.1182/blood-2015-06-651331
54. Baran W, Oehrl S, Ahmad F, Dobel T, Alt C, Buske-Kirschbaum A, et al. Phenotype, function, and mobilization of 6-sulfo LacNAc-expressing monocytes in atopic dermatitis. *Front Immunol.* (2018) 9:1352. doi: 10.3389/fimmu.2018.01352
55. Schmitz M, Zhao S, Deuse Y, Schakel K, Wehner R, Wohner H, et al. Tumoricidal potential of native blood dendritic cells: direct tumor cell killing and activation of NK cell-mediated cytotoxicity. *J Immunol.* (2005) 174:4127–34. doi: 10.4049/jimmunol.174.7.4127
56. Kunze A, Forster U, Oehrl S, Schmitz M, Schakel K. Autocrine TNF-alpha and IL-1beta prime 6-sulfo LacNAc(+) dendritic cells for high-level production of IL-23. *Exp Dermatol.* (2017) 26:314–6. doi: 10.1111/exd.13134
57. Poltorak MP, Zielinski CE. Hierarchical governance of cytokine production by 6-sulfo LacNAc (slan) dendritic cells for the control of psoriasis pathogenesis. *Exp Dermatol.* (2017) 26:317–8. doi: 10.1111/exd.13170

58. Aloulou M, Ben Mkaddem S, Biarnes-Pelicot M, Boussetta T, Souchet H, Rossato E, et al. IgG1 and IVIg induce inhibitory ITAM signaling through FcgammaRIII controlling inflammatory responses. *Blood.* (2012) 119:3084–96. doi: 10.1182/blood-2011-08-376046
59. Zarbock A, Muller H, Kuwano Y, Ley K. PSGL-1-dependent myeloid leukocyte activation. *J Leukoc Biol.* (2009) 86:1119–24. doi: 10.1189/jlb.0209117
60. Oehrl S, Prakash H, Ebling A, Trenkler N, Wolbing P, Kunze A, et al. The phosphodiesterase 4 inhibitor apremilast inhibits Th1 but promotes Th17 responses induced by 6-sulfo LacNAc (slan) dendritic cells. *J Dermatol Sci.* (2017) 87:110–5. doi: 10.1016/j.jdermsci.2017.04.005
61. Kumar NA, Cheong K, Powell DR, da Fonseca Pereira C, Anderson J, Evans VA, et al. The role of antigen presenting cells in the induction of HIV-1 latency in resting CD4(+) T-cells. *Retrovirology.* (2015) 12:76. doi: 10.1186/s12977-015-0204-2
62. Ogino T, Nishimura J, Barman S, Kayama H, Uematsu S, Okuzaki D, et al. Increased Th17-inducing activity of CD14+ CD163 low myeloid cells in intestinal lamina propria of patients with Crohn's disease. *Gastroenterology.* (2013) 145:1380–91 e1. doi: 10.1053/j.gastro.2013.08.049
63. Tufa DM, Ahmad F, Chatterjee D, Ahrenstorf G, Schmidt RE, Jacobs R. IL-1beta limits the extent of human 6-sulfo LacNAc dendritic cell (slanDC)-mediated NK cell activation and regulates CD95-induced apoptosis. *Cell Mol Immunol.* (2017) 14:976–85. doi: 10.1038/cmi.2016.17
64. Micheletti A, Costantini C, Calzetti F, Camuesco D, Costa S, Tamassia N, et al. Neutrophils promote 6-sulfo LacNAc+ dendritic cell (slanDC) survival. *J Leukoc Biol.* (2013) 94:705–10. doi: 10.1189/jlb.12 12638
65. Tufa DM, Chatterjee D, Low HZ, Schmidt RE, Jacobs R. TNFR2 and IL-12 coactivation enables slanDCs to support NK-cell function via membrane-bound TNF-alpha. *Eur J Immunol.* (2014) 44:3717–28. doi: 10.1002/eji.201444676
66. Wehner R, Lobel B, Bornhauser M, Schakel K, Cartellieri M, Bachmann M, et al. Reciprocal activating interaction between 6-sulfo LacNAc+ dendritic cells and NK cells. *Int J Cancer.* (2009) 124:358–66. doi: 10.1002/ijc. 23962
67. Jahnisch H, Wehner R, Tunger A, Kunze A, Oehrl S, Schakel K, et al. TLR7/8 agonists trigger immunostimulatory properties of human 6-sulfo LacNAc dendritic cells. *Cancer Lett.* (2013) 335:119–27. doi: 10.1016/j.canlet.2013.02.003
68. Costantini C, Calzetti F, Perbellini O, Micheletti A, Scarponi C, Lonardi S, et al. Human neutrophils interact with both 6-sulfo LacNAc+ DC and NK cells to amplify NK-derived IFN{gamma}: role of CD18, ICAM-1, and ICAM-3. *Blood.* (2011) 117:1677–86. doi: 10.1182/blood-2010-06-2 87243
69. Leyendecker A Jr, Pinheiro CCG, Amano MT, Bueno DF. The use of human mesenchymal stem cells as therapeutic agents for the *in vivo* treatment of immune-related diseases: a systematic review. *Front Immunol.* (2018) 9:2056. doi: 10.3389/fimmu.2018.02056
70. Wehner R, Wehrum D, Bornhauser M, Zhao S, Schakel K, Bachmann MP, et al. Mesenchymal stem cells efficiently inhibit the pro-inflammatory properties of 6-sulfo LacNAc dendritic cells. *Haematologica.* (2009) 94:1151–6. doi: 10.3324/haematol.2008.001735
71. Tufa DM, Ahmad F, Chatterjee D, Ahrenstorf G, Schmidt RE, Jacobs R. Brief report: HIV-1 infection results in increased frequency of active and inflammatory SlanDCs that produce high level of IL-1beta. *J Acquir Immune Defic Syndr.* (2016) 73:34–8. doi: 10.1097/QAI.0000000000001082
72. Bensinger WI, Weaver CH, Appelbaum FR, Rowley S, Demirer T, Sanders J, et al. Transplantation of allogeneic peripheral blood stem cells mobilized by recombinant human granulocyte colony-stimulating factor. *Blood.* (1995) 85:1655–8.
73. Baumeister SH, Holig K, Bornhauser M, Meurer M, Rieber EP, Schakel K. G-CSF mobilizes slanDCs (6-sulfo LacNAc+ dendritic cells) with a high pro-inflammatory capacity. *Blood.* (2007) 110:3078–81. doi: 10.1182/blood-2006-12-062984
74. Mimiola E, Marini O, Perbellini O, Micheletti A, Vermi W, Lonardi S, et al. Rapid reconstitution of functionally active 6-sulfoLacNAc(+) dendritic cells (slanDCs) of donor origin following allogeneic haematopoietic stem cell transplant. *Clin Exp Immunol.* (2014) 178:129–41. doi: 10.1111/cei.12387
75. Mager K, Wehner R, Bahr F, Oelschlagel U, Platzbecker U, Wermke M, et al. Reconstitution of 6-sulfo LacNAc dendritic cells after allogeneic stem-cell transplantation. *Transplantation.* (2012) 93:1270–5. doi: 10.1097/TP.0b013e31824fd8b4
76. Baran W, Koziol M, Wozniak Z, Banasik M, Boratynska M, Kunze A, et al. Increased numbers of 6-sulfo LacNAc (slan) dendritic cells in hand transplant recipients. *Ann Transplant.* (2015) 20:649–54. doi: 10.12659/AOT.894828
77. Thomas K, Dietze K, Wehner R, Metz I, Tumani H, Schultheiss T, et al. Accumulation and therapeutic modulation of 6-sulfo LacNAc(+) dendritic cells in multiple sclerosis. *Neurol Neuroimmunol Neuroinflamm.* (2014) 1:e33. doi: 10.1212/NXI.0000000000000033
78. Bsat M, Chapuy L, Baba N, Rubio M, Panzini B, Wassef R, et al. Differential accumulation and function of pro-inflammatory 6-sulfo LacNAc dendritic cells in lymph node and colon of Crohn's versus ulcerative colitis patients. *J Leukoc Biol.* (2015) 98:671–81. doi: 10.1189/jlb.5A1014-509RR
79. Dutertre CA, Amraoui S, DeRosa A, Jourdain JP, Vimeux L, Goguet M, et al. Pivotal role of M-DC8(+) monocytes from viremic HIV-infected patients in TNFalpha overproduction in response to microbial products. *Blood.* (2012) 120:2259–68. doi: 10.1182/blood-2012-03-418681
80. Weaver CT, Hatton RD, Mangan PR, Harrington LE. IL-17 family cytokines and the expanding diversity of effector T cell lineages. *Annu Rev Immunol.* (2007) 25:821–52. doi: 10.1146/annurev.immunol.25.022106.1 41557
81. Gunther C, Starke J, Zimmermann N, Schakel K. Human 6-sulfo LacNAc (slan) dendritic cells are a major population of dermal dendritic cells in steady state and inflammation. *Clin Exp Dermatol.* (2012) 37:169–76. doi: 10.1111/j.1365-2230.2011.04213.x
82. Lowes MA, Chamian F, Abello MV, Fuentes-Duculan J, Lin SL, Nussbaum R, et al. Increase in TNF-alpha and inducible nitric oxide synthase-expressing dendritic cells in psoriasis and reduction with efalizumab (anti-CD11a). *Proc Natl Acad Sci USA.* (2005) 102:19057–62. doi: 10.1073/pnas.0509736102
83. Brembilla NC, Senra L, Boehncke WH. The IL-17 family of cytokines in psoriasis: IL-17A and beyond. *Front Immunol.* (2018) 9:1682. doi: 10.3389/fimmu.2018.01682
84. Brunner PM, Koszik F, Reininger B, Kalb ML, Bauer W, Stingl G. Infliximab induces downregulation of the IL-12/IL-23 axis in 6-sulfo LacNac (slan)+ dendritic cells and macrophages. *J Allergy Clin Immunol.* (2013) 132:1184–93 e8. doi: 10.1016/j.jaci.2013.05.036
85. Gunther C, Blau K, Forster U, Viehweg A, Wozel G, Schakel K. Reduction of inflammatory slan (6-sulfo LacNAc) dendritic cells in psoriatic skin of patients treated with etanercept. *Exp Dermatol.* (2013) 22:535–40. doi: 10.1111/exd.12190
86. Bippes CC, Feldmann A, Stamova S, Cartellieri M, Schwarzer A, Wehner R, et al. A novel modular antigen delivery system for immuno targeting of human 6-sulfo LacNAc-positive blood dendritic cells (SlanDCs). *PLoS ONE.* (2011) 6:e16315. doi: 10.1371/journal.pone.0016315
87. Leung DY, Bieber T. Atopic dermatitis. *Lancet.* (2003) 361:151–60. doi: 10.1016/S0140-6736(03)12193-9
88. Werfel T, Allam JP, Biedermann T, Eyerich K, Gilles S, Guttman-Yassky E, et al. Cellular and molecular immunologic mechanisms in patients with atopic dermatitis. *J Allergy Clin Immunol.* (2016) 138:336–49. doi: 10.1016/j.jaci.2016.06.010
89. Yoshida K, Kubo A, Fujita H, Yokouchi M, Ishii K, Kawasaki H, et al. Distinct behavior of human Langerhans cells and inflammatory dendritic epidermal cells at tight junctions in patients with atopic dermatitis. *J Allergy Clin Immunol.* (2014) 134:856–64. doi: 10.1016/j.jaci.2014.08.001
90. Skabytska Y, Wolbing F, Gunther C, Koberle M, Kaesler S, Chen KM, et al. Cutaneous innate immune sensing of Toll-like receptor 2-6 ligands suppresses T cell immunity by inducing myeloid-derived suppressor cells. *Immunity.* (2014) 41:762–75. doi: 10.1016/j.immuni.2014. 10.009
91. Arndt J, Smith N, Tausk F. Stress and atopic dermatitis. *Curr Allergy Asthma Rep.* (2008) 8:312–7. doi: 10.1007/s11882-008-0050-6
92. Buske-Kirschbaum A, Kern S, Ebrecht M, Hellhammer DH. Altered distribution of leukocyte subsets and cytokine production in response to acute psychosocial stress in patients with psoriasis vulgaris. *Brain Behav Immun.* (2007) 21:92–9. doi: 10.1016/j.bbi.2006.03.006

93. Gschwandtner M, Schakel K, Werfel T, Gutzmer R. Histamine H(4) receptor activation on human slan-dendritic cells down-regulates their pro-inflammatory capacity. *Immunology.* (2011) 132:49–56. doi: 10.1111/j.1365-2567.2010.03336.x
94. Thangam EB, Jemima EA, Singh H, Baig MS, Khan M, Mathias CB, et al. The role of histamine and histamine receptors in mast cell-mediated allergy and inflammation: the hunt for new therapeutic targets. *Front Immunol.* (2018) 9:1873. doi: 10.3389/fimmu.2018.01873
95. Gilles S, Jacoby D, Blume C, Mueller MJ, Jakob T, Behrendt H, et al. Pollen-derived low-molecular weight factors inhibit 6-sulfo LacNAc+ dendritic cells' capacity to induce T-helper type 1 responses. *Clin Exp Allergy.* (2010) 40:269–78. doi: 10.1111/j.1365-2222.2009.03369.x
96. Moulton VR, Suarez-Fueyo A, Meidan E, Li H, Mizui M, Tsokos GC. Pathogenesis of human systemic lupus erythematosus: a cellular perspective. *Trends Mol Med.* (2017) 23:615–35. doi: 10.1016/j.molmed.2017.05.006
97. Hall JC, Casciola-Rosen L, Rosen A. Altered structure of autoantigens during apoptosis. *Rheum Dis Clin North Am.* (2004) 30:455–71 vii. doi: 10.1016/j.rdc.2004.04.012
98. Vollmer J, Tluk S, Schmitz C, Hamm S, Jurk M, Forsbach A, et al. Immune stimulation mediated by autoantigen binding sites within small nuclear RNAs involves Toll-like receptors 7 and 8. *J Exp Med.* (2005) 202:1575–85. doi: 10.1084/jem.20051696
99. Means TK, Latz E, Hayashi F, Murali MR, Golenbock DT, Luster AD. Human lupus autoantibody-DNA complexes activate DCs through cooperation of CD32 and TLR9. *J Clin Invest.* (2005) 115:407–17. doi: 10.1172/JCI23025
100. Vallin H, Perers A, Alm GV, Ronnblom L. Anti-double-stranded DNA antibodies and immunostimulatory plasmid DNA in combination mimic the endogenous IFN-alpha inducer in systemic lupus erythematosus. *J Immunol.* (1999) 163:6306–13.
101. Eloranta ML, Lovgren T, Finke D, Mathsson L, Ronnelid J, Kastner B, et al. Regulation of the interferon-alpha production induced by RNA-containing immune complexes in plasmacytoid dendritic cells. *Arthritis Rheum.* (2009) 60:2418–27. doi: 10.1002/art.24686
102. Baiu DC, Barger B, Sandor M, Fabry Z, Hart MN. Autoantibodies to vascular smooth muscle are pathogenic for vasculitis. *Am J Pathol.* (2005) 166:1851–60. doi: 10.1016/S0002-9440(10)62494-7
103. Tsokos GC, Lo MS, Costa Reis P, Sullivan KE. New insights into the immunopathogenesis of systemic lupus erythematosus. *Nat Rev Rheumatol.* (2016) 12:716–30. doi: 10.1038/nrrheum.2016.186
104. Kurts C, Panzer U, Anders HJ, Rees AJ. The immune system and kidney disease: basic concepts and clinical implications. *Nat Rev Immunol.* (2013) 13:738–53. doi: 10.1038/nri3523
105. Nimmerjahn F, Ravetch JV. Fcgamma receptors as regulators of immune responses. *Nat Rev Immunol.* (2008) 8:34–47. doi: 10.1038/nri2206
106. de Zubiria Salgado A, Herrera-Diaz C. Lupus nephritis: an overview of recent findings. *Autoimmune Dis.* (2012) 2012:849684. doi: 10.1155/2012/849684
107. Voet S, Prinz M, van Loo G. Microglia in central nervous system inflammation and multiple sclerosis pathology. *Trends Mol Med.* (2019) 25:112–23. doi: 10.1016/j.molmed.2018.11.005
108. Goverman J. Autoimmune T cell responses in the central nervous system. *Nat Rev Immunol.* (2009) 9:393–407. doi: 10.1038/nri2550
109. Mars LT, Saikali P, Liblau RS, Arbour N. Contribution of CD8 T lymphocytes to the immuno-pathogenesis of multiple sclerosis and its animal models. *Biochim Biophys Acta.* (2011) 1812:151–61. doi: 10.1016/j.bbadis.2010.07.006
110. Steinman RM, Banchereau J. Taking dendritic cells into medicine. *Nature.* (2007) 449:419–26. doi: 10.1038/nature06175
111. Calderon TM, Eugenin EA, Lopez L, Kumar SS, Hesselgesser J, Raine CS, et al. A role for CXCL12 (SDF-1alpha) in the pathogenesis of multiple sclerosis: regulation of CXCL12 expression in astrocytes by soluble myelin basic protein. *J Neuroimmunol.* (2006) 177:27–39. doi: 10.1016/j.jneuroim.2006.05.003
112. Krumbholz M, Theil D, Cepok S, Hemmer B, Kivisakk P, Ransohoff RM, et al. Chemokines in multiple sclerosis: CXCL12 and CXCL13 up-regulation is differentially linked to CNS immune cell recruitment. *Brain.* (2006) 129:200–11. doi: 10.1093/brain/awh680
113. Grip O, Bredberg A, Lindgren S, Henriksson G. Increased subpopulations of CD16(+) and CD56(+) blood monocytes in patients with active Crohn's disease. *Inflamm Bowel Dis.* (2007) 13:566–72. doi: 10.1002/ibd.20025
114. Kaser A, Zeissig S, Blumberg RS. Inflammatory bowel disease. *Annu Rev Immunol.* (2010) 28:573–621. doi: 10.1146/annurev-immunol-030409-101225
115. Brenchley JM, Price DA, Schacker TW, Asher TE, Silvestri G, Rao S, et al. Microbial translocation is a cause of systemic immune activation in chronic HIV infection. *Nat Med.* (2006) 12:1365–71. doi: 10.1038/nm1511
116. Moir S, Chun TW, Fauci AS. Pathogenic mechanisms of HIV disease. *Annu Rev Pathol.* (2011) 6:223–48. doi: 10.1146/annurev-pathol-011110-130254
117. Aukrust P, Muller F, Lien E, Nordoy I, Liabakk NB, Kvale D, et al. Tumor necrosis factor (TNF) system levels in human immunodeficiency virus-infected patients during highly active antiretroviral therapy: persistent TNF activation is associated with virologic and immunologic treatment failure. *J Infect Dis.* (1999) 179:74–82. doi: 10.1086/314572
118. Yeap WH, Wong KL, Shimasaki N, Teo EC, Quek JK, Yong HX, et al. CD16 is indispensable for antibody-dependent cellular cytotoxicity by human monocytes. *Sci Rep.* (2016) 6:34310. doi: 10.1038/srep34310
119. Lamarthee B, de Vassoigne F, Malard F, Stocker N, Boussen I, Mediavilla C, et al. Quantitative and functional alterations of 6-sulfo LacNac dendritic cells in multiple myeloma. *Oncoimmunology.* (2018) 7:e1444411. doi: 10.1080/2162402X.2018.1444411
120. Perez-Aso M, Montesinos MC, Mediero A, Wilder T, Schafer PH, Cronstein B. Apremilast, a novel phosphodiesterase 4 (PDE4) inhibitor, regulates inflammation through multiple cAMP downstream effectors. *Arthritis Res Ther.* (2015) 17:249. doi: 10.1186/s13075-015-0771-6
121. Schafer PH, Parton A, Gandhi AK, Capone L, Adams M, Wu L, et al. Apremilast, a cAMP phosphodiesterase-4 inhibitor, demonstrates anti-inflammatory activity *in vitro* and in a model of psoriasis. *Br J Pharmacol.* (2010) 159:842–55. doi: 10.1111/j.1476-5381.2009.00559.x
122. Cutolo M, Myerson GE, Fleischmann RM, Liote F, Diaz-Gonzalez F, Van den Bosch F, et al. A phase III, randomized, controlled trial of apremilast in patients with psoriatic arthritis: results of the PALACE 2 trial. *J Rheumatol.* (2016) 43:1724–34. doi: 10.3899/jrheum.151376
123. Saporito RC, Cohen DJ. Apremilast use for moderate-to-severe atopic dermatitis in pediatric patients. *Case Rep Dermatol.* (2016) 8:179–84. doi: 10.1159/000446836
124. Oehrl S, Olaru F, Kunze A, Maas M, Pezer S, Schmitz M, et al. Controlling the pro-inflammatory function of 6-sulfo LacNAc (slan) dendritic cells with dimethylfumarate. *J Dermatol Sci.* (2017) 87:278–84. doi: 10.1016/j.jdermsci.2017.06.016
125. Maier C, Ramming A, Bergmann C, Weinkam R, Kittan N, Schett G, et al. Inhibition of phosphodiesterase 4 (PDE4) reduces dermal fibrosis by interfering with the release of interleukin-6 from M2 macrophages. *Ann Rheumat Dis.* (2017) 76:1133–41. doi: 10.1136/annrheumdis-2016-210189
126. Kocieda VP, Adhikary S, Emig F, Yen JH, Toscano MG, Ganea D. Prostaglandin E2-induced IL-23p19 subunit is regulated by cAMP-responsive element-binding protein and C/AATT enhancer-binding protein beta in bone marrow-derived dendritic cells. *J Biol Chem.* (2012) 287:36922–35. doi: 10.1074/jbc.M112.402958
127. Bros M, Montermann E, Cholaszczynska A, Reske-Kunz AB. The phosphodiesterase 4 inhibitor roflumilast augments the Th17-promoting capability of dendritic cells by enhancing IL-23 production, and impairs their T cell stimulatory activity due to elevated IL-10. *Int Immunopharmacol.* (2016) 35:174–84. doi: 10.1016/j.intimp.2016.03.025
128. Al-Jaderi Z, Maghazachi AA. Utilization of dimethyl fumarate and related molecules for treatment of multiple sclerosis, cancer, and other diseases. *Front Immunol.* (2016) 7:278. doi: 10.3389/fimmu.2016.00278
129. Gavrilescu LC, Denkers EY. Interleukin-12 p40- and Fas ligand-dependent apoptotic pathways involving STAT-1 phosphorylation are triggered during infection with a virulent strain of Toxoplasma gondii. *Infect Immunity.* (2003) 71:2577–83. doi: 10.1128/IAI.71.5.2577-2583.2003
130. Wehner R, Bitterlich A, Meyer N, Kloss A, Schakel K, Bachmann M, et al. Impact of chemotherapeutic agents on the immunostimulatory properties

of human 6-sulfo LacNAc+ (slan) dendritic cells. *Int J Cancer.* (2013) 132:1351–9. doi: 10.1002/ijc.27786

131. Cavo M. Proteasome inhibitor bortezomib for the treatment of multiple myeloma. *Leukemia.* (2006) 20:1341–52. doi: 10.1038/sj.leu.2404278
132. Richardson PG, Mitsiades C, Hideshima T, Anderson KC. Bortezomib: proteasome inhibition as an effective anticancer therapy. *Annu Rev Med.* (2006) 57:33–47. doi: 10.1146/annurev.med.57.042905.122625
133. Straube C, Wehner R, Wendisch M, Bornhauser M, Bachmann M, Rieber EP, et al. Bortezomib significantly impairs the immunostimulatory capacity of human myeloid blood dendritic cells. *Leukemia.* (2007) 21:1464–71. doi: 10.1038/sj.leu.2404734

16

Regulation of Antigen Export to the Cytosol During Cross-Presentation

*Marine Gros and Sebastian Amigorena**

INSERM U932, Institut Curie, Paris, France

***Correspondence:**
Sebastian Amigorena
sebastian.amigorena@curie.fr

Cross-priming refers to the induction of primary cytotoxic $CD8^+$ T cell responses to antigens that are not expressed in antigen presenting cells (APCs) responsible for T cell priming. Cross-priming is achieved through cross-presentation of exogenous antigens derived from tumors, extracellular pathogens or infected neighboring cells on Major Histocompatibility Complex (MHC) class I molecules. Despite extensive research efforts to understand the intracellular pathways involved in antigen cross-presentation, certain critical steps remain elusive and controversial. Here we review recent advances on antigen cross-presentation, focusing on the mechanisms involved in antigen export to the cytosol, a crucial step of this pathway.

Keywords: dendritic cells, cross-presentation, cytosolic antigen export, ERAD, endosomal leakage

INTRODUCTION

Dendritic cells (DCs) play a central role in immune homeostasis by linking innate sensing to adaptive immune responses. After sampling antigens in peripheral tissues, DCs mature and migrate to lymph nodes, where they initiate adaptive immune responses by presenting processed antigens in the context of Major Histocompatibility Complex (MHC) molecules to T cells. For a long time, the generally accepted paradigm supposed that exogenous antigens were exclusively presented *via* MHC-II molecules to $CD4^+$ T cells, while endogenous cytosolic antigens, derived from self or foreign proteins, were loaded on MHC-I, thereby leading to naïve cytotoxic $CD8^+$ T cell activation. Yet, this simple assumption failed to explain how cytotoxic immune responses could be mounted against pathogens that do not readily infect DCs. This apparent contradiction was resolved by the discovery of cross-presentation, a process enabling the delivery of exogenous antigens to the MHC-I pathway for cross-priming $CD8^+$ cytotoxic T cell responses (1, 2). Since its first description over forty years ago, our understanding of the sequence of events governing antigen cross-priming has extensively increased, leading to the description of two main pathways of antigen cross-presentation, referred to as "vacuolar" and "cytosolic." While the requirement for cross-presentation in the initiation of anti-tumor immune responses is now well established (3–7), its control and the precise intracellular routes involved remain incompletely understood and, for some parts, controversial.

Here, we review the most recent advances in the analysis of antigen cross-presentation in mouse (unless stated otherwise), with a particular emphasis on the advances in understanding of antigen export to the cytosol, a crucial, yet debated, step of the cytosolic pathway.

PATHWAYS FOR ANTIGEN CROSS-PRESENTATION

In 1976, seminal work by M. Bevan showed that exogenous antigens could be presented on MHC-I molecules and prime cytotoxic immune responses, thereby unearthing a novel antigen presentation pathway that he called cross-priming (1, 2). However, the molecular mechanisms underlying cross-priming and "cross-presentation" remained elusive until the early nineties.

At that time, several lines of evidence reported that cross-presentation of bacterial antigens [i.e., the 257-264 H-2K^b-restricted epitope of ovalbumin (OVA) fused to *E. coli* Crl protein] was resistant to proteasome inhibitors (8) (suggesting lysosomal processing of the corresponding peptides), unaffected by brefeldin A (BFA) treatment (8–10) [arguing against a critical role for endoplasmic reticulum (ER)-Golgi transport] and most of the time, occurred independently from TAP, the transporter mediating peptide import into the ER (8, 11). These observations led to the first description of the "vacuolar pathway." After internalization, antigens remain confined in intracellular compartments, where they undergo lysosomal degradation, a process largely dependent on cathepsin S activity (12), and followed by loading onto post-Golgi MHC-I molecules.

Simultaneous studies with particulate, non-bacterial antigens (i.e., bead-bound OVA), showed that TAP1 deficiency in macrophages, as well as BFA treatment, abolished their ability to cross-present exogenous antigens, thereby suggesting that antigen-derived peptides must be transferred from the cytosol to the ER to bind newly synthesized MHC-I molecules (13). Additionally, cross-presentation was disrupted by proteasome inhibitors (13–16), consistent with a model in which antigens are delivered into the cytosol before proteasomal degradation and peptide import into the ER. This pathway, later termed the "cytosolic pathway," implies the export of antigens from endocytic compartments to the cytosol. The first experimental evidence of this crucial step was provided by the use of gelonin, a membrane-impermeant toxin that inactivates ribosomes when transferred to the cytosol. Macrophages phagocytosing gelonin-coated beads displayed reduced protein synthesis, indicating export of bead-bound gelonin to the cytosol (13, 14).

The aforementioned pivotal studies used mouse macrophages as models of antigen-presenting cells (APCs). It later became clear that DCs, rather than macrophages, cross-present antigens and cross-prime cytotoxic immune responses efficiently (17, 18), by means of different properties of their phagocytic pathway, including lower degradation capacity (19). When considering DCs, these cells represent a series of ontogenically and functionally diverse populations. In mice, two main resident DC subsets are found in the spleen and lymph nodes, namely Batf3-dependent CD8$^+$ XCR1$^+$ DCs (DC1s) and IRF4-dependent CD8$^-$ CD11b$^+$ DCs (DC2s) [reviewed in (20)]. At steady state, DC1s cross-present cell-associated antigens more efficiently than their DC2 counterparts, a capacity first attributed to their increased ability to capture this type of antigen (21, 22). Later experiments showed that higher cross-presentation efficacy in mouse DC1s is intrinsic and unrelated to the route of antigen uptake (23, 24), thus contrasting with the FcγR-dependent optimization of cross-presentation observed in human DC1s (25). In mouse, surface receptors, including Clec9A/DNGR-1 (26–29) or mannose receptor (MR) (30), were proposed to preferentially deliver antigens to the cross-presentation pathway, most likely through delaying delivery of their cargoes to late endosomal and lysosomal degradative compartments. DC1s also bear specialized endocytic properties that reduce/delay acidification and degradation of endocytic cargo (19, 31).

Consistent with these *in vitro* observations, mice deficient for DC1s (5), or displaying cross-presentation-defective DCs (4, 6), fail to mount cytotoxic immune responses against tumors and to control tumor development, even after treatment with checkpoint blockers. Although DC1s are best suited for cross-presentation both *in vitro* and *in vivo*, DC2s' ability to cross-present is increased by targeting antigens to DC2 specific receptors, such as FcγR (32) or DCIR2, in a stimulatory context (33), thus suggesting that both DC1 and DC2 are capable of cross-presenting antigens depending on the conditions.

The relative contributions of the cytosolic and vacuolar pathways to *in vivo* cross-presentation and cross-priming remain unclear. TAP dependency can potentially affect both pathways, as it impairs the exit of MHC-I molecules from the ER (34–37). Whether critical players in cross-presentation, such as Sec22b (4, 38, 39) or Rab43 (40), which are both required for effective cross-priming, are selectively involved in one or both pathways is unknown. The best available evidence for the cytosolic pathway being predominant in cross-priming comes from a study using mice defective for the immunoproteasome subunit LMP7. These mice show impaired cross-priming for an immunoproteasome-dependent H-Y epitope, supporting a critical role for proteasome-dependent processing, and therefore, for the cytosolic pathway *in vivo* (41). Since delivery of internalized antigens to the cytosol is very ineffective in most cell types, DCs might have developed specialized pathways to link these two subcellular compartments.

BIOLOGICAL PARAMETERS INFLUENCING ANTIGEN EXPORT TO THE CYTOSOL

Nature of Cytosolic Export-Competent Cells

By using gelonin activity or cytosolic fluorescence quantification as readouts, initial studies showed that inflammatory (14) or activated (16) mouse macrophages displayed a measurable ability to export bead-conjugated (14) or soluble (16) cargo into the cytosol. Further work revealed that soluble or complexed antigens also get access to the cytosol in steady-state bone-marrow derived DCs (BMDCs) or in a DC cell line, without prior activation (17, 18). Moreover, antigen export to the cytosol is more efficient in DCs than in macrophages, as illustrated by subcellular fractionation and subsequent western blotting (18). To assess whether DC subsets differ in their capacity to perform such transfer, Lin et al. developed a cytochrome c-based assay relying on the selective apoptosis of cells exporting exogenous cytochrome c into the cytosol (42). Only a fraction of DC1s showed susceptibility to cytochrome c-induced apoptosis, indicating a functional specialization for endosome to cytosol transport in these cells (42, 43). Notably, this cytochrome c-sensitive DC1 population strictly corresponds to the cohort of efficient cross-presenters, whereas cytochrome c-resistant DC1s cross-present antigens inefficiently and share other functional features with DC2s (42).

Nature of Antigens Exported to the Cytosol

Early microscopy observations showed that fluorescent (i.e., dextrans) or soluble (i.e., enzymatically active horseradish peroxidase: HRP) antigens gained access to the cytosol in DCs (17, 18). While 3–40 K dextrans are rapidly relocated to the cytosol, higher molecular mass dextrans (500–2,000 K) remain vacuolar (18), suggesting that antigen export to the cytosol is size-selective (18, 44). Particulate antigens, which are more efficiently cross-presented than soluble ones (14), often form large aggregates and therefore require dissociation before their translocation to the cytosol. Indeed, inhibition of vacuolar acidification abolishes the disaggregation of immune complexes and their subsequent cytosolic export (18), thus pointing to a crucial role of slightly acidic endo/phagosomal pH in this process. While some degree of degradation might favor antigen export to the cytosol due to the size-restriction of transported antigens (18), high proteolytic activity, favored by acidic pH, could destroy MHC-I-binding epitopes. In this regard, regulation of endocytic pH is of crucial importance. In DCs' endocytic compartments, incomplete assembly of v-ATPase proton pump together with Rab27a-dependent recruitment of NOX2 jointly lead to active alkalinization of luminal pH (19, 45), thereby preserving antigens from detrimental excessive degradation (46).

Export to the Cytosol and DC Activation

Aside from putative intrinsic properties of DC1s, extrinsic signals, such as Toll-Like Receptor stimulation, influence antigen export to the cytosol. Indeed, short (3–5 h) lipopolysaccharide (LPS) stimulation of BMDCs increases the proportion of cells displaying exogenous HRP in their cytosol (47). A possible explanation for the observed LPS-mediated increase in antigen export may reside in the requirement for TRIF in this process (48). Until recently, absence of quantitative reliable antigen export assays based on endotoxin-free reagents impeded detailed analysis of the role of DC activation in antigen transport to the cytosol. Recently published export assays should overcome this limitation (49).

Kinetics of Antigen Export to the Cytosol in DCs

Kinetics studies showed that HRP appeared in BMDC cytosol only 15 min after internalization (17). Rapid egress suggests that antigens are exported from early endosomes (50), as supported by microscopy experiments (51) or by mathematical modeling (52). The latter predicts that 20 min after internalization, cytosolic export of yeast-derived antigen competes with degradation associated with maturation of the endocytic compartment. Thus, only a tiny fraction of, at least, non-complexed antigens released after this time point might contribute to cross-presentation. Cytosolic translocation of HRP immune complexes appears after 60 min, and reaches a plateau after 6 h (18). Similar findings were reported for cytosolic egress of antigens associated to beads (53, 54). Additionally, these two studies provided compelling evidence that ER-mediated delivery of MHC-I loading machinery to the phagosome rendered this compartment competent for cross-presentation (55) following TAP-mediated import of cytosolic peptides (53, 54). While the relative contributions of ER and plasma membrane to the formation of cross-presentation-competent phagosomes remain debated (39, 56), Houde et al. postulated that an ER transporter, Sec61, might be involved in the translocation of antigens from the phagosomal lumen to the cytosol (53). This hypothesis was later experimentally supported by several studies detailed in the next section.

MOLECULAR MECHANISMS OF ANTIGEN EXPORT TO THE CYTOSOL

ERAD Transporter-Dependent Hypothesis

Existence of a transporter mediating antigen export to the cytosol naturally imposes conformational constraints on the translocated antigen. Indeed, antigens are unlikely to be transported in their native structure, considering the narrow diameter of known transporter pores, and are therefore expected to undergo an unfolding step before translocation. Supporting this idea, fixed OVA is less efficiently translocated into the cytosol than structurally flexible one (57). Moreover, during unfolding, reduction of disulfide bonds by GILT, a phagolysosomal thiol reductase constitutively expressed in APCs, is essential for cytosolic export of viral disulfide-rich antigens and subsequent cross-presentation (58) (**Figure 1**, left panel).

Although the requirement for protein unfolding suggests that antigens gain access to the cytosol through a transporter, the nature of the channel mediating this process remains controversial. Studies attempting to answer this question reported interactions between unfolded OVA and members of the ER-associated degradation (ERAD) machinery in ER-associated compartments (59), consistent with previous findings (53, 54). This observation led to the hypothesis that the ERAD machinery, mediating retro-translocation of misfolded proteins from the ER lumen to the cytosol, potentially through the trimeric Sec61 channel, could also operate from endocytic compartments during cross-presentation. The first functional insights into ERAD contributions to antigen export to the cytosol, came from studies using exotoxin A (ExoA), a bacterial toxin binding to the cytosolic N-terminal domain of Sec61α, and resulting in channel closure (60, 61). ExoA treatment reversed the ICP47-mediated inhibition of TAP, the latter resulting from the translocation of exogenously delivered ICP47 to the cytosol and its subsequent interaction with the cytosolic side of TAP (62). This finding, associated with the observed decrease in OVA cross-presentation following ExoA treatment (62, 63) or siRNA-mediated silencing of Sec61 (48, 59), strongly pointed to Sec61 being the channel controlling antigen export to the cytosol (**Figure 1**, left panel). In line with this hypothesis, the expression of the Sec61α, β and γ subunits is increased in DC1s, as compared to DC2s, correlating with their specific cross-presenting ability (64).

However, it has been extremely difficult to address the precise contribution of Sec61 in antigen cross-presentation and retrotranslocation from endo/phagosomes, as this channel also mediates co-translational import of proteins, including MHC-I, into the ER. To shed some light on this issue, Zehner et al. used a intrabody-based approach aiming to retain Sec61 in the ER and thereby prevent its recruitment to endocytic

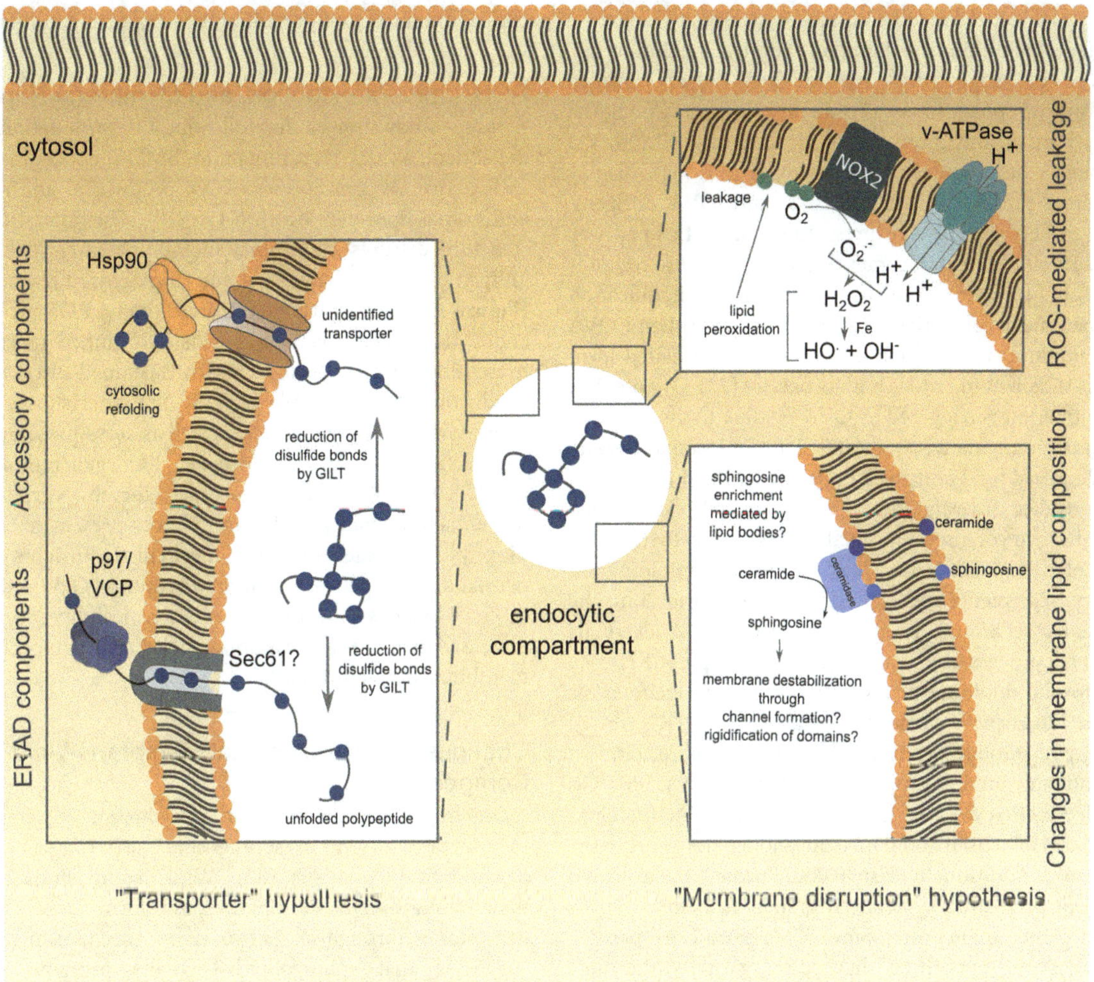

FIGURE 1 | Schematic representation of the current understanding of antigen export to the cytosol during cross-presentation. The transporter hypothesis is depicted on the left side of the figure, with complexes involved grouped according to known (for ERAD) or supposed (Hsp90 with unknown transporter) interactions. The alternative membrane disruption hypothesis is depicted on the right side of the figure. The ROS-mediated leakage part has been confirmed experimentally, while modification of endo/phagosome lipid composition, suggested by biophysical studies, is speculative and lacks functional relevance in antigen export to the cytosol.

compartments (48). Expression of the anti-Sec61 intrabody in BMDCs impairs antigen export to the cytosol and OVA cross-presentation, consistent with a role for Sec61 outside the ER, possibly in endosomes. Still, the involvement of Sec61 itself in ERAD-dependent retrotranslocation remains unclear and fraught with technical issues [reviewed in (65)]. Additionally, recent work has shown that sustained inhibition of Sec61 with a specific toxin, mycolactone, has no effect on antigen export to the cytosol, and indirectly reduces OVA cross-presentation through downregulation of other players in the pathway, including MHC-I (66). While Sec61 involvement in cytosolic antigen translocation needs further clarification, other ERAD components, such as Hrd1 and Derlin-1, might be alternative candidates.

Hrd1, an ER-resident ubiquitin ligase tagging ERAD substrates, exhibits six transmembrane domains, which is enough to form a channel (67, 68). siRNA-mediated depletion of Hrd1 in DCs results in decreased antigen export to the cytosol and cross-presentation, as well as impaired MHC-II presentation (48). These alterations in antigen presentation pathways might be caused by Hrd1 silencing-mediated ER stress and therefore require further investigation. On the other hand, the protease Derlin-1 (Der1), comprising four transmembrane domains, cannot form a channel but could possibly function as an accessory subunit of the export channel (69) by trapping ERAD substrates and rerouting them for cytosolic degradation (70). Yet, antigen cross-presentation is not perturbed by Der1 silencing in both murine BMDCs (48) and human monocyte-derived DCs (71), thus excluding a putative role for Der1 in antigen export to the cytosol.

To date, the best evidence available suggests that ERAD might control antigen transfer to the cytosol through the activity of the AAA ATPase p97. P97 forms an hexameric ring and is thought to provide the energy necessary for passage of proteins through the retrotranslocating channel (72). Exogenous addition of p97 to isolated phagosomes loaded with luciferase leads to luciferase release, whereas addition of a dominant negative version of p97 fails to do so (62), suggesting a role for the ATPase in antigen translocation from phagosomes (**Figure 1**, left panel). Along the same lines, human and mouse DCs silenced for p97 (59, 71) or expressing a dominant negative form of p97 (62), display impaired cross-presentation of MelanA and OVA antigens, respectively, whereas p97 overexpression enhances this pathway (73). P97 is recruited to endosomes following mannose receptor (MR)-poly-ubiquitination. This post-translational modification proves to be crucial for antigen export to the cytosol and OVA cross-presentation as expression of a mono-ubiquitinated form of the MR is sufficient to reduce both processes (73). Of note, MR poly-ubiquitination is triggered by OVA binding to the receptor, and is negatively regulated by the ESCRT (Endosomal Sorting Complex Required for Transport)-I protein TSG-101 (73).

Several studies investigating the role of p97 in antigen export to the cytosol used the luciferase enzyme to monitor this intracellular event (62, 74). Following unfolding in endocytic compartments and subsequent translocation into the cytosol, luciferase would need to be refolded to exert its functionality, a process likely mediated by the chaperone Hsp90. Indeed, cytosolic refolding of exogenous unfolded luciferase is compromised in Hsp90β-silenced human DCs or in DCs treated with the Hsp90 inhibitor radicicol (74). Furthermore, Hsp90α deficiency not only inhibits cross-presentation in mouse BMDCs, but also decreases cytosolic translocation of OVA, therefore implying that Hsp90 itself could mediate antigen transport to the cytosol (43, 57). Additionally, Hsp90 could protect the exported antigens from premature cytosolic degradation, before Hsp70-mediated targeting to the proteasome (57) (**Figure 1**, left panel).

The "transporter hypothesis" has, so far, garnered the most experimental support, as the main conduit for antigen export. However, it still raises important questions. Given the high degree of substrate selectivity during ERAD [reviewed in (65)], the use of a unique transporter translocating a wide variety of antigens seems unlikely. Moreover, this hypothesis fails to explain how large, non-protein molecules, such as dextrans, can be transferred to the cytosol in absence of ubiquitination, the latter being a pre-requisite for ERAD-mediated translocation. Altogether, these observations do not exclude a role for ERAD in antigen export to the cytosol, but rather suggest the contribution of additional mechanisms.

Alternative Hypothesis: Rupture of the Antigen-Containing Compartment

The first descriptions of the cytosolic pathway for cross-presentation supposed that antigens could escape endocytic compartments through membrane rupture. This hypothesis, at that time termed "indigestion model," relies on the observation that large particles are more efficiently cross-presented than small ones, and could thus be responsible for phagosomal overload, leading to membrane disruption and efficient antigen leakage to the cytosol (14). Despite intensive use of this pathway for cytosolic delivery of antibodies or bioactive proteins conjugated with endosomolytic peptides (75–77), evidence of its contribution to cross-presentation were lacking, until recently.

ROS, Lipid Peroxidation, and Membrane Rupture

A recent study showed that following LPS stimulation, VAMP8-dependent NOX2 recruitment to BMDC endosomes resulted in Reactive Oxygen Species (ROS) production and subsequent endosomal lipid peroxidation (78, 79). This alteration of lipid structure disrupts endosomal membrane integrity, leading to antigen escape to the cytosol and OVA cross-presentation (78) (**Figure 1**, upper right panel). Interestingly, ROS production in endocytic compartments is intrinsically linked to cells' cross-presenting ability. Indeed, DCs show sustained and stronger ROS production than macrophages (19), the latter subset increasing phagosomal ROS production, as well as cross-presentation, only after activation (17, 19). Moreover, ROS generation is higher in DC1 than in DC2 phagosomes, thereby correlating with the enhanced ability of DC1s to cross-present antigens (31). Biophysical studies provided mechanistic insights into lipid peroxidation-dependent membrane rupture. Oxidized lipid-rich artificial bilayers show higher water permeability (80), as well as increased membrane curvature, associated with micellization and membrane destabilization (81).

Changes in Endolysosomal Membrane Lipid Composition

Aside from lipid peroxidation, enrichment in ceramide, and to a greater extent in sphingosine, also triggers membrane permeability to solutes (82). While some studies proposed that sphingosine-based lipids could form large channels in membranes through an "all or none" mechanism (83), others suggested that sphingolipids actually promote membrane permeabilization by a graded process involving rigidification of membrane domains and subsequent creation of local structural defects (82, 84) (**Figure 1**, lower right panel). Sphingosine synthesis results from ceramide deacetylation by two ceramidases, encoded by the Asah1 and Asah2 genes, and respectively functioning at acid or neutral pH. Notably, the expression of both enzymes is higher in DC1s than in DC2s (immgen.org), suggesting that ceramide conversion into membrane-disrupting sphingosine could be increased in DC1 endocytic compartments. This DC1-specific enrichment in sphingosine could possibly be mediated by lipid bodies, which have also been proposed to destabilize some ER or phagosomal membrane domains during their formation, thereby causing leakage of the content of these compartments (85). Along the same line, BMDCs deficient for Igtp, a GTPase controlling accumulation of lipid bodies, show a selective defect for cross-presentation (86). Moreover, intracellular accumulation of lipid droplets correlates with cross-presentation efficiency, as DC1s display significantly higher amounts of these organelles than DC2s (86). However, pharmacological interference with lipid body formation fails to influence antigen export to the cytosol in the context of saponin adjuvant-based cross-presentation (87). Thus, the precise role of lipid bodies in cross-presentation and cytosolic antigen leakage remains to be specified.

Compensatory Mechanisms for Endocytic Membrane Rupture

Although several lines of evidence point to a contribution of endocytic membrane disruption and subsequent antigen leakage into the cytosol, this model has been repeatedly dismissed owing to its presumable lack of regulation and ensuing cell toxicity. Indeed, links between endocytic leakage and cell death were reported in different systems. Silica crystal-dependent phagosomal rupture, for example, leads to cytosolic release of intraluminal cathepsin B, which in turn activates the NLRP3 inflammasome, resulting in pyroptosis (88). Hydroxychloroquine-mediated cathepsin release from lysosomes can also trigger caspase activation and apoptosis (89), suggesting a requirement for control mechanisms to contain damaging consequences of leakage.

In this regard, the ESCRT machinery, formerly known for its key role in viral budding or cytokinetic abscission (90, 91), was recently identified as a core component of biological membrane repair following damage (92–96). A role for the ESCRT-I protein TSG101 in antigen export to the cytosol and cross-presentation has been previously suggested (73). However, increased cytosolic export observed following TSG101 silencing had been attributed to TSG101-dependent inhibition of MR poly-ubiquitination, required for cytosolic antigen translocation. Yet, considering the dispensable role of ubiquitination in antigen export to the cytosol (43) and the fact that TSG101 is also required for ESCRT-III-mediated repair of endolysosomal membranes (95, 96), defects in endocytic membrane repair, concomitant with TSG101 depletion, may have also contributed to the observed increased export phenotype (73). Yet, the possible involvement of ESCRT-III in controlling antigen export to the cytosol has not been investigated so far.

CONCLUSION

Identification of several critical players in antigen cross-presentation, such as Sec22b (4), or Rab43 (40), and their subsequent validation in conditional knock-out mouse pre-clinical models established a major role for this pathway in different types of immunes responses, including anti-tumor immune responses. Yet, the way antigens gain access to the cytosol during cross-presentation is far from being entirely resolved. Export to the cytosol is not only the last event in the pathway that remains largely obscure, but it is also a rate-limiting step in the process (52, 97). Identifying the molecular mechanism involved will certainly provide relevant targets to manipulate antigen cross-presentation for vaccination and immunotherapy purposes.

AUTHOR CONTRIBUTIONS

MG and SA designed, prepared and wrote the manuscript.

ACKNOWLEDGMENTS

The authors thank Dr. Philippe Benaroch and Dr. Marianne Burbage for critical reading and feedback on the manuscript. This work benefitted from data assembled by the Immgen consortium.

REFERENCES

1. Bevan MJ. Cross-priming for a secondary cytotoxic response to minor H antigens with H-2 congenic cells which do not cross-react in the cytotoxic assay. *J Exp Med.* (1976) 143:1283–8.
2. Bevan MJ. Minor H antigens introduced on H-2 different stimulating cells cross-react at the cytotoxic T cell level during *in vivo* priming. *J Immunol.* (1976) 117:2233–8.
3. Sharma MD, Rodriguez PC, Koehn BH, Baban B, Cui Y, Guo G, et al. Activation of p53 in immature myeloid precursor cells controls differentiation into Ly6c+CD103+ monocytic antigen-presenting cells in tumors. *Immunity* (2018) 48:91–106.e6. doi: 10.1016/j.immuni.2017.12.014
4. Alloatti A, Rookhuizen DC, Joannas L, Carpier J-M, Iborra S, Magalhaes JG, et al. Critical role for Sec22b-dependent antigen cross-presentation in antitumor immunity. *J Exp Med.* (2017) 214:2231–41. doi: 10.1084/jem.20170229
5. Hildner K, Edelson BT, Purtha WE, Diamond M, Matsushita H, Kohyama M, et al. Batf3 deficiency reveals a critical role for CD8alpha+ dendritic cells in cytotoxic T cell immunity. *Science* (2008) 322:1097–100. doi: 10.1126/science.1164206
6. Theisen DJ, Davidson JT, Briseño CG, Gargaro M, Lauron EJ, Wang Q, et al. WDFY4 is required for cross-presentation in response to viral and tumor antigens. *Science* (2018) 362:694–9. doi: 10.1126/science.aat5030
7. Roberts EW, Broz ML, Binnewies M, Headley MB, Nelson AE, Wolf DM, et al. Critical role for CD103(+)/CD141(+) dendritic cells bearing CCR7 for tumor antigen trafficking and priming of T cell immunity in melanoma. *Cancer Cell* (2016) 30:324–36. doi: 10.1016/j.ccell.2016.06.003
8. Song R, Harding CV. Roles of proteasomes, transporter for antigen presentation (TAP), and beta 2-microglobulin in the processing of bacterial or particulate antigens via an alternate class I MHC processing pathway. *J Immunol.* (1996) 156:4182–90.
9. Pfeifer JD, Wick MJ, Roberts RL, Findlay K, Normark SJ, Harding CV. Phagocytic processing of bacterial antigens for class I MHC presentation to T cells. *Nature* (1993) 361:359–62. doi: 10.1038/361359a0
10. Harding CV, Song R. Phagocytic processing of exogenous particulate antigens by macrophages for presentation by class I MHC molecules. *J Immunol.* (1994) 153:4925–33.
11. Bertholet S, Goldszmid R, Morrot A, Debrabant A, Afrin F, Collazo-Custodio C, et al. Leishmania antigens are presented to CD8+ T cells by a transporter associated with antigen processing-independent pathway *in vitro* and *in vivo*. *J Immunol.* (2006) 177:3525–33. doi: 10.4049/jimmunol.177.6.3525
12. Shen L, Sigal LJ, Boes M, Rock KL. Important role of cathepsin S in generating peptides for TAP-independent MHC class I crosspresentation *in vivo*. *Immunity* (2004) 21:155–65. doi: 10.1016/j.immuni.2004.07.004
13. Kovacsovics-Bankowski M, Rock KL. A phagosome-to-cytosol pathway for exogenous antigens presented on MHC class I molecules. *Science* (1995) 267:243–6.
14. Reis e Sousa C, Germain RN. Major histocompatibility complex class I presentation of peptides derived from soluble exogenous antigen by a subset of cells engaged in phagocytosis. *J Exp Med.* (1995) 182:841–51.
15. Oh YK, Harding CV, Swanson JA. The efficiency of antigen delivery from macrophage phagosomes into cytoplasm for MHC class I-restricted antigen presentation. *Vaccine* (1997) 15:511–8.

16. Norbury CC, Hewlett LJ, Prescott AR, Shastri N, Watts C. Class I MHC presentation of exogenous soluble antigen via macropinocytosis in bone marrow macrophages. *Immunity* (1995) 3:783–91.
17. Norbury CC, Chambers BJ, Prescott AR, Ljunggren HG, Watts C. Constitutive macropinocytosis allows TAP-dependent major histocompatibility complex class I presentation of exogenous soluble antigen by bone marrow-derived dendritic cells. *Eur J Immunol.* (1997) 27:280–8. doi: 10.1002/eji.1830270141
18. Rodriguez A, Regnault A, Kleijmeer M, Ricciardi-Castagnoli P, Amigorena S. Selective transport of internalized antigens to the cytosol for MHC class I presentation in dendritic cells. *Nat Cell Biol.* (1999) 1:362–8. doi: 10.1038/14058
19. Savina A, Jancic C, Hugues S, Guermonprez P, Vargas P, Moura IC, et al. NOX2 controls phagosomal pH to regulate antigen processing during crosspresentation by dendritic cells. *Cell* (2006) 126:205–18. doi: 10.1016/j.cell.2006.05.035
20. Guilliams M, Ginhoux F, Jakubzick C, Naik SH, Onai N, Schraml BU, et al. Dendritic cells, monocytes and macrophages: a unified nomenclature based on ontogeny. *Nat Rev Immunol.* (2014) 14:571–8. doi: 10.1038/nri3712
21. Iyoda T, Shimoyama S, Liu K, Omatsu Y, Akiyama Y, Maeda Y, et al. The CD8+ dendritic cell subset selectively endocytoses dying cells in culture and *in vivo*. *J Exp Med.* (2002) 195:1289–302. doi: 10.1084/jem.20020161
22. den Haan JM, Lehar SM, Bevan MJ. CD8(+) but not CD8(-) dendritic cells cross-prime cytotoxic T cells *in vivo*. *J Exp Med.* (2000) 192:1685–96. doi: 10.1084/jem.192.12.1685
23. Schnorrer P, Behrens GMN, Wilson NS, Pooley JL, Smith CM, El-Sukkari D, et al. The dominant role of CD8+ dendritic cells in cross-presentation is not dictated by antigen capture. *Proc Natl Acad Sci USA.* (2006) 103:10729–34. doi: 10.1073/pnas.0601956103
24. Pooley JL, Heath WR, Shortman K. Cutting edge: intravenous soluble antigen is presented to CD4 T cells by CD8- dendritic cells, but cross-presented to CD8 T cells by CD8+ dendritic cells. *J Immunol.* (2001) 166:5327–30. doi: 10.4049/jimmunol.166.9.5327
25. Flinsenberg TWH, Compeer EB, Koning D, Klein M, Amelung FJ, van Baarle D, et al. Fcγ receptor antigen targeting potentiates cross-presentation by human blood and lymphoid tissue BDCA-3+ dendritic cells. *Blood* (2012) 120:5163–72. doi: 10.1182/blood-2012-06-434498
26. Ahrens S, Zelenay S, Sancho D, Hanč P, Kjær S, Feest C, et al. F-actin is an evolutionarily conserved damage-associated molecular pattern recognized by DNGR-1, a receptor for dead cells. *Immunity* (2012) 36:635–45. doi: 10.1016/j.immuni.2012.03.008
27. Hanč P, Fujii T, Iborra S, Yamada Y, Huotari J, Schulz O, et al. Structure of the complex of F-Actin and DNGR-1, a C-type lectin receptor involved in dendritic cell cross-presentation of dead cell-associated antigens. *Immunity* (2015) 42:839–49. doi: 10.1016/j.immuni.2015.04.009
28. Zelenay S, Keller AM, Whitney PG, Schraml BU, Deddouche S, Rogers NC, et al. The dendritic cell receptor DNGR-1 controls endocytic handling of necrotic cell antigens to favor cross-priming of CTLs in virus-infected mice. *J Clin Invest.* (2012) 122:1615–27. doi: 10.1172/JCI60644
29. Sancho D, Joffre OP, Keller AM, Rogers NC, Martínez D, Hernanz-Falcón P, et al. Identification of a dendritic cell receptor that couples sensing of necrosis to immunity. *Nature* (2009) 458:899–903. doi: 10.1038/nature07750
30. Burgdorf S, Kautz A, Böhnert V, Knolle PA, Kurts C. Distinct pathways of antigen uptake and intracellular routing in CD4 and CD8 T cell activation. *Science* (2007) 316:612–6. doi: 10.1126/science.1137971
31. Savina A, Peres A, Cebrian I, Carmo N, Moita C, Hacohen N, et al. The small GTPase Rac2 controls phagosomal alkalinization and antigen crosspresentation selectively in CD8(+) dendritic cells. *Immunity* (2009) 30:544–55. doi: 10.1016/j.immuni.2009.01.013
32. den Haan JMM, Bevan MJ. Constitutive versus activation-dependent cross-presentation of immune complexes by CD8(+) and CD8(-) dendritic cells *in vivo*. *J Exp Med.* (2002) 196:817–27. doi: 10.1084/jem.200 20295
33. Neubert K, Lehmann CHK, Heger L, Baranska A, Staedtler AM, Buchholz VR, et al. Antigen delivery to CD11c+CD8- dendritic cells induces protective immune responses against experimental melanoma in mice *in vivo*. *J Immunol.* (2014) 192:5830–8. doi: 10.4049/jimmunol.13 00975
34. Chefalo PJ, Grandea AG, Van Kaer L, Harding CV. Tapasin–/– and TAP1–/– macrophages are deficient in vacuolar alternate class I MHC (MHC-I) processing due to decreased MHC-I stability at phagolysosomal pH. *J Immunol.* (2003) 170:5825–33. doi: 10.4049/jimmunol.170.12.5825
35. Day PM, Esquivel F, Lukszo J, Bennink JR, Yewdell JW. Effect of TAP on the generation and intracellular trafficking of peptide-receptive major histocompatibility complex class I molecules. *Immunity* (1995) 2: 137–47.
36. Van Kaer L, Ashton-Rickardt PG, Ploegh HL, Tonegawa S. TAP1 mutant mice are deficient in antigen presentation, surface class I molecules, and CD4–8+ T cells. *Cell* (1992) 71:1205–14.
37. Merzougui N, Kratzer R, Saveanu L, van Endert P. A proteasome-dependent, TAP-independent pathway for cross-presentation of phagocytosed antigen. *EMBO Rep.* (2011) 12:1257–64. doi: 10.1038/embor.2011.203
38. Cebrian I, Visentin G, Blanchard N, Jouve M, Bobard A, Moita C, et al. Sec22b regulates phagosomal maturation and antigen crosspresentation by dendritic cells. *Cell* (2011) 147:1355–68. doi: 10.1016/j.cell.2011.11.021
39. Nair-Gupta P, Baccarini A, Tung N, Seyffer F, Florey O, Huang Y, et al. TLR signals induce phagosomal MHC-I delivery from the endosomal recycling compartment to allow cross-presentation. *Cell* (2014) 158:506–21. doi: 10.1016/j.cell.2014.04.054
40. Kretzer NM, Theisen DJ, Tussiwand R, Briseño CG, Grajales-Reyes GE, Wu X, et al. RAB43 facilitates cross-presentation of cell-associated antigens by CD8α+ dendritic cells. *J Exp Med.* (2016) 213:2871–83. doi: 10.1084/jem.20160597
41. Palmowski MJ, Gileadi U, Salio M, Gallimore A, Millrain M, James E, et al. Role of immunoproteasomes in cross-presentation. *J Immunol.* (2006) 177:983–90. doi: 10.4049/jimmunol.177.2.983
42. Lin ML, Zhan Y, Proietto AI, Prato S, Wu L, Heath WR, et al. Selective suicide of cross-presenting CD8+ dendritic cells by cytochrome c injection shows functional heterogeneity within this subset. *Proc Natl Acad Sci USA.* (2008) 105:3029–34. doi: 10.1073/pnas.0712394105
43. Imai T, Kato Y, Kajiwara C, Mizukami S, Ishige I, Ichiyanagi T, et al. Heat shock protein 90 (HSP90) contributes to cytosolic translocation of extracellular antigen for cross-presentation by dendritic cells. *Proc Natl Acad Sci USA.* (2011) 108:16363–8. doi: 10.1073/pnas.1108372108
44. Mant A, Chinnery F, Elliott T, Williams AP. The pathway of cross-presentation is influenced by the particle size of phagocytosed antigen. *Immunology* (2012) 136:163–75. doi: 10.1111/j.1365-2567.2012.03558.x
45. Jancic C, Savina A, Wasmeier C, Tolmachova T, El-Benna J, Dang PM-C, et al. Rab27a regulates phagosomal pH and NADPH oxidase recruitment to dendritic cell phagosomes. *Nat Cell Biol.* (2007) 9:367–78. doi: 10.1038/ncb1552
46. Accapezzato D, Visco V, Francavilla V, Molette C, Donato T, Paroli M, et al. Chloroquine enhances human CD8+ T cell responses against soluble antigens *in vivo*. *J Exp Med.* (2005) 202:817–28. doi: 10.1084/jem.20051106
47. Gil-Torregrosa BC, Lennon-Duménil AM, Kessler B, Guermonprez P, Ploegh HL, Fruci D, et al. Control of cross-presentation during dendritic cell maturation. *Eur J Immunol.* (2004) 34:398–407. doi: 10.1002/eji.2003 24508
48. Zehner M, Marschall AL, Bos E, Schloetel J-G, Kreer C, Fehrenschild D, et al. The translocon protein Sec61 mediates antigen transport from endosomes in the cytosol for cross-presentation to CD8(+) T cells. *Immunity* (2015) 42:850–63. doi: 10.1016/j.immuni.2015.04.008
49. Lu Q, Grotzke JE, Cresswell P. A novel probe to assess cytosolic entry of exogenous proteins. *Nat Commun* (2018) 9:3104. doi: 10.1038/s41467-018-05556-z
50. Burgdorf S, Schölz C, Kautz A, Tampé R, Kurts C. Spatial and mechanistic separation of cross-presentation and endogenous antigen presentation. *Nat Immunol.* (2008) 9:558–66. doi: 10.1038/ni.1601
51. Hotta C, Fujimaki H, Yoshinari M, Nakazawa M, Minami M. The delivery of an antigen from the endocytic compartment into the cytosol for cross-presentation is restricted to early immature dendritic cells. *Immunology* (2006) 117:97–107. doi: 10.1111/j.1365-2567.2005.02270.x
52. Howland SW, Wittrup KD. Antigen release kinetics in the phagosome are critical to cross-presentation efficiency. *J Immunol.* (2008) 180:1576–83. doi: 10.4049/jimmunol.180.3.1576
53. Houde M, Bertholet S, Gagnon E, Brunet S, Goyette G, Laplante A, et al. Phagosomes are competent organelles for antigen cross-presentation. *Nature* (2003) 425:402–6. doi: 10.1038/nature01912
54. Guermonprez P, Saveanu L, Kleijmeer M, Davoust J, Van Endert P, Amigorena S. ER-phagosome fusion defines an MHC class I

cross-presentation compartment in dendritic cells. *Nature* (2003) 425:397–402. doi: 10.1038/nature01911

55. Gagnon E, Duclos S, Rondeau C, Chevet E, Cameron PH, Steele-Mortimer O, et al. Endoplasmic reticulum-mediated phagocytosis is a mechanism of entry into macrophages. *Cell* (2002) 110:119–31. doi: 10.1016/S0092-8674(02)00797-3
56. Touret N, Paroutis P, Terebiznik M, Harrison RE, Trombetta S, Pypaert M, et al. Quantitative and dynamic assessment of the contribution of the ER to phagosome formation. *Cell* (2005) 123:157–70. doi: 10.1016/j.cell.2005.08.018
57. Kato Y, Kajiwara C, Ishige I, Mizukami S, Yamazaki C, Eikawa S, et al. HSP70 and HSP90 differentially regulate translocation of extracellular antigen to the cytosol for cross-presentation. *Autoimmune Dis.* (2012) 2012:745962. doi: 10.1155/2012/745962
58. Singh R, Cresswell P. Defective cross-presentation of viral antigens in GILT-free mice. *Science* (2010) 328:1394–8. doi: 10.1126/science.1189176
59. Imai J, Hasegawa H, Maruya M, Koyasu S, Yahara I. Exogenous antigens are processed through the endoplasmic reticulum-associated degradation (ERAD) in cross-presentation by dendritic cells. *Int Immunol.* (2005) 17:45–53. doi: 10.1093/intimm/dxh184
60. Schäuble N, Cavalié A, Zimmermann R, Jung M. Interaction of *Pseudomonas aeruginosa* exotoxin A with the human Sec61 complex suppresses passive calcium efflux from the endoplasmic reticulum. *Channels Austin Tex.* (2014) 8:76–83. doi: 10.4161/chan.26526
61. Koopmann JO, Albring J, Hüter E, Bulbuc N, Spee P, Neefjes J, et al. Export of antigenic peptides from the endoplasmic reticulum intersects with retrograde protein translocation through the Sec61p channel. *Immunity* (2000) 13:117–27. doi: 10.1016/S1074-7613(00)00013-3
62. Ackerman AL, Giodini A, Cresswell P. A role for the endoplasmic reticulum protein retrotranslocation machinery during crosspresentation by dendritic cells. *Immunity* (2006) 25:607–17. doi: 10.1016/j.immuni.2006.08.017
63. Goldszmid RS, Coppens I, Lev A, Caspar P, Mellman I, Sher A. Host ER-parasitophorous vacuole interaction provides a route of entry for antigen cross-presentation in Toxoplasma gondii-infected dendritic cells. *J Exp Med.* (2009) 206:399–410. doi: 10.1084/jem.20082108
64. Dudziak D, Kamphorst AO, Heidkamp GF, Buchholz VR, Trumpfheller C, Yamazaki S, et al. Differential antigen processing by dendritic cell subsets *In vivo*. *Science* (2007) 315:107–11. doi: 10.1126/science.1136080
65. Römisch K. A case for Sec61 channel involvement in ERAD. *Trends Biochem Sci.* (2017) 42:171–9. doi: 10.1016/j.tibs.2016.10.005
66. Grotzke JE, Kozik P, Morel J D, Impens F, Pietrosemoli N, Cresswell P, et al. Sec61 blockade by mycolactone inhibits antigen cross-presentation independently of endosome-to-cytosol export. *Proc Natl Acad Sci USA.* (2017) 114:E5910–19. doi: 10.1073/pnas.1705242114
67. Schoebel S, Mi W, Stein A, Ovchinnikov S, Pavlovicz R, DiMaio F, et al. Cryo-EM structure of the protein-conducting ERAD channel Hrd1 in complex with Hrd3. *Nature* (2017) 548:352–5. doi: 10.1038/nature23314
68. Stein A, Ruggiano A, Carvalho P, Rapoport TA. Key steps in ERAD of luminal ER proteins reconstituted with purified components. *Cell* (2014) 158:1375–88. doi: 10.1016/j.cell.2014.07.050
69. Mehnert M, Sommer T, Jarosch E. Der1 promotes movement of misfolded proteins through the endoplasmic reticulum membrane. *Nat Cell Biol.* (2014) 16:77–86. doi: 10.1038/ncb2882
70. Kadowaki H, Satrimafitrah P, Takami Y, Nishitoh H. Molecular mechanism of ER stress-induced pre-emptive quality control involving association of the translocon, Derlin-1, and HRD1. *Sci Rep.* (2018) 8:7317. doi: 10.1038/s41598-018-25724-x
71. Ménager J, Ebstein F, Oger R, Hulin P, Nedellec S, Duverger E, et al. Cross-presentation of synthetic long peptides by human dendritic cells: a process dependent on ERAD component p97/VCP but Not sec61 and/or Derlin-1. *PLoS ONE* (2014) 9:e89897. doi: 10.1371/journal.pone.0089897
72. Ye Y, Meyer HH, Rapoport TA. Function of the p97-Ufd1-Npl4 complex in retrotranslocation from the ER to the cytosol: dual recognition of nonubiquitinated polypeptide segments and polyubiquitin chains. *J Cell Biol.* (2003) 162:71–84. doi: 10.1083/jcb.200302169
73. Zehner M, Chasan AI, Schuette V, Embgenbroich M, Quast T, Kolanus W, et al. Mannose receptor polyubiquitination regulates endosomal recruitment of p97 and cytosolic antigen translocation for cross-presentation. *Proc Natl Acad Sci USA.* (2011) 108:9933–8. doi: 10.1073/pnas.1102397108
74. Giodini A, Cresswell P. Hsp90-mediated cytosolic refolding of exogenous proteins internalized by dendritic cells. *EMBO J.* (2008) 27:201–11. doi: 10.1038/sj.emboj.7601941
75. Akishiba M, Takeuchi T, Kawaguchi Y, Sakamoto K, Yu H-H, Nakase I, et al. Cytosolic antibody delivery by lipid-sensitive endosomolytic peptide. *Nat Chem.* (2017) 9:751–61. doi: 10.1038/nchem.2779
76. El-Sayed A, Futaki S, Harashima H. Delivery of macromolecules using arginine-rich cell-penetrating peptides: ways to overcome endosomal entrapment. *AAPS J.* (2009) 11:13–22. doi: 10.1208/s12248-008-9071-2
77. Li M, Tao Y, Shu Y, LaRochelle JR, Steinauer A, Thompson D, et al. Discovery and characterization of a peptide that enhances endosomal escape of delivered proteins *in vitro* and *in vivo*. *J Am Chem Soc.* (2015) 137:14084–93. doi: 10.1021/jacs.5b05694
78. Dingjan I, Verboogen DR, Paardekooper LM, Revelo NH, Sittig SP, Visser LJ, et al. Lipid peroxidation causes endosomal antigen release for cross-presentation. *Sci Rep.* (2016) 6:22064. doi: 10.1038/srep22064
79. Dingjan I, Paardekooper LM, Verboogen DRJ, von Mollard GF, Ter Beest M, van den Bogaart G. VAMP8-mediated NOX2 recruitment to endosomes is necessary for antigen release. *Eur J Cell Biol.* (2017) 96:705–14. doi: 10.1016/j.ejcb.2017.06.007
80. Wong-Ekkabut J, Xu Z, Triampo W, Tang I-M, Tieleman DP, Monticelli L. Effect of lipid peroxidation on the properties of lipid bilayers: a molecular dynamics study. *Biophys J.* (2007) 93:4225–36. doi: 10.1529/biophysj.107.112565
81. Agmon E, Solon J, Bassereau P, Stockwell BR. Modeling the effects of lipid peroxidation during ferroptosis on membrane properties. *Sci Rep.* (2018) 8:5155. doi: 10.1038/s41598-018-23408-0
82. Contreras F-X, Sot J, Alonso A, Goñi FM. Sphingosine increases the permeability of model and cell membranes. *Biophys J.* (2006) 90:4085–92. doi: 10.1529/biophysj.105.076471
83. Siskind LJ, Kolesnick RN, Colombini M. Ceramide channels increase the permeability of the mitochondrial outer membrane to small proteins. *J Biol Chem.* (2002) 277:26796–803. doi: 10.1074/jbc.M200754200
84. Jiménez-Rojo N, Sot J, Viguera AR, Collado MI, Torrecillas A, Gómez-Fernández JC, et al. Membrane permeabilization induced by sphingosine: effect of negatively charged lipids. *Biophys J.* (2014) 106:2577–84. doi: 10.1016/j.bpj.2014.04.038
85. Ploegh HL. A lipid-based model for the creation of an escape hatch from the endoplasmic reticulum. *Nature* (2007) 448:435–8. doi: 10.1038/nature06004
86. Bougnères L, Helft J, Tiwari S, Vargas P, Chang BH-J, Chan L, et al. A role for lipid bodies in the cross-presentation of phagocytosed antigens by MHC class I in dendritic cells. *Immunity* (2009) 31:232–44. doi: 10.1016/j.immuni.2009.06.022
87. den Brok MH, Büll C, Wassink M, de Graaf AM, Wagenaars JA, Minderman M, et al. Saponin-based adjuvants induce cross-presentation in dendritic cells by intracellular lipid body formation. *Nat Commun.* (2016) 7:13324. doi: 10.1038/ncomms13324
88. Hornung V, Bauernfeind F, Halle A, Samstad EO, Kono H, Rock KL, et al. Silica crystals and aluminum salts activate the NALP3 inflammasome through phagosomal destabilization. *Nat Immunol.* (2008) 9:847–56. doi: 10.1038/ni.1631
89. Boya P, Gonzalez-Polo R-A, Poncet D, Andreau K, Vieira HLA, Roumier T, et al. Mitochondrial membrane permeabilization is a critical step of lysosome-initiated apoptosis induced by hydroxychloroquine. *Oncogene* (2003) 22:3927–36. doi: 10.1038/sj.onc.1206622
90. Carlton JG, Caballe A, Agromayor M, Kloc M, Martin-Serrano J. ESCRT-III governs the Aurora B-mediated abscission checkpoint through CHMP4C. *Science* (2012) 336:220–5. doi: 10.1126/science.1217180
91. Garrus JE, von Schwedler UK, Pornillos OW, Morham SG, Zavitz KH, Wang HE, et al. Tsg101 and the vacuolar protein sorting pathway are essential for HIV-1 budding. *Cell* (2001) 107:55–65. doi: 10.1016/S0092-8674(01)00506-2

92. Olmos Y, Hodgson L, Mantell J, Verkade P, Carlton JG. ESCRT-III controls nuclear envelope reformation. *Nature* (2015) 522:236–9. doi: 10.1038/nature14503
93. Vietri M, Schink KO, Campsteijn C, Wegner CS, Schultz SW, Christ L, et al. Spastin and ESCRT-III coordinate mitotic spindle disassembly and nuclear envelope sealing. *Nature* (2015) 522:231–5. doi: 10.1038/nature14408
94. Jimenez AJ, Maiuri P, Lafaurie-Janvore J, Divoux S, Piel M, Perez F. ESCRT machinery is required for plasma membrane repair. *Science* (2014) 343:1247136. doi: 10.1126/science.1247136
95. Skowyra ML, Schlesinger PH, Naismith TV, Hanson PI. Triggered recruitment of ESCRT machinery promotes endolysosomal repair. *Science* (2018) 360:eaar5078. doi: 10.1126/science.aar5078
96. Radulovic M, Schink KO, Wenzel EM, Nähse V, Bongiovanni A, Lafont F, et al. ESCRT-mediated lysosome repair precedes lysophagy and promotes cell survival. *EMBO J.* (2018) 37:e99753. doi: 10.15252/embj.201899753
97. Moore MW, Carbone FR, Bevan MJ. Introduction of soluble protein into the class I pathway of antigen processing and presentation. *Cell* (1988) 54:777–85.

Permissions

All chapters in this book were first published by Frontiers; hereby published with permission under the Creative Commons Attribution License or equivalent. Every chapter published in this book has been scrutinized by our experts. Their significance has been extensively debated. The topics covered herein carry significant findings which will fuel the growth of the discipline. They may even be implemented as practical applications or may be referred to as a beginning point for another development.

The contributors of this book come from diverse backgrounds, making this book a truly international effort. This book will bring forth new frontiers with its revolutionizing research information and detailed analysis of the nascent developments around the world.

We would like to thank all the contributing authors for lending their expertise to make the book truly unique. They have played a crucial role in the development of this book. Without their invaluable contributions this book wouldn't have been possible. They have made vital efforts to compile up to date information on the varied aspects of this subject to make this book a valuable addition to the collection of many professionals and students.

This book was conceptualized with the vision of imparting up-to-date information and advanced data in this field. To ensure the same, a matchless editorial board was set up. Every individual on the board went through rigorous rounds of assessment to prove their worth. After which they invested a large part of their time researching and compiling the most relevant data for our readers.

The editorial board has been involved in producing this book since its inception. They have spent rigorous hours researching and exploring the diverse topics which have resulted in the successful publishing of this book. They have passed on their knowledge of decades through this book. To expedite this challenging task, the publisher supported the team at every step. A small team of assistant editors was also appointed to further simplify the editing procedure and attain best results for the readers.

Apart from the editorial board, the designing team has also invested a significant amount of their time in understanding the subject and creating the most relevant covers. They scrutinized every image to scout for the most suitable representation of the subject and create an appropriate cover for the book.

The publishing team has been an ardent support to the editorial, designing and production team. Their endless efforts to recruit the best for this project, has resulted in the accomplishment of this book. They are a veteran in the field of academics and their pool of knowledge is as vast as their experience in printing. Their expertise and guidance has proved useful at every step. Their uncompromising quality standards have made this book an exceptional effort. Their encouragement from time to time has been an inspiration for everyone.

The publisher and the editorial board hope that this book will prove to be a valuable piece of knowledge for researchers, students, practitioners and scholars across the globe.

List of Contributors

Sebastian Montealegre and Peter M. van Endert
Institut National de la Santé et de la Recherche Médicale, Unité 1151, Paris, France
Université Paris Descartes, Faculté de Médecine, Paris, France
Centre National de la Recherche Scientifique, UMR8253, Paris, France

Felix Wagner, Ulrike Hölig, Friederike Wilczkowski and Maximilian Kießler
Institute of Immunology, Faculty of Medicine Carl Gustav Carus, Technische Universität Dresden, Dresden, Germany

Ioana Plesca
Institute of Immunology, Faculty of Medicine Carl Gustav Carus, Technische Universität Dresden, Dresden, Germany
Department of Radiotherapy and Radiation Oncology, University Hospital Carl Gustav Carus, Technische Universität Dresden, Dresden, Germany

Ulrich Sommer and Armin Jarosch
Institute of Pathology, University Hospital of Dresden, Dresden, Germany

Gunnar Folprecht and Martin Bornhäuser
Partner Site Dresden, National Center for Tumor Diseases (NCT), Dresden, Germany
Partner Site Dresden, German Cancer Consortium (DKTK), and German Cancer Research Center (DKFZ), Heidelberg, Germany
Department of Medicine I, University Hospital Carl Gustav Carus, Technische Universität Dresden, Dresden, Germany

Rebekka Wehner and Marc Schmitz
Institute of Immunology, Faculty of Medicine Carl Gustav Carus, Technische Universität Dresden, Dresden, Germany
Partner Site Dresden, National Center for Tumor Diseases (NCT), Dresden, Germany
Partner Site Dresden, German Cancer Consortium (DKTK), and German Cancer Research Center (DKFZ), Heidelberg, Germany

Katharina Flecke and Maia Arsova
Institute of Immunology, Faculty of Medicine Carl Gustav Carus, Technische Universität Dresden, Dresden, Germany
Department of Medicine I, University Hospital Carl Gustav Carus, Technische Universität Dresden, Dresden, Germany

Antje Tunger
Institute of Immunology, Faculty of Medicine Carl Gustav Carus, Technische Universität Dresden, Dresden, Germany
Partner Site Dresden, National Center for Tumor Diseases (NCT), Dresden, Germany

Andreas Bogner
Department of Gastrointestinal, Thoracic, and Vascular Surgery, University Hospital Carl Gustav Carus, Technische Universität Dresden, Dresden, Germany

Christoph Reißfelder
Department of Surgery, Mannheim University Medical Centre, University of Heidelberg, Mannheim, Germany

Jürgen Weitz
Partner Site Dresden, National Center for Tumor Diseases (NCT), Dresden, Germany
Partner Site Dresden, German Cancer Consortium (DKTK), and German Cancer Research Center (DKFZ), Heidelberg, Germany
Department of Gastrointestinal, Thoracic, and Vascular Surgery, University Hospital Carl Gustav Carus, Technische Universität Dresden, Dresden, Germany

Fareed Ahmad and Knut Schäkel
Department of Dermatology, University Hospital of Heidelberg, Heidelberg, Germany

Esther G. C. Troost and Mechthild Krause
Department of Radiotherapy and Radiation Oncology, University Hospital Carl Gustav Carus, Technische Universität Dresden, Dresden, Germany
Partner Site Dresden, National Center for Tumor Diseases (NCT), Dresden, Germany
Partner Site Dresden, German Cancer Consortium (DKTK), and German Cancer Research Center (DKFZ), Heidelberg, Germany
OncoRay – National Center for Radiation Research in Oncology, Dresden, Germany
Institute of Radiooncology – OncoRay, Helmholtz-Zentrum Dresden-Rossendorf, Dresden, Germany

Michael P. Bachmann
Partner Site Dresden, National Center for Tumor Diseases (NCT), Dresden, Germany
Partner Site Dresden, German Cancer Consortium (DKTK), and German Cancer Research Center (DKFZ), Heidelberg, Germany
Department of Radioimmunology, Institute of Radiopharmaceutical Cancer Research, Helmholtz Center Dresden-Rossendorf, Dresden, Germany

Daniela Aust and Gustavo Baretton
Institute of Pathology, University Hospital of Dresden, Dresden, Germany
Partner Site Dresden, National Center for Tumor Diseases (NCT), Dresden, Germany
Partner Site Dresden, German Cancer Consortium (DKTK), and German Cancer Research Center (DKFZ), Heidelberg, Germany

Denise van Uden, Karin Boomars and Mirjam Kool
Department of Pulmonary Medicine, Erasmus MC, Rotterdam, Netherlands

Rajkumar Noubade, Sonia Majri-Morrison and Kristin V. Tarbell
Department of Inflammation and Oncology, Amgen Research, Amgen Inc., South San Francisco, CA, United States

Edione Cristina dos Reis, Vinícius Nunes Cordeiro Leal, Jaíne Lima da Silva Soares, Fernanda Pereira Fernandes, Dhêmerson Souza de Lima and Alessandra Pontillo
Laboratory of Immunogenetics, Department of Immunology, Institute of Biomedical Sciences/ICB, University of São Paulo/USP, São Paulo, Brazil

Bruna Cunha de Alencar
Laboratory of Immune System Cell Biology, Department of Immunology, Institute of Biomedical Sciences/ICB, University of São Paulo/USP, São Paulo, Brazil

Rafael Tibúrcio, Sara Nunes, Ivanéia Nunes, Mariana Rosa Ampuero, Icaro Bonyek Silva and Reinan Lima
Gonçalo Moniz Institute, Oswaldo Cruz Foundation, Salvador, Brazil
Federal University of Bahia, Salvador, Brazil

Natalia Machado Tavares and Cláudia Brodskyn
Gonçalo Moniz Institute, Oswaldo Cruz Foundation, Salvador, Brazil
Federal University of Bahia, Salvador, Brazil
Instituto Nacional de Ciência e Tecnologia (INCT) iii Instituto de Investigação em Imunologia, São Paulo, Brazil

Manuela Schönfeld, Ulla Knackmuss, Parul Chandorkar, Cornelia Lass-Flörl, Wilfried Posch and Doris Wilflingseder
Division of Hygiene and Medical Microbiology, Medical University of Innsbruck, Innsbruck, Austria

Paul Hörtnagl
Central Institute for Blood Transfusion and Immunological Department, Medical University of Innsbruck, Innsbruck, Austria

Thomas John Hope
Department of Cell and Molecular Biology, Feinberg School of Medicine, Northwestern University, Chicago, IL, United States

Arnaud Moris
Sorbonne Université, INSERM, CNRS, Center for Immunology and Microbial Infections - CIMI-Paris, Paris, France
Institute for Integrative Biology of the Cell (I2BC), CEA, CNRS, Université Paris-Sud, Université Paris-Saclay, Gif-sur-Yvette, France

Rosa Bellmann-Weiler
Department of Internal Medicine II, Medical University of Innsbruck, Innsbruck, Austria

David M. Knipe
Department of Microbiology and Immunobiology, Harvard Medical School, Boston, MA, United States

Neal DeLuca
Department of Microbiology and Molecular Genetics, University of Pittsburgh School of Medicine, Pittsburgh, PA, United States

Beatrice Schuler-Thurner, Stefanie Gross, Jan Dörrie and Niels Schaft
Department of Dermatology, Universitätsklinikum Erlangen, Friedrich-Alexander-Universität Erlangen-Nürnberg, Erlangen, Germany

Christian Bach
Lab for Immunogenetics, Universitätsklinikum Erlangen, Erlangen, Germany

Anette Rohrhofer
Institute of Clinical Microbiology and Hygiene, University Hospital Regensburg, Regensburg, Germany

Melanie Werner-Klein
Chair of Immunology, Regensburg Center for Interventional Immunology (RCI), University of Regensburg, Regensburg, Germany

Barbara Schmidt
Institute of Clinical and Molecular Virology, Friedrich-Alexander-Universität Erlangen-Nürnberg, Erlangen, Germany
Institute of Clinical Microbiology and Hygiene, University Hospital Regensburg, Regensburg, Germany
Institute of Medical Microbiology and Hygiene, University of Regensburg, Regensburg, Germany

Philipp Schuster
Institute of Medical Microbiology and Hygiene, University of Regensburg, Regensburg, Germany

Jan B. Boscheinen and Sabrina Thomann
Institute of Clinical and Molecular Virology, Friedrich-Alexander-Universität Erlangen-Nürnberg, Erlangen, Germany

Arthur Baruel Zaneti, Marcio Massao Yamamoto, Fernando Bandeira Sulczewski, Bianca da Silva Almeida, Higo Fernando Santos Souza and Natália Soares Ferreira
Department of Parasitology, Institute of Biomedical Sciences, University of São Paulo, São Paulo, Brazil

Denicar Lina Nascimento Fabris Maeda, Natiely Silva Sales and Luís Carlos de Souza Ferreira
Department of Microbiology, Institute of Biomedical Sciences, University of São Paulo, São Paulo, Brazil

Daniela Santoro Rosa
Department of Microbiology, Immunology and Parasitology, Federal University of São Paulo (UNIFESP/EPM), São Paulo, Brazil
Institute for Investigation in Immunology (iii)-INCTiii, São Paulo, Brazil

Silvia Beatriz Boscardin
Department of Parasitology, Institute of Biomedical Sciences, University of São Paulo, São Paulo, Brazil
Institute for Investigation in Immunology (iii)-INCTiii, São Paulo, Brazil

Shafaqat Ali
Institute of Medical Microbiology and Hospital Hygiene, University of Düsseldorf, Düsseldorf, Germany
Cluster of Excellence EXC 1003, Cells in Motion, Münster, Germany

Ritu Mann-Nüttel, Anja Schulze, Lisa Richter and Stefanie Scheu
Institute of Medical Microbiology and Hospital Hygiene, University of Düsseldorf, Düsseldorf, Germany

Judith Alferink
Cluster of Excellence EXC 1003, Cells in Motion, Münster, Germany
Department of Psychiatry, University of Münster, Münster, Germany

Andrea Musumeci, Konstantin Lutz, Elena Winheim and Anne Barbara Krug
Institute for Immunology, Biomedical Center, Ludwig-Maximilian-University, Munich, Germany

Julia Koerner and Dennis Horvath
Division of Immunology, Department of Biology, University of Konstanz, Konstanz, Germany

Marcus Groettrup
Division of Immunology, Department of Biology, University of Konstanz, Konstanz, Germany
Biotechnology Institute Thurgau at the University of Konstanz, Kreuzlingen, Switzerland

Jean-Charles Cancel, Karine Crozat, Marc Dalod and Raphaël Mattiuz
CNRS, INSERM, Centre d'Immunologie de Marseille-Luminy, Turing Center for Living Systems, Aix Marseille University, Marseille France

Thiago A. Patente, Mariana P. Pinho, Aline A. Oliveira, Gabriela C. M. Evangelista and Patrícia C. Bergami-Santos
Laboratory of Tumor Immunology, Department of Immunology, Institute of Biomedical Sciences, University of São Paulo, São Paulo, Brazil

José A. M. Barbuto
Laboratory of Tumor Immunology, Department of Immunology, Institute of Biomedical Sciences, University of São Paulo, São Paulo, Brazil
Discipline of Molecular Medicine, Department of Medicine, Faculty of Medicine, University of São Paulo, São Paulo, Brazil

Thomas Döbel
Department of Dermatology, Heidelberg University Hospital, Heidelberg, Germany
Dermatology Branch, National Institute of Arthritis and Musculoskeletal and Skin Diseases, Bethesda, MD, United States

Index

www.ingramcontent.com/pod-product-compliance
Lightning Source LLC
LaVergne TN
LVHW082205200926
848484LV00008B/2214